Handbook of Experimental Pharmacology

Volume 121

Springer
Berlin
Heidelberg
New York
Barcelona
Budapest
Hong Kong
London
Milan
Paris
Santa Clara
Singapore
Tokyo

Drug-Induced Hepatotoxicity

Contributors

S. Anuras, M.Z. Badr, A.S. Basile, S.A. Belinsky, L.M. Blendis
R.G. Cameron, J.G. Conway, F.A. de la Iglesia, M.U. Dianzani
E. Farber, G. Feuer, R.J. Fingerote, P.E. Ganey, A.K. Ghoshal
K.G. Ishak, Y. Israel, E.A. Jones, K. Kitani, C.D. Klaassen
J.S. Leeder, G.A. Levy, I.R. Mackay, D.K. Monteith, A.B. Okey
B.K. Park, M. Pirmohamed, W.F. Pool, E.A. Roberts, E. Rubin
R.W. Sallie, D.C. Snover, R.G. Thurman, F. Trevisani, D.H. Van Thiel
R.R. Varma, R.M. Walker, J.B. Watkins III, P.G. Welling
T.F. Woolf, H.J. Zimmerman, M.J. Zuckerman

Editors

R.G. Cameron, G. Feuer, and F.A. de la Iglesia

With a Foreword by M. James Phillips

Springer

Professor Ross G. Cameron, M.D., Ph.D.
University of Toronto
Department of Pathology
Division of Experimental Pathology
Medical Sciences Building
1 King's College Circle
Toronto, Ontario, Canada M5S 1A8

Professor George Feuer, Ph.D.
University of Toronto
Department of Clinical Biochemistry
Banting Institute, Room 521, 100 College Street
Toronto, Ontario, Canada M5G 1L5

Felix A. de la Iglesia, M.D.
Parke-Davis Pharmaceutical Research Division
Department of Pathology and Experimental Toxicology
Warner Lambert Company
2800 Plymouth Road
Ann Arbor, MI 48105, USA

With 88 Figures and 62 Tables

ISBN-13: 978-3-642-64657-7 e-ISBN-13: 978-3-642-61013-4
DOI: 10.1007/978-3-642-61013-4

Library of Congress Cataloging-in-Publication Data. Drug-induced hepatotoxicity/contributors, S. Anuras ... [et al.]; editors, R.G. Cameron, G. Feuer, and F. de la Iglesia. p. cm.—(Handbook of experimental pharmacology; v. 121) Includes bibliographical references and index. ISBN 978-3-642-64657-7
ISBN 978-3-642-64657-7 1. Hepatotoxicology. 2. Drugs—Toxicology. I. Anuras. S. II. Cameron, R.G. (Ross G.), 1949– . III. Feuer, George, 1921– . IV. De la Iglesia, Felix A., 1939– . V. Series. [DNLM: 1. Liver Diseases—chemically induced. 2. Drug Therapy—adverse effects. W1 HA51L v. 121 1996/WI 700 D7941 1996] QP905.H3 vol. 121 [RC848.H48] 615'.1 s—dc20 [616.3'62] DNLM/DLC for Library of Congress 95-45927

Softcover reprint of the hardcover 1st edition 1996

Cover design: Springer-Verlag, Design & Production

Typesetting: Best-set Typesetter Ltd., Hong Kong

SPIN: 10474332 27/3136/SPS – 5 4 3 2 1 0

Foreword

The advances in science and medicine we are now experiencing are unprecedented and exciting. Life expectancy is prolonged, and quality of life is much improved. We learn of fabulous new discoveries made at the bench or the bedside every week. Many diseases have been totally eliminated, others can be significantly improved by new therapeutic formulations. Much of the success can be attributed to a better understanding of disease processes and the specific targeting of new and more effective medications.

As is the case in many areas of successful human endeavour, there can be a downside. In the case of drugs and chemicals it is their adverse effects which are of concern. Of course, every effort is made to devise medications that are safe, and the need to elucidate and understand mechanisms are crucial, yet adverse effects remain a problem. They can be unpredictable and diverse. Drugs have been shown to induce virtually the whole gamut of human liver pathology from acute fulminant hepatitis to chronic active hepatitis to cirrhosis and even malignancy. Hence the possibility of adverse drug effects must be considered in the differential diagnosis of many patients with liver disease. This is well recognized and is very important; indeed, removal of the offending agent can often lead to reversal of the adverse effect. This is an area of hepatology where we can really make a difference.

The clinicians, scientists, pharmacologists, toxicologists, pathologists and others who contributed to this book are not bystanders admiring the momentous medical advances we see on all sides, but are at the forefront of making those advances in their own fields of study. Each of the contributors is a well-known national and international expert in toxicologic and drug-induced liver disease.

This book contains the most up-to-date information on all the important aspects of drug-induced hepatotoxicity and is the last word on the subject. The volume will be necessary reading for students, practitioners and scientists for years to come.

I extend sincere congratulations to the editors and contributors on setting a new standard of excellence in this field.

Department of Pathology, University of Toronto
Toronto, Ontario, Canada

M. James Phillips

Preface

The application of therapeutic agents in medicine is an irreplaceable approach in the management of human disease. Given the complexity of some of these diseases, multidrug treatments are increasing, with a higher probability of adverse effects in different organs or systems. The liver is a major organ with a central role in the metabolism of drugs; consequently, it receives the largest number of toxic insults. Hepatic adverse reactions are recognizable, and their study is therefore essential for understanding health risks that exposure to drugs may represent. These were the main reasons for us to assemble this volume.

A previous volume (Vol. 16) in this series which addressed hepatotoxicity appeared in 1976 thanks to the efforts of Drs. H. Zimmerman and I. MacKay. This exemplary précis set the tone of excellence for future volumes in this area. During the past two decades many new therapeutic agents have been discovered, representing significant advances. Many scientific communications have since appeared, characterizing the clinical and biomolecular mechanisms of liver responses to different drugs. These achievements included the development of several animal models, definition of in vitro cell systems and molecular analysis of drug metabolism mechanisms. The role of multiple species of cytochrome P450 has emerged, and genetic susceptibility as well as pathological-biochemical mechanisms of cell injury have been elucidated.

It is for these purposes that an international array of expert contributors was assembled. Since the literature on liver cell reactions to chemicals, and toxins is immense, we concentrated on the most recent knowledge base of pharmacologic agents in hepatotoxicity, focusing on as many therapeutic categories as possible. This was an ambitious plan, but we realized that some areas were to be missed, not purposely, but for the mere reason of timeliness and the great deal of energy required to make it an overall, extremely comprehensive treatise. Fortunately, some of the few missing areas are being covered by specialized volumes that have appeared only very recently. We feel that this volume, as presented, will satisfy most of our demanding hepatologist colleagues, and that it could be viewed as a useful window into the field of drug-induced hepatotoxicity.

Our gratitude goes to many supporters that provided expert advice. In particular, we acknowledge Dr. Pedro Cuatrecasas whose encouragement was the main thrust to complete this work. It was also a great pleasure working with Mrs. Doris Walker from Springer-Verlag. An unexpected dividend of this work were the positive interactions with the contributors and the cementing of a long-existing scientific and personal relationship between us.

Toronto, Ontario, Canada
Ann Arbor, Michigan, USA

ROSS G. CAMERON, GEORGE FEUER
FELIX A. DE LA IGLESIA

List of Contributors

ANURAS, S., Department of Internal Medicine, Texas Tech University Health Sciences Center, School of Medicine, Lubbock, TX 79430, USA

BADR, M.Z., University of Missouri-Kansas City, M3-102, 2411 Holmes Street, Kansas City, MO 64108-2792, USA

BASILE, A.S., Laboratory of Neuroscience, National Institutes of Diabetes, Digestive and Kidney Diseases (NIDDK), National Institutes of Health, Building 8, Room 111, Bethesda, MD 20892, USA

BELINSKY, S.A., Inhalation Toxicology Research Institute, P.O. Box 5890, Albuquerque, NM 87185, USA

BLENDIS, L.M., Department of Medicine, Toronto Hospital, 621 University Avenue, Toronto, Ontario, Canada M5G 2C4

CAMERON, R.G., Department of Pathology, University of Toronto, The Toronto Hospital, 621 University Avenue, Toronto, Ontario, Canada M5G 2C4

CONWAY, J.G., CIIT, P.O. Box 12137, Research Triangle Park, NC 27709, USA

DE LA IGLESIA, F.A., Department of Pathology and Experimental Toxicology, Parke-Davis Pharmaceutical Research Division, Warner Lambert Company, 2800 Plymouth Road, Ann Arbor, MI 48105, USA

DIANZANI, M.U., Department of Experimental Medicine and Oncology, Section of General Pathology, University of Torino, Corso Raffaello 30, I-10125 Torino, Italy

FARBER, E., Department of Pathology and Biochemistry, University of Toronto, Medical Sciences Building, Toronto, Ontario, Canada M5S 1A8. Current address: Department of Pathology and Cell Biology, Jefferson Medical College, Thomas Jefferson University, 1020 Locust Street, Philadelphia, PA 19107-6799, USA

FEUER, G., Department of Clinical Biochemistry, University of Toronto, Banting Institute, Room 521, 100 College Street, Toronto, Ontario, Canada M5G 1L5

FINGEROTE, R.J., University of Toronto, Toronto General Hospital, Norman Urquhart Wing 10-151, 621 University Avenue, Toronto, Ontario, Canada M5G 2C4

GANEY, P.E., Division of Medicine, Life Sciences Building, Michigan State University, East Lansing, MI 48864, USA

GHOSHAL, A.K., Department of Pathology, Medical Sciences Building, University of Toronto, 1 King's College Circle, Toronto, Ontario, Canada M5S 1A8

ISHAK, K.G., George Washington University, Department of Hepatic and Gastrointestinal Pathology, Armed Forces Institute of Pathology, Washington, DC 20306-6000, USA

ISRAEL, Y., Department of Pathology, Anatomy and Cell Biology, Jefferson Medical College, Thomas Jefferson University, Room 275, 1020 Locust Street, Philadelphia, PA 19107, USA

JONES, E.A., Liver Diseases Section, National Institute of Diabetes and Digestive and Kidney Diseases, National Institutes of Health, Bldg. 10, Rm. 4D-52, Bethesda, MD 20892, USA

KITANI, K., Radioisotope Research Institute, Faculty of Medicine, University of Tokyo, 7-3-1 Hongo, Bunkyo-ku, Tokyo 113, Japan, and National Institute for Longevity Sciences, 36-3 Gengo, Morioka-cho, Obu-shi, Aichi 474, Japan

KLAASSEN, C.D., Department of Pharmacology, Toxicology and Therapeutics, University of Kansas Medical Center, Kansas City, KS 66160-7417, USA

LEEDER, J.S., Division of Clinical Pharmacology and Toxicology, Research Institute, The Hospital for Sick Children, 555 University Avenue, Toronto, Ontario, Canada M5G 1X8

LEVY, G.A., University of Toronto, Toronto General Hospital, Norman Urquhart Wing 10-151, 621 University Avenue, Toronto, Ontario, Canada M5G 2C4

MACKAY, I.R., Centre for Molecular Biology and Medicine, Monash University, Wellington Road, Clayton, Victoria, 3168 Australia

MONTEITH, D.K., Department of Pathology and Experimental Toxicology, Parke-Davis Pharmaceutical Research Division, Warner Lambert Company, 2800 Plymouth Road, Ann Arbor, MI 48105, USA

OKEY, A.B., Department of Pharmacology, The University of Toronto, Medical Sciences Building, Toronto, Ontario, Canada M5S 1A8

PARK, B.K., Department of Pharmacology and Therapeutics, The University of Liverpool, P.O. Box 147, Liverpool L69 3BX, Great Britain

PIRMOHAMED, M., Department of Pharmacology and Therapeutics, The University of Liverpool, P.O. Box 147, Liverpool L69 3BX, Great Britain

POOL, W.F., Department of Pharmacokinetics and Drug Metabolism, Parke-Davis Pharmaceutical Research Division, Warner Lambert Company, 2800 Plymouth Road, Ann Arbor, MI 48105, USA

ROBERTS, E.A., Divisions of Gastroenterology/Nutrition and Clinical Pharmacology and Toxicology, The Hospital for Sick Children, and University of Toronto, 555 University Avenue, Toronto, Ontario, Canada M5G 1X8

RUBIN, E., Department of Pathology, Anatomy and Cell Biology, Jefferson Medical College, Thomas Jefferson University, 1020 Locust Street, Philadelphia, PA 19107, USA

SALLIE, R.W., Liver Diseases Section, National Institute of Diabetes and Digestive and Kidney Diseases, National Institutes of Health, Bethesda, MD 20892, USA

SNOVER, D.C., Department of Laboratory Medicine and Pathology, University of Minnesota Hospital, 420 Delaware Street SE, Minneapolis, MN 55455, USA

THURMAN, R.G., Laboratory of Hepatobiology and Toxicology, Department of Pharmacology, The University of North Carolina, CB#7365, Faculty Laboratory Office Building, Chapel Hill, NC 27599-7365, USA

TREVISANI, F., Oklahoma Transplant Institute, Baptist Medical Center of Oklahoma, 3300 Northwest Expressway, Oklahoma City, OK 73112, USA

VAN THIEL, D.H. Oklahoma Transplant Institute, Baptist Medical Center of Oklahoma, 3300 Northwest Expressway, Oklahoma City, OK 73112, USA

VARMA, R.R., Hepatology Unit, Division of Gastroenterology, Medical College of Wisconsin, Froedtert Memorial Lutheran Hospital, 9200 W. Wisconsin Avenue, Milwaukee, WI 53226, USA

WALKER, R.M., Parke-Davis Research Institute, Sheridan Park, Speakman Drive, Mississauga, Ontario, Canada L5K 1B4

WATKINS III, J.B., Medical Sciences Program, Indiana State University School of Medicine, Bloomington, IN 47405, USA

WELLING, P.G., Department of Pharmacokinetics and Drug Metabolism, Parke-Davis Pharmaceutical Research Division, Warner Lambert Company, 2800 Plymouth Road, Ann Arbor, MI 48105, USA

WOOLF, T.F., Department of Pharmacokinetics and Drug Metabolism, Parke-Davis Pharmaceutical Research Division, Warner Lambert Company, 2800 Plymouth Road, Ann Arbor, MI 48105, USA

ZIMMERMAN, H.J., George Washington University, Armed Forces Institute of Pathology, Department of Hepatic Pathology, Washington, DC 20306-6000, USA

ZUCKERMAN, M.J., Division of Gastroenterology, Texas Tech University Health Sciences Center, 4800 Alberta Avenue, El Paso, TX 79905, USA

Contents

CHAPTER 1

Orientation in Liver Toxicity by Drugs
E. Farber. With 1 Figure 1

A. Introduction 1
B. Agents and Processes 1
C. Responses to Injury as Multitier or Multigrid Patterns 2
I. Quantitative Versus Qualitative Changes 3
II. Patterns of Liver Toxicity 4
1. Tier One: Patterns of Interactions of Agents with Liver 4
2. Tier Two: Patterns of Biological Responses to Cell Injury 8
3. Tier Three: Cellular and Intracellular Responses 10
4. Tier Four: Cellular and Tissue Physiology 19
D. Conclusion 21
References 21

CHAPTER 2

Clinical Studies and Role of Necrosis in Hepatotoxicity
R.G. Cameron and L.M. Blendis. With 7 Figures 25

A. Zonal Necrosis as a Response to Acetaminophen 25
I. Zonality: Specific Hepatocytes Die as a Group 25
II. Ethanol Plus Acetaminophen: Extension of Zone of Necrosis 28
III. Constitutive Bases of Zonal Responses 30
1. Perivenous Localization of Acetaminophen-Metabolizing enzyme CYP 2E1 32
IV. Zonal Hepatocellular Necrosis: Historical Perspective 33
B. Regeneration in Response to Zonal Necrosis of Acetaminophen Overdose 33
I. Regeneration of Periportal and Mid-zonal Hepatocytes to Restore the Perivenous Zone 33

C. Clinical Implications of "Adaptive" Perivenous Necrosis 38
References 39

CHAPTER 3

Subcellular Biochemical and Pathological Correlates in Experimental Models of Hepatotoxicity
G. FEUER and F.A. DE LA IGLESIA. With 5 Figures 43

A. Introduction 43
B. Organization of the Liver Cell 44
C. Liver Cell Injury 45
D. Subcellular Organelle Pathology 46
I. Endoplasmic Reticulum 46
1. Membrane Structure 46
2. Cytochrome P450 System 48
3. Proliferation and Induction 48
4. Structure-Activity Relationships 50
5. Membrane-Bound Phospholipids 51
II. Golgi Apparatus 52
III. Intracellular Membrane Dynamics 54
IV. Mitochondria..................................... 55
V. Lysosomes 56
VI. Peroxisomes 57
E. Biochemical Pathology of Subcellular Changes 59
I. Cell Respiration 59
II. Protein Metabolism 60
III. Lipid Metabolism 61
IV. Bile Secretion 62
F. Latent Hepatotoxicity Models 63
G. Conclusions 64
References 65

CHAPTER 4

Molecular Biology of Hepatic Drug Reactions
R.W. SALLIE and E.A. JONES. With 6 Figures 75

A. Introduction 75
B. General Considerations 75
C. DNA Damage 77
I. Drugs and DNA Metabolism 77
II. DNA Replication and Repair Pathways 78
D. Inhibition of DNA Replication 79
I. Inhibition of DNA Polymerases 79
II. Inhibition of DNA Ligase 80

III. Chain Termination 81
IV. Inhibition of DNA Repair 81
V. Alterations in Purine/Pyrimidine Metabolism 83
VI. Alterations in DNA Processing Post Synthesis 83
E. Damage to RNA 84
F. Interference with Protein Synthesis 85
G. Apoptosis 86
H. Future Developments 92
I. Summary and Conclusions 93
References 94

CHAPTER 5

In Vitro Models of Liver Toxicity
R.G. THURMAN, P.E. GANEY, S.A. BELINSKY, J.G. CONWAY, and M.Z. BADR. With 4 Figures 99

A. Introduction 99
I. Metabolism of Foreign Compounds Can Cause Zone-Specific Hepatotoxicity 99
II. Advantages and Disadvantages of Whole Cell Models 100
B. Techniques Used to Study Zone-Specific Hepatotoxicity in the Isolated Perfused Liver 101
I. Metabolite Measurements in Tissue and Perfusate 103
II. Microlight Guides 104
III. Miniature Oxygen Electrodes 105
IV. Trypan Blue Exclusion 106
C. Applying In Vitro Models to the Study of Liver Toxicology 106
I. Monooxygenation in Periportal and Pericentral Zones of the Liver Lobule 106
II. Conjugation Reactions in Periportal and Pericentral Regions of the Liver Lobule 107
1. Sulfation 107
2. Glucuronidation 109
III. Oxygen as a Determinant of Zone-Specific Hepatotoxicity 111
D. Conclusions 113
References 113

CHAPTER 6

Cytochromes P450 and Liver Injury
J.S. LEEDER and A.B. OKEY. With 4 Figures 119

A. Drug Biotransformation, Cytochromes P450 and the Liver 119
I. Drug Biotransformation by the Liver 119
II. General Drug Biotransformation Processes 119

III. Phase I Reactions . . . 120
IV. Introduction to the Cytochromes P450 . . . 120
B. Cytochromes P450 and Drug Biotransformation . . . 121
I. Human Hepatic Cytochromes P450 . . . 121
II. Sources of Variability in P450 Expression and Activity . . . 125
1. P450 Genetics and Polymorphisms . . . 126
2. P450 Induction . . . 127
3. P450 Inhibition . . . 129
4. Liver Disease: Effects on Drug Biotransformation . . . 130
II. Reaction Mechanism . . . 130
III. Drug Biotransformation and Drug Toxicity . . . 132
1. Cytochrome P450 and Bioactivation . . . 132
2. Activation/Detoxification Balance . . . 132
3. "Probe Drugs" for Determining P450 Activities in Humans In Vivo . . . 134
C. Mechanisms of P450-Mediated Liver Injury . . . 135
I. Reactive Metabolites . . . 135
1. Noncovalent Interactions . . . 136
2. Covalent Adduct Formation . . . 137
II. P450s as Targets of Immune Effectors . . . 138
D. Specific Drugs/P450s and Liver Injury . . . 139
I. Acetaminophen . . . 139
II. Halothane . . . 141
III. Tienilic Acid . . . 142
IV. Dihydralazine . . . 143
V. Diclofenac . . . 144
E. Conclusions . . . 144
References . . . 145

CHAPTER 7

Mechanisms of Drug-Induced Cholestasis
J.B. WATKINS III and C.D. KLAASSEN . . . 155

A. Definition of Cholestasis . . . 155
B. Mechanisms of Canalicular Bile Formation . . . 156
I. Transport of Bile Acids . . . 156
II. Transport of Inorganic Ions and Glutathione . . . 157
III. Other Mechanisms . . . 157
C. Mechanisms of Cholestasis . . . 158
I. Alterations in Basolateral Membrane Function . . . 158
II. Alterations in Canalicular Membrane Function . . . 158
III. Alterations in Intracellular Events . . . 159
1. Binding to Intracellular Proteins and Conjugation Enzymes . . . 159
2. Cytoskeleton . . . 159

IV. Permeability Changes in the Biliary Tree 160
1. Altered Permeability of the Junctional Complex 161
2. Altered Permeability of the Canalicular Membrane 161
3. Alterations in Membrane Proteins 162
4. Alterations in Membrane Composition and Function ... 164
D. Drugs and Other Chemicals Inducing Cholestasis 165
I. α-Naphthylisothiocyanate 165
II. Androgenic and Estrogenic Steroids 166
III. Bile Acids 168
IV. Chlorpromazine and Other Phenothiazines 169
V. Cyclosporine 170
VI. Miscellaneous Cholestatic Agents 170
References 171

CHAPTER 8

Fatty Liver and Drugs
M.U. DIANZANI. With 1 Figure 185

A. General Mechanisms for Fatty Liver 185
B. Drugs Provoking Fatty Liver 187
I. Drugs Provoking Fatty Liver by Increasing
FFA Supply to the Liver 187
II. Drugs Provoking Fatty Liver
by Intrahepatic Mechanisms 188
1. Drugs Increasing Intrahepatic FFA Synthesis 188
2. Drugs Provoking Fatty Liver by Decreasing
Fatty Acid Oxidation. 192
3. Drugs Blocking Lipoprotein Secretion 192
III. Drugs Decreasing Fat Infiltration in the Liver 200
References 202

CHAPTER 9

Choline Deficiency: An Important Model for the Study of Hepatotoxicity
A.K. GHOSHAL. With 2 Figures 211

A. Introduction 211
B. Hepatotoxicity by Dietary Manipulation – Not by Addition
but by Depletion 212
C. Absence of Choline in an Otherwise Complete Diet –
An Excellent Model for the Study of Liver Cell Death
and Liver Cancer 213

I. Choline Deficiency Model and Cell Death ... 215
II. Choline Deficiency and Liver Cancer ... 216
D. Lipotrope Deficiency Versus Choline Deficiency ... 217
E. Step by Step Development of Liver Aberration ... 217
F. Hypothesis of Choline Deficiency Induced Hepatocarcinoma ... 218
G. Conclusions ... 218
References ... 218

CHAPTER 10

Immune Mechanisms and Liver Toxicity
I.R. MACKAY. With 3 Figures ... 221

A. Introduction and Overview of Drug-Mediated Hepatotoxicity ... 221
B. Functional Aspects of the Immune System ... 222
I. Immune Repertoire ... 222
II. Major Histocompatibility Complex ... 223
III. Afferent Limb of the Immune Response ... 224
IV. Efferent Limb of the Immune Response ... 225
V. Regulation and Dysregulation of Immune Responses ... 226
C. Genetic Determinants of Adverse Drug Reactions ... 227
D. Liver in Relation to Adverse Drug Reactions ... 228
I. Intrahepatic Metabolism of Drugs by Microsomal Enzymes ... 228
1. Cytochrome P450 Oxidases (CYP450) ... 228
2. UDP Glucuronosyl Transferases ... 228
3. Carboxyl Esterases ... 228
II. Intrahepatic Immune Processes ... 229
1. Initiation of Immune-Mediated Drug Reactions in the Liver ... 229
2. Regulatory and Dysregulation of Intrahepatic Immune Reactions ... 229
III. Infrequency of Hepatic Hypersensitivity Drug Reactions ... 230
IV. Immunopathology of Hepatic Hypersensitivity Drug Reactions ... 230
V. Drug-Altered Neoantigen – The Halothane Paradigm ... 232
1. Halothane Hepatitis ... 232
2. Immunological Investigations of Halothane Hepatitis ... 233
3. Detection of Antibodies to TFA Conjugates ... 233
VI. Native Liver Antigens – The Liver-Kidney Microsomal (LKM) System ... 234
1. Hepatitis with Anti-LKM-2 ... 235
2. Identification of LKM as Cytochrome P450 Species ... 235

3. Antibodies to CYP 1A2 in Drug-Induced Hepatitis 236
4. Inhibition of Enzyme Function by Anti-LKM 237
5. Origins of Anti-LKM Reactivity 237
VII. Drug-Induced Hepatitis with Reactions to Autoantigens ... 238
E. Experimental Models of Drug-Induced Immune-Mediated Disease 239
F. Laboratory Investigation of Immune-Mediated Hepatic Drug Reactions 240
I. General Laboratory Investigations 240
II. Drug-Specific Immunological Investigations 240
1. Detection of T-Cell-Mediated Reactions 241
III. Pharmacological Idiosyncrasy 242
References 242

CHAPTER 11

Hepatic Encephalopathy

A.S. Basile 249

A. Introduction 249
I. Clinical Manifestations of Hepatic Encephalopathy 249
II. Neuropathological Changes in Hepatic Encephalopathy ... 251
1. Anatomy 251
2. Electrophysiology 251
B. Involvement of Neurotoxins in the Pathogenesis of Hepatic Encephalopathy 252
I. Ammonia 253
1. Glial Interactions 253
2. Electrophysiological Changes 254
3. Changes in Oxidative Metabolism 256
4. Summary 256
II. Synergistic Neurotoxins 257
C. Neurotransmitter Involvement in the Pathogenesis of Hepatic Encephalopathy 258
I. γ-Aminobutyric Acid 258
1. Electrophysiology 258
2. Neurochemistry and Pharmacology 258
3. Behavior 260
4. Summary 260
II. Excitatory Amino Acids 261
III. Aromatic Amino Acids and Monoamine Neurotransmitters 263
D. Conclusions 265
References 265

CHAPTER 12

Liver Drug Reactions and Pregnancy

F. TREVISANI and D.H. VAN THIEL . . . 273

A. The Liver in Normal Pregnancy . . . 273
I. Liver Histology . . . 273
II. Liver Perfusion and Function . . . 274
B. Effects of Pregnancy on the Risk of Experiencing a Drug-Induced Hepatic Injury . . . 276
I. Specific Pre-Marketing Risk/Benefit Evaluation of Drugs . . 276
II. Risk of Exposure to Hepatotoxic Drugs . . . 276
III. Pharmacokinetics . . . 278
1. Absorption . . . 278
2. Distribution . . . 278
3. Hemodynamics and Drug Clearance . . . 279
4. Maternal-Placental-Fetal Unit . . . 279
IV. Liver Vulnerability . . . 280
C. Liver Drug Reactions Occurring During Pregnancy . . . 282
I. Antibiotics . . . 282
II. Antiemetics . . . 283
III. Anesthetics and Analgesics . . . 283
IV. Anticonvulsants . . . 284
V. Other Agents . . . 284
D. Clinical Presentation and Diagnostic Approach to Hepatic Injury in Pregnancy . . . 285
E. Treatment . . . 286
F. Prevention . . . 287
References . . . 288

CHAPTER 13

Pediatric Hepatic Drug Reactions

E.A. ROBERTS . . . 293

A. Classification of Drug Hepatotoxicity . . . 293
B. Specific Drugs Causing Hepatotoxicity in Children . . . 294
I. Acetaminophen . . . 294
II. Phenytoin . . . 296
III. Valproic Acid . . . 297
IV. Isoniazid . . . 301
V. Halothane . . . 302
VI. Carbamazepine . . . 303
VII. Phenobarbital . . . 304
VIII. Antineoplastic Drugs . . . 304
IX. Pemoline . . . 306

X. Sulfonamides ... 306
XI. Aspirin ... 307
XII. Propylthiouracil ... 307
XIII. Erythromycin ... 308
XIV. Methotrexate ... 308
XV. Estrogens: Oral Contraceptive Pill ... 310
XVI. Ketoconazole ... 310
XVII. Haloperidol ... 310
XVIII. Amiodarone ... 310
XIX. Nitrofurantoin ... 311
XX. Retinoids ... 311
XXI. Azathioprine ... 311
XXII. Cocaine ... 312
References ... 312

CHAPTER 14

Reye's Syndrome
R.R. Varma ... 323

A. Introduction ... 323
B. Clinical Features ... 324
C. Laboratory Features ... 326
D. Diagnostic Criteria for Population Surveys ... 327
E. Liver Morphology ... 328
F. Brain Morphology ... 328
G. Liver Histology and Electron Microscopy in Reye's Syndrome ... 329
H. Pathophysiology ... 330
I. Aspirin and Reye's Syndrome ... 332
J. Animal Models ... 334
K. Reye's Syndrome in Adults ... 335
L. Treatment ... 335
M. Sequelae ... 336
References ... 337

CHAPTER 15

Drug Hepatotoxicity in the Elderly
K. Kitani. With 7 Figures ... 341

A. Introduction ... 341
B. Clinical Information ... 341
I. Idiosyncratic Hepatotoxicity: The Swedish Experience ... 341
II. Dose-Dependent Hepatotoxicity ... 343

C. Age-Related Alterations in Hepatic Detoxifying Functions: Discrepancies Between Human and Animal Data . . . 343
I. Phase I Drug Metabolism . . . 344
II. Phase II Metabolism . . . 346
1. Glucuronidation and Sulfation: Acetaminophen Conjugation . . . 346
2. Glutathione *S*-Transferases . . . 347
III. Oxidant and Antioxidant Variables . . . 350
1. Lipid Peroxidation . . . 351
2. Glutathione . . . 351
3. Antioxidant Enzymes . . . 351
D. Morbidity and Frailty as Major Factors for Lowered Drug Clearances in the Elderly: A Possible Role in Hepatotoxicity . . . 353
E. Adverse Drug Reactions in the Liver in Old Animals: Mini Review . . . 354
I. Hepatocyte Susceptibility to Chlorpromazine and Erythromycin Estolate . . . 355
II. Acetaminophen Hepatotoxicity: An Example of Variability of the Results in Studies Using Rodents . . . 355
III. Ethanol Metabolism in the Liver and Its Hepatotoxicity: Another Controversy . . . 358
IV. Hepatotoxicities by Other Toxicants . . . 361
F. Conclusions and Suggestions for Future Studies . . . 361
References . . . 362

CHAPTER 16

Effect of Liver Disease on Drug Metabolism and Pharmacokinetics
P.G. WELLING and W.F. POOL. With 6 Figures . . . 367

A. Introduction . . . 367
B. Function and Structure of the Liver . . . 368
C. Types and Severity of Liver Disease . . . 369
I. Changes in Hepatic Function . . . 369
II. Changes in Hepatic Vasculature . . . 369
III. Changes in Renal Function . . . 370
IV. Ascites . . . 370
D. Pharmacodynamic Factors . . . 370
E. Pharmacokinetic Factors . . . 371
I. Linear Pharmacokinetic Models . . . 371
1. One-Compartment Model, Intravenous Dosing . . . 371
2. First-Order Absorption and Elimination . . . 373
3. Repeated Dosing with Linear Pharmacokinetics . . . 374
II. Nonlinear Pharmacokinetic Models . . . 376

III. Impact of Liver Disease 377
1. Distribution Volume 379
2. Elimination Half-Life 379
3. Protein Binding 380
4. Presystemic Clearance 380
F. Markers of Liver Disease Relevant to Drug Metabolism and Pharmacokinetics 381
G. Examples of Effects of Liver Disease on the Pharmacokinetics of Some Drug Therapeutic Classes 382
I. Cardiovascular Agents 383
II. Drugs Acting on the Central Nervous System 384
III. Antimicrobial Agents 385
IV. Other Drugs 386
H. Conclusions 387
References 388

CHAPTER 17

Liver Reactions to Tacrine
T.F. WOOLF, W.F. POOL, R.M. WALKER, and D.K. MONTEITH. With 2 Figures 395

A. Introduction 395
B. Clinical Experience 395
C. Metabolism of Tacrine in Humans 397
D. Preclinical Toxicology 399
E. Metabolism of Tacrine in Animals 401
F. Cytotoxicity Studies 402
G. In Vitro Metabolism Studies 403
H. Conclusions 405
References 406

CHAPTER 18

Mechanisms of Hypertransaminemia
M. PIRMOHAMED and B.K. PARK. With 7 Figures 411

A. Introduction 411
B. Overview of Liver Transaminase Monitoring 411
I. Significance of the Different Tests Used to Monitor Liver Function 411
II. Spectrum of Drug-Induced Hepatotoxicity and Hypertransaminemia 413

III. Clinical Correlates of Transaminase Measurement 414
1. Sensitivity and Specificity of Hypertransaminemia 414
2. Correlation Between Severity of Hepatic Injury and Degree of Hypertransaminemia 415
3. Clinical Significance of Minor Degrees of Hypertransaminemia 416
C. Classification of the Causes of Hypertransaminemia 419
D. Mechanisms of Acute Hepatic Injury Leading to Hypertransaminemia 419
I. Role of Drug Metabolism 419
II. Evidence for the Formation of Chemically Reactive Metabolites 421
III. Acute Chemical Hepatotoxicity 422
1. Acetaminophen Hepatotoxicity 422
2. Carbon Tetrachloride Hepatotoxicity 424
IV. Acute Idiosyncratic Hepatotoxicity 425
1. Metabolic Idiosyncrasy Causing Hypertransaminemia ... 425
2. Immune-Mediated Drug-Induced Hypertransaminemia 426
E. Mechanisms of Chronic Hepatic Injury Causing Hypertransaminemia 431
I. Chronic Chemical Hypertransaminemia 431
II. Chronic Idiosyncratic Drug-Induced Hypertransaminemia 432
F. Diagnosis of Drug-Induced Hypertransaminemia 433
I. Distinction Between Drug- and Non-Drug-Induced Etiologies 433
II. Distinction Between Direct and Immune-Mediated Acute Idiosyncratic Toxicity 433
G. Conclusions 434
References 435

CHAPTER 19

Diagnostic Tools and Clinical Pathology

D.C. Snover 441

A. General Features and Clinical Evaluation of Drug-Induced Liver Diseases 441
B. General Mechanisms of Drug Reactions 442
I. Toxic Reactions 442
II. Idiosyncratic Reactions 443
III. Tumor Formation 443
IV. Vascular Reactions 444
V. Interactions 445

C. General Biochemical and Histological Types of Drug Reactions . . . 445
I. Hepatocellular Reactions . . . 445
II. Cholestatic Reactions . . . 447
III. Mixed Hepatocellular-Cholestatic . . . 448
IV. Tumors . . . 448
V. Vascular Lesions . . . 448
D. Clinical Evaluation and Diagnosis of Hepatic Drug Reactions . . . 449
I. History . . . 450
II. Laboratory Findings . . . 450
III. Histopathological Findings . . . 451
E. Some Specific Illustrative Drug Reactions . . . 451
I. Unsuspected Acetaminophen Overdose Caused by Consumption of Nyquil . . . 451
II. Suspected Fatal Isoniazid Toxicity Disproven by Autopsy Examination . . . 452
III. Toxicity Due to Health Food ("Hot Stuff") . . . 452
F. Summary of the Clinical Approach to Drug Toxicity . . . 453
References . . . 453

CHAPTER 20

Antimicrobial Drugs
H.J. ZIMMERMAN and K.G. ISHAK. With 7 Figures . . . 457

A. Antibiotics . . . 457
I. Aminoglycosides . . . 457
II. Cephalosporins . . . 457
III. Chloramphenicol . . . 457
IV. Clindamycin . . . 458
V. Colimycin . . . 458
VI. Erythromycin . . . 459
VII. Fusidic Acid . . . 460
VIII. Roxithromycin . . . 460
IX. Tetracyclines . . . 461
X. Troleandomycin . . . 461
XI. Penicillin . . . 462
B. Synthetic Antimicrobials . . . 463
I. Organic Arsenicals . . . 463
II. Quinolones . . . 467
III. Sulfonamides . . . 468
IV. Sulfamethoxazole-Trimethoprim . . . 468
V. Sulfasalazine . . . 468
VI. Sulfones . . . 468
VII. Nitrofurantoin . . . 469
VIII. Furazolidone . . . 469

C. Antituberculous Drugs . . . 469
I. *p*-Aminosalicylic Acid . . . 469
II. Isoniazid . . . 470
III. Rifampin . . . 470
D. Antifungal Agents . . . 471
I. Griseofulvin . . . 471
II. Ketoconazole . . . 471
III. Other Imidazoles . . . 471
IV. Flucytosine . . . 471
E. Antiviral Agents . . . 472
F. Antiprotozoal Agents . . . 472
I. Anthelmintics . . . 472
References . . . 473

CHAPTER 21

Hepatotoxicity of Cardiovascular Drugs
R.G. CAMERON, F.A. DE LA IGLESIA, and G. FEUER. With 9 Figures . . . 477

A. Introduction . . . 477
B. α-Methyldopa . . . 478
I. Hepatitis . . . 479
II. Fatty Change . . . 481
III. Hepatic Necrosis . . . 482
IV. Cholestasis . . . 482
V. Cirrhosis . . . 483
C. Amiodarone . . . 483
I. Alcoholic-Type Hepatitis . . . 484
II. Phospholipid Fatty Liver . . . 487
III. Reye's Syndrome-Like Disease . . . 488
D. Aprindine . . . 488
I. Hepatitis . . . 488
E. Hydralazine and Dihydralazine . . . 489
I. Hepatitis . . . 490
F. Papaverine . . . 491
I. Hepatitis . . . 492
G. Procainamide . . . 492
I. Hepatitis . . . 492
II. Cholestasis . . . 493
H. Quinidine . . . 493
I. Hepatitis . . . 494
II. Granulomatous Hepatitis . . . 494
I. Lipid-Regulating Agents . . . 495
I. Classes of Lipid-Regulating Agents . . . 495
II. Hyperlipoproteinemia and Liver Structure . . . 496
III. Nicotinic Acid . . . 498

IV. Fibrates ... 498
V. Statins ... 500
J. Miscellaneous Cardiovascular Drugs ... 501
K. Modulation of Hepatotoxicity ... 502
L. Conclusions ... 502
References ... 504

CHAPTER 22

Analgesic Hepatopathy
M.J. ZUCKERMAN and S. ANURAS ... 515

A. Introduction ... 515
B. Acetaminophen ... 515
I. Epidemiology ... 515
1. Incidence of Hepatotoxicity ... 515
2. Hepatotoxicity in Alcoholics ... 516
3. Hepatotoxicity in Therapeutic Settings ... 517
II. Pathogenesis ... 518
1. Hepatotoxic Dose and Blood Level ... 518
2. Mechanism ... 518
3. Factors Influencing Hepatotoxicity ... 519
III. Clinical Manifestations and Laboratory Findings ... 519
1. Clinical Course ... 519
2. Pathology ... 520
3. Prognosis ... 521
IV. Treatment ... 522
1. General Management ... 522
2. Specific Therapy ... 523
3. Fulminant Hepatic Failure ... 524
V. Prevention ... 525
C. Nonsteroidal Antiinflammatory Drugs ... 526
I. Epidemiology ... 526
II. Pathogenesis ... 529
III. Clinical Manifestations and Laboratory Findings ... 531
1. General Observations ... 531
2. Specific NSAIDs ... 532
IV. Treatment ... 534
V. Prevention ... 535
D. Narcotic Analgesics ... 536
References ... 537

CHAPTER 23

Steroids and Other Hormones
H.J. ZIMMERMAN and K.G. ISHAK. With 7 Figures ... 543

A. Gonadal Steroids and Their Derivatives ... 543
B. Anabolic Steroids ... 543
I. Cholestasis ... 544
1. Structural Characteristics of Icterogenic Steroids ... 544
2. Incidence ... 544
3. Clinical Features ... 545
4. Biochemical Features ... 546
5. Histopathology ... 546
6. Prognosis ... 546
7. Mechanism ... 547
II. Peliosis Hepatis ... 548
III. Neoplasms ... 549
1. Nodular Regenerative Hyperplasia ... 549
2. Hepatocellular Adenoma ... 549
3. Hepatic Carcinoma ... 550
4. Other Neoplasms ... 550
C. Female Sex Hormones and the Contraceptive Steroids ... 551
I. Estrogenic Hormones and Related Drugs ... 551
II. Progestational Steroids ... 552
III. Adverse Effects of Contraceptive Steroids on the Liver ... 553
IV. Syndrome of Contraceptive Steroid Jaundice ... 554
1. Clinical Features ... 554
2. Biochemical Features ... 554
3. Histologic Characteristics ... 554
4. Prognosis ... 554
5. Susceptibility ... 554
V. Tumors Associated with Oral Contraceptives ... 555
1. Hepatocellular Adenoma ... 555
2. Focal Nodular Hyperplasia ... 558
3. Hepatocellular Carcinoma ... 558
VI. Vascular Lesions ... 560
1. Effect on Hemangiomas and Related Lesions ... 560
2. Sinusoidal Dilatation ... 560
3. Peliosis Hepatis ... 560
4. Hepatic Vein Thrombosis ... 561
5. Rupture of the Liver ... 562
6. Other Vascular Changes ... 563
VII. Disturbed Porphyrin Metabolism ... 563
VIII. Mechanisms of Injury by Contraceptive Steroids ... 563
IX. Cholelithiasis ... 564
D. Drugs Related to Sex Hormones ... 565
I. Antiestrogens ... 565
1. Clomiphene ... 565
2. Cyclofenil ... 565
3. Tamoxifen ... 565

II. Antihypophysial Drugs 565
1. Danazol 565
2. Octreotide 566
E. Glucocorticoids 566
F. Oral Hypoglycemic Agents 566
I. Sulfonylureas 566
II. Clinical Syndrome 567
III. Prognosis 568
IV. Biguanide 569
V. Other Oral Hypoglycemic Agents 569
G. Antithyroid Drugs 569
I. Form of Injury 570
II. Clinical Features 570
III. Prognosis 570
IV. Mechanism 571
V. Comment 571
References 571

CHAPTER 24

Hepatotoxicity of Immunomodulating Agents
R.J. Fingerote and G.A. Levy 581

A. Introduction 581
B. Immunostimulatory Agents 582
I. Classification 582
1. Immune-System-Derived Biologicals 583
2. Immunostimulatory Pharmaceutical Agents 583
II. Hepatotoxicity of Specific Immunostimulatory Agents 583
1. Interleukin-2 583
2. Interferons 585
C. Immunosuppressive Agents 588
I. Classification 588
1. Antilymphocyte Products 589
2. Immunophilin-Binding Agents 589
3. Cytotoxic Agents 589
4. Sterols 590
5. Immunosuppressive Antibiotics 590
6. Arachidonic Acid Metabolites 590
II. Hepatotoxic Effects
of Specific Immunosuppressive Agents 591
1. Methotrexate 591
2. Corticosteroids 594
3. Azathioprine 595

4. Cyclosporine 598
5. FK-506 601
D. Conclusion 602
References 602

CHAPTER 25

Alcohol-Induced Liver Injury
Y. Israel and E. Rubin 611

A. Epidemiology 611
B. Liver Dysfunction in Alcoholic Liver Disease 612
I. Hemodynamic Alterations 612
II. Liver Failure 613
C. Alcoholic Liver Injury: Morphological Studies 615
I. Hepatocytes 615
II. Inflammation 616
III. Collagen Deposition 616
IV. Nonparenchymal Cells (EM Studies) 616
1. Ito Cells 616
2. Endothelial Cells 616
3. Kupffer Cells 616
D. Clustering 617
I. Fatty Liver 617
II. Alcoholic Hepatitis 617
III. Alcoholic Cirrhosis 617
E. Pathogenesis of Alcohol-Induced Liver Injury 617
I. Liquid Diet Model 617
II. Cytochrome P450 2E1 618
III. Acetaldehyde Adducts 619
IV. Hepatocyte Ballooning and Hepatomegaly 620
V. Hepatic Oxygen Consumption 621
VI. Liver Hypoxia 622
VII. Intragastric Infusion Model 623
VIII. Modulation of Alcohol-Induced Liver Injury 624
IX. Glutathione 626
X. Micropig Model of Alcoholic Liver Injury 627
XI. Baboon Model of Alcoholic Liver Injury 627
References 628

CHAPTER 26

Antiepileptic Drugs
H.J. Zimmerman and K.G. Ishak. With 10 Figures 637

A. Phenytoin 637
I. Type of Hepatic Injury 637
II. Clinical Manifestations 638
III. Biochemical Features 640
IV. Histopathology 640
V. Prognosis 641
VI. Mechanism 643
VII. Other Hydantoins 645
1. Mephenytoin 645
2. Acetylurea Derivatives 645
3. Oxazolidinediones 646
4. Barbiturates and Primidone 646
B. Carbamazepine 646
I. Susceptibility 646
II. Clinical Features 647
III. Biochemical Features 647
IV. Histopathology 648
V. Prognosis 648
VI. Mechanism 648
C. Valproic Acid 649
I. Incidence of Injury 649
II. Susceptibility 650
III. Clinical Features 650
IV. Biochemical Features 652
V. Histopathology 652
VI. Prognosis 654
VII. Mechanism of Injury 654
VIII. Prevention 657
References 657

Subject Index 663

CHAPTER 1

Orientation in Liver Toxicity by Drugs

E. FARBER

A. Introduction

It is generally well appreciated that virtually all drugs, no matter what organ, tissue, or process is being affected, exert some effects which are irrelevant to their major therapeutic role. In many instances, these irrelevancies manifest undesirable or toxic effects on the host. The liver is no exception in this aspect of drug therapeutics. However, because of its size, its very diverse role in many aspects of host metabolism and its most active role in the metabolism of xenobiotics, the liver becomes far more vulnerable to the "irrelevancies" than does almost any other organ or tissue. The liver plays a very large special role in drug toxicity, far beyond its susceptibility as a target for drug therapy. A wide variety of drugs, of almost every chemical structure, are subject to metabolic detoxification by the liver. The type and degree of these metabolic activities are major determinants in the quantitative and qualitative design of drug therapy. However, this important role of the liver is a "double-edge sword." Since the liver often converts original drugs to water-soluble forms for excretion, it must of necessity convert many an "inactive" compound to an "active" one during this process. The "active" ones are the vehicles for toxicity in many instances. As outlined in this volume, there are many other aspects to drug metabolism which are documented and highlighted. An important basic conceptual aspect in many of these facets can be epitomized by the phrase – "agents versus processes."

B. Agents and Processes

A concept very important in any discussion of cell injury and the responses of the liver to such injury is that of agents and of processes, as separate viewpoints. Toxic manifestations of exposure of a drug or chemical are often the result of the mutual interaction between the agent and the target cells and tissues. Chemicals act on the liver, the liver acts on the chemical, and each in turn is subject to major modulation by diet, by other drugs, and by the physiological or pathological setting in which the interactions take place (e.g., FARBER and FISHER 1979, 1980; MCDANELL and MCLEAN 1985; ROE 1985). This holistic orientation, as opposed to a reductionist one, makes analysis as well as synthesis difficult. Nevertheless, it is essential if we are to understand and in turn to suggest ways of minimizing the toxicological consequences of exposure to drugs or chemicals.

If this integrative orientation is valid, then at least three critical aspects come to mind: (1) the physicochemical nature of the drug and its metabolism in the liver; (2) the state of receptivity of the liver and its modulation; and (3) the qualitative and quantitative responses of the host liver. The first aspect takes us too far afield from the focus of this introductory article and will be handled throughout this monograph as specific drugs are discussed. The second and third aspects, but especially the third, will receive the major emphasis here.

A common approach in current research is to attempt to explain the type of injury and the responses to each injury by emphasis on the agent itself. Although it is axiomatic and well appreciated that a thorough knowledge of the properties, metabolism, and immediate biochemical or metabolic consequences of an active drug is most desirable, it is becoming evident that this approach is far too limited to explain responses to injury. In chronic diseases such as cirrhosis and cancer development, despite a great diversity in the physicochemical properties of different agents, the response patterns of the liver are remarkably similar. Thus, a diversity of input is associated often with a commonality of output or response. This is also now becoming evident in acute responses such as in the induction of cell death. This orientation is gaining recognition because of the realization of the multistep nature of some acute response patterns seen in liver injury. For example, necrosis of liver cells with many agents, such as nitrosamines and acetaminophen, is multistep in nature and can often be prevented even many hours after an initial biochemical or metabolic injury (YING et al. 1980, 1981).

In this context, it should be emphasized that the so-called "pathological" reaction to the alterations in cell biochemistry or cell biology associated with many types of cell injury is not at all pathological in the etymological sense, i.e., it is *not* abnormal. Rather, it is a normal or physiological response to a perturbation in the cell and/or tissue. It can be shown that the response is programmed genetically, to be called upon when the organism or its component parts are stressed in certain ways. It is axiomatic that life on the planet Earth can only have developed, evolved, and "progressed" under conditions permitting living beings to function reasonably well in a hostile environment. It is not unreasonable to suggest that perhaps as muh as 5% or 10% of genetic inheritance could be related to these survival functions.

C. Responses to Injury as Multitier or Multigrid Patterns

The response to virtually all environmental perturbations leading to cell or tissue injury cannot be understood in terms of a single level of organization, even at the cell and tissue level. At least four tiers or grids can now be identified and perhaps more will become evident in the future.

I. Quantitative Versus Qualitative Changes

Before discussing each tier or grid in some detail, it is appropriate to highlight a feature that underlines virtually all aspects of the study of how the liver responds to drug injury – the quantitative versus the qualitative. One of the most difficult aspects in biology, including pathology and toxicology generally, is the relation between different quantitative levels of biochemical, physiological, or structural changes induced by an agent and the cellular or tissue consequences in biological terms. This may be best illustrated by an example (Fig. 1). The exposure of a rat to a single dose of dimethylnitrosamine (DMN) leads to methylation of DNA, RNA, protein, and probably many other cell components and finally to liver cell death. DMN must be metabolized by the microsomal monooxygenase (cytochrome P450) system before it becomes active both chemically and biologically. As seen in Fig. 1, the degree of methylation is continuous and proportional to the dose, beginning with the smallest. The degree of DNA "damage," as measured by sucrose gradient analysis of size, is also proportional to the dose, but only up to about 10 mg/kg body weight, after which it plateaus. The appearance of cell death is also discontinuous. No detectable cell death by any criteria is found until a dose of 13 mg/kg body weight is administered. The degree of cell death is proportional to the dose

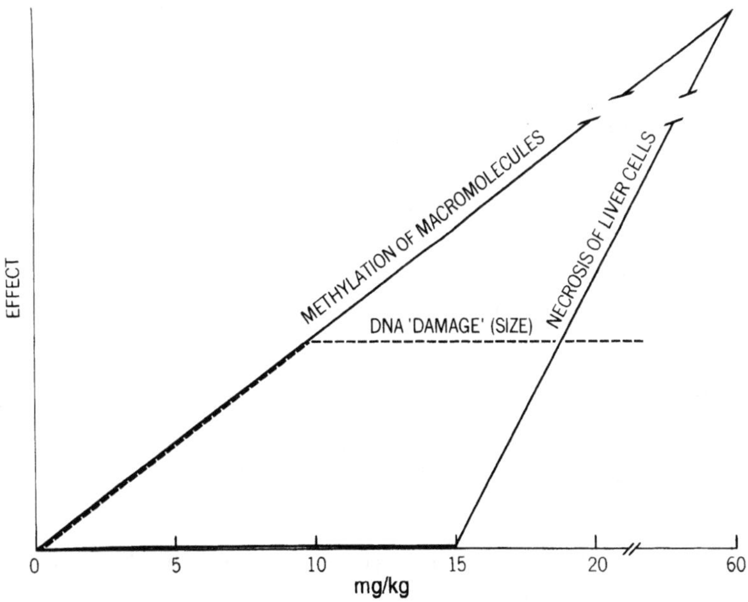

Fig. 1. Schematic representation of the dose responses of three different effects of DMN in rat liver: methylation of a macromolecule, induction of DNA damage as measured by strand breaks in alkali (DNA size), and the induction of liver cell necrosis. Note especially the sharp onset of necrosis when the dose is increased from about 12 to 15 mg/kg. Even a small decrease in the generation of the active moiety or moieties of DMN by the liver could result in a striking loss of a new qualitative effect, necrosis

administered above this threshold level. As is also evident from Fig. 1, the same dose dependence is not seen with every endpoint of cell injury.

We cannot explain this phenomenon in any molecular, biochemical, or cell biological terms at this time. Does the discontinuity in cell response reflect a similar discontinuity at some molecular level or is the relationship more subtle?

This multiplicity is also evident in the liver responses to another hepatoxin, CCl_4. This agent induces at least three discrete tissue responses in the liver: cell death, fatty change (steatosis), and ballooning or dilatation of the smooth and rough endoplasmic reticulum (POPP et al. 1978). Hepatocyte necrosis is seen with extremely small doses and the dose-response curves are different for each of the three discrete endpoints.

II. Patterns of Liver Toxicity

1. Tier One: Patterns of Interactions of Agents with Liver
(CAMERON et al. 1979)

a) *Pattern 1: Harmless and Efficacious*

Drug
or + liver → harmless and efficacious
Chemical

Drug Metabolism (phase I)
or + liver ——————→ harmless and efficacious
Chemical and/or conjugation

This is the desirable pattern and seems to apply to many therapeutically effective agents. Presumably, the conjugation with glucuronic acid, sulfate, cysteine, glycine, or other dietary and cellular constituents does not interfere significantly with the therapeutic efficacy.

b) *Pattern 2: Genesis of Metabolic Imbalance*

Drug Metabolic deficiency or
or → metabolite(s) → imbalance, e.g., ATP, UTP, PO_4, NAD
Chemical

A few compounds, either artifacts of man or naturally occurring, can induce major metabolic imbalances, including deficiencies. Examples of these in the experimental field are the methionine analogue ethionine, inducing ATP deficiency by excessive trapping of adenine, galactosamine, inducing UTP deficiency by trapping uracil, and fructose, inducing alterations in phosphate and ATP. Each of these in turn induces a spectrum of pathological reactions, including fatty liver with ATP deficiency and necrosis with UTP deficiency.

The analysis of the mechanism of induction of the metabolic imbalance has suggested novel or unexpected ways of preventing or curing the experimental disease. For example, with each of the different ways of inducing ATP deficiency, the deficiency can be readily prevented or cured by supplying adenine or, preferably, a nontoxic adenine precursor such as inosine. With UTP, liver cell damage including necrosis can be easily prevented by the administration of uridine, even several hours after inducing the drop in UTP. These are excellent illustrations of the potential of this approach for this general type of liver injury in humans.

c) Pattern 3: Activation of Toxic Metabolites

Drug	Metabolism		Cell	
or	⟶	activated	⟶	Toxic steatosis,
Chemicals			constituents	ballooning,
				necrosis, etc.

Many drugs and other chemicals are metabolized to activated or highly reactive derivatives, which then interact with cellular constituents to produce chemical or biochemical damage and occasionally cellular or tissue damage. An important model for this type of interaction is the interaction of the liver with carbon tetrachloride. Carbon tetrachloride is activated first in the hepatic microsomes to a free radical, which then mediates numerous toxic effects, including membrane damage to the endoplasmic reticulum (ER), diffuse fatty change or steatosis, disaggregation of the polysomes, ballooning of hepatocytes, and liver cell necrosis in zone 3. These acute effects, in particular the fatty change, the cystic dilatation of the ER, and cell death, are clearly distinct and separate response to the hepatotoxin.

An important aspect of this pattern is that the active derivatives of some drugs and chemicals can be trapped in sulfhydryl-containing compounds, such as glutathione (GSH), and in this way prevented from interacting with other cell constituents. Glutathione levels may be depleted, for example, by diethylmaleate or by diet. As has been shown by several groups, administration of compounds such as acetaminophen or bromobenzene produces in the case of GSH depletion an increased covalent binding of activated derivatives to cellular macromolecules, leading to cell damage. Conversely, increasing GSH concentration by the administration of methionine protects the liver against these toxic compounds.

This pattern is potentially very useful, not only for preventing or modulating acute toxic manifestations of drugs or environmental chemicals, but also in the genesis of chronic effects. For example, as discussed below, activated forms of some carcinogens can also be trapped and thereby "neutralized" by suitable liver constituents such as GSH.

Drug	Metabolism	+ GSH	S-Chemical
or	⟶ activated		
chemical		–GSH	Damage

It should be recalled that cell death is a multistep process, one of the late steps common to many situations being an activation of phospholipase A by an increase in Ca^{2+} levels. This in turn breaks down membrane phospholipids resulting in irreversible loss of membrane integrity, with a major influx of Ca^{2+} and Na^{+}, loss of K^{+}, etc.

d) *Pattern 4: Induction of Enzymes and Increase of SER*

	Short-term	
Drugs, toxic agents, → chemicals, etc.	SER → + Enzymes	metabolism
	Long-term	
Drugs, toxic agents,→ chemicals, etc.	SER →	metabolism

A consistent and prominent response of the liver cell to drugs and chemicals is an increase of the smooth endoplasmic reticulum (SER). Following exposure to a large number of different compounds, including steroids, polycyclic aromatic hydrocarbons, anesthetic agents, and insecticides, a proliferation of SER is evident which is accompanied by an increased activity of drug-metabolizing enzymes, especially the microsomal mono-oxygenases.

In addition to the short-term induction, leading to an increase in both membranes and enzyme activities, a long-term phenomenon occurs in which there is a dissociation between many of the enzyme activities and the membranes. In chronic liver disease, including chronic exposure to environmental agents such as dieldrin and other genotoxic hepatocarcinogens, and to hepatitis B virus, one observes the production of excessive amounts of smooth ER, seen in H&E preparations as abundant "ground glass" cytoplasm. This change may be accompanied by a decrease, not an increase, in the concentration of many ER enzymes, leading to what has been called "hypoactive hypertrophic ER." We are of the opinion that this change might be an important sign of the genesis of resistant cells which are considered to play a key role in carcinogenesis (see below).

e) *Pattern 5: Carcinogenesis*

The first four patterns are general ones affecting either all the hepatocytes or all hepatocytes in certain zones of all the liver acini. This pattern, pattern 5, is of a totally different nature. It seems to affect only a very small minority of hepatocytes and these apparently at random.

Drug or Chemical	→	Activated →	Permanent genetic cell change
			↓
		Cancer ← ← ← ←	New hepatocytes

The carcinogenic process can be divided into very different phases. The first phase, or initiation, is usually short and involves the interaction of the active derivative with DNA or other macromolecules, leading to an essentially permanent cellular change resembling a somatic mutation. The second phase is a slow, progressive, cellular evolution, resembling a differentiation process involving the appearance of new cell populations in succession from preneoplastic to premalignant, and then malignant.

The chemical carcinogen becomes activated in the liver to an electrophilic reactant which then causes widespread chemical and biochemical damage. Many cells repair this molecular damage and occasional cells die. This initiation event induces a large array of different changes in various cells, only a few of which are functionally suited for selective growth as precursors for the next phase of cellular evolution. One altered phenotype which serves as a functional basis for selection is the property of carcinogen resistance. About $1/10^6$ of the original hepatocytes are induced with this phenotype by a single dose with the initiating carcinogen diethylnitrosamine and about $1/10^8$ of the original hepatocytes show this carcinogen-resistant property following the carcinogen aflatoxin B_1 (FARBER and SARMA 1987).

If cell replication occurs prior to repair of the molecular damage in these altered cells, there is fixation of the damage in the daughter cells. These focal areas of altered phenotype are identifiable by a number of positive and negative histochemical markers, namely positive-staining for γ-glutamyl-transpeptidase and negative-staining for glucose-6-phosphatase and ATPase.

The funtional property of these altered hepatocytes of resistance to the cytotoxic and cytoinhibitory effects of liver toxins and carcinogens can be utilized as a basis for selective growth of these cells relative to the surrounding "carcinogen-sensitive" cells. What then is the mechanism for the resistance of these altered cells to hepatotoxins? Hepatocyte ("hyperplastic") nodules derived from these focal lesions demonstrate several alterations in the uptake and metabolism of hepatotoxins and carcinogens which may represent the bases for this resistance. In vitro, nodule cells demonstrate a striking resistance to the cytotoxic effects of aflatoxin B_1, relative to normal and to surrounding liver.

The vast majority of preneoplastic lesions, i.e., the hundreds of foci and many of the hepatocyte nodules, undergo a maturation or remodeling towards phenotypically normal liver. A small number of preneoplastic nodular lesions persist and in several months cancers arise. Metastasis is quite frequent, commonly in the lung. In some cases, the cancer can be seen to arise within an hepatocyte nodule. An important point is that one or only very few cancers develop, irrespective of the carcinogen used. The carcinogenic process then seems to be a probability phenomenon in that, despite the exposure of all liver cells to the carcinogen, only a proportion of these cells develop into foci. Of these foci, only a few nodules persist to serve as precursors for the ultimate evolution of cancer. There appears to be a continual selection of smaller and smaller numbers of cells, each with an increasingly greater probability of development into cancer.

An important feature is the long latent period or time lag between the initial appearance of a cellular reaction to the carcinogen, or the appearance of preneoplastic lesions, and the appearance of recognizable cancer. This delay of the appearance of cancer, which lasts for many months to years in animals and at least 15–25 years in humans, has important survival values for the species, as the peak of the appearance of malignancy is prolonged past the reproductive period. The host factors responsible for delaying the rate of cellular evolution to malignancy are as yet unknown. In the liver model, the application of a selection pressure for carcinogen-altered cells greatly accelerates the rate of cellular evolution to malignancy. A similar phenomenon is evident in man, in which a continued or repeated exposure to a carcinogen, or carcinogens as in the case of occupational exposure, decreases the latent period for cancer development. A knowledge of the environmental conditions that confer a selective growth advantage on initiated cells in tissues other than liver could be of great value in controlling malignant development in that tissue.

Finally, it is important to point out that the preneoplastic phase of liver carcinogenesis, which lasts for 50% or more of the time taken to develop cancer, is a form of adaptive hyperplasia (FARBER and SARMA 1987; FARBER 1990; FARBER and RUBIN 1991). The availability of a small population of cells with a new resistance phenotype can enable the mature sensitive hepatocytes to be replaced by new resistant ones and thus has survival value for the host under adverse conditions. We think this is one way in which adaptation to carcinogens or carcinogenic stimuli has occurred in a positive way during evolution (FARBER and SARMA 1987; FARBER 1990; FARBER and RUBIN 1991). The preneoplastic phase of liver carcinogenesis would then represent a flexible, adaptive response that could play an important role in the survival of the species. Once the reproductive period is over, whether or not cancer develops is of no major consequence to survival of the species, seemingly a major force in selecting the direction of evolution.

2. Tier Two: Patterns of Biological Responses to Cell Injury

It has been known for over 25 years that the liver (and many other tissues or organs to different degrees) are by no means passive targets for the effects of drugs and chemicals. Rather, the liver is highly responsive at several levels of organization to a large number of xenobiotics including chemicals designed for therapeutic purposes (drugs) (Table 1). The liver responds with the produc-

Table 1. Response of living organisms to xenobiotic agents

A. Xenobiotic microorganisms: viruses, bacteria, protozoa, etc.
   1. Phagocytosis
   2. Inflammation
   3. Immune systems

B. Xenobiotic chemicals

   General
   1. Reversible enzyme induction (general)
   2. Constitutive enzyme induction (focal)
   3. Heat shock proteins
   4. Acute reactive proteins

   Genotoxic
   1. Metabolizing enzymes (general)
   2. DNA repair enzymes, e.g., "adaptive response" (alkyltransferase)
   3. Clonal adaptation

Table 2. Some patterns of biological responses to cell injury

I. General or zonal
   A. Production of new protein patterns
      1. Heat shock proteins
      2. Acute reactive proteins (see KUSHNER et al. 1982)
   B. Hypertrophy – induction of enzymes and membranes
      1. Acute
         a) Induction of many enzymes (microsomal, etc.) plus other cell constituents (e.g., glutathione and several phase 1 and phase 2 components)
         b) Production of membranes
      2. Chronic
         a) Production of membranes
         b) New patterns of induction of enzymes and other constituents – e.g., decrease in phase 1 and increase in many phase 2 components
         c) "Ground-glass" cells
   C. Hyperplasia – caused by some enzyme inducers, lead nitrate, etc.

II. Focal
   A. Hyperplasia
   B. Carcinogenesis – rare mutation-like change plus selection generating new resistant hepatocyte population

tion of many enzymes and other proteins utilized both intracellularly and for secretion. Although our knowledge and understanding of these patterns is certainly not exhaustive or complete, we are beginning to delineate some overall patterns. Based upon our current understanding and with some extrapolation to liver from tissues and cells generally [e.g., in the case of "heat shock proteins" (SCHLESSINGER et al. 1982)], a reasonable resumé of some of the highlights is presented in Table 2. Two references in particular are worth nothing, as they give a comprehensive review of several aspects of these patterns (SCHULTE-HERMANN 1974, 1979). It is not surprising and in fact desirable to have an overlap between the responses in the different tiers.

3. Tier Three: Cellular and Intracellular Responses

A third level of response concerns the whole cell and its organelles. Included in this grouping are irreversible responses such as cell death, as well as many reversible ones.

a) Irreversible Response: Cell Death

Physiologically, cell death is most easily characterized by a change in membrane properties. In in vitro preparations of isolated cells, the dead ones readily become visible by accumulating dyes such as trypan blue while viable cells do not. Also, dying or dead cells show accumulations of Ca^{2+} and Na^{+} with loss of K^{+}. Thus, they manifest some severe alterations in cell membrane function as an index of cell death. Despite the obvious severe physiological disturbance, the cells may not appear abnormal for several hours, even by electron microscopy. However, within several hours, obvious changes begin to appear in the cells indicative of self-digestion or autolysis and it is at this time that we can recognize that tissue cells have died at some time previously. This series of morphological changes that ensue following cell death we call necrosis.

As predictable, mitochondria undergo swelling and lose their capacity for oxidative generation of ATP, membranes of the endoplasmic reticulum show progressive dilatation with destruction, and the tissues often become increasingly acid if they contain carbohydrates that can be broken down by glycolysis to pyruvic and lactic acid without their further oxidation to CO_2 and water. However, the changes that are most useful are those in the nucleus. Depending upon the type of cell and the etiological agent, the nucleus of a dead cell becomes shrunken and dark-staining (condensation of DNA or chromain) (pyknosis, adjective: pyknotic), shows fragmentation into many small pieces (karyorrhexis), or shows progressive loss of staining (karyolysis).

The cell cytoplasm shows a loss of basophilia, as the ribosomes and their RNA get broken down, with an increasing loss of any cytoplasmic detail. This is often seen as a progressive eosinophilic staining of the dead cells. The breakdown of the tissue constituents releases many soluble components from cells into the blood including enzymes. The increase in serum levels of enzymes is a very useful diagnostic indicator of cell death. The delay in the appearance of necrosis poses a diagnostic problem. For example, if an individual dies of acute coronary artery occlusion within a few hours of onset, no evidence of cell death and necrosis may be found. If the person lived for 12h or longer, one can easily see evidence of localized necrosis.

α) Apoptosis Versus Necrosis

We all realize that cell death is an important variable in several phases of cell and tissue toxicity. Despite the obvious importance of cell death to our understanding of many pathological conditions including those relating to cancer, this pathobiological process remains poorly understood. However, a current source of major confusion relates to the term "*apoptosis*," as compared and contrasted with "*necrosis*." "Apoptosis" and "necrosis" are considered to represent quite different types or examples of cell death (Wyllie et al. 1980).

I have recently re-read, very carefully, many of the published articles on apoptosis, programmed cell death, necrosis, etc., and can state that there is no field of basic cell biology and cell pathology relating to toxicology that is more confusing and more unintelligible than is the area of *apoptosis versus necrosis* (see Farber 1994). If any degree of clarity is to develop in our understanding of the fundamental principles underlying cell death of any type, it is encumbent upon us to re-think "from square one" the scientific analysis of how cells die and how we assess cell death in a reasonably rational manner.

Before comparing, briefly, these two presumed different processes, it is important to point out that there are two fundamental aspects of cell death that are quite separate but are often "lumped" together: (1) *the process of cell death* and (2) *the series of structural-biochemical changes that transpire in cells and tissues after some of the cells die*, i.e., *the postmortem autolytic changes*. These two processes are quite different and discrete physiologically but unfortunately are not often handled separately in the analysis of either apoptosis or necrosis. Almost all our assays for cell death of any kind rely mainly on the structural and physiological changes the dead cells undergo *after they die*. Thus, mainly if not exclusively, they assay for "postmortem" changes, not the process or processes involved in the death of the cell. The antemortem changes leading to cell death and the postmortem changes are radically different, since the former are "active" and often adaptive while the latter appear to be passive.

Some of the major sources for the confusion concerning the seemingly different types of cell death are as follows: (1) morphological characterization, (2) cell variation, (3) programmed versus unprogrammed cell death, and (4) cell death as an active, not a passive process.

1. The designation of "apoptosis" as a special form of cell death is scientifically unjustified. The "shrinkage necrosis" characterized in part by the nuclear and cytoplasmic changes that are reputed to be characteristic can be found in many different mammalian organs or tissues during the classical process of necrosis. It is easy to see, even on casual examination, "single cell necrosis" indistinguishable from the so-called apoptosis, in many tissues in which necrosis has been induced by toxic xenobiotics, including various chemotherapeutic agents, as well as by microorganisms and ischemic and other environmental perturbations. For example, carbon tetrachloride is a potent toxic agent for the rat liver, inducing "classical" zonal necrosis in zone 3 of the liver acinus. Examination of the liver with even a moderate degree of necrosis readily reveals single cell necrosis, especially at the periphery of the major lesion, that by itself would be designated as apoptotic. Very small doses of carbon tetrachloride that do *not* induce zonal necrosis do induce single cell necrosis in zone 3 that again could be designated as apoptosis.

In the morphological assessment of apoptosis, a critical property of different cells is overlooked. Comparisons are repeatedly made with so-called coagulative necrosis, as described by Trump and associates (e.g., TRUMP et al. 1965, 1981, 1984). Most of the comparisons are between dead, autolyzing, and putrefying liver undergoing postmortem change in vitro or after ischemia and the apoptotic cells. The comparisons are entirely the structural changes that transpire in cells and tissues *after* they die. The process of cell death is totally ignored in all of these studies. The types and rates of changes that occur postmortem, either in the living organism or after death of the organism, vary very widely with the type of cell, with the etiological agent, with the pathological process under study, and with the physiological condition of the tissues prior to death.

2. It is appreciated by developmental cell biologists as well as by cell pathologists that cells vary widely in their responses to physiological and pathological environmental modulations, including of course their reactions to cytotoxic xenobiotics and hormones. This variation encompasses both the processes of cell death and the morphological and other changes that follow the death of cells, the postmortem autolytic changes. At one extreme are some lymphocytes (and perhaps other cells in the thymus) that often show a fairly short period of cell death and an inordinately rapid set of postmortem changes, the latter being designated as "apoptosis." Lymphocytes often show advanced postmortem changes ("apoptosis") within 2–3h (e.g., HUGON and BORGERS 1966). At the other end of the spectrum are rat liver hepatocytes, when cell death is induced by cytotoxic nitrosamines, such as dimethylnitrosamine and diethylnitrosamine. They often show morphological characteristics of necrosis (usually zone 3 necrosis) in hepatocytes only after 36–48h, even though the nitrosamines undergo their complete metabolic conversion to highly reactive derivatives by 4–8h (YING et al. 1980, 1981). Most cells in the various tissues and organs, including liver cells exposed to many different xenobiotics, fall somewhere between the two extremes in this spectrum.

Also, the same cells may show wide variations both in the process of cell death and in the postmortem changes depending upon the nature of the initiating agent. For example, with carbon tetrachloride, no reports have appeared to suggest that the induction of cell death in the liver can be inhibited or prevented by treatments as rapid as a few minutes *after* the parenteral administration of the CCl_4. Treatments immediately *before* its administration [e.g., cycloheximide, diphenyl-*p*-phenylenediamine (DPDD), diethyl-dithiocarbamate (DEDTC), and other compounds] can be very effective in preventing cell death (POPP et al. 1978). In contrast to the very short duration of the process of cell death is the relatively long period (12–24h) before the structural postmortem autolytic changes become readily apparent. With dimethylnitrosamine or diethylnitrosamine, the processes of cell death in the same zone, zone 3, in the same species and the same strain, last at least 4 and 8h, respectively (YING et al. 1980). This is followed by a relatively long period (48–72h or longer) of postmortem change.

Also, the nature of the postmortem changes varies considerably with the cell and the initiating agent or perturbation. Classically, dead cells may undergo pyknosis (nuclear condensation), karyorrhexis (nuclear breakup), or karyolysis (progressive loss of nuclear material). Until the biochemical bases for these changes are studied and understood, it is impossible to state that the nuclear condensation, including the inconstant nucleosomal laddering effect, seen in so-called apoptosis, is anything but a minor variant falling within this spectrum of changes (e.g., AMENTA et al. 1993). In addition, the same initiating agent can induce varying morphological changes in the same cell type at the same time. This can be readily seen with CCl_4 as mentioned and with thioacetamide (LEDDA-COLUMBANO et al. 1991).

It is obvious that the popular selection of some (as yet unknown) types of lymphocytes and thymocytes as typical cells for the study of apoptosis introduces an enormous bias and distortion in any objective analysis of the processes of cell death and of postmortem changes in many biological phenomena, be they physiological or pathological. This is clearly illustrated by the study of cell death in the small intestine of the rat or mouse induced by a variety of cytotoxic treatments. Inhibitors of DNA synthesis, such cytosine arabinoside ("ara C"), and some alkylating agents such as nitrogen mustard, as well as X-rays, induce clear-cut morphological changes in the cells lining the crypts. These changes have been interpreted for a long time as acute lethal effects on the proliferating mucosal epithelial cells.

The process is more complex than appeared. These agents have at least two effects on the intestinal mucosa. One effect, seen with all three types of agents, is a rapid induction of cell death in some of the lymphocytes in the submucosa (VERBIN et al. 1971, 1973). This cell death appears within a few hours and is followed shortly by phagocytosis of the dead lymphocytes by the mucosal epithelial cells. This is considered to be necrosis or, if you like, "apoptosis" (WYLLIE et al. 1980). A second effect, seen with X-rays and with mitogen mustard, is a slower one, in which the mucosal epithelial cells disappear and the villi become atrophic. How this occurs is not known. Thus, in a classical example of cell death with necrosis, the target cells are some lymphocytes in the submucosa which undergo cell death and subsequent postmortem changes followed by phagocytosis by other cells, all within a few hours.

This is considered to be an example of "apoptosis," similar or analogous to what happens in many different types of cells, including skeletal muscle cells, during developmental programmed cell death. Since no mechanisms for such changes are understood, the conclusions with regard to similarities are entirely speculative and highly problematical from the point of view of the cell pathologist as well as the molecular biologist.

The topic of "lymphocytes" and "apoptosis" is further complicated by the presence of at least two different responses of "lymphocytes" to the same agents inducing inhibition of protein synthesis. Inhibitors of protein synthesis, such as cycloheximide and tenuazonic acid, at doses that inhibit protein synthesis at about 90%, rapidly induce cell death followed quickly by postmortem change in "some lymphocytes" in many lymph nodes and in Peyer's patches (Verbin et al. 1971). The same inhibitors in the same dosage do *not* induce cell death in lymphocytes in the intestinal submucosa and in some bone marrow cells but rather protect these cells against cell death induced by inhibitors of DNA synthesis, an alkylating agent (nitrogen mustard) of X-rays (Verbin et al. 1973; Ben-Ishay and Farber 1975). Thus seemingly similar cells, "lymphocytes" of undetermined type, can respond quite differently to the same metabolic disturbance induced by the same agent.

Clearly, until these various responses and some inkling of mechanisms of cell death and postmortem autolytic change are clarified, it is foolhardy to introduce yet another term for an unknown portion of the response spectrum of cells in the mammalian organism.

3. It is now frequently stated that apoptosis, unlike necrosis, is "programmed" cell death. Necrosis is presumably unprogrammed.

Unfortunately, the terms "programmed" and "unprogrammed" are used in different contexts and in some ways that are ill defined and confusing. There are at least three different meanings for the term "programmed."

1. Programmed cell death refers to very selective cell death that is seen regularly and predictably during normal embryologic development and during maturation of organisms, tissues, or organs (e.g., Lockshin et al. 1984). This use is completely logical, rational, and meaningful at the phenomenological level. Whether there are genes or a specific genetic pattern for the occurrence of the cell death at the right time and in the right location is, of course, often implied but incorrectly so (e.g., see Williams and Smith 1993; Barinaga 1994). It is equally plausible theoretically that some other highly reproducible event or series of events during development might be the actual trigger or stimulus for a derivative cell death. The finding of a gene that codes for a protein that participates in either the process of cell death or the postmortem autolytic changes that follow should not be confused with a gene or set of genes that is or are *responsible* for the specific cell death, if such exist. This process of selective cell death might perhaps be better referred to as "*developmentally programmed*" cell death. I would anticipate that the biochemical sequences leading to death of a cell and the sequences during the postmortem phase would be highly variable from cell to cell or tissue to tissue, since the biochemical *pattern* of every type of cell is obviously unique.

2. A second use of the word programmed appears to relate to a reproducible sequence of cellular properties that play an active role in the genesis of cell death induced by a wide variety of xenobiotic chemicals and microorganisms and by other environmental modulations. The mechanisms underlying such programs are unknown, even though, again, it is *not* valid to consider this as gene-determined unless the gene can be shown to code for the *program*, and not simply for one of the protein components in the sequence. This form of cell death could easily be a reflection of predictable biochemical patterns of types of cells that follow automatically from one or more specific perturbations initiating that particular process of cell death. Naturally, since the genome is

one important arm of the determinants of the phenotype of all cells, it must play at least an indirect role in the process: This form of cell death is often called *pathological.* Perhaps it should be designated as "*biochemically programmed*" cell death (e.g., COHEN and BARNER 1954; FARBER et al. 1971). It could involve zones or regions of an organ or tissue or individual scattered cells or clusters of cells ("focal"). For example, the liver (and other organs) may show zonal cell death, scattered individual cell death, or scattered focal collections of cells undergoing cell death. The designation of zonal or focal as "necrosis" and of individual as "apoptosis" has yet to be justified by any very careful comparisons at different levels of organization including the whole cell and the organ or tissue.

An obvious problem that has not been studied is the mistaken notion that single dead cells in sinusoids of the liver accompanied by evidence of phagocytosis of cell debris by hepatocytes represent hepatocytes that have undergone "apoptosis" (e.g., LEDDA-COLUMBANO et al. 1992). An equally likely or perhaps more likely possibility is that the dead cells are lymphocytes or other cells from the hematolymphopoietic system that become trapped and secondarily phagocytosed by the intact liver cells.

3. A third form of "programmed" cell death, perhaps better designated as "*physiologically programmed,*" is seen in organs or tissues that undergo temporary hyperplasia and then return to their "resting physiological" level of cell turnover (SCHULTE-HERMANN 1974, 1979; BURSCH et al. 1984). The return of the liver to its physiological cell level after hyperplasia with diet or with selective mitogenic xenobiotics is a favorite object of current study for "programmed cell death" or "apoptosis." Whether so-called "apoptosis" can *quantitatively* account for the degree of cell loss remains to be established.

There are no doubt other forms of cell death that might fit into the "programmed" category. The use of the term "programmed" obviously implies that there are forms of cell death that are "unprogrammed." Whether this is so or not remains to be established. The major subject for comparison with "programmed" cell death is either tissue undergoing postmortem autolytic change in vitro in the incubator or following occlusion of blood supply to induce an infarct. How "unprogrammed" the cell death is in the latter instance is totally unknown, only surmised intuitively. Intuition is a dangerous basis for making conclusions in biological systems. The remarkable protective effects of proteolytic preparations administered to patients even 1 h or more *after* coronary artery occlusion indicate the probable presence of a "programmed" sequence of changes before the myocardial cells die. Intuition would probably discourage such exciting developments.

I think it behooves critical scientific investigators to be much more specific and detailed in their studies of cell death as "programmed" or "unprogrammed." Also, a clear-cut separation of cell death and postmortem changes in cells or at least a recognition of the existence of the two quite separate processes, coupled with a respect for the many biochemical differences between cells, would no doubt assist in the rational analyses of cell death as an important component of many biological systems. Included in such analyses should be the likelihood that the biochemical changes seen under these many conditions are quite different.

4. It is frequently assumed, without evidence, but based on intuition, that the death of cells under most circumstances, is passive, not active. This assumption is certainly implied frequently when cell death is induced by exogenous environmental influences, such as xenobiotic chemicals and microorganisms or by physiological compromises such as ischemia. Cell death is considered to be an unfortunate consequence of a "pathological process."

This nonbiological antiquated view of cell death (and of many other so-called pathological changes) ignores completely the possible role of cell death in physiological maintenance and adaptation. It is easy to propose that many instances of cell death have survival value for the organism. If this were so, it would be anticipated that cells, tissues, and organisms have evolved mechanisms to remove "seriously injured" cells and to restore the system. With respect to long-term processes such as the development of cancer via carcinogenesis, it has been shown that some of the early so-called pathological tissue responses are adaptively beneficial to the organism with clear-cut survival value (FARBER 1990; FARBER and RUBIN 1991). It can be easily seen that the induction of cell death followed by removal and replacement has much greater survival value than does the accumulation of injured cells that could progressively and seriously interfere with the physiological performance of that organism, organ, or tissue.

There are now many examples in which RNA and protein synthesis, presumably leading to the appearance of new proteins or increased levels of proteins already present, play critical roles in the pathogenesis of cell death (e.g., see LIEBERMAN et al. 1970; FARBER 1971; FARBER et al. 1971; POPP et al. 1978; YING et al. 1980; VERBIN et al. 1973; MCDANELL and MCLEAN 1985). This has been described in prokaryotes, bacteria, by COHEN and BARNER where unbalanced cell death in *E. coli* was shown to be an active, not a passive, process (COHEN and BARNER 1954, 1975; COHEN 1966). It cannot be assumed, as is often done in discussions of apoptosis, that "ordinary" cell death or "necrosis" is a passive process while the presumed special form of cell death, "apoptosis," is active. The data available so far, although by no means exhaustive, indicate that many forms of cell death, regardless of their particular morphological appearance, are active in that enzyme induction and perhaps other forms of active responses occur as common and essential components of the process of cell death.

Thus, it cannot be concluded that the concept of "apoptosis" adds new insights into the problem of cell death from the point of view of the experimental cell pathologist. Since I personally have no experience in developmental biology, I am in no position to judge whether the concept of "apoptosis" is particularly valuable in normal development. However, the concept does not seem to have any value for cell pathology, for our understanding of disease, or in bridging the gap between the "normal" and the so-called "pathological."

b) Reversible Response

a*) Change in Cell Size*

i) Atrophy. This is manifested as a decrease in the average size of the cells. The changes seen are virtually all cytoplasmic, such as in the endoplasmic reticulum and in mitochondria, and involve losses in proteins, RNA, and phospholipids with no loss in the DNA per cell. This is frequently associated with no loss or with the apparent increase in selected pigments, such as hemosiderin and lipofuscin. Such changes appear to be the basis for the old designation "brown atrophy."

ii) Hypertrophy. A general increase in the size of the hepatocytes is seen frequently in responses to many drugs. These may involve the nucleus, or one or more of the cytoplasmic organelles.

Nucleus: Normally, the maturation of liver is associated with the progressive increase in ploidy of hepatocytes leading to tetraploid or octaploid nuclei or even nuclei with a complement of 16nDNA. These changes in turn are associated with increasingly larger nuclei. With some xenobiotics, such as the widespread plant pyrrolizidine alkaloids, e.g., lasiocarpine, the hepatocytes show a striking megalocytosis, due presumably to DNA replication without cell division (SAMUEL and JAGO 1975). Nuclear "hypertrophy" is a common response of hepatocytes to many xenobiotics, especially in some species such as the mouse. Similar responses do occur in the human but are less striking than in some animals.

Endoplastic reticulum (ER): One of the most common responses of the liver to many drugs, toxic xenobiotics, and some viruses is proliferation of the ER (see Sect. C.II.1.d). Patients who become hepatitis B carriers show this in its chronic form. This type of response may have a special relevance to the genesis of hepatocellular carcinoma.

Mitochondria: Proliferation of mitochondria is seen in response to some drugs. A recent example is the rapid and vigorous proliferation of mitochondria in hepatocytes in rats treated with the antihistaminic methapyrilene (REZNIK-SCHULLER and LIJINSKY 1982). How this change may relate to the liver carcinogenic effect of this drug is not clear.

Peroxisomes ("microbodies"): A common response of the liver to several different hypolipidemic agents (clofibrate, nafenopin, etc.) used clinically to lower blood cholesterol and/or triglycerides is the proliferation of peroxisomes. This is associated with increased activities of peroxisomes enzymes. A similar response of the liver is seen on exposure to some plasticizers such as the substituted phthalates.

β) Accumulations and Storages

i) Tryglceride (TF) Accumulation in Liver ("Fatty Liver"). The liver plays a major role in the synthesis and secretion of serum proteins. If a block occurs between sites of synthesis of TG in the ER and of secretion at the cell surface, TG accumulates in ER or the Golgi apparatus. Such a block may be due to the interference with synthesis of constituents needed to package TG for secretion as very low density lipoproteins (VLDLs). These include protein, polysaccharide, phospholipids, and cholesterol. This is an excellent example of the dynamics of a disease process in which the morphological changes can be accounted for largely in pathophysiological terms.

ii) Glycogen. At least seven different types of glycogen storage diseases are known. These include the nonlysosomal type I (von Gierke's) form in which the liver is a major site. This form is associated with a deficiency of glucose-6-phosphatase.

iii) Iron. Siderosis of the liver, with iron overload, is seen in response to repeated blood transfusions. A much more serious form of iron storage, hemachromatosis, is associated with a slowly progressive cell damage in the liver and an increased risk of developing hepatocellular carcinoma.

iv) α_1-Antitrypsin. Some individuals with low or absent levels of normal α_1-antitrypsin (AAT) in the blood show liver accumulation of this glycoprotein. The deficiency in some instances is due not to a failure to synthesize the protein, but rather to a defect in intracellular transport or secretion. The accumulation of ATT in hepatocytes is not infrequent in liver cancer. About 10% of individuals with pulmonary emphysema have an AAT deficiency.

γ) Changes in General Metabolic Pathways

It is virtually axiomatic that many responses of the liver to injury will involve, to major or minor degrees, either decreases or even increases in such fundamental activities as (1) protein synthesis, (2) RNA synthesis, (3) DNA synthesis, (4) energy production and levels of ATP and other nucleotides, and (5) glycolysis.

i) Protein Synthesis. Inhibition of the overall synthesis of protein by as much as 90% for many hours has relatively few consequences in most cells in vivo. A few show dramatic effects. A few examples are shown below.

Diptheria toxin: The toxin (a protein) is split at the cell surface and one split product enters and inhibits protein synthesis. This may be one basis for the generalized toxemia seen in diptheria.

Lymphoid organs: Inhibition of protein synthesis causes rapid cell death in some populations of cells in the lymphoreticular system. Especially sensitive are germinal centers of follicles and some cells in the thymus. The exact nature of the affected cells, whether of a so-called stem cell type or of B or T cells, remains unknown.

Mitoses: Inhibition of protein synthesis arrests the cell cycle before mitosis early in G_2; therefore, cells later in the cycle complete the cycle, whereas the others are arrested in G_2; Thus, within 1 or 2h, the body becomes devoid of all mitotic figures, including the liver during regeneration.

Liver: The liver shows a progressive accumulation of TG, first in the ER, and then by coalescence throughout the cytoplasm. On return of protein synthesis, the TG becomes packaged in VLDLs and secreted.

General: The effects of inhibition of protein synthesis on the ribosomes depend upon the site of inhibition. In most cases, the rough ER shows extensive loss of ribosomes. The free ribosomes often show reproducible alterations in structure with eventual loss of function, usually by 24h.

ii) RNA Synthesis. As with protein synthesis, we do not know in most instances the effects of specific inhibition of synthesis of any single type of RNA. Overall, the nucleolus shows extensive damage when RNA synthesis is inhibited. This takes one of two forms: (1) so-called segregation of the normal components so that they separate out in regions instead of being intertwined, and (2) diffuse breakup and scattering of the nucleolus into many pieces. Each can be fairly rapidly restored in the absence of new proteins. Thus, the defect is related somehow to the way in which the normal components are organized. The functional consequences to the cell of such lesions are not understood. In the human, it is seen in its most dramatic form in *Amanita* poisoning. One of the toxic agents, a cyclic peptide, α-amanatin, is a very potent inhibitor of the synthesis of RNA in many tissues including liver and kidney. Whether this biochemical lesion is the cause of the severe toxicity of *Amanita* is not known.

iii) Focal Cytoplasmic Degeneration. The use of the electron microscope has uncovered a very common form of cell injury, called focal cytoplasmic degeneration. Many causes for cell injury induce irreversible damage to one or more cytoplasmic components. The latter include endoplasmic reticulum (ER) [smooth (S) and rough (R)], mitochondria, peroxisomes, etc. Such localized areas of cell damage are engulfed by lysosomes which segregate the injured structures (autophagy). The lysosomes in turn hydrolyze the proteins, nucleic acid, lipids, carbohydrates, and other constituents in the damaged organelles. Any undigested material either accumulates or is often excreted by the cell. Virtually all cytoplasmic components can participate in this type of focal damage with the notable exception of the plasma membrane. This membrane and the nucleus do not seem to be dispensable to a significant degree and thus are two of the key sites in the cell that are essential for cell integrity.

4. Tier Four: Cellular and Tissue Physiology

One of the most important levels of integration in the understanding of responses to injury is the physiological or functional one. Among the basic response patterns of the liver to injury are those shown below.

a) *Cholestasis*

One of the commonest responses to drugs is the modulation of the secretion of bile. Cholestasis is one of the most striking changes seen under many circumstances. A recent survey of this can be found in Phillips and Poucell (1986). A variety of different forms or types of cholestasis are known. These include cholestasis with cholangitis, cholestasis without cholangitis, cholangiolar cholestasis, canalicular cholestasis, syndromatic cholestasis, subcellular cholestasis, and subclinical cholestasis (Phillips and Poucell 1986). Drug-related cholestatic conditions are largely concerned with intrahepatic forms including changes in liver cell and canalicular functions. The possible alterations by drugs of the paracellular pathway of flow of some bile constituents have been given serious consideration as has the dysfunction of pericanalicular microfilaments. These and other functional and structural alterations are rational current hypotheses for drug-induced cholestasis.

b) *Inflammation*

Like any other living tissue, the liver is a site for a variety of different types of acute and chronic inflammation. Since liver cell necrosis is a relatively common form of response to injury, one not infrequently observes an acute inflammatory reaction to the necrotic tissue. Recent studies indicate that several different mediators play important roles in these types of reactions including vasoactive amines, components of the complement system, and other plasma protein-derived agents, leukocyte organelles, prostaglandins, leukotrienes, and others. One reaction that is often considered to be important is the lymphoid response, especially in viral hepatitis. Included in this group are some putative autoimmune reactions (e.g., Chisari et al. 1979). Although a popular subject for speculation, there is little "solid" evidence with which to place in perspective the possible importance of these special responses in the pathogenesis of disease and in the biology of drug-induced injury. A critical scientific approach appears to be indicated.

c) *Fibrosis*

One of the most serious responses of the liver to injury is fibrosis with disorganization of the basic architecture leading to cirrhosis. The past decade or so has seen an expanding interest in the factors that accompany the increasing development of fibrosis and their possible modulation in the prevention of cirrhosis (e.g., Rojkind and Dunn 1979; Popper and Stern 1979; Stern 1979; Popper and Martin 1982).

The relationship between the different types of collagen synthesized and hepatic fibrosis and cirrhosis coupled with the increasing emphasis on patterns and inducers of collagen breakdown is receiving increasing attention. In addition, liver proteoglycans and glycoproteins and their relationship to specific cell types such as fibroblasts, Ito cells and myofibroblasts, and hepatocytes and a variety of peptide growth factors and modifiers are now being implicated in one or more aspects of fibrogenesis. These studies should lead to a better understanding of the molecular events associated with fiber formation and fibrosis.

An area that is critical, but remains poorly understood, is the nature of the influences that determine whether injured liver cells will "proliferate" to form a reasonably normal regenerated organ or will somehow stimulate a fibroblastic response. The determinants of biological options in this sequence of patterns to chronic injury are major challenges for the future, since their elucidation may offer new and exciting tools to the physician in preventing the undesirable responses to such injury.

D. Conclusion

In summary, it is evident from this cursory view of hepatic responses to injury that this is an area of physiology and pathology that needs much more in depth study. Given the importance of the liver in normal physiology and its many responses to injury, increasing studies of mechanisms of disease at biochemical and molecular levels, correlated with changes in cell and tissue structure and function, could make an important contribution to the development of better drugs and therapeutic regimens in liver disease.

References

Amenta JS, Sargus MJ, Baccino FM, Sacchi C, Bonelli C (1993) Cell death induced in L-cells by treatment with thymidine: staging the process and relationship to apoptosis. In Vitro Cell Dev Biol 29A:855–861

Barinaga M (1994) Research news: cell suicide: by ICE, not fire. Science 263:754

Ben-Ishay Z, Farber E (1975) Protective effects of an inhibitor of protein synthesis, cycloheximide, one bone marrow damage induced by cytosine arabinoside or nitrogen mustard. Lab Invest 33:478–490

Bursch W, Lauer B, Timmermann-Trosiener I, Schuppler BG, Schulte-Hermann R (1984) Controlled death (apoptosis) of normal and putative preneoplastic cells in rat liver following withdrawal of tumor promoters. Carcinogenesis 5:453–458

Cameron R, Murray RK, Farber E, Sharma RN (1979) Some patterns of response of liver to environmental agents. Ann NY Acad Sci 329:39–47

Chisari FV, Milich DR, Tiallais P (1984) Hepatitis B virus infection: a model for immunologically mediated hepatocellular injury. In: Keppler D, Popper H, Bianchi L, Ruetter W (eds) Mechanisms of hepatocyte injury and death. MTP Press, Lancaster (Chap 28)

Cohen SS (1966) Introduction to the biochemistry of D-arabinosyl nucleosides. Prog Nucleic Acid Res 5:1–88

Cohen SS, Barner HD (1954) Studies on unbalanced growth in *Escherichia coli*. Proc Natl Acad Sci USA 40:885

Cohen SS, Barner HD (1975) The death of bacteria as a function of unbalanced growth. Pediatrics 16:704

Farber E (1971) Biochemical pathology. Annu Rev Pharmacol 17:71–96

Farber E (1990) Clonal adaptation during carcinogenesis. Biochem Pharmacol 39:1837–1846

Farber E (1994) Programmed cell death: necrosis versus apoptosis. Mod Pathol 7:605–609

Farber E, Fisher MM (eds) (1979) Toxic injury of the liver, part A. Dekker, New York
Farber E, Fisher MM (eds) (1980) Toxic injury of the liver, part B. Dekker, New York
Farber E, Rubin H (1991) Cellular adaptation in the origin and development of cancer. Cancer Res 51:2751–2761
Farber E, Sarma DSR (1987) Biology of disease: hepatocarcinogenesis: a dynamic cellular perspective. Lab Invest 56:4–22
Farber E, Verbin RS, Lieberman M (1971) Cell suicide and cell death. In: Aldridge WN (ed) Mechanisms of toxicity. MacMillan, London, pp 163–170
Hugon J, Borgers M (1966) Ultrastructural and cytochemical studies on karyotic bodies in the epithelium of the duodenal crypt of whole body x-irradiated mice. Lab Invest 15:1528–1543
Kushner I, Volanakis JE, Gervurz H (eds) (1982) C-reactive protein and the plasma response to injury. Ann N Y Acad Sci 389:36
Ledda-Columbano GM, Coni P, Curto M, Giacomini L, Faa G, Oliviero S, Piacentini M, Columbano A (1991) Induction of two different modes of cell death, apoptosis and necrosis, in rat liver after a single dose of thioacetamide. Am J Pathol 139:1099–1110
Ledda-Columbano GM, Coni P, Faa G, Manenti G, Columbano A (1992) Rapid induction of apoptosis in rat liver by cycloheximide. Am J Pathol 140:545–549
Lieberman MW, Verbin RS, Landay M, Liang H, Farber E, Lee T-N, Starr R (1970) A probable role for protein synthesis in intestinal epithelial cell damage induced in vivo by cytosine arabinoside, nitrogen mustard or x-irradiation. Cancer Res 30:942–951
Lockshin RA, Zakeri-Milovanoviu Z (1984) Nucleic acids in cell death. In: Davies I, Sigel DC (eds) Cell ageing and cell death. Cambridge University Press, Cambridge, p 243
McDanell RE, McLean AEM (1985) Role of nutritional states in drug metabolism and toxicity. In: Sidransky H (ed) Nutritional pathology. Dekker, New York, Chap 8
Phillips MJ, Poucell S (1986) Cholestasis: surgical pathology mechanisms and new concepts. In: Farber E, Phillips MJ (eds) The pathogenesis of liver diseases. Williams and Wilkins, Baltimore, Chap 5
Popp JA, Shinozuka H, Farber E (1978) The protective effects of diethydithiocarbamate and cycloheximide in the multiple hepatic lesions induced by carbon tetrachloride in the rat. Toxicol Appl Pharmacol 45:549–564
Popper H, Martin GR (1982) Fibrosis of the liver: the role of the ectoskeleton. In: Popper H, Schaffner F (eds) Progress in liver diseases, vol 7, Chap 8. Greene and Stratton, New York
Popper H, Stern R (1979) Reactions of the liver to injury: fibrosis. In: Farber E, Fisher MM (eds) Toxic injury of the liver, part A. Dekker, New York, Chap 6
Reznik-Schuller HM, Lijinsky WL (1982) Ultrastructural changes in the liver of animals treated with methapyrilene and some analogs. Ecotoxicol Environ Safety 6:328–335
Roe DA (1985) Pathological changes associated with drug-induced malnutrition. In: Sidransky H (ed) Nutritional pathology. Dekker, New York, Chap 9
Rojkind M, Dunn MA (1979) Hepatic fibrosis. Gastroenterology 76:849–863
Samuel A, Jago MV (1975) Localization of the cell cycle of the antimitotic action of the pyrrolizidene alkaloid, lasiocarpine and its metabolite, dehydroheliotridine. Chem Biol Interact 10:185–197
Schlessinger MJ, Ashburner M, Tissieres A (eds) (1982) Heat shock: from bacterial to man. Cold Spring Harbor Laboratory, New York
Schulte-Hermann R (1974) Induction of liver growth by xenobiotic compounds and other stimulus. CRC Crit Rev Toxicol 3:97–158
Schulte-Hermann R (1979) Reactions of the liver to injury: adaptation. In: Farber E, Fisher M (eds) Toxic injury of the liver, part A. Dekker, New York, Chap 9
Stern R (1979) Experimental aspects of hepatic fibrosis. In: Popper H, Schaffner F (eds) Progress in liver diseases, vol 6, Chap 9. Greene and Stratton, New York

Trump BF, Goldblatt PJ, Stowell RE (1965) Studies on necrosis of mouse liver in vitro. Ultrastructural alterations in the mitochondria of hepatic parenchymal cells. Lab Invest 14:343–373
Trump BF, Berezesky IK, Osornio-Vargas AR (1981) Cell death and the disease process. The role of calcium. In: Bowen ID, Lockshin RA (eds) Cell death in biology and pathology. Chapman and Hall, London, pp 209–242
Trump BF, Berezesky IK, Sato I, Laiho KV, Phelps PC, DeClaris N (1984) Cell calcium, cell injury and cell death. Environ Health Perspect 57:218
Verbin RS, Longnecker DS, Ling H, Farber E (1971) Some observations on the acute histopathologic effects of cycloheximide in vivo. Am J Pathol 62:111–126
Verbin RS, Diluiso G, Liang H, Farber E (1972) The effects of cytosine arabinoside upon proliferating epithelial cells. Cancer Res 32:1476–1488
Verbin RS, Diluiso G, Farber E (1973) Protective effects of cycloheximide against 1-β-D-arabinofuranosylcytosine-induced intestinal lesions. Cancer Res 33:2086–2093
Williams GT, Smith CA (1993) Molecular regulation of apoptosis: genetic control on cell death. Cell 74:777
Wyllie AH, Kerr JFR, Currie AR (1980) Cell death: the significance of apoptosis. Int Rev Cytol 68:251–306
Ying TS, Sarma DSR, Farber E (1980) The sequential analysis of liver cell necrosis. Am J Pathol 99: 159–174
Ying TS, Sarma DSR, Farber E (1981) Role of acute hepatic necrosis in the induction of early steps in liver carcinogenesis by diethylnitrosamine. Cancer Res 41:2096–2102

CHAPTER 2

Clinical Studies and Role of Necrosis in Hepatotoxicity

R.G. Cameron and L.M. Blendis

Zonal hepatocellular necrosis, which is a response to chemicals including drugs and a phenomenon often seen in clinical pathology and the laboratory, is the subject of this short treatise. The critical analysis of the liver biopsies of over 40 patients with acetaminophen overdose has served as the basis of specific hypotheses concerning the responses of the liver to certain forms of injury namely: (1) zone 3 (perivenous) hepatocytes die as a unit, and this phenomenon is physiologic or adaptive; and (2) recovery is also a coordinated response involving removal of the dead hepatocytes (and toxic metabolites) and regeneration of new hepatocytes to reconstitute this zone 3 unit.

Several important observations are also made concerning the profound negative effects of co-existing ethanol toxicity on the extent of hepatic necrosis and course of recovery in 20 patients with acetaminophen plus ethanol overdose. It was found that exposure to alcohol led to an extension of hepatocellular necrosis beyond the zone 3 unit, and that there was a delay of regeneration and recovery.

A. Zonal Necrosis as a Response to Acetaminophen

I. Zonality: Specific Hepatocytes Die as a Group

Critical evidence for this hypothesis can be found by examining the hepatic response of patients to exposures to acetaminophen alone of nonfatal overdoses at a wide range of exposure levels, i.e., from 150 to 1000 mg/kg body weight and from 10 to 50 g total dose (Table 1). The location and proportion of hepatocytes which die (Fig. 1) is always the same irrespective of the dose (Table 1). This was a consistent finding not only in these six patients (Table 1) but also in biopsies of six other patients with acetaminophen overdose (Cameron et al. 1995). Serial sections of a block of tissue of whole liver removed at transplant of one of these patients revealed that the perivenular necrosis was a continuous "sleeve" up to the length of about 50 hepatocytes in 20-step sections that were examined (Fig. 2). Electron microscopic examination (Fig. 3) revealed a sharp margin between healthy mid-zone hepatocytes and dead zone 3 hepatocytes. This sharp demarcation line between perivenular necrotic hepatocytes and intact mid-zone hepatocytes after

Table 1. Extent of necrosis in relation to dose of acetaminophen

Patient[a]	ACM dose[b] (mg/kg)	ACM dose[b] (g)	Serum ACM level[c]	Necrosis[d] (%)
#1 Fa Pr	150	10	469	30
#2 Ja Ne	300	25	2046	40
#3 Mi Mi	400	25	985	40
#4 Ro Ir	400	30	–	40
#5 Ag Ko	600	30	934	40
#6 Ta Ma	1000	50	666	40

ACM, acetaminophen.
[a] Patients are identified by an assigned number and by parts of their names.
[b] Milligrams per kilogram body weight of ACM overdose, or total dose in grams (g).
[c] Micromoles per liter at 12–14h after overdose.
[d] Percentage of hepatocellular necrosis in liver biopsy measured by quantitative image analysis.

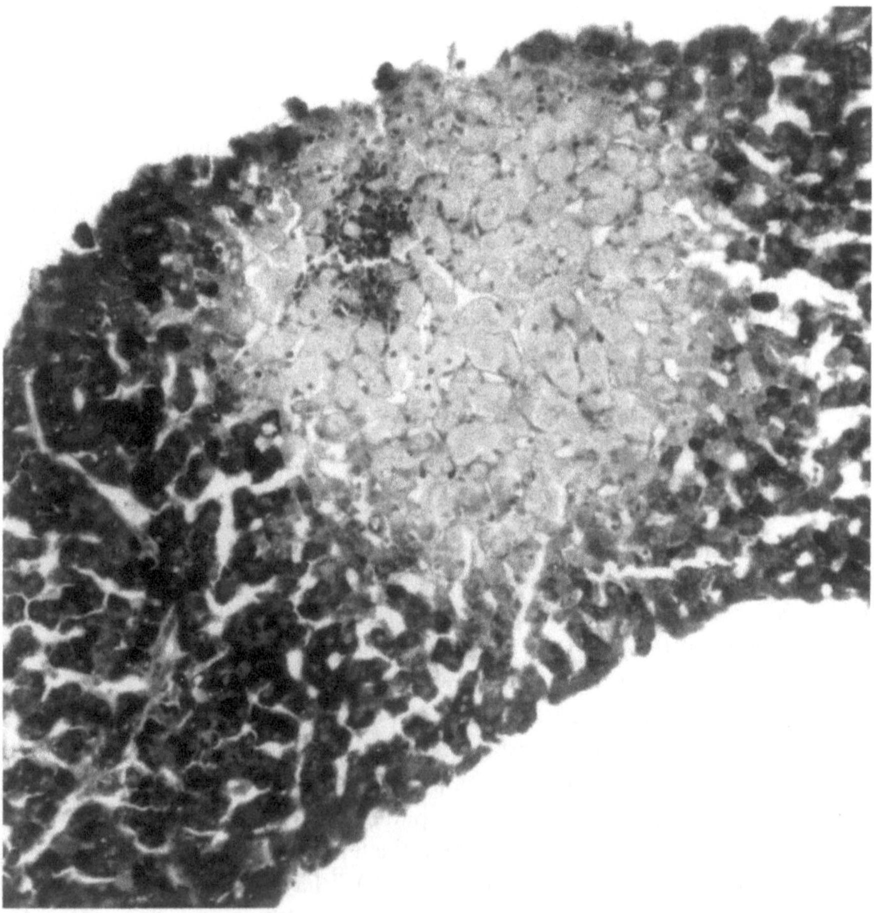

Fig. 1. Photomicrograph of liver biopsy of patient #6 (Ta Ma) showing complete necrosis of perivenular hepatocytes (*pale area*) and complete sparing of mid-zone and periportal hepatocytes (*dark areas*) at day 2 after acetaminophen overdose of 1000mg/kg body wt. Periodic acid Schiff stain, ×200)

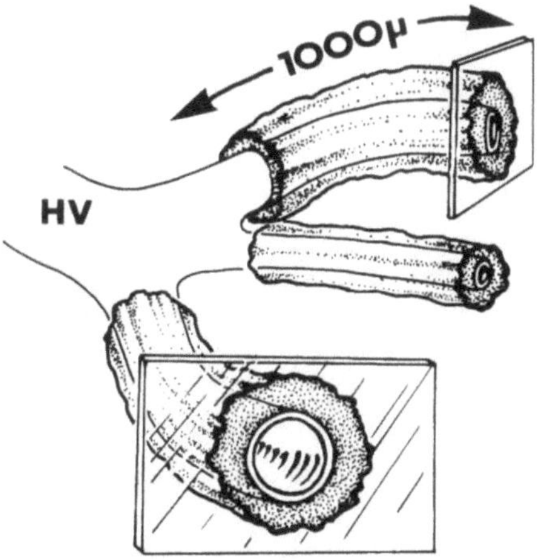

Fig. 2. Line drawing of terminal branches of hepatic veins representing the "sleeve" pattern of necrosis of perivenular hepatocytes. Twenty serial step sections at 50-μm intervals of liver removed at transplant of patient #19 (Sh Jo) always showed perivenous zonal necrosis, suggesting that the hepatic necrogenic response was as a sleeve around the terminal hepatic venules

Table 2. Clinical response to acetaminophen overdose

Patient	AST[a] (IU/l)	PT[a] (s)	Encephalopathy stage[b]	Discharge date	Outcome
#1 Fa Pr	2442	16	I	Day 6[c]	Recovery
#2 Ja Ne	7660	18	II	Day 8	Recovery
#3 Mi Mi	4455	17	II	Day 6	Recovery
#4 Ro Ir	4830	18	II	Day 6	Recovery
#5 Ag Ko	8240	16	II	Day 6	Recovery
#6 Ta Ma	10212	22	II	Day 18	ATN, Recovery

AST, serum aspartate aminotransaminase; PT, prothrombin time; ATN, acute tubular necrosis.
[a] AST and PT are peak values, which were on days 3,3,2,3, 2 and 3 for patients #1–#6, respectively.
[b] Stage I is characterized by mild confusion; stage II has drowsiness and lethargy (Basile, Chap. 11, this volume).
[c] Days (6) after day of overdose.

acetaminophen overdoses is most likely related to the expression of specific enzymes for the activation of acetaminophen to its cytotoxic derivative which occur virtually exclusively in the hepatocytes of the perivenous zone, as discussed below.

The clinical response to acetaminophen overdose (Table 2) is also indicative of the adaptive nature of the hepatic response: patients regain liver function within 4–5 days of the drug overdose (Table 3) and show a complete clinical recovery by day 6 (Table 2 and Donaldson et al. 1994).

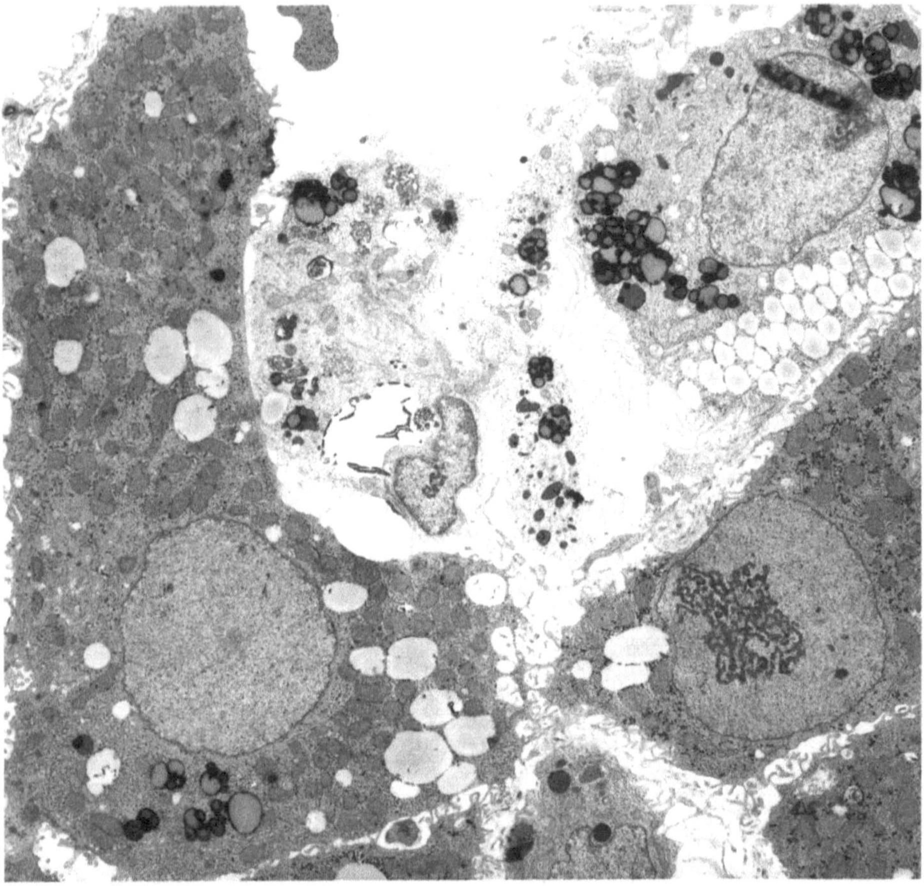

Fig. 3. Electron micrograph of liver biopsy of patient #4 (Ro Ir), showing the sharp margin between healthy hepatocytes of the mid-zone (*bottom*) and dead hepatocytes of the perivenous zone (*center*) at day 4 after 400 mg/kg body wt. of acetaminophen. Mild microvesicular steatosis is seen in hepatocytes of both zones, ×4000

II. Ethanol Plus Acetaminophen: Extension of Zone of Necrosis

The examination of liver biopsies of patients with both acetaminophen overdose and a history of recent excessive ethanol intake (Table 4) shows clearly that whenever there is evidence of ethanol toxicity, e.g., steatosis, there is an extension of the acetaminophen-induced zone 3 "unit" necrosis to include the mid-zone or zone 2 (Fig. 4). This response was consistent in the biopsies of all 20 chronic alcoholic patients with both alcohol and acetaminophen overdose but without fibrosis or cirrhosis. There was a profound loss of liver function (Table 5) in association with the extension of necrosis to involve both zones 3 and 2, i.e., necrosis of 60%–80% of all hepatocytes, which was manifest by acute loss of hepatic synthetic function (prothrombin) and hepatic coma (Table 5). Recovery to normal liver function after acetaminophen overdose was greatly delayed, or did not occur, when there was co-existing acute ethanol toxicity (Tables 5, 6) even at relatively low dose acetaminophen exposures (Tables 4–6), as reported also by KAYSEN et al. (1985), LESSER et al. (1986) and SEEFF et al. (1986).

Table 3. Hepatocyte loss and recovery as monitored by liver (function) tests

	Patient	Day					
		1	2	3	4	5	6
A. PT[a]	#1 Fa Pr	14	16	16	16		
	#2 Ja Ne	13	15	18	25	12	11
	#3 Mi Mi	12	17	16	14	12	12
	#4 Ro Ir		17	18		12	
	#5 Ag Ko		16	14	11		
	#6 Ta Ma	13	17	22	16	12	
B. AST[b]	#1 Fa Pr	77	243	2442	2050	1442	257
	#2 Ja Ne	108	186	7660	3550	1080	158
	#3 Mi Mi	51	4455	1766	683	296	122
	#4 Ro Ir		184	4830	2071	352	
	#5 Ag Ko	10160	8240	938	270	84	50
	#6 Ta Ma	72	377	10212	6500		58

[a] PT is one measure of loss and recovery of liver synthetic function towards normal coagulation of 10–12s prothrombin time by day 4 or 5 after the overdose.
[b] AST is an index of hepatocellular necrosis which peaks by 48–72h after the overdose.

Table 4. Extent of necrosis after exposure to both acetaminophen and ethanol[a]

Patient[a]	ACM dose (mg/kg body wt.)	ACM dose (g)	Serum ACM level (μmol/l)	Hepatocellular necrosis (%)	Ethanol toxicity (% fat)[b]
#7 Ra Ch	30[c]	3	45	80	90
#8 Cl Du	50[c]	4	66	70	90
#9 Ju Ma	50[c]	3		40	20
#10 Jo Wa	150	8	352	70	50
#11 Do Wa	200	10	137	40	90
#12 Ja Sh	200	15	115	80	90
#13 Ma Sh	200	10	276	90	20
#14 Wa Sh	210	16	140	60	80
#15 Al Ro	240	18	–	50	50
#16 Ja Mc	250	15	–	60	60
#17 El Fe	300	15	700	80	50
#18 Je Jo	2000	100	++++	60	60

[a] History of recent excessive ethanol intake.
[b] Percentage of living hepatocytes with macrovesicular steatosis.
[c] Doses are in the therapeutic range.

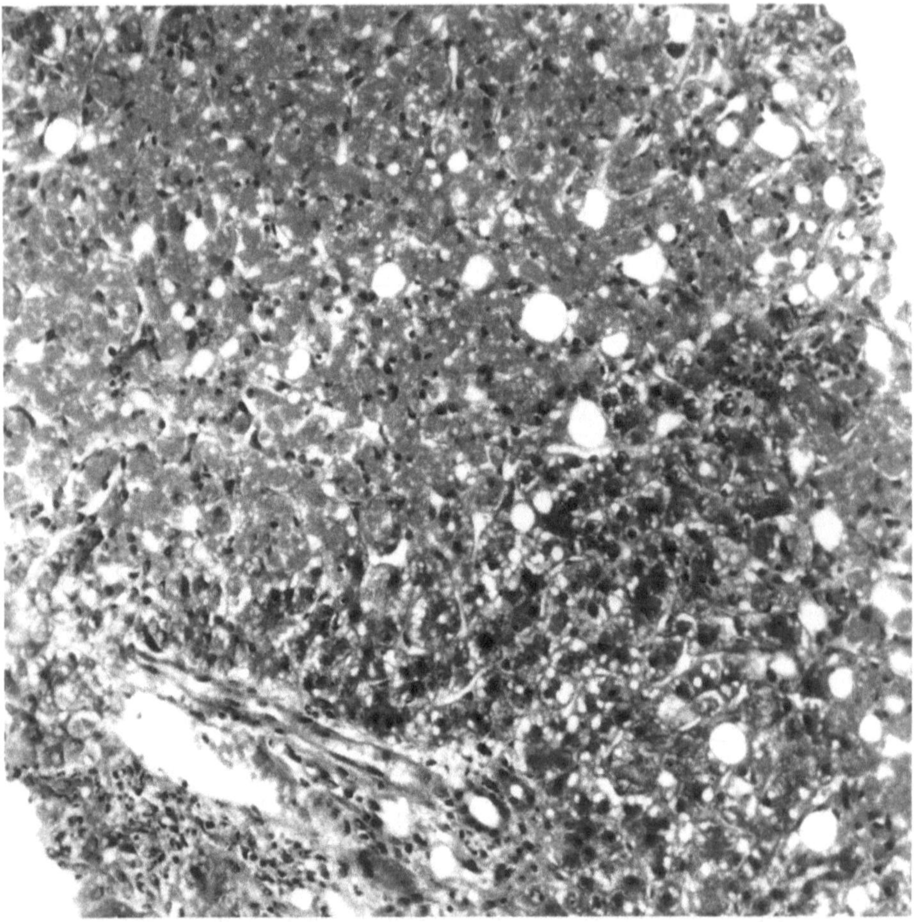

Fig. 4. Photomicrograph of liver biopsy of patient #14 (Wa Sh), showing necrosis involving not only all of the perivenous hepatocytes (*top and center*) but also most of the mid-zonal hepatocytes (*center*) with sparing of periportal hepatocytes (*bottom*) at day 2 after acetaminophen 210mg/kg body wt. plus acute ethanol. Macrovascular and microvascular steatosis is evident in many hepatocytes in all zones. H&E, ×200

III. Constitutive Bases of Zonal Responses

The liver has been shown to have multiple repeating units with "metabolic zonation" (GEBHARDT 1992) with respect to glucose metabolism (NOVIKOFF 1959; JUNGERMANN and KATZ 1989), drug metabolic enzymes (BARON et al. 1982; GEBHARDT 1992), bile formation (GUMUCIO 1983; GEBHARDT 1992), glutamine and glutamate metabolism (GEBHARDT 1992) and cholesterol and bile acid biosynthesis (GEBHARDT 1992). In addition, within these units (lobules or acini), there are gradients of blood-borne factors such as oxygen (RAPPAPORT et al. 1954; LAMERS et al. 1987; JUNGERMANN and KATZ 1989;

Table 5. Clinical response to acetaminophen plus ethanol

Patient	AST[a] (IU/l)	PT[a] (s)	Encephalopathy stage[b]	Discharge date[c]	Outcome[d]
#7 Ra Ch	19038	31	III	Day 4	Died
#8 Cl Du	15710	40	III	Day 25	Died
#9 Ju Ma	2976	17	II	Day 36	Recovered
#10 Jo Wa	5073	22	III	Day 14	Died
#11 Do Wa	13680	50	IV	Day 11	Died
#12 Ja Sh	4960	33	III	Day 12	Died
#13 Ma Sh	16700	60	IV	Day 4	Died
#14 Wa Sh	23800	30	III	Day 26	Recovered
#15 Al Ro	4884	24	III	Day 8	Recovered
#16 Ja Mc	12809	40	III	Day 18	ATN, Recovered
#17 El Fe	8730	72	IVa	Day 30	Coma[d] Recovered
#18 Je Jo	6340	70	III	Day 13	Recovered

ATN, acute tubular necrosis; AST, serum aspartate aminotransferase; PT, prothrombin time.
[a] AST and PT are peak values, which were on days 2 or 3.
[b] Stage III is characterized by somnolence with rousability; stage IVa is coma with loss of response to painful stimuli (Basile, Chap. 11, this volume).
[c] Days after day of overdose until discharge (or death).
[d] Patient #17 was 12 days in coma.

Table 6. Hepatocyte loss and recovery after acetaminophen plus ethanol

	Patient	Day 2	4	6	8	10
A. PT[a] (s)	#8 Cl Du	40	28	22	22	20
	#10 Jo Wa	22	18	13	15	14
	#11 Do Wa	50	30	23	20	16
	#14 Wa Sh	30	25	14	11	11
	#16 Ja Mc	40	22	17	14	12
	#17 El Fe	53	28	15	12	12
	#18 Je Jo	70	70	15	13	12
B. AST[b] (IU/l)	#8 Cl Du	15710	1374	143	94	77
	#10 Jo Wa	5073	191	45	52	47
	#11 Do Wa	13680	1052	283	93	68
	#14 Wa Sh	23800	7030	111	43	42
	#16 Ja Mc	12809	1371	431	56	36
	#17 El Fe	6450	2150	179	98	119
	#18 Je Jo	904	6340	1090	169	60

AST, serum aspartate aminotransferase; PT, prothrombin.
[a] PT is one measure of loss and recovery of liver synthetic function towards normal of 10–12 s by day 8–10 after the acetaminophen overdose plus ethanol.
[b] AST is an index of hepatocellular necrosis which peaks by 48–72 h after the acetaminophen overdose plus ethanol.

WAGENAAR et al. 1993; THURMAN et al., Chap. 5, this volume), solutes (GUMACIO 1983) and growth factors (JUNGERMANN and KATZ 1989; GEBHARDT 1992). The histopathologic response of zone 3 necrosis was not accompanied by any vascular lesions such as thromboses or arteritis which might further accentuate constitutive oxygen gradients. The distribution of maximum concentrations of multiple cytochrome P450 isozymes appears to exactly correspond to those hepatocytes of the perivenous zone 3 "sleeve" that are lost in the necrotic response to acetaminophen (Figs. 1, 2), suggesting that the zonation of the drug metabolic network is a major factor contributing to the zonal necrosis response (GEBHARDT 1992; LEEDER and OKEY, Chap. 6, this volume), and that in fact the zone 3 necrosis is an integral part of the metabolic response to high levels of toxicants.

1. Perivenous Localization of Acetaminophen-Metabolizing Enzyme CYP 2E1

Most enzymes of the cytochrome P450 family are predominantly expressed in perivenous hepatocytes of human liver, including CYP 1A2 and CYP 2E1, as shown in immunohistochemical and in situ hybridization studies (TSUTUMI et al. 1989; MCKINNON et al. 1991), as dense perivenous rings of protein or mRNA "expression" corresponding to similar perivenous "rings" of necrosis after acetaminophen (Fig. 1). Acetaminophen at toxic doses is metabolized by CYP 2E1 (RAUCY et al. 1989) to *N*-acetyl-*p*-benzoquinone imine (NAPQI), which binds to glutathione (MITCHELL et al. 1974; DAHLIN et al. 1984; KETTERER 1986), or to macromolecules when glutathione is depleted by more than 30% (GILLETTE 1981; LAUTERBURG and VELEZ 1988; RUMORE and BLAIKLOCK 1992). Ethanol both induces CYP 2E1 in perivenous and mid-zone hepatocytes of human liver as shown in the immunohistochemical studies of TSUTSUMI et al. (1989). In our study, prior exposure to alcohol led to two major consequences, firstly, there was perivenous hepatocellular necrosis in response to much lower dose exposures to acetaminophen (Table 4), and, secondly, there was extensive necrosis of hepatocytes outside of the strict confines of this perivenous "sleeve" (Fig. 2), involving the mid-zone hepatocytes (Fig. 4). One possible mechanism of both of these responses to alcohol exposure prior to acetaminophen is by means of the induction of CYP 2E1 in zone 3 and mid-zone hepatocytes (TSUTSUMI et al. 1989). Repeated exposure of hepatocytes containing high levels of CYP 2E1 to ethanol would lead to the generation of high levels of reactive metabolites (GUENGERICH et al. 1991; TSUTSUMI et al. 1993; GONZALEZ and GELBOIN 1994; ISRAEL, Chap. 25, this volume). These reactive metabolites of alcohol bind to glutathione and this whole process depletes glutathione (DAHLIN et al. 1984; KETTERER 1986; SLATTERY et al. 1987). Exposure of these hepatocytes with glutathione depletion to acetaminophen and induction of CYP 2E1 would lead to a sharp increase in formation of NAPQI, the toxic metabolite of acetaminophen, and to greatly increased covalent binding of NAPQI to target macromolecules in the absence of glutathione, followed by enhanced hepatocellular toxicity (Dietz et al. 1984; Roberts et al. 1987; Lieber et al. 1990; Patten et al. 1993).

IV. Zonal Hepatocellular Necrosis: Historical Perspective

Since 1966, a large number of histopathologic studies of livers of patients with acetaminophen overdose (Davidson and Eastham 1966; Boyd and Bereczky 1966) have documented as the hepatic response a sharply circumscribed perivenous (zone 3) necrosis similar to that depicted in Figs. 1 and 2 (Clark et al. 1973; Portmann et al. 1975; Seeff et al. 1986; Pessayre 1993; Zuckerman and Anuras, Chap. 22, this volume). Perivenous zonal necrosis is also the response illicited by a variety of other chemicals (Zimmerman 1978) including bromobenzene, carbon tetrachloride, dimethylnitrosamine (Lee et al. 1993), diethylnitrosamine and thioacetamide (see Gebhardt 1992 for references). Periportal zonal necrosis is rarely seen as a response to drug or chemical "overdose" except with allyl alcohol exposure (Zimmerman 1978; Gebhardt 1992; Thurman et al., Chap. 5, this volume). A series of recent studies have shown that allyl alcohol undergoes rapid uptake and oxidation and depletes glutathione in the periportal region preferentially (see Gebhardt 1992 for references). It is also possible that preferential induction of specific cytochrome P450 isozymes in periportal hepatocytes by allyl alcohol is contributing to periportal necrosis. Similarly, β-napthoflavone induces CYP IA1 and CYP IA2 proteins and mRNAs in periportal hepatocytes but without periportal necrosis (Wolf et al. 1984).

B. Regeneration in Response to Zonal Necrosis of Acetaminophen Overdose

Inherent to the overall response to acetaminophen overdose is the complete reconstitution of the zone of perivenous hepatocytes and their function, which involves replication of zone 1 (periportal) and zone 2 (mid-zonal) hepatocytes to yield sufficient hepatocytes to restore the perivenous zone, and differentiation of these hepatocytes to fit their metabolic (zonal) functions.

I. Regeneration of Periportal and Mid-zonal Hepatocytes to Restore the Perivenous Zone

In response to acetaminophen-induced perivenous zonal necrosis, which involves 30%–40% of all hepatocytes, periportal and mid-zonal hepatocytes can be seen to replicate (simultaneously), as shown in Figs. 5 and 6. This is in contrast to post-hepatectomy or after dimethylnitrosamine (Lee et al. 1993), in which a wave of DNA synthesis and cell proliferation passes sequentially from periportal to mid-zonal to perivenous hepatocytes. In patients with follow-up biopsies 1 week later, normal architecture is evident in the perivenous zone. In

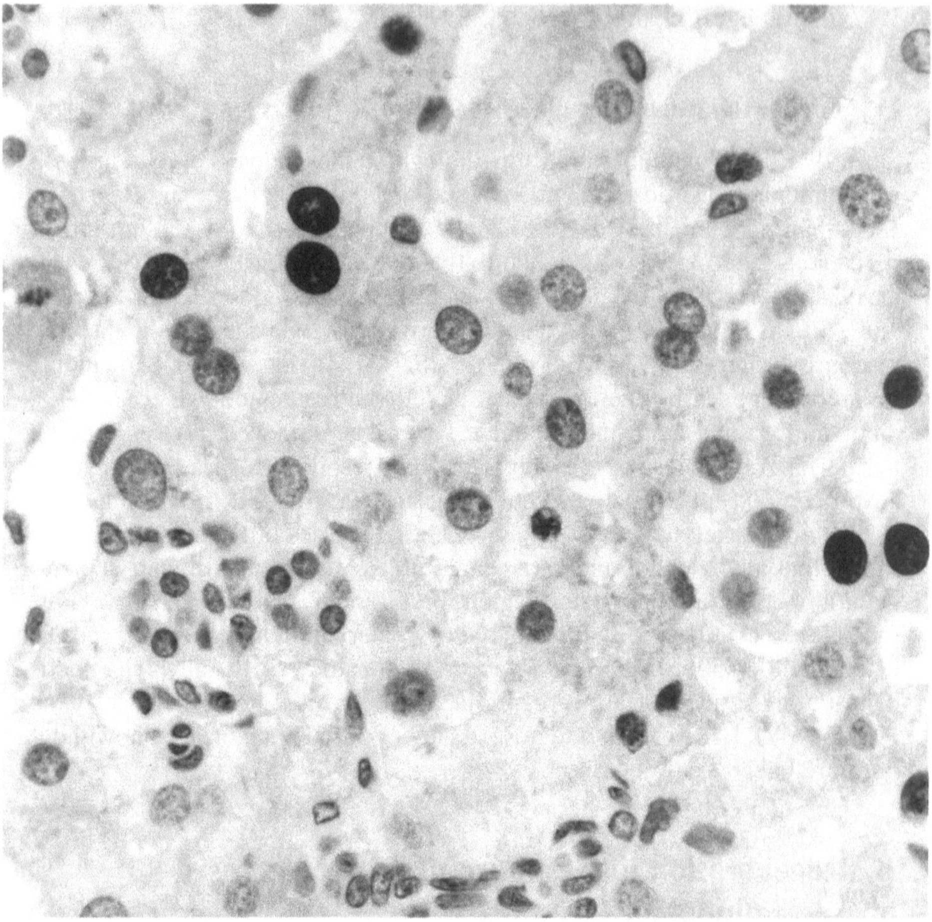

Fig. 5. Photomicrograph of liver section of biopsy of patient #6 (Ta Ma), also shown in Fig. 1, stained by the immunoperoxidase method with antibodies to proliferating cell nuclear antigen or PCNA according to Koukoulis et al. (1992) to mark hepatocytes in DNA synthesis (*dark nuclei*). Six hepatocytes next to the portal tract (*bottom*) are in DNA synthesis and one is in mitosis, ×500

patients with ethanol plus acetaminophen overdose and with mid-zonal necrosis in addition to perivenous necrosis, there are many fewer hepatocytes to regenerate (Table 4). The proportion of living hepatocytes which are seen to be undergoing active DNA synthesis and mitoses shows a wide range, with 10%–26% in DNA synthesis or 5%–8% in mitoses (Tables 7, 8). Thus, if restitution is to take place, the process is considerably delayed until a small number of hepatocytes can replicate many times to replace a much larger mass of necrosed cells. An intriguing aspect of this reconstitution is that the periportal and mid-zonal hepatocytes replace perivenous hepatocytes, which have a very different metabolic phenotype. Four patients in our study

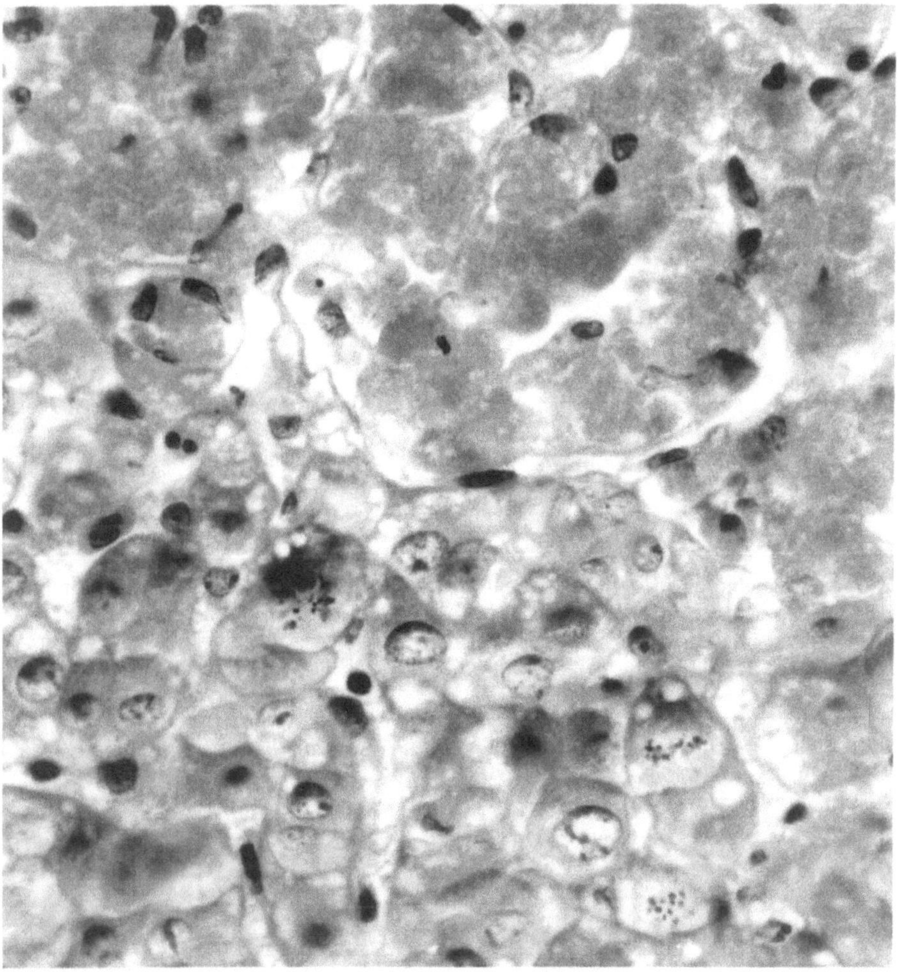

Fig. 6. Photomicrograph of liver section adjacent to region shown in Fig. 5 of patient #6 (Ta Ma). Three hepatocytes of the mid-zone (*bottom*) are in mitosis, revealing that regeneration of hepatocytes occurs in mid-zone and periportal zones simultaneously, not sequentially. This figure also shows that in the necrotic zone (*top*) hepatocytes die but sinusoidal lining cells remain intact to preserve the architectural frameworks of this region. H&E, ×500

had multiple acetaminophen overdoses at intervals of months or years. Each time the hepatic response was identical (despite major variation in the overdose) with respect to the degree of perivenous necrosis and the rate of recovery of liver function in 4 or 5 days, suggesting that periportal cells did indeed reconstitute the original zonal phenotype as part of the regenerative response to the previous overdose. This suggests that the "necrotic response" by the individual liver and perivenular region is "fixed" for that individual, regardless of the degree of acetaminophen overdose and insult.

Table 7. Regeneration of periportal and mid-zone hepatocytes in response to necrosis after exposure to acetaminophen

Patient	Date of biopsy[a]	Necrosis (%)	Rate of DNA synthesis (%)[b]	Rate of mitosis (%)[c]
#1 Fa Pr	Day 3	30	NA[b]	6
#2 Ja Ne	Day 2	30	13	12
#3 Mi Mi	Day 2	40	35	21
#3 Mi Mi	Day 9[d]	–	3	0
#4 Ro Ir	Day 3	40	NA	10
#5 Ag Ko	Day 2	40	25	28
#6 Ta Ma	Day 2	40	31	11

NA, tissue not available.
[a] Days following overdose.
[b] Percentage of intact hepatocytes with PCNA positivity measured with method of Koukoulis et al. (1992).
[c] Number of hepatocytes in mitosis/100 hepatocytes in section.
[d] Second biopsy, follow-up, in same patient.

Table 8. Regeneration of intact hepatocytes of periportal or mid-zonal regions in response to necrosis after exposure to both acetaminophen and ethanol

Patient	Date of biopsy[a]	Necrosis (%)	Rate of DNA synthesis (%)[b]	Rate of mitosis (%)[c]
#7 Ra Ch	Day 3	80	60	10
#8 Cl Du	Day 7	70	NA[b]	15
#10 Jo Wa	Day 3	70	21	1
#14 Wa Sh	Day 3	60	65	7
#15 Al Ro	Day 3	50	20	8
#17 El Fe	Day 4	80	90	5
#18 Je Jo	Day 3	80	26	8
#18 Je Jo	Day 14[d]	–	6	1

NA, tissue not available to assess PCNA.
[a] Days following overdose.
[b] Percentage of surviving hepatocytes showing PCNA positivity as in Table 7.
[c] Percentage of intact hepatocytes in mitoses as in Table 7.
[d] Second biopsy in same patient.

This process is also very different from post-surgical hepatectomy regeneration, in which hepatocytes of remaining lobes must reconstitute every zone and not just the perivenous zone. In addition, after partial surgical hepatectomy, not only hepatocytes but vascular and biliary cells and structures have to be replaced. With acetaminophen-induced perivenous necrosis, hepatocytes are lost without collapse and sinusoidal architecture remains intact (Figs. 6, 7), awaiting the replacement of hepatocytes. Important factors in this adoption, by regenerated zone 1 and 2 hepatocytes, of the zone 3 phenotype could be environmental such as oxygen levels, or aspects of metabolic

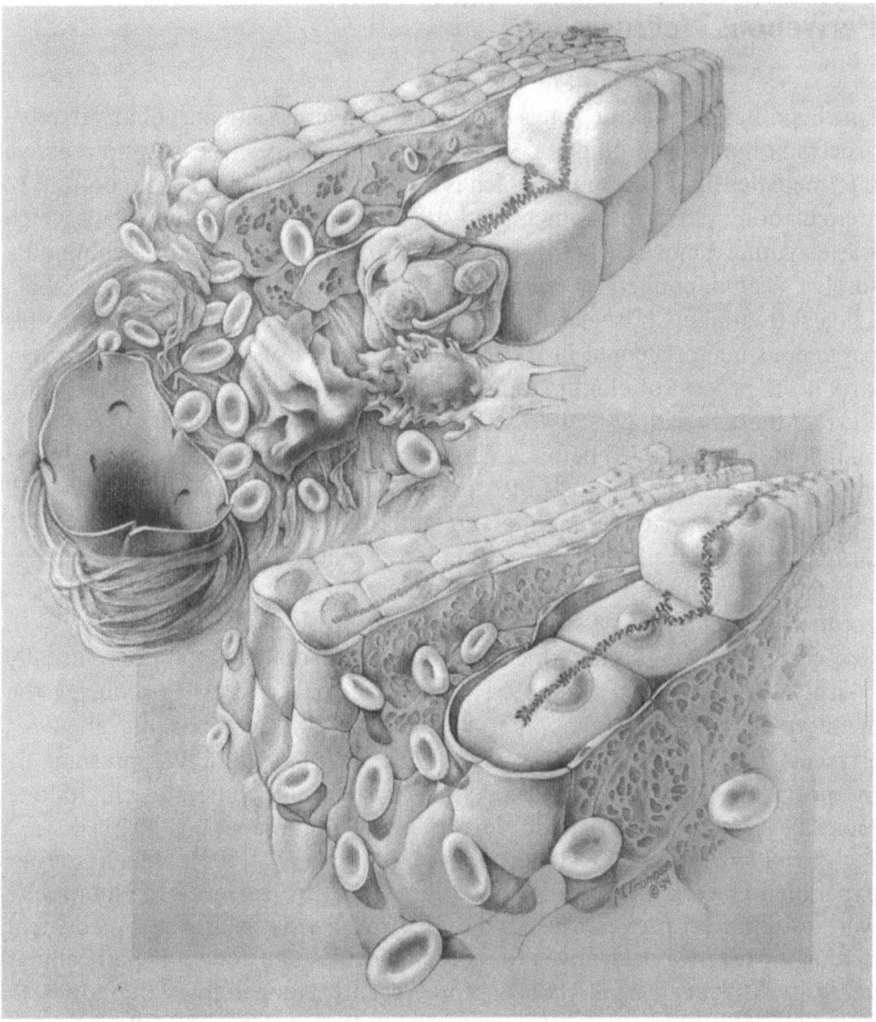

Fig. 7. Artist's rendering of perivenular hepatocellular necrosis (*top left*) and the process of regeneration which follows (*bottom right*) in response to acetaminophen overdose. Necrosis seems to spare the sinusoidal cells including the endothelium and Kupffer cells, and collapse does not occur. Phagocytic cells including PMNs and macrophages are often seen in the perivenous zone soon after hepatocellular necrosis. Bile canalicular channels are depicted as normal in intact hepatocytes, and restored completely after regeneration. Sizes of cells are magnified by about ×500

zonation including bile formation, glucose levels or cholesterol and bile acid content. The local sinusoidal cells that remain intact in spite of loss of hepatocytes could serve as a "conditioning" substratum to new hepatocyte differentiation.

C. Clinical Implications of "Adaptive" Perivenous Necrosis

One hypothesis is that the zones of perivenous necrosis are part of an adaptive process in the liver to bind and sequester large volumes of toxic and reactive intermediates akin to a sump, which is defined as a chamber at the bottom of a circulation system into which fluid drains before recirculation or in which wastes gather before disposal. Patients with perivenous necrosis commonly survive acetaminophen overdose and reconstitute their perivenous zone. Clinical treatment strategies (drugs, inhibitors, etc.) designed to prevent this perivenous necrosis could in fact delay the process of regeneration, particularly if the process of elimination of toxic metabolites is also interfered with. Current therapy with *N*-acetylcysteine, however, does lead to binding of toxic metabolites as discussed below. In contrast, with ethanol and acetaminophen overdose, mid-zonal necrosis also occurs and is accompanied by delays in restitution of normal liver architecture and liver function. Clinical treatments designed to prevent mid-zonal necrosis would seem critical. Histologic examination of these livers reveals that necrosis of mid-zone hepatocytes is occurring synchronously with perivenous necrosis and is evident by 48h (day 2). Clinical therapies which provide precursors to glutathione, usually *N*-acetylcysteine (Vale et al. 1981), have had some success in reducing the acute toxicity of acetaminophen in the first 24h (Rumack et al. 1981; Prescott 1981; Janes and Routledge 1992; Sheiner et al. 1992), presumably by providing an excess of exogenous cysteine to generate glutathione molecules which bind to toxic derivatives of acetaminophen (Miller and Jollow 1986; Ketterer 1986; Vermeulen et al. 1992). Much earlier experimental work in mouse liver had shown that critical levels of glutathione were essential to prevent acetaminophen toxicity as measured by covalent binding of reactive derivatives to macromolecules and zone 3 hepatocellular necrosis (Mitchell et al. 1974). More recently, longer term therapy with *N*-acetylcysteine for not only the first 24h but for the duration of clinical signs of liver failure has met with success (Harrison et al. 1991; Lewis and Paloucek 1991; Smilkstein et al. 1991). In our study, we observe that hepatocytes continue to die as measured by continual release of serum transaminase or AST (Tables 3, 6) up to day 5 after acetaminophen alone and even until day 8 after acetaminophen plus ethanol. Clinical therapy to provide glutathione in excess could be beneficial clinically in the prevention of necrosis particularly of mid-zone hepatocytes that are involved in the regeneration of liver (Fig. 6) and restoration of liver function to optimal levels. The choline deficiency model of hepatotoxicity (Ghazarian et al. 1994; Chaps. 1 and 9, this volume) is instructive in the sequential analysis of hepatocellular necrosis which is found to occur as a multistep process over days and even weeks as long as the chemical imbalance is present. In all our patients, the serum acetaminophen level is undetectable within 48h after the overdose and yet evidence of acetaminophen-associated necrosis is present up to 1 week later (Table 6). The acetaminophen molecule is metabolized within 2 days, but it is possible that toxic by-products can persist in the liver for much longer. That necrosis is not a direct result of chemical insult is suggested by analysis of the CD model in which necrosis develops as a distant resultant of multiple synchronous chemical reactions as follows: liver triglycerides accumulate within 8h after the start of a CD diet, nuclear membrane lipid peroxidation is detected within 24h, DNA alterations by 48h, increased phospholipase A_2 activity at 72h and hepatocellular necrosis not until 5 days after a CD diet (GHOSHAL, Chap. 9, this volume). Necrosis is ongoing at 5 days from the initial chemical insult in our patients as well. If it were possible to identify and characterize key rate-limiting steps in the induction of necrosis of human liver particularly of mid-zone hepatocytes, further rational therapy, in addition to glutathione supplements, could be developed.

Subcellular mechanisms leading to hepatocellular necrosis have been postulated to include plasma membrane lysis, phospholipase A_2 activity and influx of calcium as critical events (FARBER and GERSHON 1984; Chaps. 1 and 9, this volume). Subnecrogenic dose exposures to acetaminophen do lead to dilatation of rough endoplasmic reticulum (RER) and changes in sizes of mitochondria (PHILLIPS et al. 1987; FEUER and DE LA IGLESIA, Chap. 3, this volume). Mitochondria RER complexes contain specific cytochrome P450s (PICKETT et al. 1981) and glutathione (HWANG et al. 1992) so that these EM changes could represent a structural manifestation of the metabolic response to acetaminophen (RAUCY et al. 1989).

Acknowledgements. Thanks to Drs. Al Jones and Doug Schmucker at UCSF and the library staff at VA Hospital, San Francisco, for their help. Also thanks to Lori Cutler for excellent work on the manuscript, to Paul Schwartz for the photography and Meagan Thompson for the art.

References

Baron J, Redick JA, Guengerich FP (1982) Effect of 3-methylcholanthrene, β-naphthoflavone and phenobarbital on the 3-methylcholanthrene-inducible cytochromes P450 within centrilobular, midzonal and periportal hepatocytes. J Biol Chem 256:5931–5937

Boyd EM, Bereczky GM (1966) Liver necrosis from paracetamol. Br J Pharmacol 26:606–614

Cameron RG, Blendis LM, Tu G, Israel Y (1995) The deleterious effects of alcohol on necrogenic and regenerative response of human liver to acetaminophen overdose. Hepatology (to be submitted)

Clark R, Thompson RPH, Borirakchanyavat V, Widdop B, Davidson AR, Goulding R, Williams R (1973) Hepatic damage and death from overdose of paracetamol. Lancet I:66–70

Dahlin DC, Mirva GT, Lu AYH, Nelson SD (1984) N-acetyl-p-benzoquinone imine: a cytochrome P450-mediated oxidation product of acetaminophen. Proc Natl Acad Sci USA 81:1327–1331

Davidson DGD, Eastham WN (1966) Acute liver necrosis following overdose of paracetamol. Br Med J 2:497–499

Dietz AJ, Carlson JD, Wahbakhabil SK, Nygard G (1984) Effects of alcoholism on acetaminophen pharmacokinetics in man. J Clin Pharmacol 24:205–208
Donaldson BW, Gopinath R, Wanless IR, Phillips MJ, Cameron R, Roberts EA, Greig PD, Levy F, Blendis L (1994) The role of transjugular liver biopsy in fulminant liver failure: relation to other prognostic indicators. Hepatology 18:1370–1376
Farber JL, Gerson RJ (1984) Mechanisms of cell injury with hepatotoxic chemicals. Pharmacol Rev 36:72s
Gebhardt R (1992) Metabolic zonation of the liver: regulation and implications for liver function. Pharmacol Ther 53:275–354
Ghazarian DM, Ghoshal AK, Farber E (1994) In vivo free radical generation in the rat liver by a choline devoid diet and its role in relation to phospholipase A_2 activation. Proc Am Assoc Cancer Res 35:609 (abstract)
Gillette JR (1981) An integrated approach to the study of chemically reactive metabolites of acetaminophen. Arch Intern Med 141:375–379
Gonzalez FJ, Gelboin HV (1994) Role of human cytochrome P450 in the metabolic activation of chemical carcinogens and toxins. Drug Metab Rev 26:165–183
Guengerich FP, Kim D-H, Iwasaki M (1991) Role of human cytochrome P450 III E1 in the oxidation of many low molecular weight cancer suspects. Chem Res Toxicol 4:168–179
Gumucio JJ (1983) Functional and anatomic heterogeneity in the liver acinus: impact on transport. Am J Physiol 244:G578–G582
Harrison PM, Wendon JA, Gimson AES, Alexander GJM, Williams R (1991) Improvement by acetylcysteine of hemodynamics and oxygen transport in fulminant hepatitis. N Engl J Med 324:1852–1857
Hwang C, Sinskey AJ, Lodish HF (1992) Oxidized redox state of glutathione in the endoplasmic reticulum. Science 257:1496–1502
Janes J, Routledge PA (1992) Recent developments in the management of paracetamol (acetaminophen) poisoning. Drug Safety 7:170–177
Jungermann K, Katz N (1989) Functional hepatocellular heterogeneity. Pharmacol Rev 69:708–764
Kaysen GA, Pond SM, Roper MH, Austin KF (1985) Combined hepatic and renal injury in alcoholics during therapeutic use of acetaminophen. Arch Intern Med 145:2019–2023
Ketterer B (1986) Detoxification reactions of glutathione and glutathione transferases. Xenobiotics 16:957–973
Koukoulis G, Rayner A, Tan KC, Williams R, Portmann B (1992) Immunolocalization of regenerating cells after submassive liver necrosis using PCNA staining. J Pathol 166:359–368
Lamers WH, Gaasbeek Janzen JW, te Kortschot A, Charles R, Moorman AFM (1987) The development of enzymic zonation in liver parenchyma is related to the development of the acinar architecture. Differentiation 35:228–235
Lauterburg BH, Velez ME (1988) Glutathione deficiency in alcoholics: risk factor for paracetamol hepatotoxicity. Gut 29:1153–1157
Lee VM, Cameron RG, Archer MC (1993) The role of hepatocyte heterogeneity in the initiation of hepatocarcinogenesis. Carcinogenesis 14:1403–1408
Lesser PB, Vietti MM, Clark WD (1986) Lethal enhancement of therapeutic doses of acetaminophen by alcohol. Dig Dis Sci 31:103–105
Lewis RK, Paloucek FP (1991) Assessment and treatment of acetaminophen overdose. Clin Pharmacol 10:765–774
Lieber CS (1990) Interaction of ethanol with drugs, hepatotoxic agents, carcinogens and vitamins. Alcohol Alcohol 25:157–176
McKinnon RA, de la Hall P, Quattrochi LC, Tukey RH, McManus ME (1991) Localization of CYP1A1 and CYP1A2 mRNA in normal human liver and in hepatocellular carcinoma by *in situ* hybridization. Hepatology 14:848–856
Miller MG, Jollow DJ (1986) Acetaminophen hepatotoxicity studies on the mechanism of cystamine protection. Toxicol Appl Pharmacol 83:115–125

Mitchell JR, Thorgeirsson SS, Potter WZ, Jollow DJ, Keiser H (1974) Acetaminophen-induced hepatic injury: protective role of glutathione in man and rationale for therapy. Clin Pharmacol Ther 16:676–684
Novikoff AB (1959) Cell heterogeneity within the hepatic lobule of the rat (staining reaction). J Histochem Cytochem 7:240–244
Patten CJ, Thomas PE, Guy RL, Lee M, Gonzalez FJ, Guengerich FP, Yang CS (1993) Cytochrome P450 enzymes involved in acetaminophen activation by rat and human liver microsomes and their kinetics. Chem Res Toxicol 6:511–518
Pessayre D (1993) Physiopathologie des hépatopathis médicomenteuses. Gastroenterol Clin Biol 17:H3–H17
Phillips MJ, Poucell S, Patterson J, Valencia P (1987) The liver: an atlas and text of ultrastructural pathology. Raven, New York
Pickett CB, Rosenstein NR, Jeter RL (1981) The physical association between rat liver mitochondria and rough endoplasmic reticulum. II. Possible role RER-MT complexes play in the biosynthesis of cytochrome P450. Exp Cell Res 132: 225–234
Portmann B, Talbot IC, Day DW, Davidson AR, Murray-Lyon IM, Williams R (1975) Histopathological changes in the liver following a paracetamol overdose: correlation with clinical and biochemical parameters. J Pathol 117:169–181
Prescott L (1981) Treatment of severe acetaminophen poisoning with intravenous acetylcysteine. Arch Intern Med 141:386–389
Rappaport AM, Borowy ZJ, Lougheed WM, Lotto WN (1954) Subdivision of hexagonal liver lobules into a structural and functional unit: role in hepatic physiology and pathology. Anat Rec 119:11–34
Raucy JL, Lasher JM, Lieber CS, Black M (1989) Acetaminophen activation by human liver cytochromes P450 IIE1 and P450 1A2. Arch Bioch Biophys 271:270–283
Roberts DW, Pumford NR, Potter DW, Benson RW, Hinson JA (1987) A sensitive immunochemical assay for acetaminophen-protein adducts. J Pharmacol Exp Ther 241:527–533
Rumack BH, Peterson RC, Koch GG, Amara IA (1981) Acetaminophen overdose: 662 cases with evaluation of oral acetylcysteine treatment. Arch Intern Med 141: 380–385
Rumore MM, Blaiklock RG (1992) Influence of age-dependent pharmacokinetics and metabolism on acetaminophen hepatotoxicity. J Pharm Sci 81:203–207
Seeff LB, Cuccherini BA, Zimmerman HJ, Adler E, Benjamin SB (1986) Acetaminophen hepatotoxicity in alcoholics: a therapeutic misadventure. Ann Intern Med 104:399–404
Sheiner P, de Majo W, Levy GA (1992) Acetylcysteine and fulminant hepatic failure. Hepatology 15:552–554
Slattery JT, Wilson JM, Kalhorn TF, Nelson SD (1987) Dose-dependent pharmacokinetics of acetaminophen: evidence of glutathione depletion in humans. Clin Pharmacol Ther 41:413–418
Smilkstein MJ, Bronstein AC, Linden C, Augenstein WL, Kulig KW, Rumack BH (1991) Acetaminophen overdose: a 48-hour intravenous *N*-acetylcysteine treatment protocol. Ann Emerg Med 20:1058–1063
Tsutsumi M, Lasher JM, Shimizer M, Rosman AS, Lieber CS (1989) The intralobular distribution of ethanol-inducible P450 IIE1 in rat and human liver. Hepatology 10:437–446
Tsutsumi M, Takada A, Wong J-S, Takase S (1993) Genetic polymorphisms of cytochrome P450 2E1 related to the development of alcoholic liver disease. Hepatology 18:272 (abstract)
Vale JA, Meredith TJ, Goulding R (1981) Treatment of acetaminophen poisoning: the use of oral methionine. Arch Intern Med 141:394–396
Vermeulen NP, Bessems JG, Van de Straat R (1992) Molecular aspects of paracetamol-induced hepatotoxicity and its mechanism-based prevention. Drug Metab Rev 24:367–407

Wagenaar GTM, Chamuleau RAFM, de Hann JG, Maas MAW, de Boer PAJ, Marx F, Moorman AFM, Frederiks WM, Lamers WH (1993) Experimental evidence that the physiological position of the liver within the circulation is not a major determinant of zonation of gene expression. Hepatology 18:1144–1153

Zimmerman HJ (1978) Drug hepatotoxicity – the adverse effects of drugs and other chemicals on the liver. Appleton-Century Crofts, New York

CHAPTER 3

Subcellular Biochemical and Pathological Correlates in Experimental Models of Hepatotoxicity

G. FEUER and F.A. DE LA IGLESIA

A. Introduction

Side effects of drugs often result from impairment of liver function or structural damage to hepatocytes. To evaluate toxic interactions, the assessment of adverse changes manifesting in basic parameters of hepatic activities is important. Clinical observations in humans and experimental investigations in animals have frequently revealed impairment of liver function. This chapter will survey the relevant studies and update the approaches concerning the intrinsic relationship which exists between structural and support tissue or cell components and functional, metabolic or enzymatic parameters of hepatocytes responding to toxic drug effects.

Many reports have been published characterizing basic parameters of cellular function and structure to evaluate toxic effects on the liver (ANTHONY et al. 1978; BOLENDER et al. 1978; DAVID and UERLINGS 1983; DE LA IGLESIA et al. 1982a,b; DE PIERRE and ERNSTER 1977; MARZELLA and TRUMP 1991; STAUBLI and HESS 1975; WEIBEL et al. 1969). A practical goal has been to define early changes that reflect impairment of hepatic function and thus apply them as potential diagnostic tools for assessing the toxic or nontoxic characteristics of drugs, food additives, pesticides or environmental chemicals. In particular, the aim was to develop reliable, sensitive and rapid biochemical-morphological correlations that could be used as primary screening tests for detecting adverse cellular changes (CORNELIUS 1991; DE LA IGLESIA et al. 1982a,b; FEUER et al. 1974; KODAVANTE and MEHENDALE 1991).

Subcellular organelles participate in toxic reactions that affect cell respiration, drug metabolism, biotransformation or organelle biosynthesis. Structural-functional modifications occur frequently in the endoplasmic reticulum (ER) caused by foreign compounds, and this membranous organelle is exquisitely sensitive to compensatory or harmful actions (BERGER et al. 1987). Thus, improvement in the prediction of toxicity by certain methods can lead to more accurate evaluations and mechanistic interpretation of changes in hepatic function. We will emphasize the application of combined, correlative microscopic and biochemical techniques that are important for establishing toxic or nontoxic properties of a test compound with prognostic potential for side effects in humans (MIKHAEL and KACEW 1985).

B. Organization of the Liver Cell

Advances in ultrastructural morphology of the hepatocyte have revealed very fine details of subcellular organization and point to the uniqueness of hepatocyte disposition. Subcellular structures include membranous and particulate compartments, such as the nucleus and nucleolus, plasma membrane, membranes of the bile canaliculi, mitochondria, lysosomes, rough and smooth ER, Golgi complexes and peroxisomes. The liver cell has been considered as the fundamental functional elementary unit in controlling metabolic homeostasis,

Table 1. Compartmentalized view of organelles within liver cells, including the population parameters, enzymatic markers and their primary function with subsequent alterations

Organelle	Population, markers	Functions	Alterations
Plasma membrane 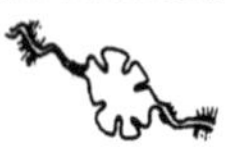	$0.12\,m^2/cm^3$ Adenosine triphosphatase	Intake, transport, elimination, secretion	Enzyme leakage, cholestasis
Rough endoplasmic reticulum 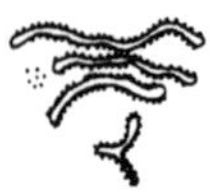	$3\,m^2/g$ Glucose-6-phosphatase, azo reductases	Protein synthesis, phospholipid metabolism	Dilatation, degranulation, concentric lamellae
Smooth endoplasmic reticulum 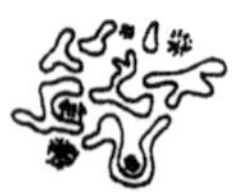	$6\,m^2/g$ Cytochrome P450 system	Drug metabolism	Proliferation, dilataion
Golgi apparatus 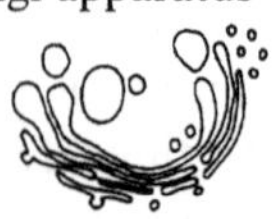	$0.7\,m^2/g$ Thiamine pyrophosphatase	Lipoprotein metabolism, secretion	Hypertrophy
Mitochondria 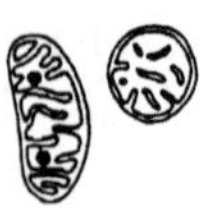	$378 \times 10^9/cm^3$ Succinic dehydrogenase	Cell respiration, fatty acid metabolism	Swelling, oxidative stress
Peroxisomes 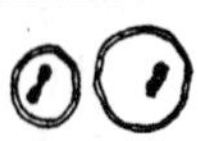	$189 \times 10^9/cm^3$ Catalase, fatty acid oxidases	Peroxidation, fatty acid metabolism	Proliferation, oxidative stress
Lysosomes 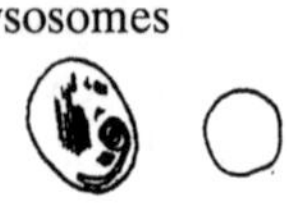	$66 \times 10^9/cm^3$ Phosphatases, cathepsin, glucuronidase	Autophagy, catabolism, storage	Accumulation, excess storage, phospholipidosis

and presents itself as a repeating unit throughout the parenchyma (MIYAI 1991). Hepatocytes evolve while traversing along the cords of the liver lobule, and acquire or express different functions, including the synthesis and activity of enzymes involved in oxidative xenobiotic metabolism and multidrug resistance (BRALET et al. 1994; LAMERS et al. 1989; ZAJICEK et al. 1985). Regional anatomical and functional diversity is apparent within the liver lobule (MARZELLA and TRUMP 1991; RAPPAPORT 1979); the properties of various compartments composed by the aggregate of a certain type of subcellular organelle are responsible for various liver functions. The various membranes and subcellular organelles contribute to metabolic regulation, and foreign compounds can impair their functions, eventually interfering with the maintenance of closely regulated metabolic controls. These subcellular compartments can be individually isolated and the subcellular organelles show clearly defined enzyme properties that provide respiratory, excretory of other metabolic functions (Table 1).

The internal structure of the hepatocyte is quite similar from cell to cell and from species to species. Liver parenchymal cells show some qualitative interspecies differences in structure or function or in the number and composition of subcellular organelles (GUMUCIO and CHIANALE 1988). Peroxisomes show structural differences between species in the distribution of purine-metabolizing enzymes, and there are differences in the total membrane surface of the endoplasmic reticulum from humans, dogs and rats (DE LA IGLESIA et al. 1982).

C. Liver Cell Injury

Traditionally, liver cell injury was assessed by evaluating basic structural changes observed by light microscopy, establishing ultrastructural alterations by electron microscopy, or by measuring tissue or serum enzyme activities or other biochemical endpoints. Thus the diagnosis of liver cell damage could be based on presumptive correlates of descriptive morphology or biochemistry (CORNELIUS 1991; DENK 1973; DHAMI et al. 1981; PHILLIPS et al. 1986; SWEENEY and DIARIO 1991). Quantitative morphological and clinical biochemical measurements can be correlated to define the degree of injury (ROHR et al. 1976; WEIBEL et al. 1969). The most frequent hepatic manifestations related to adverse drug effects are cholestasis, hepatitis and necrosis (LUDWIG 1979). Alterations of functional tests are not necessarily linked or integrated, representing a fundamental disadvantage since several structural and functional changes are frequently concomitant in damaged cells. Current morphofunctional quantitative correlative methodology facilitates the assessment of mechanisms causing cellular alterations, but these studies are not frequent (FRANKE 1990). Expansion of a multipronged methodology should be pursued to better correlate experimental animal data with similar clinical findings in humans (DHAMI et al. 1979).

D. Subcellular Organelle Pathology

Histochemical and biochemical assays are tools for detecting changes in subcellular organelles caused by foreign compounds. Enzyme markers include: adenosine triphosphatase for plasma membrane and bile canaliculi; inosine diphosphatase for rough ER and nuclear membranes; glucose-6-phosphatase, inorganic pyrophosphatase and azoreductase for both rough and smooth ER; thiamine pyrophosphatase for Golgi apparatus; cytidine monophosphatase, α-glycerophosphatase, other nonspecific acid phosphatases, cathepsin, β-glucuronidase and arylsulfatase for lysosomes; and succinic dehydrogenase for mitochondria (CHAMLIAN et al. 1992; KODAVANTE and MEHENDALE 1991). The role of peroxisomes is known in cholesterol and purine metabolism, and catalase can be used to measure increased activity, since this constitutive enzyme accompanies the proliferation of these organelles (BIERI et al. 1988; LOCK et al. 1989). In certain cases morphological alterations are found representing neoformation or the occurrence of spurious densities in the peroxisome matrix, observable in patients with hepatitis, idiopathic jaundice or hyperlipoproteinemia (DE LA IGLESIA et al. 1982).

I. Endoplasmic Reticulum

Considering the action of drugs on the liver cell and their interaction with subcellular structures, the most important organelle appears to be the ER, which shows adaptive or toxic responses to foreign compounds (CONNEY 1986) (Table 2). The adaptive response is also recognized as induction, since it includes increased enzyme activity and membrane proliferation. Many drugs, insecticides, pesticides, polycyclic aromatic hydrocarbons and food additives cause adaptive hepatomegaly, proliferation of the smooth ER and increased activity of cytochrome P450 enzymes (BOCK et al. 1994; FRANK et al. 1982; SCHULTE-HERMANN 1974; UBLEY and MEHENDALE 1989). These membrane-bound enzymes can sometimes metabolize their own inducers at a faster rate (GILLETTE et al. 1972; KOYMANS et al. 1993).

1. Membrane Structure

The ER of the hepatocyte has two structurally and functionally discrete membrane populations based on structural characteristics: the rough and the smooth fractions. The rough ER is characterized by ribosome-studded membranes arranged in characteristic parallel strands interspersed among other organelles in the hepatocyte cytoplasm (MIYAI 1991). The smooth-surfaced portion of the ER contains the cytochrome P450 enzymes involved in the metabolism of endogenous and exogenous substrates. In the early postnatal period dramatic changes occur in the volume and disposition of the ER (DE LA IGLESIA et al. 1976; ROHR et al. 1971), with the density of rough ER membranes increased with a vectorial flowing-off to the smooth membrane component. Protein transport across ER membranes can be divided into initiation and

Table 2. Morphological and functional characteristics of the ER membrane reacting to drugs[a]

Hepatic reaction	Morphological features	Structural composition	Enzyme activity
High induction	Greatly proliferated, large surface increase	Highly unsaturated, increased load	Greatly increased
Low induction	Moderately proliferated, increased surface	Unsaturated	Increased
No effect	Normal surface and volume	Slightly unsaturated, normal load	Unchanged
Low toxicity	Dilatation, unchanged surface	Saturated, some change in load	Slight decrease
High toxicity	Disarray, dilatation, decreased surface	Highly saturated, decreased load	Greatly decreased

[a] These characteristics represent the aggregate of reactions from the literature correlating morphology, morphometry, biochemistry and enzymology of ER membranes. Morphological features include descriptive changes and morphometric evaluations of ER volume and surface. Structural composition refers to phospholipid composition and synthesis, and ratio or load of enzyme activity per unit membrane surface area. Enzyme activity covers oxidative metabolism, phosphatases and cytochrome P450 content.

actual transfer phases and may play a role in hepatocyte injury (RAPOPORT 1991). In the normal liver, the process of smooth ER development occurs postnatally and is closely regulated. The ability of the liver to generate membranes varies with age, and an unexplained decrease in ER volume density occurs in older animals (SCHMUCKLER 1976). The distribution of cytochrome P450 in the liver lobule changes with age (RATANASAVANH et al. 1991).

A morphometric study of human hepatocytes revealed two distinguishable types of smooth ER membrane after drug treatment (JEZEQUEL et al. 1974; JORI et al. 1969). Type 1 adult membranes and type 2 newly formed membranes appeared to have different biological features. Diazepam-induced stimulation caused no change in the synthesis of type 1 membranes, whereas type 2 membranes showed significant proliferative responses. Phenobarbital or phenytoin, well-known inducers of enzyme activity, failed to stimulate differentially either type 1 or type 2 membranes (GONZALEZ 1989; LINDAMOOD 1991).

The ER compartments make up most of the hepatocyte volume, and provide a large membrane surface area available for metabolic interactions (FEUER et al. 1972). The total ER membrane surface of human liver is approximately 24000 m^2 compared to 160–200 m^2 in rat liver (DE LA IGLESIA et al. 1982b). Functionally, the ER membranes are the major sources of protein and phospholipid biosynthesis needed for membrane integrity as well as the major site for the metabolism of endogenous substances and foreign compounds (GUENGERICH et al. 1982).

2. Cytochrome P450 System

This enzyme system metabolizes many foreign compounds including drugs (CROFTS et al. 1994; KOYMANS et al. 1993), endogenous substrates, steroids, fatty acids (CONNEY 1986) and ethanol (COON et al. 1984). The system consists of three essential components: a flavoprotein enzyme: NADPH-cytochrome *c* reductase, a hemoprotein: cytochrome P450, and phospholipid. Phospholipids are essential for the catalytic activity of the enzyme system; substrate specificity resides in the hemoprotein part, which exists in different forms with varying molecular weights, immunological properties, and catalytic activity toward various substrates (GUENGERICH 1989). The activity of these hemoproteins is genetically controlled and therefore differentially influenced by various inducers (ULLRICH 1977; DANNAN et al. 1983).

ER membranes containing the family of cytochrome P450 subtypes show strong interindividual variation and interspecies differences (WRIGHTON and STEVENS 1992). Cytochrome P450 dependent drug-metabolizing enzymes reside in a fluid environment by virtue of their position within ER membranes. These membrane enzymes involved in hydroxylation processes with common functional needs for NADPH cofactor requirements are inhibited by SKF 525A in vitro, and show competitive inhibition between various substrates in vivo (HALPERT et al. 1994; NETTER 1982; TESTA and JENNER 1981). Membrane proliferation is substrate specific, and different inducers stimulate the synthesis of different cytochrome P450 species (DANNAN et al. 1983). The interaction of xenobiotics and cytochrome P450 can disrupt heme biosynthesis (DRUMMOND and KAPPAS 1982; MARKS et al. 1988), influence steroid receptors (FEUER et al. 1985) and cause changes in ER function eventually reflected in other organelles due to interdependencies on membrane synthesis. The subject of cytochrome P450 is dealt in more detail in another chapter of this volume.

3. Proliferation and Induction

ER membranes are very sensitive to toxicants or inducers, reacting with rapid changes in enzyme activity, disposition and volume (GONZALEZ 1989; NEBERT 1979; STAUBLI et al. 1969). Responding to several exogenous substances, membrane proliferation proceeds at an exaggerated rate many times over the normal rate of synthesis (BOLENDER and WEIBEL 1973). Regional lobular differences in enzyme induction have been found following phenobarbital administration; centrilobular hepatocytes showed a fivefold increase in cytochrome P450 compared to periportal hepatocytes (GUMUCIO and CHIANALE 1988). However, there seems to be no difference in the potential for hepatocytes from all three lobular zones to synthesize SER membranes once the xenobiotic stimulus is recognized (KANAI et al. 1993). The membrane proliferation caused by xenobiotics may be accompanied by an adaptive synthesis of drug-metabolizing enzymes, although occasionally the proliferation may be exclusive of enzyme induction. Some of these aspects of membrane proliferation and the de novo enzyme synthesis have been studied in human liver (JEZEQUEL et al. 1974). The hypofunctional ER consists of "empty" membranes due to low cytochrome P450 content and morphological pseudohypertrophic state (DREW and PRIESTLY 1978; FEUER and DIFONZO 1992; SCHAFFNER and POPPER 1969). The rough ER is only slightly affected, and drug-metabolizing enzymes, cytochrome P450, protein and phospholipid content of microsomal membranes are increased significantly (CONNEY 1986). The absolute and relative increase in phospholipids may be particularly important, since these molecules play a role in the interaction between the hydrophobic and hydrophilic sites of the different components of the lipoprotein membrane (DIFONZO et al. 1983).

Parallel with the inductive action on drug-metabolizing enzymes, the de novo membrane-bound phospholipid synthesis is also raised. The effects include increased phosphatidylcholine and lysophosphatidylcholine contents, and stimulation of *S*-adenosyl-L-methionine: microsomal phosphatidylethanolamine methyl transferase activity (DE PIERRE and ERNSTER 1977; DHAMI et al. 1979; FEUER et al. 1980). Drugs can increase significantly and selectively the distribution of unsaturated fatty acids in phospholipids from rough and smooth ER membranes (FEUER et al. 1994) (Fig. 1). Cobalt protoporphyrin inhibits heme oxygenase indirectly, causing decreased catalytic activity of microsomal enzymes (DRUMMOND and KAPPAS 1982; SARDANA and KAPPAS 1987).

Inducers of drug metabolism can modify either the therapeutic action of drugs or the hepatotoxic reactions. Detailed studies of the action of hypnotic

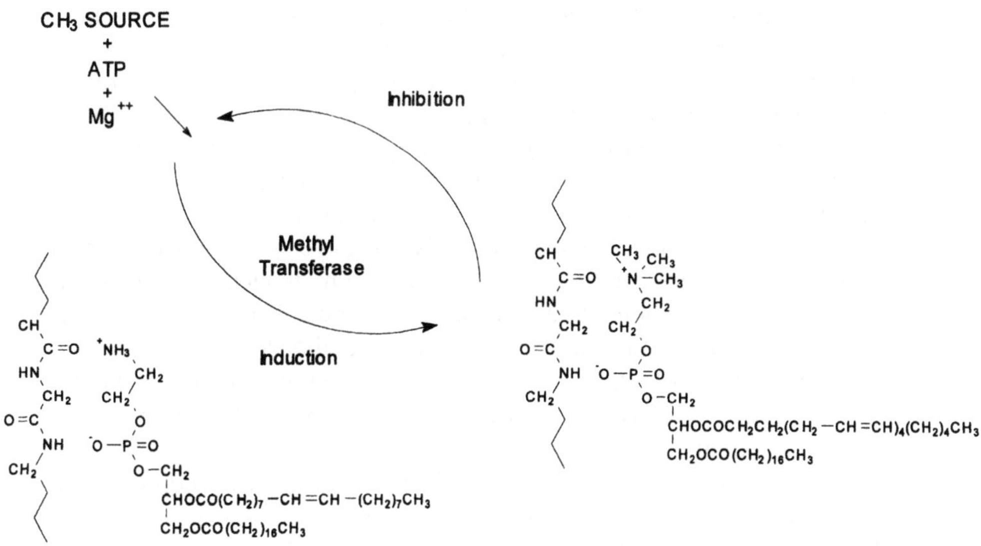

Fig. 1. Schematic representation of the underlying molecular mechanism in the process of induction by methyl transfer reactions. As a result of enhanced synthesis, phosphatidylcholine contains more unsaturated fatty acid components. Hepatotoxicants cause synthesis inhibition and increased fatty acid saturation. (Modified from DE LA IGLESIA et al. 1982b)

inducers showed that barbiturates exert the greatest action on hexobarbital oxidase; 4-methylcoumarin on coumarin 3-hydroxylase; butylated hydroxytoluene on butylated hydroxytoluene oxidase; and nicotine on nicotine oxidase. These results suggest that different cytochrome P450 species are involved and a possible correlation may exist between enzyme induction and the structural similarity of inducer to substrate (FEUER et al. 1980). Induction of UDP-glucuronyltransferase after administration of phenobarbital, methylcholantrene, pregnenolone-16 α-carbonitrile and polychlorobiphenyls to rats leads to decreased thyroxine with subsequent effects on the thyroid gland (BARTER and KLAASSEN 1994; MCCLAIN et al. 1988). Because of toxic insult to the ER, characteristic morphological changes include dilatation or vesiculation of cisternae and modification of the ribosome-membrane relationship (FARISS et al. 1994; MONTEITH et al. 1995). Glutathione provides protection to the ER against lipid peroxidation (BURK 1983). The loss of membrane-associated ribosomes constitutes an early indicator of protein synthesis inhibition or of interaction of intercalating agents with nucleic acids (LE BOT et al. 1988). Whether the membrane effects of hepatotoxicants and inducers represent specific reactions to these compounds or a more general cellular response is not yet known.

4. Structure-Activity Relationships

Although there is a wide diversity of compounds that induce drug metabolism in the liver, there have been very few studies correlating the structural features with the effects on ER activity and membrane integrity (FRANKE 1990). These studies can contribute to the elucidation of critical steps in the mechanisms of enzyme induction, although it may represent a significant task in view of the many different cytochrome P450 variants (CROFTS et al. 1994; KOYMANS et al. 1993). Attempts to establish specific structural requirements have employed polycyclic aromatic hydrocarbons, barbiturates, organohalogen compounds, polyalkyl phenols, and coumarins (CONNEY 1986; FEUER et al. 1980). In the case of coumarins, no correlation was established between the induction effect and the lipid solubility of the inducer. The potent inducing ability of 4-methylcoumarin is attributed to a specific molecular configuration that results in the optimal conformation for triggering drug-metabolizing enzyme synthesis (WALD and FEUER 1971). In integrated morphofunctional studies, coumarin behaves as a hepatotoxicant, whereas 4-methylcoumarin displays inducing activity. The extent of the inducing effect produced by 4-methylcoumarin was not as pronounced as that elicited by phenobarbital. These findings raised the possibility that methyl groups from different moieties may participate in the initial reactions leading to enzyme induction. Among pairs of non-methylated and methylated analogues, methyl derivatives caused a greater induction of drug-metabolizing enzymes (FEUER et al. 1973) (Fig. 2). Dietary methyl-group deficiency reduces liver phospholipid content, enhances methyl transferase activity and increases the incorporation of methyl groups from

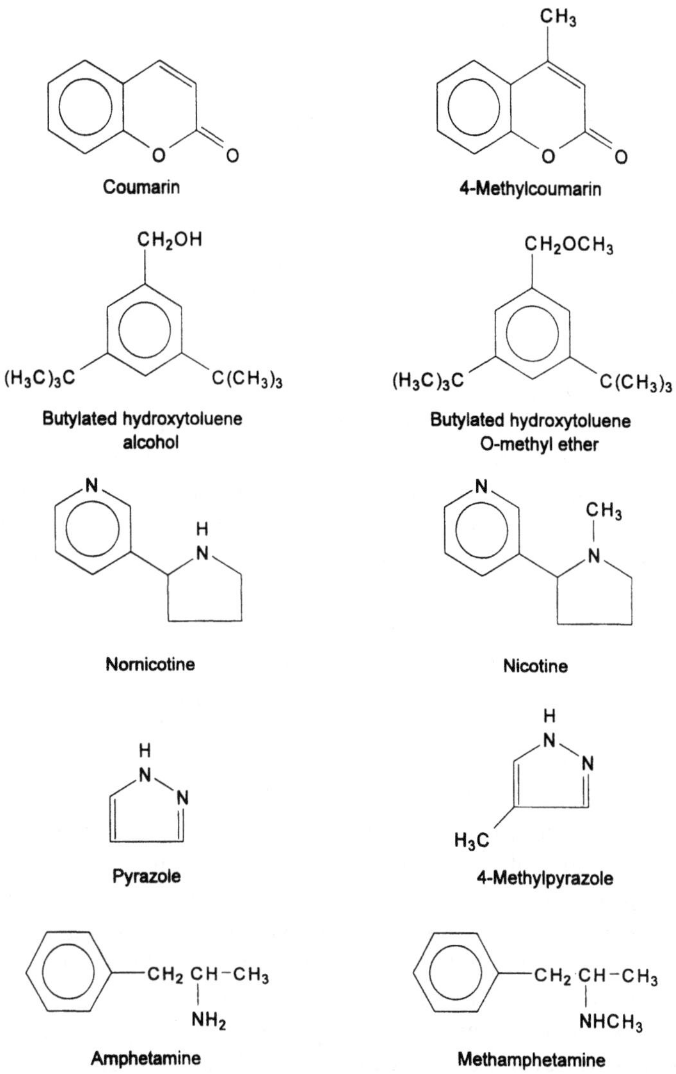

Fig. 2. Molecular pairs with methylated derivatives that affect hepatic drug metabolism

nicotine into individual phospholipids. The administration of drugs increases the utilization of alternate methyl groups for the synthesis of microsomal phospholipids when naturally available donors are reduced (GHOSHAL and FARBER 1993).

5. Membrane-Bound Phospholipids

Lipid changes within the liver cell are prompt indicators of xenobiotic action. Experimental manipulations leading to altered protein or phospholipid synthesis caused changes in the induction of drug-metabolizing enzymes (FEUER et al. 1980). The action of various xenobiotics on the ER can influence protein or lipid composition and even lipid-protein interactions, thus interfering with structural and functional responses. Alteractions of membrane lipids by hepatotoxicants include decreased phospholipid content and measurable effects on membrane surface (Feuer et al. 1994; Ilyas et al. 1978). It is possible that, under subnormal conditions of synthesis, qualitatively different or insufficient amounts of phospholipids would result in low-quality ER membranes with consequent potential hepatic side effects. In systemic phospholipidosis, changes in the relative proportions and quantity of phospholipids resulted in impaired microsomal enzyme activity, and decreased phosphatase activities may have evoked clinical symptoms (de la Iglesia et al. 1974, 1975a,b).

Actinomycin D reduced drug-metabolizing enzyme and methyl transferase activities in parallel with the synthesis of total and selected individual phospholipids in microsomes. Choline- or methionine-deficient diets, or diets high in methionine, decreased drug metabolism and the synthesis of membrane-bound phospholipids, particularly phosphatidylcholine. The addition of small amounts of methionine to the normal diet stimulated both drug metabolism and phospholipid synthesis, indicating that the induction of de novo synthesis of membrane proteins and of phospholipids by drugs are intrinsically related (Dhami et al. 1979; Feuer et al. 1980). Transfer of methyl groups from labeled methionine is increased at 30–60 min post-treatment, and overall phospholipid changes can be detected within 1–2 h, whereas drug-metabolizing activity is increased only 16–20 h after the exposure. Since the phospholipid composition of ER membranes determines the basic activity of drug-metabolizing enzymes, and changes in phosphatidylethanolamine and phosphatidylcholine influence the induction or inhibition processes, the altered organization and stability of ER membranes serves as a toxicity marker.

From the foregoing it can be concluded that: (a) the action of foreign compounds on the drug-metabolizing capacity of the liver cell is related to microsomal phospholipid biosynthesis by means of specific methyl transfer reactions, (b) some drugs can act as methyl donors in the synthesis of phospholipids, and methyl transfer could be an essential but nonspecific reaction, (c) in the induction process, synthesis of membrane-bound phosphatidylcholine may be an obligatory step in the ER proliferation, (d) the structural phospholipid changes caused by drugs represent early steps in the mechanism of proliferation and induction, since incorporation of methyl group from methylated drugs occurs shortly after compound administration and (e) the adverse effect of hepatotoxicants may also be directly related to phospholipid changes, leading to further compromise of the structrual integrity and deterioration of the phospholipid-dependent function in the ER.

II. Golgi Apparatus

The Golgi apparatus is a complex subcellular organelle associated with the biosynthesis, assembly and secretion of macromolecules needed for membrane differentiation (HIGGINS and HUTSON 1984). The role of the Golgi apparatus in various intracellular processes has been studied in functional-ultrastructural experiments in isolated, structurally intact organelles (MATSUURA and TASHIRO 1979; MOSCARELLO et al. 1978). This organelle occupies about 130–150 μm^3 or 2.5%–3% of the liver cell cytoplasm with 1.5 m^2 surface/g liver and can expand significantly upon drug-induced injury (STURGESS and DE LA IGLESIA 1972). The Golgi complex is sensitive to the effects of endogenous or exogenous substances, resulting in atrophy or buildup of membranes with modified synthesis and secretion of glycoproteins and lipoproteins (FRANKE et al. 1994). These alterations may result in abnormal assembly of membrane proteins or in the integrity of the lipid components (STURGESS and MOSCARELLO 1976). The Golgi apparatus is also the site for the attachment of sugar moieties to macromolecules by specific glycosyltransferase enzymes. The sugar side chain determines the biological activity and antigenic properties of the secretory product. Galactosyltransferase and sialyltransferase exist in different areas of the membrane and may respond independently to various drugs and chemicals (DAHAN et al. 1994). The Golgi apparatus is associated with the transport and sorting of secretory products to the cell surface by interaction with microfilaments and microtubules (FARQUAR 1985; GRIFFITH and SIMONS 1986). Age-dependent changes and the interrelationship of Golgi development and ER synthesis were shown by means of quantitative microscopy in livers from humans and experimental animals (DE LA IGLESIA et al. 1976).

The structural integrity of the Golgi apparatus is largely dependent on protein synthesis provided by the rough ER; perturbation of Golgi function can occur without clear-cut structural changes; and intramembrane changes can be studied by cleaving the membrane bilayer to reveal the inner membrane structure. The order of arrangement of these intramembrane particles may provide insights into enzyme activity, such as glycosyltransferase. Injury to the Golgi apparatus by drugs or their metabolites may alter the number of active membrane sites and influence the nature and amount of glycoproteins or lipoproteins produced. Alterations of glycoprotein secretion, such as plasma glycoproteins and mucins, are implicated in pathological and genetic disorders. Enlargement or hypertrophy of the Golgi complex has been observed in human liver due to amyloidosis, toxic hepatitis and other conditions, including drug-induced cholestasis, alcoholism and malnutrition. Atrophy or degeneration may occur during starvation, viral hepatitis and choline or protein deficiency (STURGESS 1978). Coumarin or 4-methylcoumarin treatments caused quantitative microscopic changes in the Golgi membranes in experimental animals (DE LA IGLESIA et al. 1975). The mechanism by which Golgi membranes proliferate is not known.

Preceding kidney injury by aminonucleoside, early and significant stimulation of glycoprotein assembly, increased glycosyltransferase activity and associated structural changes of the Golgi apparatus took place in liver parenchymal cells (STURGESS et al. 1974). The cisternae containing low-density lipoproteins were distended, indicating that blockade occurred between the Golgi apparatus and the cell surface. The aminonucleoside effects on the ER membranes were small, and the initial dilatation of the Golgi apparatus with membrane proliferation took place within 12h. Puromycin inhibited protein synthesis and caused specific functional and structural changes in the Golgi apparatus that persisted long after protein synthesis returned to normal (STURGESS et al. 1974). Structurally, the Golgi apparatus showed atrophic changes, with degeneration of the cisternae, formation of membranous whorls and irregular dilatation (STURGESS et al. 1974). The mechanism of these changes appears to be due to puromycin binding to Golgi membranes and reduced glycosyltransferase activity. Puromycin also affected the incorporation of amino acids into proteins and protein assembly in the rough ER. Cycloheximide, another inhibitor of protein synthesis, also produced degenerative changes in the Golgi apparatus by binding to membranes and causing functional impairment. The mechanism of the cycloheximide lesion was different from that observed with puromycin. Puromycin inhibits glycosyltransferase activity, whereas cycloheximide competitively inhibits galactose transfer onto acceptor molecules.

III. Intracellular Membrane Dynamics

Given the extent of membrane synthesis and the amound of membrane infolded and accumulated in a single hepatocyte, a high degree of dynamic membrane turnover rate is expected to occur and to have modulating influences in the liver response to drugs. The rate of the accumulation of ER membranes in the normal developing liver cell is constant and related to normal turnover rates of other subcellular organelles. From quantitative morphological data. ER membranes appear to increase at a rate of 17 cm^2/h from the postnatal period to maturity, when further renewal of membranes or de novo assembly of membranes is maintained at steady state levels. Turnover rate for individual membrane components is rapid, with half-lives between 20 and 50 cm^2/h for membrane lipids and 40–140 cm^2/h for structural proteins (DALLNER and ERICSSON 1976). Drugs such as aminonucleoside cause rapid proliferation of Golgi membranes at a rate approaching 400 cm^2/h (STURGESS et al. 1974). Phenobarbial treatment of rats increases the rate of membrane assembly in hepatocytes from 16 to 320 cm^2/h at the peak of the induction phase. Cessation of drug treatment changes the rate to a seemingly rapid catabolic phase characterized by the elimination of membranes at a rate of about 330 cm^2/h until normal levels are reached (BOLENDER and WEIBEL 1973; STAUBLI et al. 1969).

Under basic normal conditions or during development, membrane assembly appears to have different dynamics following processes controlled by different regulatory mechanisms than those involved in the response to foreign compounds or pathological conditions. Membrane turnover is reflected in differences in fatty acid composition of microsomes from fetal or neonatal developing liver as compared to the adult. In addition, selective rates of assembly of various membranes take place, and in the mature rat the Golgi apparatus reaches steady state in terms of total membrane complement before the smooth or rough ER (STURGESS and DE LA IGLESIA 1972). Subcellular morphometry allowed the in situ study of drug effects on the individual membrane components of hepatocytes, establishing more precisely defined drug-membrane interactions. The results of these interactions may be associated with a similar pattern of membrane-mediated drug effects through a common pathway, or associated with a unique response of the hepatocyte due to specific effects on target organelles by virtue of their lipid or protein composition.

IV. Mitochondria

Hepatocytes are rich in mitochondria that occupy about 20% of the cell volume in the fetus. The average adult liver cell contains $378.10^9/cm^3$ mitochondria, occupying between 1000 and $1400\,\mu m^3$ cytoplasmic volume. This significant mitochondrial population appears to be constant within hepatocytes from several species (DAVID 1977; DE LA IGLESIA et al. 1981; HESS et al. 1973; KEMMER and HANEFELD 1977; LOUD 1968; WEIBEL et al. 1969). The inner mitochondrial membrane is involved in oxidative phosphorylation and in the regulation of electron transport and provides the basis for respiratory mechanisms essential to cell survival. Thus, impairment of oxidative phosphorylation can cause dramatic changes in mitochondrial volume and shape. Oxygen levels are depleted and mitochondrial electron transport is inhibited in ischemia due to acute cell injury (CANNON et al. 1991). This toxic event can be caused by drugs and results in early structural modifications of mitochondria, loss of potassium and calcium, alterations in fatty acid composition and changes in structural phospholipids (DONNELLY et al. 1994; WOODS et al. 1977). The specific effects of mitochondrial poisons have been delineated with some compounds (BURCHAM and HARMAN 1991). Liver mitochondria seem to have a metabolic advantage over other organs, such as the adrenal, to compensate for these effects (VERNETTI et al. 1993). Nucleoside analogues with antiviral activity cause specific mitochondrial toxicity; and exert their effects by interacting with mitochondrial DNA by chain termination or internalization (PARKER and CHENG 1994) (Fig. 3). The fluorinated nucleoside analogue FIAU, or fialuridine, accumulates in the mitochondrial genome of several species, resulting in fraudulent DNA (RICHARDSON et al. 1994). These effects become manifest systemically in insidious, protracted liver dysfunction, lactic acidosis, persistent neuropathy or pancreatitis which are followed by liver transplantation or lethal outcome (MACILWAIN 1994). Methods to detect mitochondrial damage are available (ABBOTT et al. 1994); rhodamine 123 is a marker for mitochondrial membrane integrity and can be quantitatively assessed by confocal fluorescence cytometry (MONTEITH et al. 1995). Similarly, 2′,7′-dichlorodihydrofluorescein diacetate

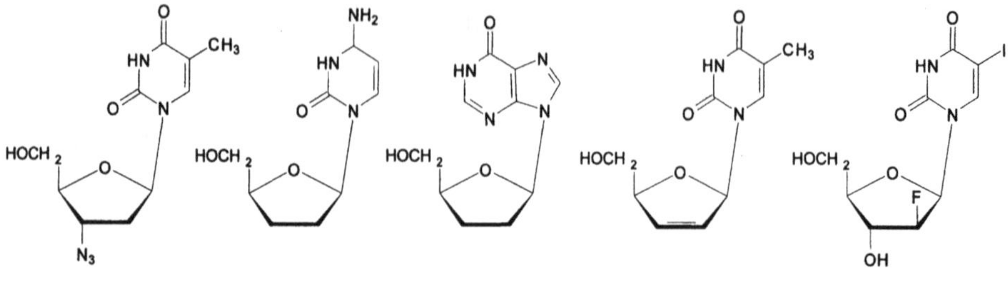

Fig. 3. Antiviral nucleosides known to cause mitochondrial toxicity by reversible DNA chain termination (*) or internalization into the mitochondrial DNA, replacing thymidine bases (**)

is useful for the study of mitochondrial hydroperoxides (BABO and CHARBONNEAU 1994).

Enlargement or hypertrophy of mitochondria is found in chronic alcoholism, dietary deficiencies and essential fatty acid deficiency, with drugs that interfere with copper metabolism, hypolipidemic agents, ethionine, orotic acid or cortisone (SMITH and ORD 1983). The increase in mitochondrial volume was attributed to a decreased number of mitochondria by fusion of preexisting ones associated with defects in the respiratory system, or to exaggerated demands on fatty acid metabolism (KIMBERG and LOEB 1972). Mitochondrial failure due to fialuridine was only increased (PARKER and CHENG 1994). Quantitative microscopic data are lacking which indicate the extent or degree of regional disposition of mitochondrial alterations. Morphometric studies showed a 33% decrease in the number of mitochondria per cell, concomitant with a 700% increase in peroxisomes after hypolipidemic treatment. These changes may indicate a triage in organelle biogenesis (MCGUIRE et al. 1994).

V. Lysosomes

Lysosomes represent the disposal compartment of the cell with the main purpose of degradation and elimination of exogenous or endogenous substances and their metabolites. These membrane-bound organelles are specialized structures, complementary to the ER and Golgi apparatus, and contain a variety of potent hydrolytic enzymes. The primary catabolic function of lysosomal enzymes is directed toward the degradation and solubilization of substances, particularly when they reach a certain colloid state (MARZELLA and TRUMP 1991).

The average hepatocyte may contain up to 200–300 lysosomes, varying considerably in shape, size and appearance, occupying about 1% of the cell volume. The volume density of the lysosome compartment may increase under pathologic conditions. A quantitative increase in lysosomes has been described in human liver following long-term oral contraceptive administration

(STAHL et al. 1977). Lysosomes resembling myeloid bodies appear in large quantities in drug-induced phospholipidosis. Lysosome accumulation occurs after intoxication with various drugs or ethanol in humans and in experimental animals. The development of these abnormal secondary lysosomes may represent impaired catabolic processes resulting from reduced enzyme activity due to excess drug or metabolites entering the cell, or from the lack of specific enzymes that degrade unusual phospholipid moieties tightly bound to membranes (DE LA IGLESIA et al. 1975). With aging, lysosomes accumulate degraded or auto-oxidized fat products, resulting in deposition of lipofuscin or ceroid (MIYAI 1991).

VI. Peroxisomes

Peroxisomes within liver cells constitute discrete membrane-bound subcellular organelles of 0.4–0.6 μm in diameter, containing many oxidative enzymes, including catalase, amino acid oxidase and urate oxidase. Peroxisomes show marked species differences in internal structure and enzyme composition. Catalase is present in the peroxisome matrix, whereas the dark crystalline core seen in some species contains urate oxidase. Peroxisome metabolism reduces oxygen to hydrogen peroxide at the expense of substrate oxidation and provides a compartment for catalase for subsequent reduction of hydrogen peroxide to water by two different routes. Peroxisomes have been extensively characterized by correlated morphological and biochemical studies (BARRASS et al. 1993; DE LA IGLESIA et al. 1982b; GIBSON and LAKE 1993; LOCK et al. 1989; RUMSBY et al. 1994).

There are significant interspecies differences in the peroxisome response to chemicals (GRAY and DE LA IGLESIA 1984; REDDY and LALWANI 1984; RODRICKS and TURNBULL 1987; STERNLIEB 1979). Quantitative microscopic studies showed between 500 and 700 peroxisomes in the cytoplasm of normal hepatocytes, and the human liver cell may contain up to 1000 peroxisomes (DE LA IGLESIA et al. 1981; WEIBEL et al. 1969). When hypolipidemic drugs are administered to rodents, a rapid florid proliferation ensues and the number of peroxisomes increases up to tenfold or more concurrent with increased particle-bound catalase activity. Hypolipidemic stimulation of peroxisome biogenesis has been studied in detail, and the initial rate of peroxisome synthesis approximates 216 organelles per hepatocyte per day during the initial 3 days of drug exposure. The biogenesis rate slows down to 75 peroxisomes per cell per day at steady state. The number of peroxisomes and peroxisome population ratios including enzyme activity changes significantly during drug treatment in periportal liver cells compared to centrilobular hepatocytes (DE LA IGLESIA et al. 1992; LINDAUER et al. 1994).

Lipid-regulating agents of the fibrate type alter the lipoprotein profile and serum lipid composition in dyslipidemic patients (DUJOVNE and HARRIS 1989) (Fig. 4). Curiously, peroxisome proliferation is not found in humans; therefore they are considered unresponsive (DE LA IGLESIA et al. 1981; KEMMER and

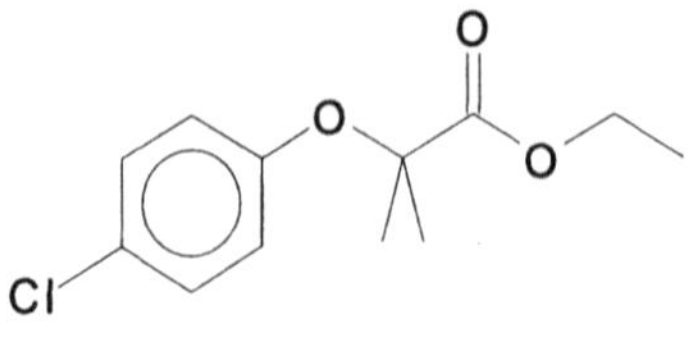

Clofibrate

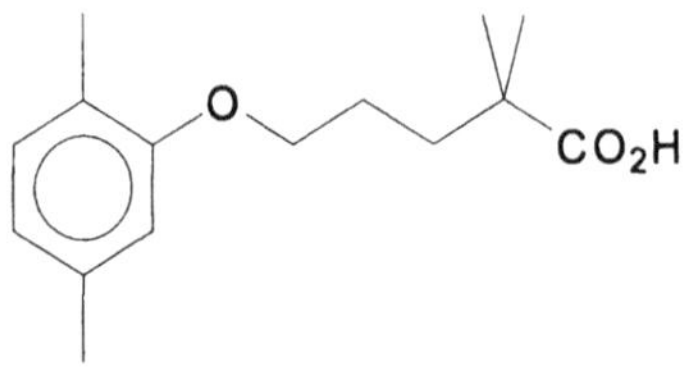

Gemfibrozil

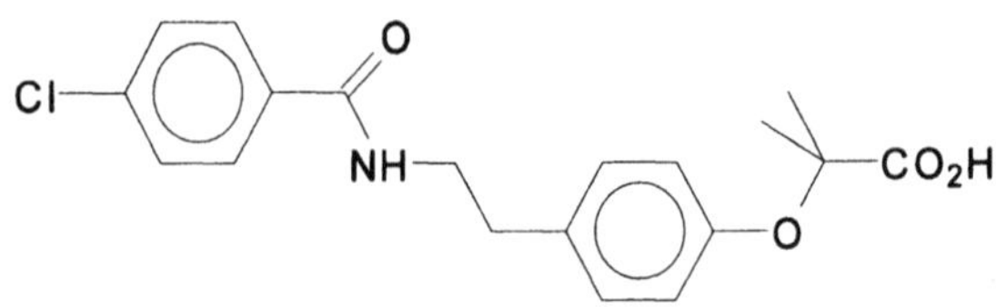

Bezafibrate

Fig. 4. Structure of prototypical lipid-regulating agents of the fibrate family widely used in the treatment of dyslipidemias

Hanefield 1977). Since most peroxisome proliferators cause liver tumors in rodents, the relevance of peroxisome proliferation to humans receiving hypolipidemics long-term is not clear (de la Iglesia and Farber 1982; Reddy and Lalwani 1984). Hypolipidemics cause the formation of 8-hydroxyguanosine and 5-hydroxy-methyl-2′-deoxyuridine in rodent liver (Srinivasan and Glauert 1990; Takagi et al. 1993). However, no direct correlation has been established between accumulation of these compounds and hepatic tumor formation. Structure-activity and functional relationship studies have indicated a correlation between the degree of peroxisome proliferation and high-density lipoprotein synthesis (McGuire et al. 1992; Stable and Hess 1975) (Fig. 6).

Peroxisomes are altered in ferrets with experimental Reye's syndrome after receiving aspirin (Gray et al. 1983), but similar findings have not been corroborated in humans affected with this condition. Deficits of peroxisomes related to drug action have been reported, but not assessed quantitatively (Sternlieb and Quintana 1982). In the cerebrohepatorenal syndrome, peroxisomes are absent in liver cells (Goldfischer 1979).

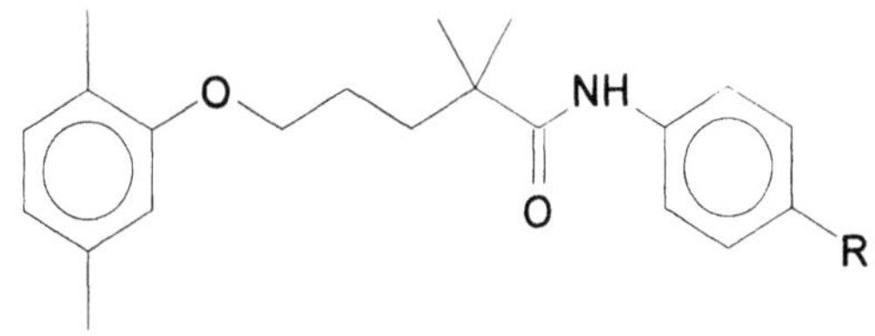

R_1: $CH{=}CHC(O)OC_2H_5$

R_2: $CH_2C(O)OC_2H_5$

R_3: $CH{=}CHSO_2NH_2$

R_4: COOH

Fig. 5. Structure of aryloxyalkanoic amides with differential effects in peroxisomes: propenoic (*R1*), benzeneacetic (*R2*), pentanamide (*R3*), benzoic acid (*R4*) chains. These experimental compounds were useful for establishing relationships between peroxisome proliferation and lipoprotein metabolism

The development of peroxisome proliferation may be the result of a receptor-ligand interaction, since the organelles do not contain genomic elements for autoreplication. The activation process may take place and the receptor has been localized in the nucleus (RAO and REDDY 1987; REDDY and LALWANI 1984). In addition, a nafenopin-binding protein has been identified in the cytosolic fraction. The dissimilarity and chemical heterogeneity of the hypolipidemic moieties lend credence to the idea that changes in binding may modulate the cell or the peroxisome response independently. A peroxisome proliferator response element was found in cytochrome P450 4A6, similar to elements found in genes regulating the enzymes of the peroxisomal β-oxidation pathway (JOHNSON et al. 1994). Peroxisome assembly may be dependent on the import of structural proteins into the matrix (MOTLEY et al. 1994).

E. Biochemical Pathology of Subcellular Changes

The action of hepatotoxic compounds on the liver cell is associated with impairment of basic biochemical processes regardless of the nature of the injurious event. Some of these effects only modify biochemical function, some cause specific functional changes in subcellular organelles, whereas some are more complex and involve many structures and their corresponding biochemical function. Examples of these complex activities are alterations of bile secretion and changes in hepatic blood flow. Sodium deoxycholate causes choleresis and defects in bile canaliculi subsequent to increased secretion of bile and enhanced arterial blood flow. Conjugated bile salts may exert a similar effect though to a lesser degree (FEUER and DIFONZO 1992).

I. Cell Respiration

The alteration of cell respiration is a common cellular response to most toxic actions due to oxygen deprivation, resulting in oxidative stress (DHAUNSI et al. 1994; DONNELLY et al. 1994; FUJII et al. 1994; VERNETTI et al. 1993). The initial morphological sign due to hypoxia or ischemia is cloudy swelling or hydropic degeneration, consisting of a granular appearance of the cytoplasm with light microscopy, and dilatation and disruption of mitochondria with electron microscopy. A dynamic view can be obtained in fluorescence tracing studies using rhodamine and following the time course of reduced transport across he membrane (BABO and CHARBONNEAU 1994; MONTEITH et al. 1995). Morphological changes are associated with reversible denaturation of cellular proteins and associated enzyme activities, especially those participating in oxidative processes. As a result of the reduced oxygen tension in the cell, oxidative phosphorylation falls and the ATP content of the cell decreases rapidly. The injury to mitochondria and other membranes is followed by an influx of sodium, calcium and water into the cell. Precipitation of proteins in the presence of calcium may cause the cloudy appearance of the cytoplasm. Accumulation of water may be so excessive that vesicles are formed in the cytoplasm. Thus, hydropic degeneration represents an advanced step of hepatic cell injury. Mitochondrial damage can be assessed in rat liver by measuring the activity of mitochondria-bound carnitine acyltransferase activity. This enzyme responds to the detrimental action of some hypolipidemics, observed in patients with clofibric acid and in animals with clofibrate (KAHONEN and YLIKAHRI 1979; MANAUTOU et al. 1994; VOSS and KEMMER 1978). The basic mechanism for this adverse effect is not known, although it is reproducible in vitro with isolated mitochondria (WOODS et al. 1977).

II. Protein Metabolism

Cellular alterations of protein metabolism or inhibition of hepatic protein synthesis reduce lipoprotein production and subsequent lipid secretion. Toxin conjugation can inhibit protein synthesis (YAZDI and MURPHY 1994). Decreased availability of apolipoproteins is the most frequent cause of toxic fatty liver. The blockade can occur at various sites along the sequence of reactions involved in protein synthesis. Cycloheximide and emetin affect translation, aflatoxin B binds strongly to DNA, α-amanitin blocks RNA polymerase, D-galactosamine acts by sequestering uridine triphosphate, and dimethylnitrosamine alters both nuclear and cytoplasmic nucleic acids by methylation. Orotic acid fatty liver is due to the formation of inadequate lipoprotein moieties due to an interference with glycosylation. Ethionine blocks protein synthesis by decreasing the availability of ATP and inhibiting methyl transfer reactions, causing a failure of the intracellular transport and secretion of lipids (DIANZANI 1976; SHINOZUKA et al. 1971). Abnormal protein elements accumulate in the liver in various pathologic conditions (SABESIN et al. 1977). Mallory bodies represent a cytoplasmic lesion indicative of preceding hepatic injury, and several drugs can cause their formation (JENSEN and GLUUD 1994a,b). The significance of this lesion eludes investigators; it could represent defective protein synthesis with persistence of abnormal elements in the hepatocyte cytoplasm. Profound and prolonged depletion of cytochrome P450 by metalloporphyrins provides an unusual opportunity not only to study drug metabolism activity, but as a tool for organelle-directed effects (DRUMMOND and KAPPAS 1982; FEUER et al. 1985).

III. Lipid Metabolism

The amount of lipid in hepatocytes represents the balance between synthesis, utilization and secretion; thus structural changes become manifest in conditions of abnormal lipid metabolism. Lipid accumulation follows the impairment of ER function, since it is the principal site for lipid synthesis and production of apoproteins needed for lipoprotein assembly. Lipoprotein particles are transported to the Golgi complex, where they are assembled before release (DAHAN et al. 1994). Several hepatotoxic compounds including CCl_4, chloroform, phosphorus and puromycin induce fatty liver by inhibition of protein synthesis. These chemicals increase free fatty acid flux into hepatocytes as a consequence of increased lipase activity modulated by the intracellular level of cyclic AMP. Fatty liver can be caused by epinephrine and norepinephrine, which stimulate synthesis of cyclic AMP; caffeine and theophylline reduce cyclic AMP metabolism and also cause fatty liver. The hepatic release of fatty acids can be prevented by the administration of adenine, affecting the levels of serum free fatty acids that mediate membrane interactions (SALTIEL et al. 1991).

Alcohol intake leads to hepatic triglyceride accumulation and hyperlipidemia by increasing fatty acid mobilization from adipose tissue stores or from dietary sources. Alcohol also affects fatty acid synthesis and esterification of fatty acids to triglycerides, with altered lipoprotein production. Fatty acid oxidation by mitochondria and lipoprotein secretion from the cell is decreased. Reduced mitochondrial function due to alcohol consumption is modulated by *S*-adenosyl-*l*-methionine (GARCIA-RUIZ et al. 1995). The adequate production of lipoproteins can be impaired by abnormal phospholipid synthesis due to low lipotropic levels. Lipotropic deficiency results in accumulation of triglycerides even if the rate of fatty acid production and uptake is normal. Choline-deficient fatty liver is due to failed intracellular transport and secretion of lipids with a concomitant defect in ER membranes and other subcellular organelles involved in lipoprotein biosynthesis (KANO-SUEOKA and NICKS 1993). Intracellular trafficking of high-density lipoproteins involves lysosomes and endosomes (JÄCKLE et al. 1993), participating in the development of functional changes. The changes with choline deficiency are reversed by the administration of precursors, such as methionine, choline or betaine, sources of essential methyl groups for methyl transfer reactions (GHOSHAL and FARBER 1993). Excess methionine causes fatty change, and vitamin E deficiency enhances the lack of methyl donors; tocopherol deficiency is preventable by selenium compounds (FEUER et al. 1975).

Several conditions cause concentric whorls of ER lamellae in the hepatocyte cytoplasm. The core of these structures contains lipid droplets and subcellular elements resembling modified lysosomes, mitochondria and peroxisomes. Membrane whorls studded with ribosomes or engulfing glycogen particles are produced by toxic compounds, dimethylnitrosamine, α-naphthylisothiocyanate, ethionine and CCl_4. Concentric whorls of smooth ER are produced by acute and chronic intoxication with dimethylnitrosamine, ethionine, CCl_4 and phenobarbital (APFFEL 1978; FLAKS et al. 1976; SHINOZUKA et al. 1971). These structures may represent transient phases of regeneration, repair or degradation and elimination of membranes. Inhibition of protein synthesis, reduction of membrane enzyme activity and abnormal phospholipid production results in these membrane whorls. The altered membrane architecture may reflect asynchrony of the protein-phospholipid assembly on the membrane bilayer. Phospholipid-fatty liver and other systemic manifestations develop as a result of chronic inake of amphipathic compounds, such as coralgil (DE LA IGLESIA et al. 1974), chlorphentermine and phentermine (KACEW et al. 1977), tilorone (LÜLLMAN-RAUCH 1983), gentamicin (KACEW 1987) or amiodarone (REASOR and KACEW 1991).

IV. Bile Secretion

Obstruction of normal bile flow causes retention of biliary substances in the blood and within hepatocytes including accumulation in smaller passages observable in bile canaliculi and smaller ductules (JONES and BURWEN 1987; KAHN et al. 1989; NI et al. 1994; SIRICA et al. 1994). Cytoplasmic changes within hepatocytes include increased lysosomal activity, dilatation and fragmentation of the rough ER, and hypertrophy of smooth membranes and Golgi apparatus. Cholestasis may result from impaired cellular processes related to contractility changes in microtubules (ARIAS et al. 1993; DEGOTT et al. 1992; THIBAULT et al. 1992; TSUKADA and PHILLIPS 1993). The alterations of the ER and mitochondria may be secondary to the detergent action of accumulated bile acids (DIFONZO et al. 1983). Changes in the biliary duct system are also secondary phenomena to the subcellular lesion, and cholestasis due to primary hepatocellular damage results in defects of bile acid oxidation and in bile composition (RADOMINSKA et al. 1993; SIMON et al. 1977; WILTON et al. 1994). Manganese and bilirubin cause cholestasis related to altered metabolic patterns (DENK 1973).

Several agents can cause cholestasis in experimental models: α-naphthylisothiocyanate produces ductular cell proliferation, disorganization of the ER, loss of ribosomes and changes in drug-metabolizing enzymes or bile acid metabolism. In chlorpromazine-induced cholestasis, the drug interacts with the lipid bilayer, inhibiting Na^+/K^+-ATPase and adenylcyclase (PLAA and PRIESTLY 1976; PHILLIPS et al. 1986; OELBERG and LESTER 1986). Anabolic and hormone steroids cause cholestasis with canalicular dilatation and reduction of microvilli (ISAK and ZIMMERMAN 1987; KREEK 1987; VORE et al. 1989). On the other hand, other steroids provide protection (DURHAM and VORE 1986).

The initiating event in cholestasis appeared related to the production of hypoactive hypertrophic smooth ER membranes (SCHAFFNER and POPPER

1969). Thus, the reduced activity of 7 and 17 cholesterol ring hydroxylation to form dihydroxy and trihydroxy bile salts may lead to excess formation of monohydroxy bile salts with subsequent bile stagnation due to the low micellar action. Following simultaneous administration of cobalt chloride and phenobarbital to rats, cholestasis did not appear to be associated with the hypoactive hypertrophic smooth ER, nor could this be reproduced by the addition of lithocholic acid (DREW and PRIESTLY 1978). The reduced cytochrome P450 content and decreased aniline hydroxylase and aminopyrine-*N*-demethylase activities did not point towards a universal, hypofunctional smooth ER, while rough ER effects were predominant.

Quantitative stereologic analysis of cobalt chloride exposed rat liver also showed significantly decreased volume density of smooth ER and increased rough-surfaced ER membranes within hepatocytes, while phenobarbital elevated smooth ER and decreased rough ER volume densities (DE LA IGLESIA et al. 1994a,b). The cobalt chloride effect was arrested by phenobarbital. Structural and functional correlates of ER membranes revealed changes predominantly in rough ER membranes, with significantly decreased glucose-6-phosphatase activity per unit surface area, but no changes in cytochrome P450 or aminopyrine-*N*-demethylase activity. Thus, the induction of chemically induced cholestasis may be related to hypoactive rough ER membranes (DIFONZO et al. 1983; FEUER and DIFONZO 1992).

F. Latent Hepatotoxicity Models

Hepatic cell injury due to drugs is a common phenomenon; thus there is a need to pursue the development of predictive animal models (ZIMMERMAN 1990). This approach can be gleaned from the observation that experimental animals become resistant to the hepatotoxic action of CCl_4 following a second administration due to the decrease and delayed synthesis of mixed-function oxidases, whereas stimulation by phenobarbital-type inducers enhances toxicity due to toxic free radical production (RECKNAGEL et al. 1991; SIPES et al. 1977).

In studying the response of the endoplasmic reticulum to anti-infective agents, penicillin and a cephalosporin were tested on rat microsomes ex vivo after phenobarbital induction or administration of diethyl maleate as glutathione depleter. Either penicillin or the cephalosporin reduced the response to induction, and cytochrome P450 content decreased in glutathione-depleted animals. Changes in microsomal structural protein and phospholipid paralleled the enzyme activity changes, indicating that these compounds exerted mild hepatotoxicity. Therefore, functional ER alterations may serve as useful indicators of hepatic side effects. Sex differences or hormonal control can be gleaned from these simple models. Common marmosets under phenobarbital induction or diethyl maleate-glutathione depletion responded similarly to rats. Penicillin sodium caused slight decreases in cytochrome P450 and aminopyrine-*N*-demethylase activity, with increases in glucose-6-phosphatase. Phenobarbital and penicillin together caused induction of cytochrome P450 and aminopyrine-*N*-demethylase, and increased triglyceride, phospholipid and protein content in microsomes. Cephalothin sodium caused slight decreases in cytochrome P450, aminopyrine-*N*-demethylase and glucose-6-phosphatase activities without glutathione changes in female marmosets. Phenobarbital combined with cephalothin sodium increased cytochrome P450 without changes in aminopyrine-*N*-demethylase activity in male marmosets (DE LA IGLESIA et al. 1994). These interactions included effects on drug metabolism and liver glutathione content, indicating that some metabolites might have adversely affected the cellular redox system (DONNELLY et al. 1994). These studies point to the usefulness of marmosets for predicting subclinical hepatotoxicity.

G. Conclusions

The objective of experimental hepatotoxicity models is to define mechanisms that can predict hepatic side effects in humans. It is also important to establish how these effects relate to subcellular organelle structure and function. For example, what would the mechanism of action be that causes a beneficial response on account of induction or toxic damage due to impairment of a particular cellular function? Most drugs are metabolized in the liver, leading to detoxication and, in some instances, toxic metabolites can cause cell necrosis and stimulate cell proliferation. The hepatic ER is a key organelle that mediates the interactions of drugs, rendering them water soluble, thus enhancing elimination. The integration of morphological and biochemical methods to study ER, mitochondria, Golgi apparatus and peroxisome responses reveals unsuspected effects of toxicants and facilitates the characterization of specific adaptive processes. Considering the significant role of the ER in eliciting hepatotoxicity, these aims can be achieved in practical terms. The approach should include electron microscopy to identify the subcellular target organelles and site of action; quantitative stereology to examine the dynamics of target organelle changes; and cytochemical or immunological techniques for specific phenotypic and molecular markers. In vitro approaches may include subcellular fractionation, specific enzyme studies and characterization of cytochrome P450 changes. A comprehensive evaluation of the lipid composition of subcellular organelles can reveal changes in membrane structure.

The nature of the hepatic response is modulated by extrahepatic and intrahepatic factors, intrinsic to organelle ontogeny and metabolic biotransformation. With inducers, the cellar response involves proliferation of smooth membranes, increased cytochrome P450 content and drug-metabolizing activity. In addition, increased phospholipid synthesis follows the increased methylation and production of phosphatidylcholine with increased amounts of polyunsaturated fatty acids. In contrast, hepatotoxicants alter the structure of

ER membranes, inhibit drug-metabolizing activity, decrease cytochrome P450 content and microsomal protein, lower phospholipid synthesis and reduce methylation of phosphatidylcholine. These structural-functonal differences provide a core aggregate of parameters to screen drugs for possible hepatic side effects. Usually, multiple cellular changes occur in gradual, concatenated time-related sequences. The phospholipid changes may represent early stages, followed by impairment or enhancement of drug metabolism and subsequent changes in ultrastructural morphology. The ultimate outcome of these changes is related to molecular alterations at the sites of membrane activity represented by interactions of phospholipids with proteins. Membrane fluidity seems very promising but has not been fully explored in drug-induced hepatotoxicity, particularly if hepatotoxicants influence signal transduction and messenger targets. Collectively, subcellular morphological and functional correlations provide new dimensions for establishing basic mechanisms of hepatotoxicity. Further knowledge on the early effects of toxicants and the associated membrane modulation may provide guidance to the nature and prediction of hepatotoxicity in humans.

References

Abbott MA, Kowolenko MD, Warner GL (1994) Measuring the effects of nucleoside analogues on mitochondrial DNA content using the polymerase chain reaction. Toxicol Methods 4:161–176

Anthony LE, Schmucker DL, Mooney JS, Jones AL (1978) A quantitative analysis of fine structure and drug metabolism in liver of clofibrate-treated young adult and retired breeder rats. J Lipid Res 19:154–165

Apffel CA (1978) The endoplasmic reticulum membrane system and malignant neoplasia. Prog Exp Tumor Res 22:317–362

Arias IM, Che M, Gatmaitan Z, Leveille C, Nishida T, St Pierre M (1993) The biology of the bile canaliculus. Hepatology 17:318–329

Babo S, Charbonneau M (1994) Measurement of rat mitochondrial hydroperoxides using in situ liver perfusion of 2′,7′-dichlorodihydrofluorescein diacetate. Toxicol Methods 4:224–233

Barrass NC, Price RJ, Lake BG, Orton TC (1993) Comparison of the acute and chronic effects of the peroxisome proliferators methylclofenapate and clofibric acid in rat liver. Carcinogenesis 14:1451–1456

Barter R, Klaassen CD (1994) Reduction of thyroid hormone levels and alteration of thyroid function by four representative UDP-glucuronosyltransferase inducers in rats. Toxicol Appl Pharmacol 128:9–17

Berger ML, Reynolds RC, Combes B (1987) Carbon tetrachloride-induced morphologic alterations in isolated rat hepatocytes. Exp Mol Pathol 46:245–257

Bieri F, Nemali MR, Muakessah-Kelley S et al. (1988) Increased peroxisomal enzyme mRNA levels in adult rat hepatocytes cultured in a chemically defined medium and treated with nafenopin. Toxicol In Vitro 2:235–240

Bock KW, Schrenk D, Forster A et al. (1994) The influence of environmental and genetic factors on CYP2D6, CYP1A2, and UDP-glucuronosyltransferases in man using sparteine, caffeine, and paracetamol as probes. Pharmacogenetics 4:209–218

Bolender RP, Weibel ER (1973) A morphometric study of removal of phenobarbital-induced membranes from hepatocytes after cessation of treatment. J Cell Biol 51:746–761

Bolender RP, Paumgartner D, Losa G, Muellener D, Weibel ER (1978) Integrated stereological and biochemical studies on hepatocytic membranes. I. Membrane recoveries in subcellular fractions. J Cell Biol 77:565–583
Bralet M, Branchereau S, Brechot C, Ferry N (1994) Cell lineage study in the liver using retroviral mediated gene transfer. Evidence against the streaming of hepatocytes in normal liver. Am J Pathol 144:896–905
Burcham PC, Harman AW (1991) Acetaminophen toxicity results in site-specific mitochondrial damage in isolated mouse hepatocytes. J Biol Chem 266:5049–5054
Burk RF (1983) Glutathione-dependent protection by rat liver microsomal protein against lipid peroxidation. Biochim Biophys Acta 757:21–28
Cannon JR, Harrison PJ, Rush GF (1991) The effect of fructose on adenosine triphosphate depletion following mitochondrial dysfunction and lethal cell injury in isolated rat hepatocytes. Toxicol Appl Pharmacol 108:407–416
Chamlian A, Benkoel L, Gulian JM et al. (1992) Loss of endoplasmic reticulum membrane integrity: an image analysis of the glucose-6-phophatase system in human hepatocyte. Cell Mol Biol 38:273–280
Conney AH (1986) Induction of microsomal cytochrome P450 enzymes: the first Bernard B. Brodie lecture at Pennsylvania State University. Life Sci 39:2493–2518
Coon MJ, Koop DR, Reve LE, Crump BL (1984) Alcohol metabolism and toxicity: role of cytochrome P-450. Fundam Appl Toxicol 4:134–143
Cornelius CE (1991) Liver function tests in the differential diagnosis of hepatotoxicity. In: Meeks RG, Harrison SD, Bull RJ (eds) Hepatotoxicology. CRC Press, Boca Raton, pp 181–214
Crofts F, Taioli E, Trachman J et al. (1994) Functional significance of different human CYP1A1 genotypes. Carcinogenesis 15:2961–2963
Dahan S, Ahluwalia JP, Wong L (1994) Concentration of intracellular hepatic apolipoprotein E in Golgi apparatus saccular distensions and endosomes. J Cell Biol 127:1859–1869
Dallner G, Ericsson JL (1976) Molecular structure and biological implication of the liver endoplasmic reticulum. In: Popper H, Schaffner F (eds) Progress in liver diseases. Grune and Stratton, New York, pp 35–50
Dannan GA, Guengerich FP, Kaminsky LS, Aust SD (1983) Regulation of cytochrome P450. J Biol Chem 258:1282–1288
David H (1977) Quantitative ultrastructural data of animal and human cells. Fischer, Stuttgart
David H, Uerlings I (1983) Quantitative ultrastructure of the rat liver by immersion and perfusion fixations. Exp Pathol 23:131–141
de la Iglesia FA, Farber E (1982) Hypolipidemics carcinogenicity and extrapolation of experimental results for human safety assessments. Toxicol Pathol 10:152–170
de la Iglesia FA, Feuer G, Takada A, Matsuda Y (1974) Morphologic studies on secondary phospholipids in human liver. Lab Invest 30:539–549
de la Iglesia FA, Feuer G, McGuire EJ, Takada A (1975a) Morphological and biochemical changes in the liver of various species in experimental phospholipids after diethylaminoethoxy-hexestrol treatment. Toxicol Appl Pharmacol 34:28–44
de la Iglesia FA, McGuire EJ, Feuer G (1975b) Coumarin and 4-methylcoumarin induced changes in the hepatic endoplasmic reticulum studied by quantitative stereology. Toxicology 4:305–314
de la Iglesia FA, Sturgess JM, McGuire EJ, Feuer G (1976) Quantitative microscopic evaluation of the endoplasmic reticulum in developing human liver. Am J Pathol 82:61–70
de la Iglesia FA, Pinn SM, Lucas JM, McGuire EJ (1981) Quantitative stereology of peroxisomes in hepatocytes from hyperlipoproteinemic patients receiving gemfibrozil. Micron 12:97–98
de la Iglesia FA, Lewis JE, Buchanan RA, Marcus EL, McMahon G (1982a) Light and electron microscopy of liver in hyperlipoproteinemic patients under long-term gemfibrozil treatment. Atherosclerosis 43:19–37

de la Iglesia FA, Sturgess JM, Feuer G (1982b) New approaches for the assessment of hepatotoxicity by means of quantitative functional-morphological interrelationships. In: Plaa G, Hewitt RW (eds) Toxicology of the liver. Raven, New York, pp 47–102

de la Iglesia FA, Gray RH, McGuire EJ (1992) Subcellular organelle biogenesis and dynamics in peroxisome proliferation. J Am Coll Toxicol 11:343–348

de la Iglesia FA, DiFonzo CJ, Martin RA, McGuire EJ, Feuer G (1994a) Quantitative changes of the functionally impaired endoplasmic reticulum in the rat liver (in press)

de la Iglesia FA, Martin RA, Walker RM, Feuer G (1994b) Metabolic effects of antiinfective agents on the liver of common marmosets (Callithrix jacchus) (in press)

De Pierre JW, Ernster L (1977) Enzyme topology of intracellular membranes. Annu Rev Biochem 46:201–262

Degott C, Feldmann G, Larrey D et al. (1992) Drug-induced prolonged cholestasis in adults: a histological semiquantitative study demonstrating progressive ductopenia. Hepatology 15:244–251

Denk H (1973) The chemical structure of the endoplasmic reticulum and the function of the P-450 dependent microsomal biotransformation system of the rat liver cell in experimental cholestasis. In: G Paumgarter G, Preisig R (eds) The liver, quantitative aspects of structure and function. Karger, Basel, pp 41–51

Dhami MS, de la Iglesia FA, Feuer G (1979) Effects of progesterone metabolites on fatty acids of the hepatic endoplasmic reticulum membranes. Toxicology 14:99–107

Dhami MS, de la Iglesia FA, Feuer G (1981) Phospholipids of the endoplasmic reticulum in developing liver: fatty acid content and composition. Res Commun Chem Pathol Pharmacol 32:99–111

Dhaunsi GS, Singh I, Orak JK, Singh AK (1994) Antioxidant enxymes in ciprofibrate-induced oxidative stress. Carcinogenesis 15(9):1923–1930

Dianzani MU (1976) Toxic liver injury by protein synthesis inhibitors. In: Popper H, Schaffner F (eds) Progress in liver diseases, vol 5. Grune and Stratton, New York, pp 232–245

DiFonzo CJ, Martin RA, Dhami MS, Feuer G, de la Iglesia FA (1983) Functional responses of the rat hepatic endoplasmic reticulum to treatment proposed as a model for cholestasis. Exp Pathol 23:237–243

Donnelly PJ, Walker RM, Racz WJ (1994) Inhibition of mitochondrial respiration in vivo is an early event in acetaminophen-induced hepatotoxicity. Arch Toxicol 68:110–118

Drew R, Priestly BG (1978) Failure of hypoactive hypertrophic smooth endoplasmic reticulum to produce cholestasis in rats. Toxicol Appl Pharmacol 45:191–199

Drummond GS, Kappas A (1982) The cytochrome P-450-depleted animal: an experimental model for in vivo studies in chemical biology. Proc Natl Acad Sci USA 79:2384–2388

Dujovne GA, Harris WS (1989) The pharmacological treatment of dyslipidemia. Annu Rev Pharmacol Toxicol 29:265–288

Durham S, Vore M (1986) Taurocholate and steroid glucuronides: mutual protection against cholestasis in the isolated perfused rat liver. J Pharmacol Exp Ther 237:490–495

Fariss MW, Johnsen SA, Walton LP, Mumaw VR, Ray SD (1994) Tetrahydroaminoacridine-induced ribosomal changes and inhibition of protein synthesis in rat hepatocyte suspensions. Hepatology 20:240–246

Farquar MG (1985) Progress in unravelling pathways of Golgi traffic. Annu Rev Cell Biol 1:447–488

Feuer CF, Dhami MS, de la Iglesia FA, Feuer G (1980) Association between membrane function and phospholipid composition in the hepatic endoplasmic reticulum: effect of development. In: Coon MJ, Conney AH, Estabrook RW, Gillette JR, O'Brien PJ (eds) Microsomes, drug oxidations and chemical carcinogenesis, vol 1. Academic, New York, pp 559–562

Feuer G, DiFonzo CJ (1992) Intrahepatic cholestasis: a review of biochemical-pathological mechanisms. Drug Metab Drug Interact 10:1–162
Feuer G, Cooper SD, de la Iglesia FA, Lumb G (1972) Microsomal phospholipids and drug action. Quantitative biochemical and electron microscopic studies. Int J Clin Pharmcol Ther Toxicol 5:389–396
Feuer G, Miller DR, Cooper SD, de la Iglesia FA, Lumb G (1973) The influence of methyl groups on toxicity and drug metabolism. Int J Clin Pharmacol 7:13–25
Feuer G, de la Iglesia FA, Cooper S (1974) Role of hepatic endoplasmic reticulum enzyme markers in the preliminary safety evaluations of drugs and other foreign compounds. Proceedings of the European Society for the Study of Drug Toxicity, International Congress series, vol 15: Excerpta Medica Foundation, Amsterdam, pp 142–159
Feuer G, Sosa-Lucero JC, de la Iglesia FA (1975) Effect of dietary hepatic necrosis on the metabolism of foreign compounds in rat liver. Nutr Rep Int 11:199–204
Feuer G, Dhami MS, de la Iglesia FA (1980) Association between membrane function and lipid composition in the hepatic endoplasmic reticulum: effect of progesterone derivatives. In: Coon MJ, Conney AH, Estabrook RW, Gillette JR, O'Brien PJ (eds) Microsomes, drug oxidations and chemical carcinogenesis, vol 1. Academic, New York, pp 563–566
Feuer G, Roomi MW, Stuhne-Sekalec L, Cameron RG (1985) Association between progesterone binding and cytochrome P-450 content of hepatic microsomes in the rat treated with cobalt-haem. Xenobiotica 15(5):407–412
Feuer G, Dhami MS, de la Iglesia FA (1994) Changes by progesterone derivatives in fatty acids from phosphatidylcholine and phophatidylethanolamine fractions in rat liver endoplasmic reticulum. Exp Toxic Pathol 46:169–176
Flaks B, O'Conner JA, Wilks PN (1976) Modification of toxic liver injury in the rat. III. Fine structure of hepatocytes during cycloheximide protection and autoprotection in acute ethionine intoxication. Toxicol Appl Pharmacol 35:423–436
Frank H, Haussman HJ, Remmer H (1982) Metabolic activation of carbon tetrachloride: induction of cytochrome P450 with phenobarbital or 3-methylcholanthrene and its effect on covalent binding. Chem Biol Interact 40:193
Franke H (1990) Structural alteration of liver parenchymal cells induced by xenobiotics. Exp Pathol 39:139–155
Franke H, Potratz I, Dargel R (1994) Zonal differences in lipoprotein formation in the thioacetamide-induced micronodular-cirrhotic liver. Exp Toxicol Pathol 46:503–511
Fujii Y, Johnson ME, Gores GJ (1994) Mitochondrial dysfunction during anoxia/reoxygenation injury of liver sinusoidal endothelial cells. Hepatology 20:177–185
Garcia-Ruiz C, Morales A, Colell A et al. (1995) Feeding S-adenosyl methionine attenuates both ethanol-induced depletion of mitochondrial glutatione and mitochondrial dysfunction in periportal and perivenous hepatocytes. Hepatology 21:207–214
Ghoshal AK, Farber E (1993) Choline deficiency, lipotrope deficiency and the development of liver disease including liver cancer: a new perspective. Lab Invest 68:255–260
Gibson G, Lake B (1993) Peroxisomes. Biology and importance in toxicology and medicine. Taylor and Francis, London
Gillette JR, Davis DC, Sasame HA (1972) Cytochrome P-450 and its role in drug metabolism. Annu Rev Pharmacol 12:57–84
Goldfischer S (1979) Peroxisomes in disease. J Histochem Cytochem 27:1371–1373
Gonzalez FJ (1989) The molecular biology of cytochrome P450s. Pharmacol Rev 40:244–288
Gray RH, de la Iglesia FA (1984) Quantitative microscopy comparison of peroxisome proliferation by the lipid-regulating agent gemfibrozil in several species. Hepatology 4:520–530
Gray RH, Deshmukh DR, Maassab JF, Robertson DG, de la Iglesia FA (1983) Structural and morphometric studies of liver in a ferret model of Reye's syndrome. Proc Electr Micr Soc Am 41:806–807

Griffith G, Simons K (1986) The trans Golgi network: sorting at the exit site of the Golgi complex. Science 234:438–443

Guengerich FP (1989) Characterization of human microsomal cytochrome P-450 enzymes. Annu Rev Pharmacol Toxicol 29:21–264

Guengerich FP, Cannan GA, Wright ST, Martin MV, Kaminsky LS (1982) Purification and characterization of rat liver microsomal cytochrome P-450: electrophoretic, spectral, catalytic and immunochemical properties and inducibility of eight isozymes treated with phenobarbital or beta-naphthoflavone. Biochemistry 21:6019–6030

Gumucio JJ, Chianale J (1988) Liver cell heterogeneity and liver function. In: Arias IM, Jacoby WB, Popper H, Schachter D, Shafortz DA (eds) The liver: biology and pathobiology, 2nd edn. Raven, New York, pp 931–947

Halpert JR, Guengerich FP, Bend JR, Correia MA (1994) Selective inhibitors of cytochromes P450. Toxicol Appl Pharmacol 125:163–175

Hess FA, Weibel ER, Preisig R (1973) Morphometry of dog liver: normal base-line data. Virchows Arch (Zell Pathol) 12:303–317

Higgins JA, Hutson JL (1984) The role of golgi and endoplasmic reticulum in the synthesis and assembly of lipoprotein lipids in hepatocytes. J Lipid Res 25:1295–1305

Ilyas MS, de la Iglesia FA, Feuer G (1978) The effect of phenobarbital and carbon tetrachloride on fatty acid content and composition of phospholipids from rat liver. Toxicol Appl Pharmacol 45:69–77

Isak KG, Zimmerman JH (1987) Hepatotoxic effects of the anabolic/androgenic steroids. Semin Liv Dis 7:230–236

Jäckle S, Rinninger F, Lorenzen T, Greten H, Widler E (1993) Dissection of compartments in rat hepatocytes involved in the intracellular trafficking of high-density lipoprotein particles or their selectively internalized cholesteryl esters. Hepatology 17:455–465

Jensen K, Gluud C (1994a) The Mallory body: morphological, clinical and experimental studies (part 1 of a literature survey). Hepatology 20:1061–1077

Jensen K, Gluud C (1994b) The Mallory body: theories on development and pathological significance (part 2 of a literature survey). Hepatology 20:1330–1342

Jezequel AM, Koch M, Orlandi F (1974) A morphometric study of the endoplasmic reticulum in human hepatocytes. Correlation between morphological and biochemical data in subjects under treatment with certain drugs. Gut 15:737–747

Johnson EF, Hsu M, Griffin K, Palmer CN (1994) Regulation of cytochrome P450 and other genes by the peroxisome proliferator activated receptor α. Proceedings. 6th North American Symposium of the International Society of Study of Xenobiotics Symposium, Raleigh, NC, p 14

Jones AL, Burwen SJ (1987) The canalicular bile mystique: its end is in sight. Hepatology 7:387–390

Jori A, Bianchetti A, Prestini PE (1969) Effect of contraceptive agents on drug-metabolism. Eur J Pharmacol 7:196–200

Kacew S (1987) Cationic amphiphilic drug-induced renal cortical lysosomal phospholipidosis: an in vivo comparative study with gentamicin and chlorphentermine. Toxicol Appl Pharmacol 91:469–476

Kacew S, Narbaitz R, Stevenson AJ (1977) The effects of chlorphentermine on certain metabolic parameters associated with development of rat kidney and liver. Chem Biol Interact 19:61–76

Kahn E, Markowitz J, Aiges H, Daum F (1989) Human ontogeny of the bile duct to portal space ratio. Hepatology 10:21–23

Kahonen MT, Ylikahri RH (1979) Effect of clofibrate and gemfibrozil on the activities of mitochondrial carnitine acyltransferases in rat liver. Dose-response relations. Atherosclerosis 32:47–56

Kanai A, Watanabe J, Fujimoto S, Kanamura S (1993) Quantitative analysis of smooth endoplasmic reticulum proliferation in periportal, midzonal and perivenular hepatocytes of mice after administration of phenobarbital. Exp Toxic Pathol 45:199–203

Kano-Sueoka T, Nicks ME (1993) Abnormal function of protein kinase c in cells having phosphatidylethanolamine-deficient and phosphatidyl-excess membranes. Cell Growth Differ 4:533–537
Kemmer C, Hanefeld M (1977) Ultrastructural findings in liver biopsies from patients with hyperlipoproteinemia. Zentralbl Allg Pathol 121:243–253
Kimberg DV, Loeb JN (1972) Effects of cortisone administration on rat liver mitochondria: support for the concept of mitochondrial fusion. J Cell Biol 55:625–643
Kodavante PR, Mehendale HM (1991) Biochemical methods of studying hepatotoxicity. In: Meeks RG, Harrison SD, Bull RJ (eds) Hepatotoxicology. CRC Press, Boca Raton, pp 241–326
Koymans L, Donne-op den Kelder GM, Koppele Te JM, Vermealen NPE (1993) Cytochrome P450: their active site, structure and mechanism of oxidation. Drug Metab Rev 25:325–387
Kreek MJ (1987) Female sex steroids and cholestasis. Semin Liver Dis 7:8–23
Lamers WH, Hilberts A, Furt E et al. (1989) Hepatic enzyme zonation: a reevaluation of the concept of the liver acinus. Hepatology 10:72–76
Le Bot MA, Begue JM, Kernaleguen D et al. (1988) Metabolism of doxorubicin, epirubicin and daunorubicin by human and rat hepatocytes in primary culture. In: Guillouzo A (ed) Liver cells and drugs. Libbey Eurotext, Paris, pp 365–370
Lindamood C (1991) Xenobiotic transformation. In: Meeks RG, Harrison SD, Bull RJ (eds) Hepatotoxicology. CRC Press, Boca Raton, pp 139–180
Lindauer M, Beier K, Völkl A, Fahimi HD (1994) Zonal heterogeneity of peroxisomal enzymes in rat liver: differential induction by three divergent hypolipidemic drugs. Hepatology 20:475–486
Lock EA, Mitchell AM, Elcombe CR (1989) Biochemical mechanism of induction of hepatic peroxisome proliferation. Annu Rev Pharmacol Toxicol 29:145–163
Loud AV (1968) A quantitative stereological description of the ultrastructure of normal rat parenchymal cells. J Cell Biol 37:27–46
Ludwig J (1979) Drug effects on the liver. A tabular compilation of drugs and drug-related hepatic diseases. Dig Dis Sci 24:785–796
Lüllman-Rauch R (1983) Tilorone-induced lysosomal storage mimicking the features of mucopolysaccharidosis and of lipidosis in rat liver. Virchows Arch [B] 44:355
Macilwain C (1994) Concern grows over reaction to deaths in clinical trials. Nature 369:268
Manautou JE, Hoivik DJ, Tveit A, Emeight Hart SG, Khairallah EA, Cohen SD (1994) Clofibrate pretreatment diminishes acetaminophen's selective covalent binding and hepatotoxicity. Toxicol Appl Pharmacol 129:252–263
Marks GS, McCluskey SA, Mackie JE, Riddick DS, James CA (1988) Disruption of hepatic heme biosynthesis after interaction of xenobiotics with cytochrome P450. FASEB J 2:2774–2783
Marzella L, Trump BF (1991) Pathology of the liver: functional and structural alterations of hepatocyte organelles induced by cell injury. In: Meeks RG, Harrison SD, Bull RJ (eds) Hepatotoxicology. CRC Press, Boca Raton, pp 93–138
Matsuura S, Tashiro Y (1979) Immunoelectron-microscopic studies of endoplasmic reticulum – Golgi relationships in the intracellular transport process of lipoprotein particles in rat hepatocytes. J Cell Sci 39:272–290
McClain RM, Posch RC, Bosakowski T, Armstrong JM (1988) Studies on the mode of action of thyroid gland tumor promotion in rats by phenobarbital. Toxicol Appl Pharmacol 94:254–265
McGuire EJ, Gray RH, de la Iglesia FA (1992) Chemical structure-activity relationships: peroxisome proliferation and lipid regulation in rats. J Am Coll Toxicol 11:353–361
McGuire EJ, Haskins JR, Lucas JA, de la Iglesia FA (1995) Hypolipidemic-induced quantitative microscopic changes in rat liver mitochondria. Abstracts, VII. International Congress of Toxicology 7:47-P-7

Mikhael NZ, Kacew S (1985) Adverse tissue reactions to drugs: a five year surveillance study. Hum Toxicol 4:583–590
Miyai K (1991) Structural organization of the liver. In: Meeks RG, Harrison SD, Bull RJ (eds) Hepatotoxicology. CRC Press, Boca Raton, pp 1–66
Monteith DK, Theiss JC, de la Iglesia FA (1995) Tacrine-induced subcellular and functional changes in rat and human hepatocytes in culture (in press)
Moscarello MA, Abe H, Sturgess JM (1978) Morphological and biochemical approaches to characterize the structure and function of the Golgi complex. In: Falkner F, Kretchmer N, Rossi E (eds) Modern problems in pediatrics, vol 19. Karger, Basel, pp 88–98
Motley A, Hettema E, Distel B, Tabak H (1994) Differential protein import deficiencies in human peroxisome assembly disorders. J Cell Biol 125:755–767
Nebert DW (1979) Multiple forms of inducible drug-metabolizing enzymes: a reasonable mechanism by which any organism can cope with adversity. Mol Cell Biochem 27:27–46
Netter KJ (1982) Inhibition of oxidative drug metabolism in microsomes. In: Schenkman JB, Kupfer D (eds) Hepatic cytochrome P-450 monooxygenase system. Pergamon, Oxford, pp 741–761 (International encyclopedia on pharmacological therapeutics, vol 108)
Ni Y, Lukito G, Marchal G et al. (1994) Potential role of bile duct collaterals in the recovery of the billary obstruction: experimental study in rats using microcholangiography, histology, serology and magnetic resonance imaging. Hepatology 20:1557–1566
Oelberg DG, Lester R (1986) Cellular mechanisms of cholestasis. Annu Rev Med 37:297–317
Parker WE, Cheng YC (1994) Mitochondrial toxicity of antiviral nucleoside analogues. J NIH Res 6:57–61
Phillips MJ, Poucel S, Oda M (1986) Biology of disease: mechanisms of cholestasis. Lab Invest 54:593–608
Plaa GL, Priestly BG (1976) Intrahepatic cholestasis induced by drugs and chemicals. Pharmacol Rev 28:207–273
Radominska A, Treat S, Little J (1993) Bile acid metabolism and the pathophysiology of cholestasis. Semin Liver Dis 13:219–234
Rao MS, Reddy JK (1987) Peroxisome proliferation and hepatocarcinogenesis. Carcinogenesis 8:631–636
Rapoport TA (1991) Protein transport across the endoplasmic reticulum membrane: facts, models mysteries. FASEB J 5:2792–2798
Rappaport AM (1979) Physioanatomical basis of toxic liver injury. In: Farber E, Fisher MM (eds) Toxic injury of the liver. Dekker, New York, pp 1–57
Ratanasavanh D, Beaune P, Morel F, Flinois JP, Guengerich FP, Guillouzo A (1991) Intralobular distribution and quantitation of cytochrome P-450 enzymes in human liver as a function of age. Hepatology 13:1142–1151
Reasor MJ, Kacew S (1991) Amiodarone pulmonary toxicity: morphological and biochemical features. Proc Soc Exp Biol Med 196:1–7
Recknagel RO, Glende EA, Britton RS (1991) Free radical damage and lipid peroxidation. In: Meeks RG, Harrison SD, Bull RJ (eds) Hepatotoxicity. CRC Press, Boca Raton, pp 401–436
Reddy JK, Lalwani ND (1984) Carcinogenesis by hepatic peroxisome proliferators: evaluation of the risk of hypolipidemic drugs and industrial plasticizers to humans. CRC Crit Rev Toxicol 12:1–58
Richardson RC, Engelhardt, Bowsher RR (1994) Fialuridine accumulates in DNA of dogs, monkeys and rats following long-term oral administration. Proc Natl Acad Sci USA 91:12003–12007
Rodricks JV, Turnbull D (1987) Interspecies differences in peroxisomes and peroxisome proliferation. Toxicol Ind Health 3:197–213
Rohr HP, Wirz A, Henning LC, Riede UN, Bianchi L (1971) Morphometric analysis of the rat liver cell in the perinatal period. Lab Invest 24:128–139

Rohr HP, Luthy J, Gudat F et al. (1976) Stereology: a new supplement to the study of human liver biopsy specimens. In: Schaffner F, Popper H (eds) Progress on liver diseases, vol 5. Grune and Stratton, New York, pp 24–34
Rumsby PC, Davies MJ, Price RJ, Lake BG (1994) Effect of some peroxisome proliferators on transforming growth factor-β_1 gene expression and insulin-like growth factor II/mannose-6-phosphate receptor gene expression in rat liver. Carcinogenesis 15:419–421
Sabesin SM, Frase S, Ragland JB (1977) Accumulation of nascent lipoproteins in rat hepatic Golgi during induction of fatty liver by orotic acid. Lab Invest 37:127–135
Saltiel AR, Ravetch J, Aderem AA (1991) Functional consequences of lipid-mediated protein-membrane interactions. Biochem Pharmacol 42:1–11
Sardana MK, Kappas A (1987) Dual control mechanism for heme oxygenase: Tin(IV)-protoporphyrin potently inhibits enzyme activity while markedly increasing content of enzyme protein in liver. Proc Natl Acad Sci USA 84:2464–2468
Schaffner F, Popper H (1969) Cholestasis is the result of hypoactive hypertrophic smooth endoplasmic reticulum in the hepatocyte. Lancet II:355–360
Schmuckler DL (1976) Age-related changes in hepatic fine structure: a quantitative analysis. J Gerontol 31:135–143
Schulte-Hermann R (1974) Induction of liver growth by xenobiotic compounds and other stimuli. CRC Crit Rev Toxicol 3:97–158
Shinozuka H, Lombardi B, Farber E (1971) Dynamics of injury and repairs in hepatic cells. II. Association of membrane with lipid during recovery from ethionine-induced fatty liver. Am J Pathol 63:161–178
Simon FR, Sinensky M, Kern F, Davis RA (1977) Reversal of ethinyl estradiol induced cholestasis: correlative changes in liver surface membrane structure and function. Clin Res 25:318
Sipes IG, Krishna G, Gillette JR (1977) Bioactivation of carbon tetrachloride, chloroform, and bromotrichloromethane: role of cytochrome P-450. Life Sci 20:1541–1548
Sirica A, Gainey TW, Mumaw VR (1994) Ductular hepatocytes. Evidence for a bile ductular origin in furan-treated rats. Am J Pathol 145:375–383
Smith RA, Ord MJ (1983) Mitochondrial form and function relationships in vivo: their potential in toxicology and pathology. Int Rev Cytol 83:63–134
Srinivasan S, Glauert HP (1990) Formation of 5-hydroxymethyl-2′-deoxyuridine in hepatic DNA of rats treated with γ-irradiation, diethylnitrosamine, 2-acetylaminofluorene or the peroxisome proliferator ciprofibrate. Carcinogenesis 11:2021–2024
Stahl K, Themann H, Verhagen A (1977) Ultrastructural-morphometric investigations on liver biopsies – the influence of oral contraceptives on the human liver. Arch Gynaekol 223:205–211
Staubli W, Hess R (1975) Lipoprotein formation in the liver cell. Ultrastructural and functional aspects relevant to hypolipidemic action. In: Kritchevsky D (ed) Hypolipidemic agents. Springer, Berlin Heidelberg New York, pp 229–289 (Handbook of experimental pathology, vol 41)
Staubli W, Hess R, Weibel ER (1969) Correlated morphometric and biochemical studies on the liver cell. II. Effects of phenobarbital on rat hepatocytes. J Cell Biol 42:92–112
Sternlieb I (1979) Electron microscopy of mitochondria and peroxisomes of human hepatocytes. In: Popper H, Schaffner F (eds) Progress in liver disease, vol 6. Grune and Stratton, New York, pp 81–104
Sternlieb I, Quintana N (1982) Abnormalities of human hepatocellular peroxisomes. Ann NY Acad Sci 386:530–533
Sturgess JM (1978) The Golgi apparatus. In: Lapedes DN (ed) Yearbook of science and technology. McGraw-Hill, New York, pp 209–211
Sturgess JM, de la Iglesia FA (1972) Morphometry of the Golgi apparatus in developing liver. J Cell Biol 55:524–530

Sturgess JM, Moscarello MA (1976) Alterations in the Golgi complex and glycoprotein biosynthesis in normal and diseased tissues. In: Ioachim HL (ed) Pathobiology annual. Appleton-Century-Crofts, New York, pp 1–29

Sturgess JM, de la Iglesia FA, Minaker E, Mitranic M, Moscarello MA (1974) The Golgi complex: II. The effects of aminonucleoside in ultrastructure and glycoprotein biosynthesis. Lab Invest 31:6–14

Sweeney DJ, Diario RB (1991) The isolated perfused liver as models for studying drug- and chemical-induced hepatotoxicity. In: Meeks RG, Harrison SD, Bull RJ (eds) Hepatotoxicology. CRC Press, Boca Raton, pp 215–240

Takagi A, Umemura T, Hasegawa R, Kurokawa Y (1993) Production of 8-hydroxydeoxyguanosine in rodent liver by the administration of peroxisome proliferators. In: Gibson G, Lake B (eds) Peroxisomes. Biology and importance in toxicology and medicine. Taylor and Francis, London, pp 569–618

Testa B, Jenner P (1981) Inhibitors of cytochrome P-450s and their mechanism of action. Drug Metab Rev 12:1–117

Thibault N, Claude JR, Ballet F (1992) Actin filament alteration as a potential marker for cholestasis: a study in isolated rat hepatocyte couplets. Toxicology 73:269–279

Tsukada N, Phillips JM (1993) Bile canalicular contraction is coincident with reorganization of pericanalicular filaments and colocalization of actin and myosin-II. J Histochem Cytochem 41:353–363

Ubley WS, Mehendale HM (1989) Phenobarbital-induced cytosolic cytoprotective mechanisms that offset increases in NADPH cytochrome P450 reductase activity in menadione mediated cytotoxicity. Toxicol Appl Pharmacol 99:323

Ullrich V (1977) The mechanism of cytochrome P-450 action. In: Ullrich V, Hildebrandt A, Roots T, Estabrook RW, Conney AH (eds) Microsomes and drug oxidations. Pergamon, Oxford, pp 192–201

Vernetti LA, MacDonald JR, Wolfgang GH, Dominick MA, Pegg DG (1993) ATP depletion is associated with cytotoxicity of a novel lipid regulator in guinea pig adrenocortical cells. Toxicol Appl Pharmacol 118:30–38

Vore M, Montgomery C, Durham S, Schlarman D, Elliott WH (1989) Structure-activity relationship of the cholestatic activity of dihydrotestosterone glucuronide, allo bile acids and lithocholate. Life Sci 44:2033–2040

Voss K, Kemmer C (1978) Image processing in pathology. VIII. Internal structure of mitochondria during treatment of HLP-patients with regadrin. Exp Pathol 15:311–318

Wald RW, Feuer G (1971) Molecular orbital calculations on coumarins and the induction of drug metabolizing enzymes. J Med Chem 14:1081–1085

Weibel ER, Staubli W, Gnagi HR, Hess FA (1969) Correlated morphometric and biochemical studies on the liver cell. I. Morphometric model, stereologic methods and normal morphometric data for rat liver. J Cell Biol 42:68–91

Wilton JC, Mattews GM, Burgoyne RD, Mills CO, Chipman K, Coleman R (1994) Fluorescent choleretic and cholestatic bile salts take different paths across the hepatocyte: transcytosis of glycolithocholate leads to an extensive redistribution of annexin II. J Cell Biol 127:401–410

Woods TA, Decker GL, Pedersen (1977) Antihyperlipidemic drugs – in vitro effect on the function and structure of rat liver mitochondria. J Mol Cell Cardiol 9:807–822

Wrighton SA, Stevens JC (1992) The human hepatic cytochromes P450 involved in drug metabolism. CRC Crit Rev Toxicol 22:1–21

Yazdi PT, Murphy RM (1994) Quantitative analysis of protein synthesis inhibition by transferrin-toxin conjugates. Cancer Res 54:6387–6394

Zajicek G, Oren R, Weinreb MJ (1985) The streaming liver. Liver 5:293–300

Zimmerman HJ (1990) Update of hepatotoxicity due to classes of drugs in common clinical use: non-steroidal drugs, anti-inflammatory drugs, antibiotics, antihypertensives, cardiac and psychotropic agents. Semin Liver Dis 10:322–335

CHAPTER 4

Molecular Biology of Hepatic Drug Reactions

R.W. SALLIE and E.A. JONES

A. Introduction

In a very real sense, the burgeoning discipline of "molecular biology", broadly defined, can be gainfully applied in most fields of medicine, including those relevant to the topics covered in the majority of chapters in this volume. Various aspects of the molecular biology of hepatic drug reactions, particularly those pertaining to cell damage mediated by lipid peroxidation, glutathione depletion and genetic susceptibility, are covered by other authors. This chapter is concerned predominantly with a theoretical discussion of hepatic drug reactions which are mediated, at least in part, by interference with the metabolism and processing of DNA or RNA and with the synthesis of proteins. Hepatocellular apoptosis is also discussed in this context. Wherever possible, the discussion indicates how mechanism(s) relate to overt liver disease in patients. Much of the work conducted to investigate mechanisms of drug toxicity has been carried out in animal models or in vitro systems using cultures of non-hepatocyte cell lines. The limitations and pitfalls of extrapolating from non-human data to the clinical situation are well recognised.

Although the number of drugs and xenobiotics which may injure the liver is virtually infinite, the list of established mechanisms known to mediate such damage is relatively small (Table 1). However, within the general pathways of hepatocellular injury discussed in this chapter it is clear that drugs and xenobiotics may modulate molecular events in a wide variety of ways. The precise cascade of molecular events that lead to drug or xenobiotic-induced hepatocellular injury and/or necrosis is completely understood for only a few thoroughly investigated or prototypic drugs.

B. General Considerations

From a purely pragmatic standpoint, hepatic drug reactions may be divided into those arising due to intrinsic drug toxicity and those due to idiosyncratic drug reactions. The former are both dose dependent and predictable, whereas the latter are, by definition, unpredictable and are also dose independent (KAHL 1991) (Table 2). Unfortunately, from both clinical and investigational perspectives, the vast majority of hepatic drug reactions appear to have

Table 1. General mechanisms of drug-induced molecular injury (mechanisms 1–4 discussed in this chapter)

1. Interference with DNA metabolism
2. Interference with RNA metabolism
3. Alteration in protein synthesis
4. Induction of apoptosis
5. Disturbance of haem synthesis
6. Interference with mitochondrial function
7. Plasma membrane damage
8. Alteration in post-translational modification
9. Intercalation of RNA
10. Interference with bile secretion
11. Lipid peroxidation
12. Formation of reactive species
13. Glutathione depletion
14. Peroxisome proliferation

Table 2. Intrinsic and idiosyncratic hepatotoxicity (comparison between defining characteristics of intrinsic and idiosyncratic hepatotoxins)

Characteristic	Intrinsic	Idiosyncratic
Predictable	Yes	No
Dose dependency	Yes	No
Animal models	Yes	No
In vitro models	Often	No
Latency	Constant	Highly variable
Mechanisms	Usually chemical/ metabolic	Often immunological
Genetic influence	No[a]	Yes
Example	Paracetamol	Halothane

[a] The degree of toxicity or the threshold level of exposure at which toxicity occurs may exhibit a genetic polymorphism, but toxicity invariably develops if dosage is sufficiently great.

an idiosyncratic basis (POHL 1990). This property of hepatic drug reactions diminishes the prospects for either their prevention as a result of pre-clinical studies or their early detection during clinical use. Furthermore, as a direct consequence of the infrequent occurrence and species specificity of most hepatic drug reactions, detailed molecular and genetic analysis of the factors responsible for their predisposition and mediation are usually precluded by the lack of any adequate animal model (POHL 1990). In addition, hepatic drug reactions are not usually amenable to investigation in in vitro systems. A notable exception to this generalisation, and an example that has been extensively studied in vitro is halothane hepatotoxicity (FARRELL et al. 1985; FROST et al. 1989). The problems inherent in studying hepatic drug reactions in vitro are compounded by the difficulties in maintaining normal human hepatocytes in long-term culture.

At a more practical level, molecular biological investigation of clinical hepatotoxicity is frequently hampered by a lack of adequate tissue for study. In the majority of patients in whom hepatic drug reactions occur, liver biopsy either is inappropriate or is not obtained and a paired or control biopsy is rarely available for comparative purposes. Moreover, the amount of tissue obtained is typically insufficient for both routine histology and molecular analysis. Accordingly, the effects of many drugs on the metabolism of DNA and/or RNA within the liver tend to be inferred from studies performed on either animal model or cell culture systems. In spite of their inherent limitations and uncertainties whether results obtained are directly applicable to the clinical situation, extensive non-human investigations have provided considerable insights into the ways in which drugs may cause hepatocellular injury at a molecular level.

C. DNA Damage

I. Drugs and DNA Metabolism

The general theoretical mechanisms by which drugs may interfere with DNA metabolism and function are listed in Table 3. In clinical practice the toxicity associated with drugs which interfere with DNA synthesis is much more likely to involve tissues which normally have a high cell turnover, such as the

Table 3. Drugs and DNA damage (general mechanisms by which drugs may mediate damage to DNA)

- Inhibition of DNA replication
  - Inhibition of DNA polymerases
    - Inhibition of DNA polymerase α (nuclear DNA)
    - Inhibition of DNA polymerase γ (mitochondrial DNA)
  - Inhibition of DNA ligase
  - Chain termination and pseudo chain termination
  - Alteration of purine/pyrimidine metabolism
  - Interference with nucleosome formation
  - Interference with other cofactors
- Inhibition of DNA repair
  - Inhibition of DNA polymerases
  - Inhibition of DNA ligase
- Direct damage to constitutive DNA bases
  - Intercalation of DNA
  - Alteration of DNA bases (DNA adduct formation)
  - DNA scission formation
- Alteration in purine/pyrimidine metabolism
- Alteration in post synthesis DNA processing
  - Interference with DNA methylation
  - Interference with DNA folding/unwinding
- Endogenous destruction of DNA
  - Activation of endogenous nucleases (induction of apoptosis)

intestinal mucosa or the bone marrow, rather than the liver. DNA turnover in hepatocytes has traditionally been considered to be low in normal liver. However, hepatocellular DNA may undergo rapid turnover during hepatic regeneration precipitated by hepatocellular necrosis. Consequently, susceptibility to the toxic effects of drugs may be increased in liver diseases characterised by an increased turnover of hepatocytes stimulated by a necroinflammatory process, e.g. chronic viral hepatitis or primary biliary cirrhosis. For the latter disease hepatotoxic drugs, such as methotrexate, are being increasingly used (KAPLAN and KNOX 1991). Furthermore, hepatocellular metabolism of a drug to a toxic metabolite (CHANG et al. 1992; KINSELLA et al. 1994), possibly combined with unpredictable effects of the enterohepatic circulation on clearance of the metabolite, may result in unanticipated toxicity to hepatic DNA.

II. DNA Replication and Repair Pathways

An appreciation of the ways in which drugs and other xenobiotics may interfere with DNA replication and repair is predicated on an understanding of the biochemical pathways involved in DNA synthesis and repair. Thus, it is pertinent to briefly review this process.

The molecular events leading up to the initiation of chromosomal DNA replication are presently unclear. In particular, the cellular signalling required to start replication and the preferred sites at which this occurs have not been precisely defined. In contrast, the biochemical events involved in chromosomal replication of DNA synthesis have been fairly well clarified (CUSICK et al. 1981; DEPAMPHILIS and WASSARMANN 1987) (for review see DEPAMPHILIS and WASSARMANN 1980) (Fig. 1). Central to the understanding of the biochemical complexity of DNA replication is the recognition that the two strands of mammalian DNA are anti-parallel in orientation and that all known DNA polymerases elongate the nascent DNA strands in a 5′ to 3′ direction. Consequently, mammalian DNA replication occurs in a semidiscontinuous

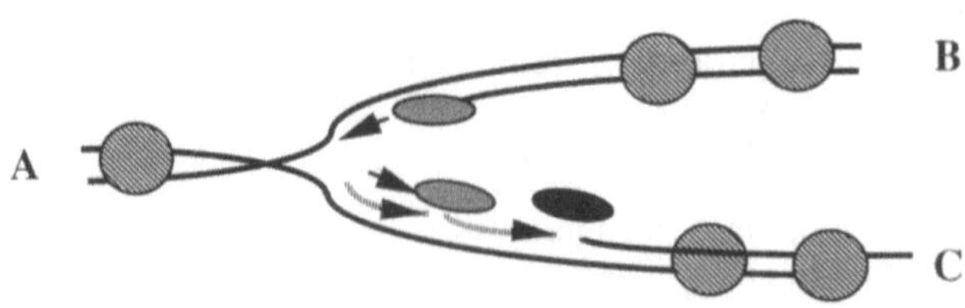

Fig. 1. DNA replication. Schematic representation of chromosomal DNA replication at the junction of the unwinding strands (*A*). DNA from strand B is copied by continuous 5′ to 3′ extension of DNA polymerase (*shaded ellipse*). DNA on strand C is copied discontinuously by repeated extension of Okazaki fragments (40–290 bases in length) (*dashed lines*), which are then joined by DNA ligases (*solid ellipse*). Nucleosomes (*shaded circles*) are found ~180 base pairs apart and function to stabilise the DNA chains. Internucleosomal DNA cleavage, mediated by nucleases activated during apoptosis, results in a characteristic ~180 base pair laddering pattern

manner (CUSICK et al. 1981). In addition to DNA polymerases, it requires the co-ordinated sequential functioning of DNA ligases, necessary concentrations of phosphorylated nucleoside substrates, appropriately presented DNA template and various protein cofactors as well as other poorly characterised factors; the DNA template itself requires properly functioning topoisomerases and gyrases (DEPAMPHILIS and WASSARMANN 1980).

During replication of the antegrade DNA arm, DNA polymerase α proceeds continuously from multiple initiation sites to extend the nascent chains by sequential addition of complementary bases. Replication of the retrograde arm requires synthesis of an RNA primer at the initiation zone, the junction of the unwinding chromosome fork. This process is rapidly followed by $5' \rightarrow 3'$ DNA polymerase α-directed synthesis of Okazaki fragments having lengths of 40–290 (mean 135) base pairs. These fragments are then joined (by the action of DNA ligase 1) to the nascent chain, which extends, discontinuously, in a 3′ to 5′ direction, along the retrograde template. Newly synthesised DNA is then stabilised by addition of nucleosomes, methylation and the action of gyrases which wind DNA into supercoiled chromatin.

The replication, as well as transcription and subsequent translation, of mitochondrial DNA, a covalently closed double-stranded molecule of ~16.5kb, is a distinct process, which is entirely independent of eukaryotic chromosomal replication (WALLACE 1992). Mitochondrial DNA is replicated bidirectionally in an asynchronous fashion exclusively by DNA polymerase γ, which is compartmentalised within mitochondria and possesses distinctive substrate specificities (ZIMMERMANN et al. 1980).

Any one of the steps involved in DNA synthesis may be inhibited by drugs and hence may be the target of drug-induced molecular toxicity.

D. Inhibition of DNA Replication

I. Inhibition of DNA Polymerases

Inhibition of DNA polymerase function as a mechanism of drug toxicity has been recognised as a consequence of the increasing use of antiviral and anti-cancer nucleoside analogues. The function of DNA polymerase α was first characterised using aphidocolin, a tetracycline obtained from *Cephalosorium aphidocolin* (HUBERMAN 1981). This compound inhibits DNA polymerase α (and β) function by competitively inhibiting the interaction between deoxycytosine triphosphate (dCTP) and the binding site of the enzyme [and non-competitively inhibiting deoxynucleotide triphosphates (dNTPs)] (HUBERMAN 1981). Many other nucleoside analogues have subsequently been found to exert inhibitory effects on this group of enzymes (KUFE et al. 1984; CHEN et al. 1991; LIN et al. 1991; KINSELLA et al. 1994). The predictable consequences of this inhibition, namely reduced DNA synthesis, impaired cell repair and inhibition of cell division, have all been extensively demonstrated in haemopoetic cell culture systems using cytosine arabinoside (ara-C) (Woodcock et al. 1979; Kufe et al. 1984) and more recently using other nucleoside analogues.

The exact nature of the toxicity mediated by these nucleoside analogues depends not only on their preferred sites of metabolism (Kinsella et al. 1994), such as phosphorylation (Chen and Cheng 1992), and local concentrations of certain canonical bases (Ayusawa et al. 1979), but also on the relative sensitivity of the different DNA polymerases to inhibition by these agents. With some drugs, such as ara-C, the inhibition is primarily directed against DNA polymerase α (Momparler et al. 1975), which results preferentially in injury to nuclear DNA with resulting chromatid breaks (Benedict et al. 1970) and chromosomal reduplication (Woodcock and Cooper 1981). Others, such as zidovudine (AZT) (Dalakas et al. 1990; Arnaudo et al. 1991) and fialuridine (FIAU), primarily inhibit DNA polymerase γ with consequent reduction in mitochondrial DNA content and function (Chen and Cheng 1992). Two major consequences of such drug-induced changes in mitochondrial metabolism, lactic acidosis (Chattha et al. 1993) and hepatic steatosis (Bach et al. 1992), result from impairment of hepatic mitochondrial metabolism of lactate and inhibition of beta oxidation of fatty acids, respectively. These phenomena have been reported after administration of AZT (Gopinath et al. 1992; Chattha et al. 1993), dideoxycytidine (ddC), dideoxyinosine (ddI) (Bissuel et al. 1994; Yarchoan et al. 1994) and, more recently, FIAU (Macilwain 1993; Brahams 1994). Nucleoside analogue-induced mitochondrial toxicity is associated not only with characteristic histological changes in the liver (microvesicular fat accumulation, ultrastructural changes in mitochondria), but also similar histological changes in skeletal muscle (Dalakas et al. 1990; Arnaudo et al. 1991), suggesting, as would be anticipated, that the mitochondrial lesion is a systemic one. Mitochondrial DNA may be more susceptible to molecular damage than nuclear DNA because (a), in contrast to nuclear DNA, mitochondrial DNA appears to lack any significant repair process, and (b) there is evidence that DNA polymerase γ preferentially incorporates some abnormal bases (Schwartz 1981).

II. Inhibition of DNA Ligase

Mammalian DNA ligase is an enzyme which exists in two forms, DNA ligase I and II. It is responsible for catalysing the formation of phosphodiester bonds between nucleotides (Modrich et al. 1973; Lehman 1974). DNA ligase I (but not DNA ligase II) activity is markedly increased during hepatic regeneration, implying a central role of DNA replication and hence repair in the response to liver damage (Johnson et al. 1987). Ara-C administration has been associated with inhibition of DNA ligase activity that may be clinically relevant (Zittoun et al. 1989), although the putative mechanism by which this occurs, reduced Okazaki fragment utilization by DNA ligase, would suggest that the inhibitory effect may not be due to a direct action of ara-C. Preliminary evidence from this laboratory suggests that FIAU is inhibitory to T4 DNA ligase (albeit derived from *E. coli*) in a dose-dependent fashion (SALLIE et al., unpublished data).

III. Chain Termination

Nucleoside analogues in which the 3′ phosphate moiety is either substituted or missing (notably the dideoxy class of compounds) act as potent chain terminators during DNA synthesis and may significantly slow DNA replication. However, not all nucleoside analogues mediate their effects by inducing chain termination and absolute chain termination, caused by physical inability to extend the nascent DNA chain, is not necessary for a drug to slow significantly or stop DNA replication. Lethal cellular injury as a consequence of functional (or pseudo) chain termination may occur by various mechanisms (Fig. 2).

IV. Inhibition of DNA Repair

DNA repair, like DNA replication, requires the co-ordinated functioning of many enzymes, including DNA polymerases α, β and probably δ, as well as DNA ligases. Accordingly, all of the agents which inhibit DNA replication will also inhibit DNA repair.

Two distinct DNA repair pathways have been characterised. Although currently controversial in mammals, short patch repair, in which ~1–4 damaged nucleosides are replaced or introduced, probably involves different enzymes from long patch repair, in which ~80–100 bases may be replaced or introduced. The exact nature of the damage inflicted on a base probably has little relevance to the type of repair process initiated. As with DNA replication, each of the steps involved in DNA repair is susceptible to inhibition and interference by drugs. Many drugs may induce DNA damage indirectly by inhibition of the basal repair of DNA damaged during normal cell division. In this context, the observation that excision repair takes 4–12 times longer in quiescent than in proliferating cells (JOHNSON et al. 1987) is of interest and may have implications for explaining the susceptibility of some cells with apparently low proliferation rates to cell death caused by DNA-injuring agents (e.g. lymphocytes and possibly hepatocytes).

Drugs may damage or alter the metabolism of constitutive DNA bases in several ways. Intercalcation, or cross-linking of two DNA strands (with hindrance to subsequent replication), is most commonly caused by ultraviolet irradiation, but may also be induced by psoralen derivatives at least in vitro, e.g. methoxypsoralen (ROUSSET et al. 1990). Adduct formation, or alteration of the constitutive bases, may be induced by a variety of drugs and environmental toxins, of which aflatoxin B1 (ESSIGMANN et al. 1982) and vinyl chloride monomer are particularly well recognised. Aflatoxin in association with hepatitis B viral infection appears to be responsible for most of the cases of

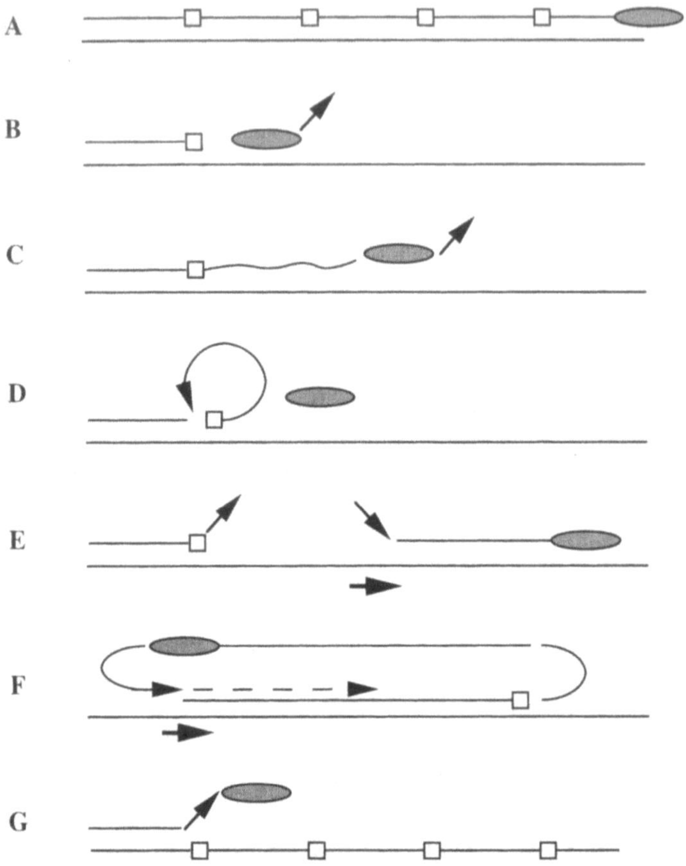

Fig. 2A–G. Nucleoside analogues and DNA damage. Potential mechanisms of nucleoside analogue (NA)-induced DNA damage, modified and extended from KUFE et al. (1984). Note NA (*open square*), DNA polymerase (*shaded ellipse*) and DNA polymerase initiation site (*arrow beneath lower DNA strand*). **A** NA incorporated with canonical bases. **B** Nucleoside chain terminates, causing polymerase to fall off and generate single-stranded DNA segments. **C** NA is non-chain terminating but destabilises the extending nascent chain and eventually causes ploymerase to fall off. **D** Incorporation of NA is associated with rapid excision repair, resulting in slowing or stuttering of the DNA polymerase. **E** NA causes DNA polymerase to fall off, resulting in single-stranded segments once polymerase reinitiates at distal site. **F** NA is associated with reinitiation and chromosomal reduplication at original initiation site, as described by WOODCOCK and COOPER (1981). **G** NA causes destabilisation of DNA polymerase incorporated normally into the opposite-strand template

hepatocellular carcinoma worldwide. Vinyl chloride monomer-associated hepatic angiosarcoma is regarded as a prototypic example of the induction of a hepatic tumour as a consequence of exposure to an industrial toxin (HAGMAR et al. 1990). DNA scission formation (or single-stranded nicking of DNA) is increasingly recognised as an important mechanism by which liver DNA is damaged by free radicals, in particular those associated with the presence of iron. The induction of strand breaks in DNA by bleomycin in association with Fe ions has been well studied (GAJEWSKI et al. 1991; KAUFMANN et al. 1992). This phenomenon suggests a mechanism by which DNA damage and subsequent malignant transformation may occur within the liver in genetic haemochromatosis and other iron-overload states. Interestingly, the proliferative response of peripheral blood lymphocytes obtained from patients with genetic haemochromatosis and other forms of iron overload is not different from that of controls (PIETRANGELO et al. 1988), suggesting that DNA repair in lymphocytes is unimpaired, perhaps due to a lower concentration of iron within these cells. DNA scission formation associated with free radicals does not only occur as a consequence of xenobiotic-metal interactions. For example, in an experimental paradigm 5-aminolevulinic acid, a haem precursor which accumulates in both drug-induced and genetically determined porphyrias, appears to combine with free Fe radicals and induces DNA strand breaks (ONUKI et al. 1994). This finding suggests a mechanism by which DNA damage may occur in porphyria.

V. Alterations in Purine/Pyrimidine Metabolism

Many drugs induce alterations in purine and pyrimidine metabolism which can result in DNA damage either directly or by inhibition of DNA repair. Well-recognised examples include hydroxyurea (JOHNSON et al. 1987) and methotrexate (SAWYER et al. 1989). Less well known are the more subtle effects of insulin (and other mitogens) which can lower purine (but not pyrimidine) pools by up to 50% (JOHNSON et al. 1987). While such reduction in purine pools is associated with a reduced efficiency of repair to previously damaged DNA in experimental paradigms (JOHNSON et al. 1987), the clinical significance of this phenomenon is unknown.

VI. Alterations in DNA Processing Post Synthesis

It is well established that regulation of eukaryotic gene expression is controlled, in part, by site specific methylation, transcriptional activity being inversely proportional to the degree of methylation (RAZIN and RIGGS 1980). Cytosine nucleoside analogues, such as 5-azacytosine and 5-fluorocytosine, when incorporated into DNA are potent inhibitors of DNA-cytosine methyltransferase (DCMT). They cause profound hypomethylation of the cognate DNA even at sites remote from incorporation of the nucleoside, with consequent alterations in both gene expression and differentiation (SANTI et al. 1983). The precise biochemical pathways mediating the reduction of DCMT have been clarified and appear to be conceptually analogous to those involved in the inhibition of thymidine synthase by 5-flurouracil (5-FU) and related compounds (STARZYK et al. 1982). The electrophilic substitution at the 5′ position of the pyrimidine heterocycle, which is thought to be responsible for the inhibition of DCMT, may also contribute to the mitochondrial toxicity induced by both perhexiline (DESCHAMPS et al. 1994) and FIAU.

Anthracyclines, as well as mitoantrone, amsacrine and eteposide (VP 16), which are widely used in clinical oncology, are inhibitors of mammalian topoisomerase II (DNA gyrase), an enzyme which supercoils DNA. These inhibitors, as well as the topoisomerase I inhibitor, camptothecin, have been shown to be potent inducers of DNA strand breaks and apoptosis in a variety of cell-culture systems (BERTRAND et al. 1993). DNA damage caused by the induction of apoptosis (which is mediated by activation of endogenous nucleases) is discussed below.

E. Damage to RNA

Drugs can alter RNA metabolism and function by many mechanisms (Table 4). Of the mechanisms involved in inhibition of RNA synthesis, inhibition of RNA polymerases I, II and III by α-amanatin, the toxin responsible for the hepatotoxicity of *Amanita* mushroom poisoning, has been extensively characterised (COCHET et al. 1974; COCHET and CHAMBON 1974). A-amanatin is a potent inhibitor of RNA polymerase III (which is responsible for synthesis of mRNAs) and to a lesser extent RNA polymerase II (which catalyses the synthesis of tRNA). Both of these enzymes are inactivated by tight 1:1 binding of α-amanatin to subunits of the cognate RNA polymerase. The K_i values of α-amanatin for RNA polymerases II and III are 10^{-8} and 10^{-5}, respectively. Binding of the toxin results in complete inhibition of RNA transcription, and, hence, protein synthesis. In amanatin poisoning, the pathological changes tend to be mild and non-specific (e.g. hepatic nuclear atypia and steatosis), but the

Table 4. Drugs and RNA damage (general theoretical mechanisms by which drugs may induce RNA damage)

Interference with RNA synthesis
Inhibition of RNA polymerases
Inhibition of RNA polymerase I (ribosomal RNA)
Inhibition of RNA polymerase II (messenger RNA)
Inhibition of RNA polymerase III (transfer RNA)
Interference with RNA polymerase promoters
Premature termination of RNA synthesis
Abnormal RNA slicing
Inhibition of ribosomal formation
Alteration in purine/pyrimidine metabolism
Alteration in post synthesis RNA processing
Inhibition of RNA cap synthesis
Intercalation of RNA
RNA adduct formation
Miscellaneous mechanisms
Enhanced RNA degradation
Induction of endogenous RNAses

biochemical changes can induce profound clinical effects, such as severe coagulopathy (due to inhibition of synthesis of liver-produced clotting factors) and hepatic encephalopathy.

The best-characterised example of direct drug-induced RNA damage is that produced by 5-FU. 5-FU is used as a single agent in the management of colorectal cancer and is frequently given by infusion into the hepatic artery when hepatic metastases are present. 5-FU and its metabolites are readily incorporated into newly synthesised RNA (DOLNICK and PINK 1983, 1985) and result in premature termination of RNA molecules (SAVANT and CLEVELAND 1992), abnormal RNA splicing (DOONG and DILNICK 1988) and, predictably, altered degradation of RNAs. These phenomena would be associated with modified base composition and the synthesis of defective proteins.

The rate at which RNA molecules are degraded, and hence the level of RNA expression, is highly variable between RNA species and is dependent upon the presence of specific motifs within the molecule, particularly within the 5′ and 3′ untranslated regions (SAVANT and CLEVELAND 1992). For example, the presence of AU-rich motifs within the 3′ untranslated region may be destabilising (SACHS 1993) and lead to enhanced degradation. Clearly, substitution of 5-FU for native bases within these regions could markedly alter RNA kinetics and hence gene expression. Other structural properties, such as the length of the poly-A tail and the presence of a methylated 5′ cap, are also functionally important (SACHS 1993). A potential mechanism of action of ribavirin is the induction of alterations in RNA cap formation, which could alter the stability of cellular RNAs (SACHS 1993). This property of ribavirin may explain the reduction in serum aminotransferase levels which commonly occurs when this drug is administered to patients with chronic hepatitis C (REICHARD et al. 1993).

F. Interference with Protein Synthesis

Clearly, damage to any of the molecular pathways "upstream" of protein translation from hepatic RNA may interfere with protein synthesis and may consequently cause hepatocellular injury or even necrosis. A-amanatin is considered the prototype of a xenobiotic which specifically inhibits hepatic protein synthesis. The specificity of the action of this hepatotoxin has led ZIMMERMANN to classify it as an "indirect hepatotoxicant". Currently, it appears to be the sole known example of an agent that causes liver injury by interferene with a single specific metabolic pathway (KAHL 1991).

In general, some of the major clinical manifestations of interference with hepatocellular synthesis of proteins encoded by nuclear DNA result from a reduction in concentrations of liver-produced plasma proteins, such as progressive coagulopathy due to low levels of clotting factors. In contrast, interference with mitochondrial protein synthesis leads to an entirely different clinical syndrome in which lactic acidosis is one of the characteristic biochemical features. Typically, in this syndrome many cytosolic synthetic and excretory functions tend to be preserved without an increase in serum bilirubin occurring until reduced energy production by mitochondria leads to hepatocellular failure. This type of clinical picture occurs, for example, in classical post-infectious Reye's syndrome.

G. Apoptosis

The term "apoptosis" ("to fall away") (KERR et al. 1972) is often used interchangeably with programmed cell death. It would probably be more correct to view apoptosis as one of the pathways (albeit possibly the most common) by which programmed cell death is effected. Differentiation of apoptosis from necrosis is critically important (Table 5).

From an evolutionary standpoint, apoptosis is likely to represent the final outcome of highly conserved biochemical pathways which form a defence system that antedates both humeral and cell-mediated immunity. Apoptosis is a mechanism by which multicellular organisms (ranging from nematode worms to mammals) isolate and destroy infected, damaged, mutant or otherwise superfluous cells whose continued viability might otherwise jeopardise the continuing viability of the whole organism (KERR et al. 1972; VAUX et al. 1994). The pathological and biochemical features of apoptosis have been reviewed extensively by KERR et al. (KERR 1971; KERR et al. 1972) and VAUX et al. have recently provided a concise synopsis of the molecular mechanisms

Table 5. Apoptosis versus necrosis (ultrastructural, histological and biochemical features that distinguish apoptosis from necrosis)

Feature	Apoptosis	Necrosis
Light microscopy	Scattered individual cells Condensed chromatin Inflammation absent	Contiguous cells Eosinophilic ghosting Exudative inflammation
Ultrastructural changes		
Chromatin	Condensed granular aggregates Confluent over nucleus or localised to crescentic caps	Marginates Aggregates loosely, eventually disappears
Nucleolus	Disperses	Evident as compact body
Nuclear membrane	Progressive convolution	Retains pore structure
Cytoplasm	Condensation of cytosol Endoplasmic reticulum may dilate Mitochondria structurally intact Organelles compacted together	Swelling of all compartments Mitochondrial matrix densities characteristic
Pathogenesis	Energy requiring Requires endonucleased	Energy independent Not enzyme mediated

thought to be operative during the early induction phase of the process (VAUX et al. 1994).

The characteristic pathological features of apoptosis in the liver (acidophilic or Councilman bodies) have been recognised in the context of viral hepatitis (especially yellow fever) for decades. However, hepatocellular apoptosis has only received significant attention comparatively recently

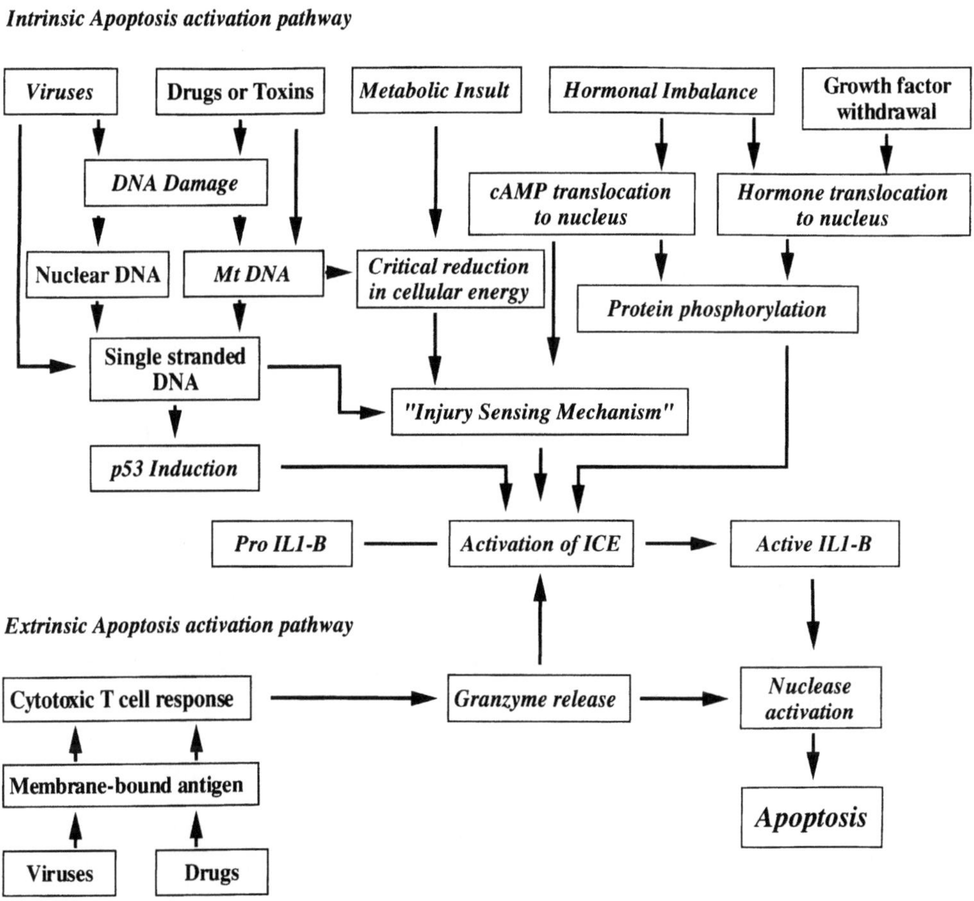

Fig. 3. Mechanisms of apoptosis. Schematic representation of the mechanisms by which apoptosis is thought to be induced, modified from concepts presented by KERR et al. (1972) and VAUX et al. (1994). While many of the pathways are established (e.g. the activation of IL 1-converting enzyme by p53 induction), many are still hypothetical (e.g. "critical reduction in cellular energy"). *Arrows* indicate the general direction or association of cause and effect and are not to be considered exclusive. For example, it is conceivable that the hypothesised, but as yet unproved, "injury-sensing mechanism" may itself activate nucleases and trigger DNA destruction. Central to induction of apoptosis by many drugs is DNA damage, resulting in intracellular single-stranded DNA and induction of p53. p53 in turn activates the interleukin 1B (*IL 1-B*)-converting enzyme (*ICE*), which catalyses the formation of active IL 1-B. Other mechanisms, such as reduction in cellular energy levels or altered protein phosphorylation, may be operative in other forms of drug hepatotoxicity

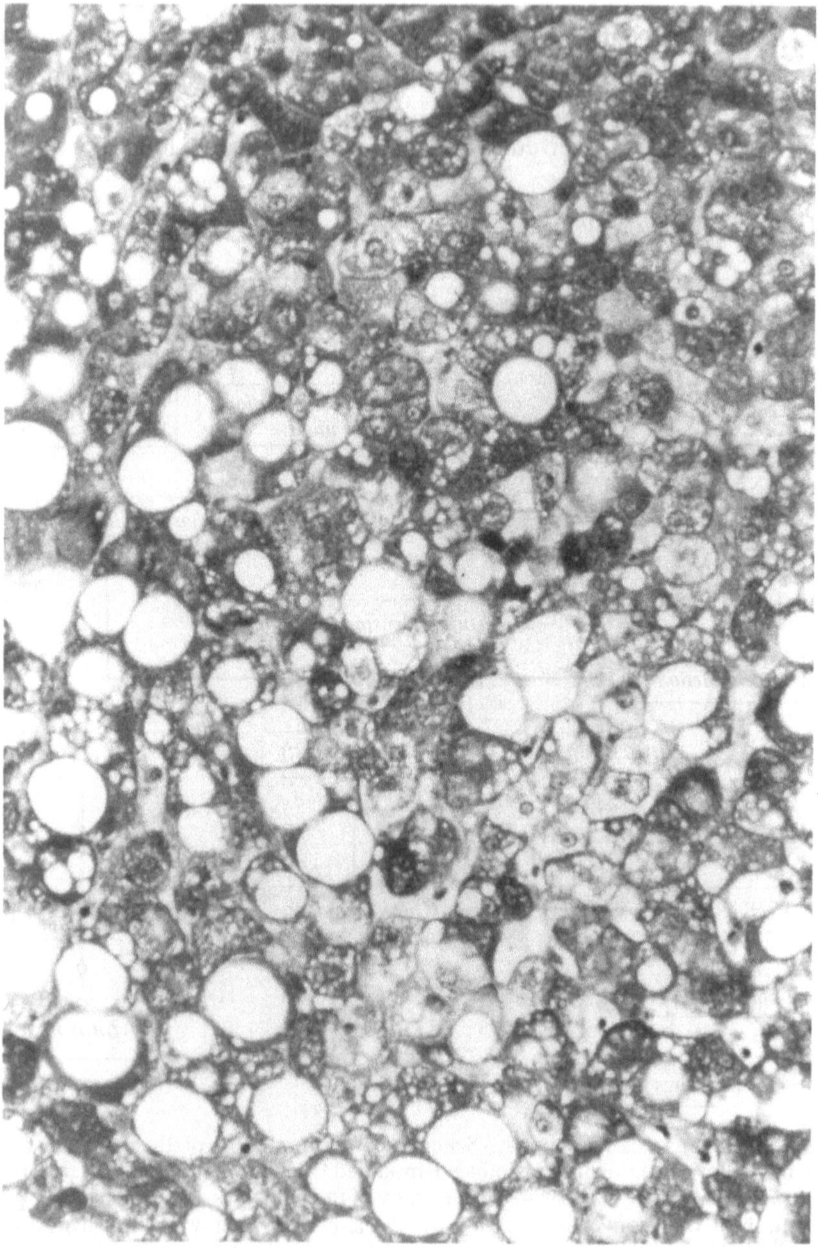

Fig. 4. Nucleoside analogues and steatohepatitis. Liver section from a patient with AZT-induced hepatotoxicity, showing marked macro- and microvesicular fatty infiltration. H&E, ×350

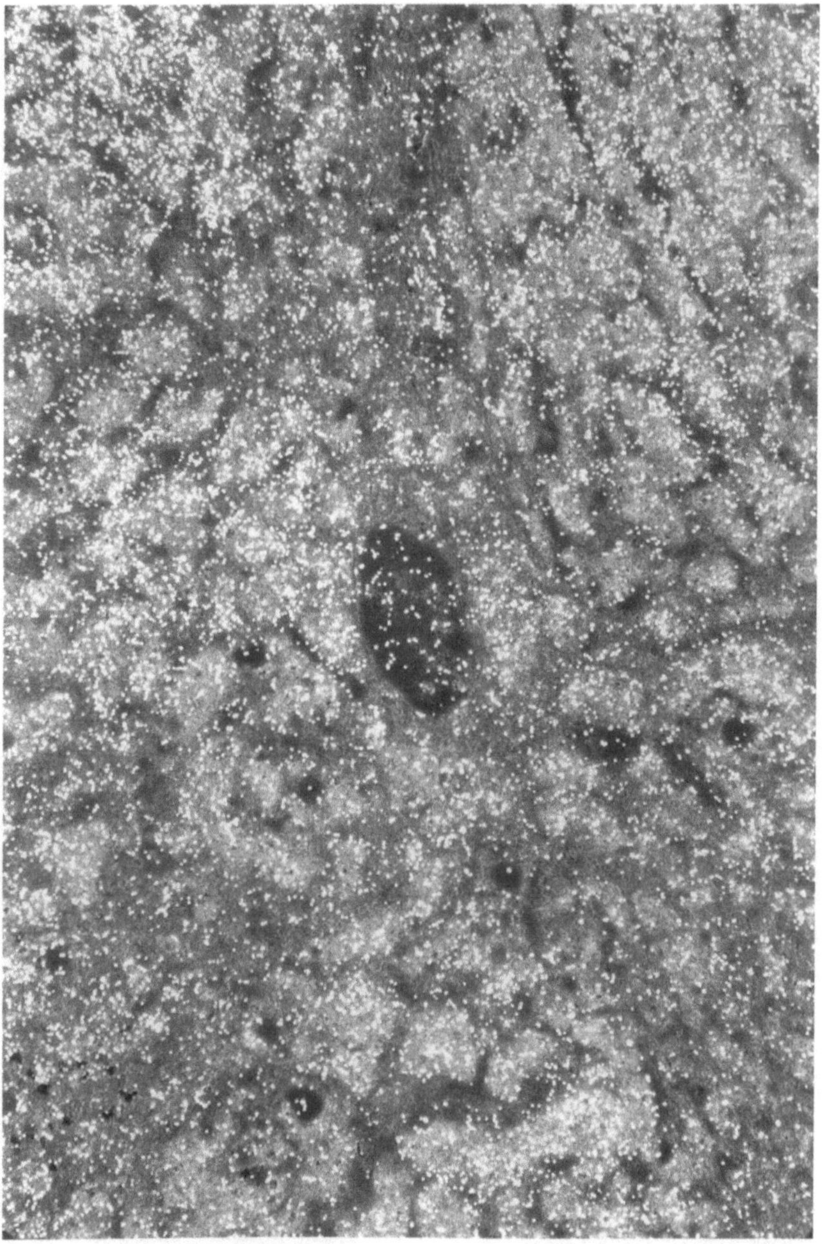

A

Fig. 5A,B. Nucleoside analogues and mitochondrial DNA. **A** In situ hybridisation for mitochondrial DNA in a patient with untreated chronic hepatitis B, centred on a hepatic venule. Silver grains represent positive signal. Note fairly even and diffuse signal throughout lobule. Darkfield illumination, ×350. **B** In situ hybridisation for mitochondrial DNA in a liver section obtained from a patient with nucleoside analogue (FIAU)-induced hepatic mitochondrial DNA damage, centred on a portal tract. Note patchy loss of mitochondrial signal between areas of bile duct proliferation. Darkfield illumination, ×350

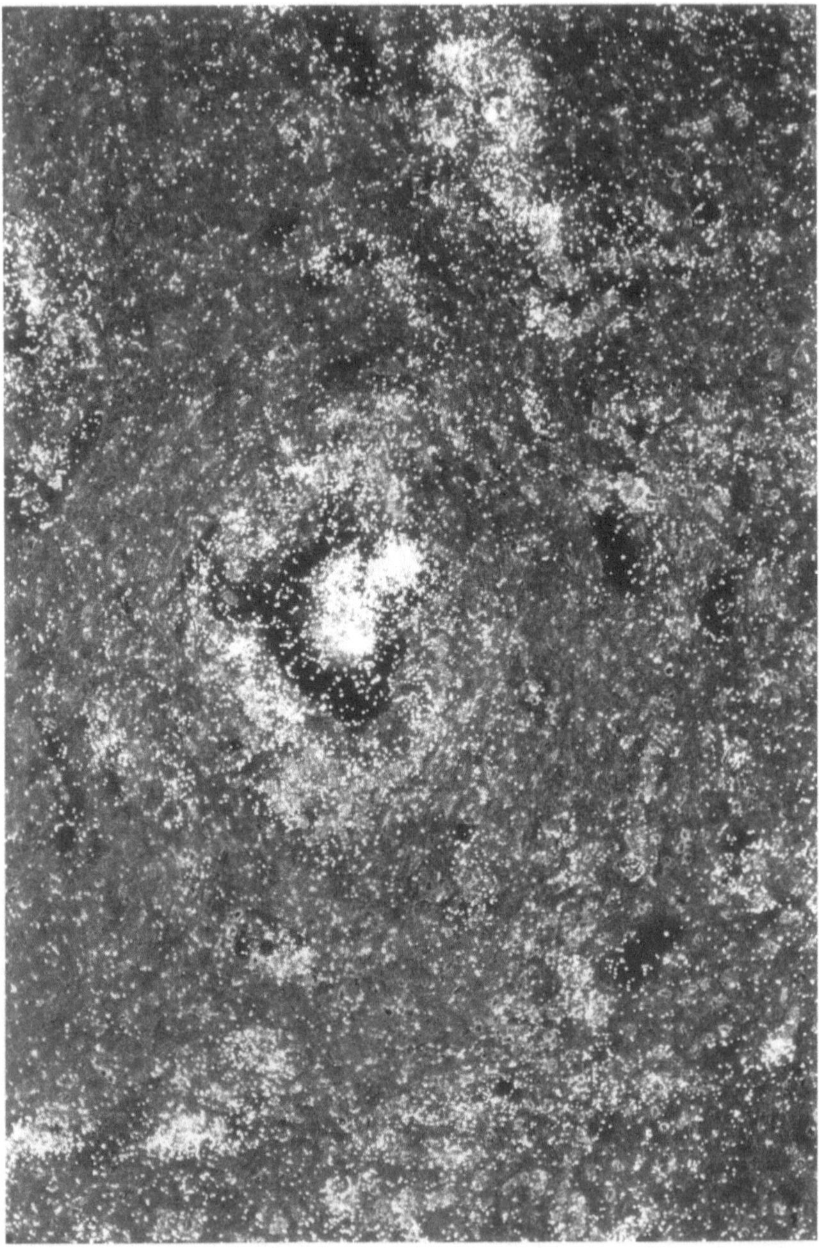

Fig. 5B

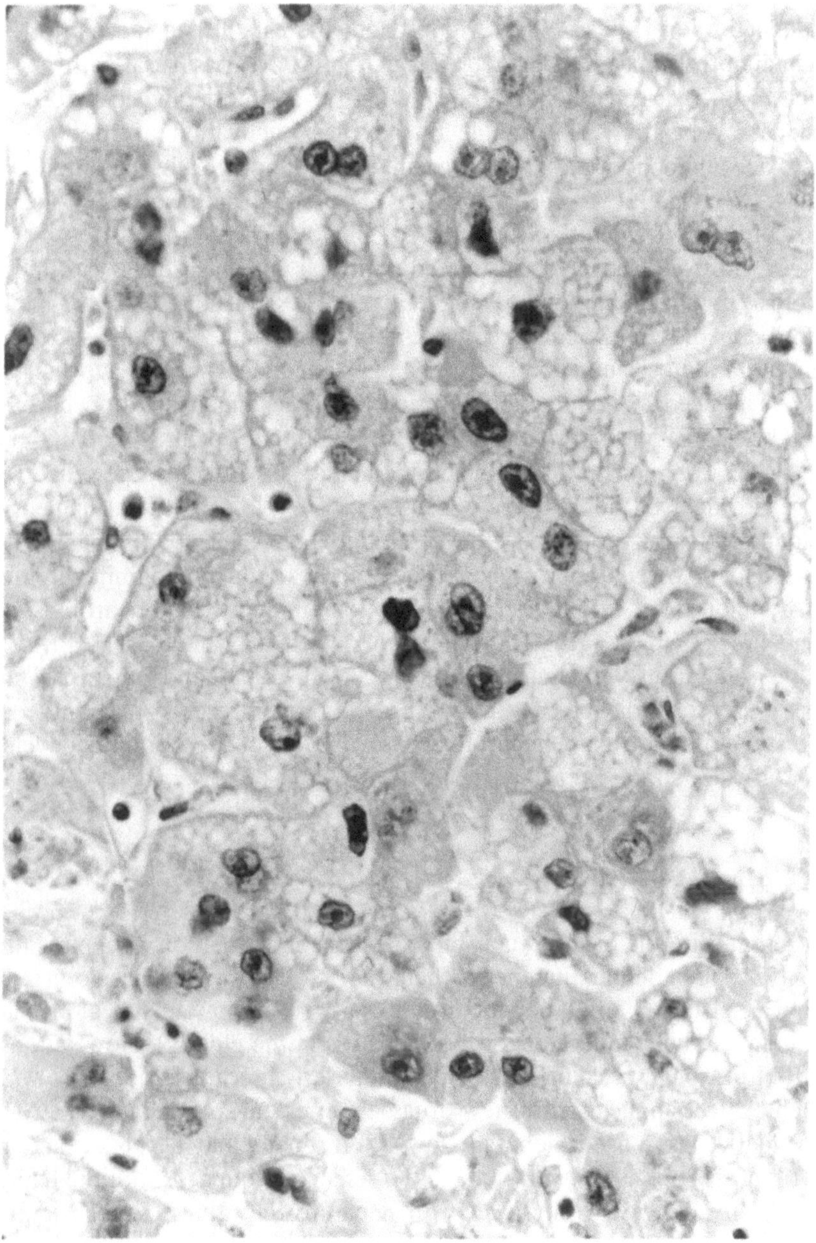

Fig. 6. Nucleoside analogues and hepatic apoptosis. In situ terminal transferase apoptosis in a liver section from a patient with FIAU-induced hepatotoxicity. Positive, dark-stained nuclei indicate the presence of intranuclear DNA fragmentation and early apoptosis. Note also presence of macro- and microvesicular fat accumulation. H&E, ×350

(FAUSTO 1993; OBERHAMMER et al. 1992, 1993), and the prevalence and relative importance of apoptosis as a mechanism of drug-induced liver injury remain to be defined. Nevertheless, it is evident from the established mechanisms by which apoptosis may be triggered (Fig. 3) that there are several pathways by which drug toxicity could theoretically induce apoptosis and lead to death of hepatocytes. It is also notable that extrinsic activation of apoptosis by cytotoxic T lymphocytes, as may occur in immunologically mediated drug toxicity (FARRELL et al. 1985), provides a potential pathway for molecular injury during idiosyncratic drug-induced hepatotoxicity.

The most extensively investigated pathways by which drugs can induce apoptosis involve induction of DNA damage (MANOME et al. 1993). While the majority of studies have focused on the ability of certain antineoplastic agents to induce apoptosis in haemopoetic cell lines, the mechanism(s) by which cell injury is induced – e.g. induction of strand breaks, chain termination, chromosomal breaks (WOODCOCK and COOPER 1981; WOODCOCK et al. 1979; KUFE et al. 1984) – are common to many nucleoside analogues. Recent experience with the severe delayed hepatotoxicity caused by FIAU, an antiviral nucleoside analogue with structural similarities to ara-C (DREW et al. 1991), suggests that the toxicity involved apoptosis consequent upon a reduction of mitochondrial DNA, inhibition of oxidative phosphorylation and induction of chromosomal strand breaks (Figs. 4–6). The type of hepatotoxicity induced by FIAU is unique in the history of clinical trials (MACILWAIN 1993), and emphasises that hepatic apoptosis may be caused by drugs. Moreover, recently published data suggest that methotrexate hepatotoxicity may be associated with the development of DNA strand breaks (SANO et al. 1991).

H. Future Developments

At present, the role of molecular biology in the investigation of hepatic drug toxicity is one of delineating the mechanisms of toxicity once it has occurred in a clinical setting. Overall, hepatic drug toxicity is a common clinical problem (and may be the commonest form of hepatitis in the elderly). However, as a result of thorough preclinical testing and phase I clinical trials prior to widespread clinical application of new drugs, the incidence of hepatotoxicity for individual drugs in use is generally low and for many may be ~1–2 reactions/ 10^4–10^5 prescriptions (SALLIE et al. 1991). As a consequence, both the experience of any individual physician with hepatotoxicity due to specific drugs and opportunities to elucidate the mechanisms of any such toxicity will be limited. Accordingly, the characterisation of the molecular mechanisms of hepatotoxicity may be most effectively undertaken by analysing material from clinically and pathologically well characterised cases at centralised or international referral centres.

As discussed above, hepatic drug reactions that do arise clinically might have been preventable had suitable animal models been available to assess the toxicity profiles of the responsible drugs. An exciting possibility, as yet unexplored, is the creation of "humanized" animal systems by the use of transgenic and gene knockout technologies. Using these approaches, animal models which can more accurately predict human drug reactions may be generated. An illustrative analogy may be the recently developed transgenic mouse which expresses the receptor for *Varicella zoster*. Use of this animal model has allowed investigation of the immunopathogenesis of human chicken pox in a manner that would not be possible in patients. It seems entirely conceivable that the same approach could be used to produce mice (or other small animals) transgenic for the recently cloned hepatitis B receptor. Such a model may facilitate more rapid and appropriate screening of antiviral compounds for treatment of hepatitis B than is currently possible using in vitro systems. It is also conceivable that animals "humanized" by being made transgenic for human immunological response or effector genes, such as those responsible for HLA or complement molecules, may provide appropriate models for studying the pathogenesis of idiosyncratic drug reactions.

While antisense technology offers potentially exciting methods of treating viral infections and neoplastic disease in the future, it has yet to be used in clinical practice. Present limitations of this approach relate to the delivery of adequate amounts of antisense molecules to target organs and to the specificity with which inhibition of the appropriate metabolic pathway occurs. Despite the theoretical specificity of antisense targeting, it is apparent from data obtained using in vitro systems that clinical toxicity resulting from non-selective inhibition of basal replicative machinery, RNA transcription or protein synthesis is to be anticipated.

It is also to be expected that more widespread application of presently available techniques of molecular biology, such as in situ hybridisation and in situ DNA labelling for detection of apoptosis, will result in a fuller understanding of the mechanisms by which drugs induce hepatotoxicity. Of particular interest is the potential use of one type of polymerase chain reaction technology, differential display (LIANG et al. 1992), to permit isolation of cDNA molecules (and hence RNA species important in the mediation of hepatotoxicity), which are either suppressed or induced by specific drugs.

I. Summary and Conclusions

While the "molecular biology" of only a few hepatic drug reactions has been completely delineated, it is evident that the discipline of molecular biology has a vast armamentarium of powerful tools that will permit further investigation, and hopefully clarification, of the mechanisms of many hepatic drug reactions which are presently incompletely understood.

The increasing use of powerful antiviral nucleoside analogues and related agents, spurred on by the threat of immunodeficiency viruses as well as the need for effective therapies for chronic viral diseases such as chronic hepatitis

B, has resulted in the recognition of two new forms of hepatic drug toxicity. These are apoptosis and toxicity caused by damage to mitochondrial DNA. As it is likely that antiviral and antineoplastic nucleoside analogues will be increasingly used in the future, increased exposure of patients to the types of toxicity induced by drugs of this class is to be anticipated. Understanding and, hopefully, preventing such toxicity in the future will be facilitated by careful investigation of the molecular mechanisms by which hepatic drug reactions are mediated.

References

Arnaudo E, Dalakas M, Shanske S et al. (1991) Depletion of muscle mitochondrial DNA in AIDS patients with zidovudine-induced myopathy. Lancet 337:508–510

Ayusawa D, Iwata K, Kozu T, Ikegami S, Seno T (1979) Increase in dATP pool in aphidicolin-resistant mutants of mouse FM3A cells. Biochem Biophys Res Commun 91:946–954

Bach N, Thiese ND, Schaffner F (1992) Hepatic histopathology in the acquired immunodeficiency syndrome. Semin Liver Dis 12:205–212

Benedict WF, Harris N, Karon M (1970) Kinetrics of 1-beta-D-arabinofuranosylcytosine-induced chromosomal breaks. Cancer Res 30:2477–2483

Bertrand R, Solary E, Jenkins J, Pommier Y (1993) Apoptosis and its modulation in human promyelocytic HL-60 cells treated with DNA topoisomerase I and II inhibitors. Exp Cell Res 207:388–397

Bissuel F, Bruneel F, Habersetzer F et al. (1994) Fulminant hepatitis with severe lactate acidosis in HIV-infected patients on didanosine therapy. J Intern Med 235:367–371

Brahams D (1994) Deaths in US fialuridine trial. Lancet 343:1494–1495

Chang CN, Doong SL, Cheng YC (1992) Conversion of 5-iodo-2-pyrimidinone-2′-deoxyribose to 5-iodo-deoxyuridine by aldehyde oxidase. Implications in hepatotropic drug design. Biochem Pharmacol 43:2269–2273

Chattha G, Arieff AI, Cummings C, Tierney LJ (1993) Lactic acidosis complicating the acquired immunodeficiency syndrome. Ann Intern Med 118:37–39

Chen CH, Cheng YC (1992) The role of cytoplasmic deoxycytidine kinase in the mitochondrial effects of the anti-human immunodeficiency virus compound, 2′,3′-dideoxycytidine. J Biol Chem 267:2856–2859

Chen CH, Vasquez-Padua M, Cheng YC (1991) Effect of anti-human immunodeficiency virus nucleoside analogs on mitochondrial DNA and its implication for delayed toxicity. Mol Pharmacol 39:625–628

Cochet MM, Chambon P (1974) Animal DNA-dependent RNA polymerases. 11. Mechanism of the inhibition of RNA polymerases B by amatoxins. Biochim Biophys Acta 353:160–184

Cochet MM, Nuret P, Courvalin JC, Chambon P (1974) Animal DNA-dependent RNA polymerases. 12. Determination of the cellular number of RNA polymerase B molecules. Biochim Biophys Acta 353:185–192

Cusick ME, Herman TM, DePamphilis ML, Wassarman PM (1981) Structure of chromatin at deoxyribonucleic acid replication forks: prenucleosomal deoxyribonucleic acid is rapidly excised from replicating simian virus 40 chromosomes by micrococcal nuclease. Biochemistry 20:6648–6658

Dalakas MC, Illa I, Pezeshkpour GH et al. (1990) Mitochondrial myopathy caused by long-term zidovudine therapy. N Engl J Med 322:1098–1105

DePamphilis ML, Wassarman PM (1980) Replication of eukaryotic chromosomes: a close-up of the replication fork. Annu Rev Biochem 49:627–666

DePamphilis ML, Wassarman PM (1987) Regulation of chromosomal replication and transcription during early mammalian development. Bioessays 7:265–271

Deschamps D, DeBeco V, Fisch C et al. (1994) Inhibition by perhexiline of oxidative phosphorylation and the beta-oxidation of fatty acids: possible role in pseudoalcoholic liver lesions. Hepatology 19:948–961

Dolnick BJ, Pink JJ (1983) 5-Fluorouracil modulation of dihydrofolate reductase RNA levels in methotrexate-resistant KB cells. J Biol Chem 258:13299–13306

Dolnick BJ, Pink JJ (1985) Effects of 5-fluorouracil on dihydrofolate reductase and dihydrofolate reductase mRNA from methotrexate-resistant KB cells. J Biol Chem 260:3006–3014

Doong SL, Dolnick BJ (1988) 5-Fluorouracil substitution alters pre-mRNA splicing in vitro. J Biol Chem 263:4467–4473

Drew WL, Miner R, King D (1991) Antiviral activity of FIAU (1-[2′deoxy-2′-fluoro-1-beta-D-arabinofuranosyl]-5-iodo-uridine) on strains of cytomegalovirus sensitive and resistant to ganciclovir. J Infect Dis 163:1388–1389

Essigmann JM, Croy RG, Bennett RA, Wogan GN (1982) Metabolic activation of aflatoxin B1: patterns of DNA adduct formation, removal, and excretion in relation to carcinogenesis. Drug Metab Rev 13:581–602

Farrell G, Prendergast D, Murray M (1985) Halothane hepatitis. Detection of a constitutional susceptibility factor. N Engl J Med 313:1310–1314

Fausto N (1993) Hepatocyte apotosis: is transforming growth factor-B1 the kiss of death? Hepatology 18:1536–1537

Frost L, Prendergast D, Farrell G (1989) Halothane hepatitis: damage to peripheral blood mononuclear cells produced by electrophilic drug metabolites is Ca(2+)-dependent. Gastroenterol Hepatol 4:1–9

Gajewski E, Aruoma OI, Dizdaroglu M, Halliwell B (1991) Bleomycin-dependent damage to the bases in DNA is a minor side reaction. Biochemistry 30:2444–2448

Gopinath R, Hutcheon M, Cheema DS, Halperin M (1992) Chronic lactic acidosis in a patient with acquired immunodeficiency syndrome and mitochondrial myopathy: biochemical studies. J Am Soc Nephrol 3:1212–1219

Hagmar L, Akesson B, Nielsen et al. (1990) Mortality and cancer morbidity in workers exposed to low levels of vinyl chloride monomer at a polyvinyl chloride processing plant. Am J Ind Med 17:553–565

Huberman JA (1981) New views of the biochemistry of eukaryotic DNA replication revealed by aphidicolin, an unusual inhibitor of DNA polymerase alpha. Cell 23:647–648

Johnson RT, Collins AR, Squires S et al. (1987) DNA repair under stress. J Cell Sci [Suppl 6]:263–288

Kahl R (ed) (1991) Toxic liver injury. In: McIntyre N, Benhamou J-P, Bircher J, Rizzetto M, Rodes J (eds) Oxford textbook of clinical hepatology. Oxford University Press, Oxford, pp 905–906

Kaplan MM, Knox TA (1991) Treatment of primary biliary cirrhosis with low-dose weekly methotrexate. Gastroenterology 101:1332–1338

Kaufmann WK, Zhang Y, Kaufman DG (1992) Inhibition by bleomycin of hepatocellular foci in the rat. Carcinogenesis 13:703–707

Kerr JF (1971) Shrinkage necrosis: a distinct mode of cellular death. J Pathol 105: 13–20

Kerr JF, Wyllie AH, Currie AR (1972) Apoptosis: a basic biological phenomenon with wide-ranging implications in tissue kinetics. Br J Cancer 26:239–257

Kinsella TJ, Kunugi KA, Vielhuber KA et al. (1994) An in vitro comparison of oral 5-iodo-2′-deoxyuridine and 5-iodo-2-pyrimidinone-2′-deoxyribose toxicity, pharmacokinetics, and DNA incorporation in athymic mouse tissues and the human colon cancer xenograft, HCT-116. Cancer Res 54:2695–2700

Kufe DW, Munroe D, Herrick D et al. (1984) Effects of 1-beta-D-arabinofuranosylcytosine incorporation on eukaryotic DNA template function. Mol Pharmacol 26:128–134

Lehman IR (1974) DNA ligase: structure, metabolism, and function. Science 186: 790–797

Liang P, Averboukh L, Keyomarsi K, Sager R, Pardee AB (1992) Differential display and cloning of messenger RNAs from human breast cancer versus mammary epithelial cells. Cancer Res 52:6966–6968

Lin TS, Luo MZ, Liu MC et al. (1991) Synthesis and anticancer and antiviral activities of various 2′- and 3′-methylidene-substituted nucleoside analogues and crystal structure of 2′-deoxy-2′-methylidenecytidine hydrochloride. J Med Chem 34:2607–2615

Macilwain C (1993) NIH, FDA seek lessons from hepatitis B drug trial deaths. Nature 364:275

Manome Y, Weichselbaum RR, Kufe DW, Fine HA (1993) Effect of Bcl-2 on ionizing radiation and 1-beta-D-arabinofuranosylcytosine-induced internucleosomal DNA fragmentation and cell survival in human myeloid leukemia cells. Oncol Res 5:139–144

Modrich P, Anraku Y, Lehman IR (1973) Deoxyribonucleic acid ligase. Isolation and physical characterization of the homogeneous enzyme from Escherichia coli. J Biol Chem 248:7495–7501

Momparler RL, Goodman J, Karon M (1975) In vitro biochemical and cytotoxicity studies with 1-beta-D-arabinofuranosylcytosine and 5-azacytidine in combination. Cancer Res 35:2853–2857

Oberhammer FA, Pavelka M, Sharma S et al. (1992) Induction of apoptosis in cultured hepatocytes and in regressing liver by transforming growth factor beta 1. Proc Natl Acad Sci USA 89:5408–5412

Oberhammer F, Bursch W, Tiefenbacher R et al. (1993) Apoptosis is induced by transforming growth factor-beta 1 and 5 hours in regressing liver without significant fragmentation of the DNA. Hepatology 18:1238–1246

Onuki J, Medeiros MH, Bechara EJ, Di MP (1994) 5-Aminolevulinic acid induces single-strand breaks in plasmid pBR322 DNA in the presence of Fe^{2+} ions. Biochim Biophys Acta 1225:259–263

Pietrangelo A, Cossarizza A, Monti D, Ventura E, Franceschi C (1988) DNA repair in lymphocytes from humans and rats with chronic iron overload. Biochem Biophys Res Commun 154:698–704

Pohl LR (1990) Drug-induced allergic hepatitis. Semin Liver Dis 10:305–315

Razin A, Riggs AD (1980) DNA methylation and gene function. Science 210:604–610

Reichard O, Yun ZB, Sonnerborg A, Weiland O (1993) Hepatitis C viral RNA titers in serum prior to, during, and after oral treatment with ribavirin for chronic hepatitis C. J Med Virol 41:99–102

Rousset S, Nocentini S, Revet B, Moustacchi E (1990) Molecular analysis by electron microscopy of the removal of psoralen-photoinduced DNA cross-links in normal and Fanconi's anemia fibroblasts. Cancer Res 50:2443–2448

Sachs AB (1993) Messenger RNA degradation in eukaryotes. Cell 74:413–421

Sallie RW, McKenzie T, Reed WD, Quinlan MF, Shilkin KB (1991) Diclofenac hepatitis. Aust N Z J Med 21:251–255

Sano H, Kubota M, Kasai Y et al. (1991) Increased methotrexate-induced DNA strand breaks and cytotoxicity following mutational loss of thymidine kinase. Int J Cancer 48:92–95

Santi DV, Garrett CE, Barr PJ (1983) On the mechanism of inhibition of DNA-cytosine methyltransferases by cytosine analogs. Cell 33:9–10

Savant BS, Cleveland DW (1992) Evidence for instability of mRNAs containing AUUUA motifs mediated through translation-dependent assembly of a > 20S degradation complex. Genes Dev 6:1927–1939

Sawyer RC, Stolfi RL, Martin DS, Balis ME (1989) Inhibition by methotrexate of the stable incorporation of 5-fluorouracil into murine bone marrow DNA. Biochem Pharmacol 38:2305–2311

Schwartz SA (1981) Preferential utilization of bromodeoxyuridine and iododeoxyuridine triphosphates by DNA polymerase gamma in vitro. Biosci Rep 1:387–398

Starzyk RM, Koontz SW, Schimmel P (1982) A covalent adduct between the uracil ring and the active site of an aminoacyl tRNA synthetase. Nature 298:136–140

Vaux DL, Haecker G, Strasser A (1994) An evolutionary perspective on apoptosis. Cell 76:777–779

Wallace DC (1992) Diseases of the mitochondrial DNA. Annu Rev Biochem 61:1175–1212

Woodcock DM, Cooper IA (1981) Evidence for double replication of chromosomal DNA segments as a general consequence of DNA replication inhibition. Cancer Res 41:2483–2490

Woodcock DM, Fox RM, Cooper IA (1979) Evidence for a new mechanism of cytotoxicity of 1-beta-D-arabinofuranosylcytosine. Cancer Res 39:1418–1424

Yarchoan R, Lietzau JA, Nguyen BY et al. (1994) A randomized pilot study of alternating or simultaneous zidovudine and didanosine therapy in patients with symptomatic human immunodeficiency virus infection. J Infect Dis 169:9–17

Zimmermann W, Chen SM, Bolden A, Weissbach A (1980) Mitochondrial DNA replication does not involve DNA polymerase alpha. J Biol Chem 255:11847–11852

Zittoun J, Marquet J, David JC, Maniey D, Zittoun R (1989) A study of the mechanisms of cytotoxicity of Ara-C on three human leukemic cell lines. Cancer Chemother Pharmacol 24:251–255

CHAPTER 5

In Vitro Models of Liver Toxicity

R.G. THURMAN, P.E. GANEY, S.A. BELINSKY, J.G. CONWAY, and M.Z. BADR

A. Introduction

I. Metabolism of Foreign Compounds Can Cause Zone-Specific Hepatotoxicity

Metabolism of foreign compounds plays an important role in the susceptibility of the liver to chemical injury (MITCHELL and JALLOW 1973). In the liver, metabolic transformation of xenobiotics usually results in detoxification; however, some nontoxic agents can be converted into toxic products. Many hepatotoxicants and hepatocarcinogens generate toxic (RECKNAGEL and GLENDE 1973; MITCHELL et al. 1973) or carcinogenic (MILLER 1970) metabolites. For instance, biotransformation of carbon tetrachloride (RECKNAGEL and GLENDE 1973), dimethylnitrosamine (MAGEE 1966), and allyl alcohol (REES and TARLOW 1967) precedes their hepatotoxicity.

Periportal and pericentral areas of the liver lobule differ in their sensitivity to many hepatotoxicants. For example, allyl compounds injure periportal regions whereas carbon tetrachloride damages pericentral areas of the liver lobule. The hepatic distribution of enzymes involved in detoxification or activation to more toxic metabolites may be a factor in the susceptibility of different regions of the liver lobule to chemically induced injury. Most enzymes of the mixed-function oxidase system, which is the major oxidative pathway for biotransformation of drugs, chemicals, and environmental pollutants, are distributed unevenly across the liver lobule. Some cytochrome P-450 isoenzymes (GOODING et al. 1978; BARON et al. 1978), in addition to the NADPH-generating enzymes glucose-6-phosphate dehydrogenase (TEUTSCH 1981), malic enzyme (TEUTSCH and REIDER 1979), and isocitrate dehydrogenase (TEUTSCH 1981), are concentrated in pericentral regions. On the other hand, glutathione (SMITH et al. 1979) and glutathione peroxidase (YOSHIMURA et al. 1977) are slightly higher in periportal areas. Other factors influencing zone-specific toxicity of some chemicals include substrate delivery and the availability of necessary cofactors. Therefore, a variety of metabolic processes involved in mechanisms of toxicity must be considered in studies of the zone-specific nature of hepatotoxicants. In vitro models such as the isolated perfused liver offer unique advantages for studying events which occur in periportal and pericentral regions of the liver lobule.

II. Advantages and Disadvantages of Whole Cell Models

Isolated hepatocytes, hepatocytes in culture, liver slices, and perfused livers have been used in studies of drug metabolism and toxicology in whole cells. Each model has advantages and disadvantages, as shown in Table 1. For example, isolated hepatocytes are convenient to use and considerable data can be generated from a single animal. Major problems with isolated hepatocytes, particularly those maintained as primary cultures, are that some enzyme activities are diminished, the lobular architecture is lost, and nonparenchymal cells are not present. Although liver slices maintain a lobular architecture, they do not make bile, and leakage of potassium is a disadvantage. In vivo studies are the most physiological, but interpretation of results is often problematic since uncontrolled changes in hormonal, circulatory, and neuronal states are complicating factors. In addition, studies in vivo usually require larger numbers of animals than in vitro models mentioned above.

One in vitro model, the isolated perfused liver, affords the unique advantage that studies can be performed under carefully controlled conditions resembling those in vivo. In addition, with this model several biochemical processes can be monitored continuously. Another important advantage is that hepatic architecture is maintained, and therefore metabolism and toxicity can be studied in distinct regions of the liver lobule and interactions can be evaluated among different cell types absent in preparations of isolated hepatocytes that may contribute to toxic effects. Moreover, the microcirculation is preserved and bile production is maintained. Disadvantages of the perfused liver are the absence of neural and hormonal signals present

Table 1. Advantages and disadvantages of various systems for studying hepatotoxicity

System	Disadvantages	Advantages
Cultured hepatocytes	Many enzyme systems revert to fetal state; cytochrome P-450 declines	Convenient; easy to collect data; reproducible
Isolated hepatocytes	Do not make bile; loss of lobular architecture	Convenient; many data points from each animal; reproducible; viable up to 24h
Liver slices	Do not make bile; leak potassium	Maintain lobular architecture; many preparations from each animal
Perfused livers	Not as efficient as hepatocytes; use more animals; decrease in some functions after 2–5h	Maintain lobular architecture; microcirculation is intact; makes bile; nearly physiological; easy to collect data; reproducible
In vivo	Excessive use of experimental animals; complex metabolic and physiological interactions; difficult to interpret data	Most physiological hormonal and neural signals are intact

in vivo and of effects of nutrients provided from the diet and peripheral tissues.

Comparative studies between drug metabolism in vivo and in perfused liver demonstrated that a good correlation exists between the two systems for many drugs (BICKEL and MINDER 1970; GARATTINI et al. 1973; VON BAHR et al. 1970a,b). The isolated perfused liver has been used in a number of in vitro studies involving interactions between intermediary metabolism, mixed-function oxidation, and toxicity that will be discussed below.

B. Techniques Used to Study Zone-Specific Hepatotoxicity in the Isolated Perfused Liver

For over a century, perfusion of isolated liver has been used to study metabolic events in intact cells. In 1855, Claude Bernard described glycogen conversion to glucose in livers perfused with tap water, and other early applications of the liver perfusion technique have been reviewed (MILLER 1973a). Surgical techniques for rat liver perfusion have also been described in detail (MILLER 1973b). Briefly, animals are anesthetized, the abdominal cavity is opened, and perfusion fluid is infused into the liver via a cannula placed in the portal vein. Perfusion must be initiated in situ since the procedure may involve potentially deleterious anoxia (SCHOLZ et al. 1969; SCHMUCKER et al. 1975). Effluent perfusate is collected via a cannula placed in the inferior vena cava.

Various fluids have been used for perfusion. Heparinized or defibrinated whole blood diluted with a buffer solution and supplemented with glucose, amino acids, albumin, vitamins, or antibiotics is frequently used (BRAUER et al. 1951; MILLER 1973a,b; MILLER et al. 1951). The use of semisynthetic media with washed erythrocytes of human (HEMS et al. 1966) or bovine (BOMBECK et al. 1968; SCHMASSEK et al. 1974) origin is also common. All of these variations, as well as perfusion fluids containing fluorocarbons, allow adequate tissue oxygenation at relatively low flow rates, and they may be adapted to either circulating or nonrecirculating systems (HEMS et al. 1966; GOODMAN et al. 1973; THURMAN et al. 1975). However, disadvantages of fluids containing red blood cells include progressive hemolysis (SCHMUCKER et al. 1975), deterioration of mixed-function oxidation, utilization of substrates and production of metabolites by red cells (GOODMAN et al. 1973), interference by hemoglobin with absorption measurements in the perfusate or intact organ, and interference with fluorescence from the liver surface (SCHOLZ et al. 1969). To avoid these problems, hemoglobin-free perfusion fluids consisting of osmotically balanced and buffered electrolyte solutions are now often used (SCHMUCKER et al. 1975; SCHOLZ et al. 1969; THURMAN et al. 1977). To compensate for the diminished capacity of these fluids to carry oxygen in comparison to blood, flow rates are elevated to provide adequate oxygenation of the tissue. With this method, rates of oxygen uptake are similar to rates obtained with blood (BRAUSER et al.

1972) or hemoglobin-free bicarbonate buffer (THURMAN and SCHOLZ 1969) used as perfusate.

Recirculating systems (BEND et al. 1978; BRAUER et al. 1951; MILLER 1973b; SCHMASSEK et al. 1973) or nonrecirculating systems (THURMAN et al. 1977) can be used for rat liver perfusion. In recirculating systems, conditions more closely approximate those in vivo, since relatively small volumes of fluid (~100ml) are recirculated and reoxygenated. However, although non-recirculating perfusion systems require large volumes of perfusate, they offer other advantages. For instance, a constant composition of influent perfusate is maintained, in contrast to recirculating systems, where the inflow fluid contains added substrates along with metabolites produced by the liver. With nonrecirculating systems, small changes in metabolites produced by the tissue are readily detected, dose-response relationships are more easily established, and different metabolic conditions in the same liver can be studied. In addition, each liver may also serve as its own control.

Direct optical measurement of metabolites in the perfusate are facilitated by the use of hemoglobin-free perfusate, and changes in fluorescence and absorption of the tissue itself may be monitored (SIES and CHANCE 1970). A number of investigators have described techniques to measure pyridine nucleotide and flavoprotein fluorescence from the liver surface (SCHOLZ et al. 1969; SCRUTTON and UTTER 1968; THEORELL et al. 1972). Flavoprotein fluorescence primarily indicates the mitochondrial redox state, whereas pyridine nucleotide fluorescence reflects the cytosolic plus mitochondrial oxidation-reduction state (SCHOLZ et al. 1969).

Spectrophotometry has been used in the whole perfused liver. The technique of direct spectrophotometric measurement of catalase H_2O_2 compound I was developed by SIES and CHANCE (1970), and the occurrence of type I and type II binding spectra of substrates to cytochrome P-450 can be monitored in the perfused liver (SIES and BRAUSER 1970). Recently, the catalase-H_2O_2 signal was effective in studies on pathways of hepatic ethanol metabolism (HANDLER et al. 1986). In addition, direct optical methods have been employed to monitor the oxidation-reduction state of cytochromes a,c,b_5, and P-450 (LÜBBERS et al. 1965; SIES and BRAUSER 1970). Perfused liver studies can use a time-sharing multichannel spectrophotometer, reflectometer, and fluorometer as described by CHANCE et al. (1975).

The period of time for which the isolated perfused liver will maintain normal metabolic functions is an important concern. Tests of viability include enzyme leakage, oxygen consumption, hepatic flow and vascular resistance, potassium levels, membrane potential, pH of the perfusate, and the continued production of bile and metabolites. With carefully controlled conditions, perfusions of 8–12h have been performed (BARTOSEK et al. 1973; JOHN and MILLER 1969); however, glucose and lipid synthesis are linear for only about 2h.

Perfusions are normally performed in the anterograde direction (portal vein to vena cava); however, livers can be perfused in the retrograde direction (vena cava to portal vein) for specific purposes. Since the oxygen gradient is reversed in retrograde perfusions, this technique is particularly beneficial in evaluating sublobular compartmentation and the effect of the oxygen tension on biochemical processes.

I. Metabolite Measurements in Tissue and Perfusate

Samples of perfusate are obtained easily to measure metabolites. Further, by ligating and removing one lobe of the liver, tissue samples can be obtained without interrupting perfusion (MILLER 1973b); however, this procedure could alter circulation to unligated lobes and therefore affect metabolic events.

Freeze-clamping with tongs chilled in liquid nitrogen is a technique for freezing livers rapidly in a particular metabolic state (WOLLENBERGER et al. 1960; KAUFFMAN et al. 1977). After extraction, standard enzymatic methods are used to measure metabolites. The effect of toxicants on metabolic pathways in sublobular regions of the liver has been evaluated with quantitative histochemical sampling techniques (LOWRY 1953) and ultramicrobiochemical assays (LOWRY 1973; KAUFFMAN and MATSCHINSKY 1986). For example, measurements of $NADP^+$ and NADPH in sublobular regions of rat livers perfused with 7-ethoxycoumarin demonstrated that cofactor supply is rate-limiting for mixed-function oxidation in both periportal and pericentral areas (BELINSKY et al. 1983). When the sugar alcohol, xylitol, was added to perfused livers of fasted rats, NADPH increased in both hepatic regions and oxidation of 7-ethoxycoumarin was stimulated (BELINSKY et al. 1983). The outcome of studies such as these has important implications for relationships between drug metabolism and nutritional status. In addition, quantitative histochemical techniques have been employed in studies identifying biochemical mechanisms of the zonal toxicity of allyl alcohol (BELINSKY et al. 1986; BADR et al. 1986). Results indicate that acrolein, the toxic metabolite of allyl alcohol, causes zone-specific injury to the liver lobule that is dependent upon oxygen tension (BADR et al. 1986). Interestingly, hepatic macrophages are involved (PRZYBOCKI et al. 1992). Further, assessment of respiration and adenine nucleotide content in sublobular regions of the liver suggests that acrolein toxicity particularly affects mitochondria (BELINSKY et al. 1986). Quantitative measurements of glutathione in sublobular regions of livers exposed to allyl alcohol demonstrated that glutathione depletion precedes mitochondrial injury.

Key enzymes participating in drug metabolism and toxicity in sublobular regions of the liver have also been assessed using ultramicrobiochemical measurements. For instance, measurement of rates of glucuronyl transferase activities in microdissected samples of periportal and pericentral zones of the rat liver lobule demonstrated that the K_m of the enzyme for 7-hydroxycoumarin was essentially the same as that determined for glucuronidation of the substrate in sublobular regions of the intact liver (CONWAY et al. 1987). Determination of the V_{max} of the enzyme from kinetic studies showed that maximal enzymatic capacity was about three times greater than maximal rates in periportal and pericentral zones of the intact perfused liver. Thus, enzyme activity is not the only rate-limiting event for glucuronidation in sublobular regions of the liver. Measurements of arylsulfatase activity in rat liver have shown that the enzyme is distributed evenly across the liver lobule (ANUNDI et al. 1986). Futile cycling between synthetic and hydrolytic enzymes involved in conjugate production may limit maximal rates of drug and toxic metabolite conjugation. In sublobular zones of human liver, studies of the distribution of synthetic and hydrolytic enzymes associated with the formation of glucuronide, sulfate, and glutathione conjugates indicate that futile cycling may play a more important role in the formation of sulfate conjugates than glucuronide conjugates (EL-MOUELHI and KAUFFMAN 1986).

The redox state of mitochondrial NAD^+ may be assessed from β-hydroxybutyrate: acetoacetate measurements in effluent perfusate. Pyridine nucleotide oxidation-reduction potentials may also be determined from metabolites measured in extracts of tissue. The basis of these calculations is the assumption that the oxidized and reduced substrates of some active pyridine nucleotide-linked dehydrogenases are in near equilibrium with the free nucleotide in specific subcellular compartments (HEMS et al. 1966; KAUFFMAN et al. 1977; WILLIAMSON et al. 1973). Similarly, alterations in $NADP^+$:NADPH ratios that are observed during mixed-function oxidation are based on changes in substrates thought to be in near equilibrium with malic enzyme, isocitrate dehydrogenase, and 6-phosphogluconate dehydrogenase (THURMAN and KAUFFMAN 1980).

II. Microlight Guides

Fluorometry of tissues has been used in living cells to determine the localization and kinetics of reduced pyridine nucleotides (CHANCE and THEORELL 1959). Light guides (tip diameters of ~5 mm) containing optical fibers were subsequently employed to measure NADH fluorescence and UV reflectance from the heart (CHANCE et al. 1974) and from the rat cerebral cortex in situ (MAYEVSKY and CHANCE 1974). With further refinement, these methods resulted in the development of microlight guides containing single strands of 25- to 80-μm-diameter fibers for the measurement of UV reflectance and NADH fluorescence from mitochondrial suspensions and hemoglobin-free perfused rat liver (JI et al. 1979). A major drawback to the original microlight guides was that they were embedded in brass plates and could not be placed on specific periportal and pericentral zones on the liver surface.

The microlight guide was subsequently modified by removing the brass plate, thus allowing placement on specific sublobular areas and noninvasive determination of local rates of mixed-function oxidation in periportal and pericentral zones in perfused liver (JI et al. 1981; LEMASTERS et al. 1986). This technique involves placement of a two-stranded, 80-μm-diameter microlight guide (Fig. 1A) on specific areas on the liver surface. One strand is connected to a light source and the other to a photomultiplier. Light from a mercury arc lamp illuminates the tissue, and the wavelengths are selected with optical filters. The adjacent strand transmits fluorescence from the tissue through selected filters prior to detection by the photomultiplier. The signal from the photomultiplier is filtered, amplified, and recorded. Treatment of the rats with phenobarbital results in periportal and pericentral regions of the lobule appearing as light and dark areas, respectively, and placement of the light guide on specific zones allows continuous fluorometric determination of the mixed-function oxidation of model compounds (JI et al. 1981). For example, measurements of fluorescence due to 7-hydroxycoumarin formation from 7-ethoxycoumarin can be obtained by illuminating tissue with light at 366 nm and measuring fluorescence at 450 nm. In addition, microlight guides have been used as a noninvasive technique to measure the conjugation of 7-hydroxycoumarin and the intracellular NADH redox state in periportal and pericentral zones of the liver lobule (see below).

III. Miniature Oxygen Electrodes

Miniature oxygen electrodes were developed in our laboratory (MATSUMURA and THURMAN 1983) to measure oxygen tension and rates of oxygen uptake in distinct regions of the liver lobule, and this method has led to new possibilities in studies of zonal hepatotoxicity. To make a miniature oxygen electrode (Fig. 1B), a 50-μm-diameter platinum wire is inserted into a glass capillary tube, the glass is pulled under heat, and the electrode tip is coated with an oxygen-

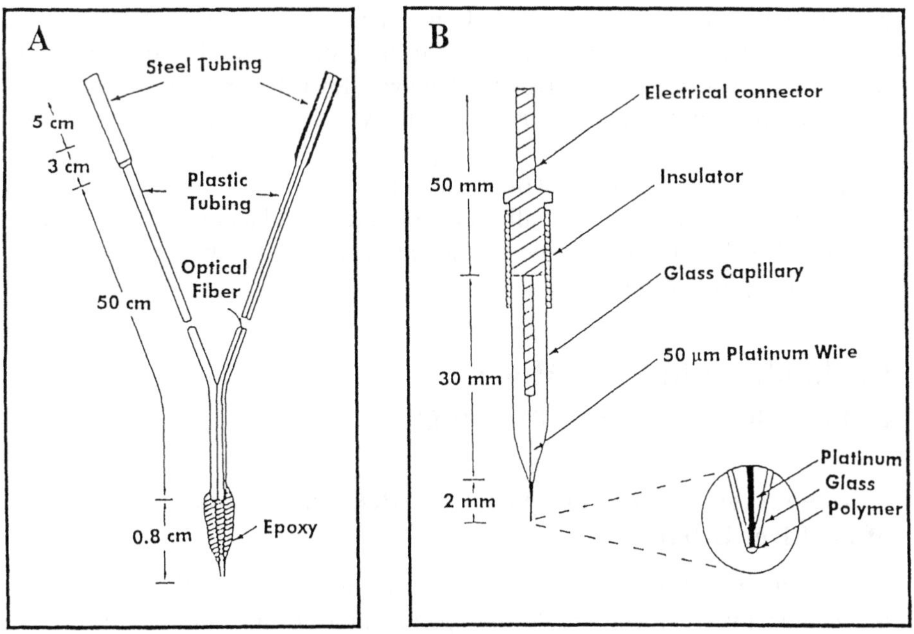

Fig. 1A,B. Schematic representations of **A** microlight guide and **B** miniature oxygen electrode. For details, see LEMASTERS et al. (1986)

permeable acrylic ester polymer. Miniature oxygen electrodes have been used to measure tissue oxygen tensions directly in periportal and pericentral zones of the liver lobule (JI et al. 1982). In addition, the miniature oxygen electrode has been used to measure rates of oxygen uptake in distinct areas of the liver lobule in perfused livers by stopping the inflow and outflow simultaneously (stopped-flow O_2 uptake technique). With the miniature oxygen electrode, rates of oxygen uptake were shown to be two- to threefold greater in periportal than in pericentral zones of the liver lobule (MATSUMURA and THURMAN 1983). Recently, this technique was used to measure rates of a variety of metabolic processes in periportal and pericentral zones based on the stoichiometric changes in rates of oxygen uptake which occur during infusion of substrate (THURMAN and KAUFFMAN 1985). Thus, local flux rates in metabolic pathways can now be measured based on alterations in regional oxygen uptake. Studies designed to examine the effects of hepatotoxicants on intermediary metabolism in different zones of the liver lobule have also employed miniature oxygen electrodes (BELINSKY et al. 1984b; see below).

IV. Trypan Blue Exclusion

In tissue culture, exclusion of trypan blue is an indicator of cell viability (KRUSE and PATTERSON 1973). More recently, trypan blue has been infused into perfused livers to detect damage to specific regions of the lobule of perfused livers (BELINSKY et al 1984c; BRADFORD et al. 1985). After trypan blue is infused, excess dye is removed and livers are perfused with paraformaldehyde. The fixed tissue is embedded in either paraffin or plastic, and sections are stained only with eosin, a cytoplasmic stain. Trypan blue can be easily detected in the nuclei of injured cells. This method was used to demonstrate that exposure of the liver to hypoxia damages downstream areas of the liver lobule: during anterograde perfusion, hepatocytes in pericentral regions were stained predominantly, whereas during perfusion in the retrograde direction periportal cells were damaged (BRADFORD et al. 1985). Moreover, when livers were injured due to hypoxia or allyl alcohol, release of lactate dehydrogenase correlated well with the degree of damage assessed by the percentage of trypan blue-positive cells.

C. Applying In Vitro Models to the Study of Liver Toxicology

I. Monooxygenation in Periportal and Pericentral Zones of the Liver Lobule

In the first study of metabolic processes in distinct regions of the liver lobule in the intact liver, cytochrome P-450-dependent mixed-function oxidation of 7-ethoxycoumarin to 7-hydroxycoumarin was measured (JI et al. 1981). Rates of

7-ethoxycoumarin O-deethylation were determined from increases in 7-hydroxycoumarin fluorescence (366 → 450 nm) measured from the liver surface with a large-tipped (2 mm diameter) light guide and 7-hydroxycoumarin measured quantitatively in the effluent perfusate. Fluorescence from many periportal and pericentral areas in several lobules can be excited and collected by light guides. Both 7-hydroxycoumarin production and fluorescence due to 7-hydroxycoumarin from the tissue increased in a stepwise manner as the concentration of 7-ethoxycoumarin infused into the liver was increased. Fluorescence of 7-hydroxycoumarin at the liver surface correlated with rates of O-deethylation of 7-ethoxycoumarin by the whole organ (JI et al. 1981). Based on this correlation, fluorescence measured with microlight guides was converted into local rates of mixed-function oxidation. During perfusions in the anterograde direction, infusion of 7-ethoxycoumarin caused increased fluorescence first in periportal areas and then in pericentral zones (JI et al. 1981). The increase in maximal fluorescence was greater in pericentral than in periportal regions in perfused livers from fed, phenobarbital-treated rats (Fig. 2). These changes in fluorescence corresponded to local rates of mixed-function oxidation of 3.6 and 7.0 μmol/g per hour in periportal and pericentral areas, respectively (BELINSKY et al. 1984a). Thus, in intact livers from phenobarbital-treated rats, rates of mixed-function oxidation of 7-ethoxycoumarin are about twofold greater in pericentral than periportal areas. Higher concentrations of cytochrome P-450 in pericentral regions are responsible, at least in part, for zonal differences in rates of 7-ethoxycoumarin O-deethylation (GOODING et al. 1978). NADPH supply is also an important determinant of rates of mixed-function oxidation in the whole organ (THURMAN et al. 1977; MOLDEUS et al. 1974; BELINSKY et al. 1980). When rats were treated with 6-aminonicotinamide to inhibit the pentose cycle, an important source of NADPH in livers from fed rats, rates of O-deethylation were diminished in both areas. Rates of mixed function oxidation in both regions of the liver lobule were also reduced by perfusion with potassium cyanide, an inhibitor of cytochrome oxidase, to inhibit NADPH supply by mitochondria (BELINSKY et al. 1984a). Therefore, both cytosolic and mitochondrial pathways clearly contribute to the generation of NADPH in periportal and pericentral zones of the liver. Further, local rates of monooxygenation in both regions of the liver are rate-limited by NADPH supply.

II. Conjugation Reactions in Periportal and Pericentral Regions of the Liver Lobule

1. Sulfation

The isolated, perfused liver is an excellent in vitro model for studies of conjugation reactions which are regulated by various metabolic factors such as substrate concentration, enzyme activity, and cofactor supply. Sulfation of phenolic substrates is a low-capacity, high-affinity system dependent upon

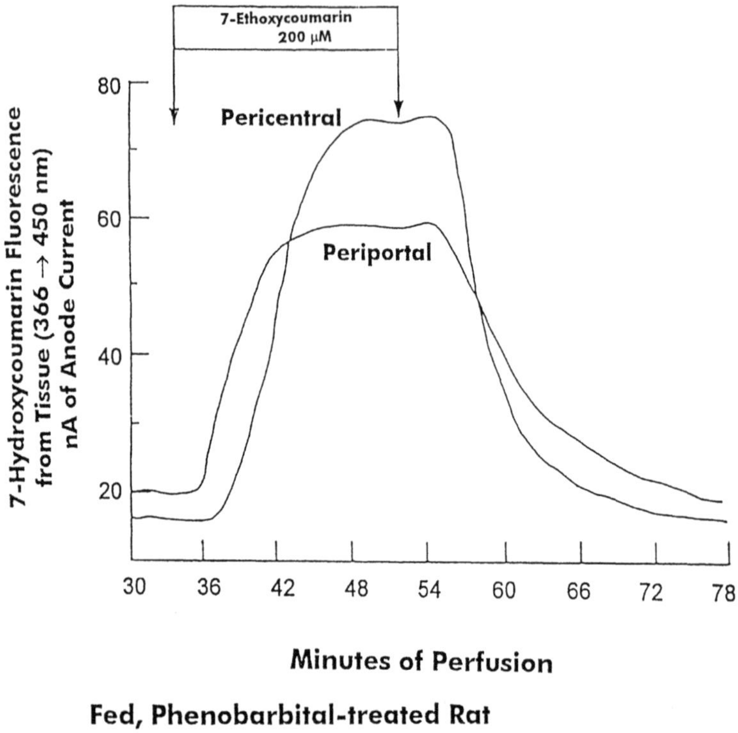

Fig. 2. Fluorescence of 7-hydroxycoumarin from periportal and pericentral areas of the liver lobule. Two microlight guides were placed on two adjacent periportal zones (1–3 mm apart) on the left lateral lobe, and the output voltages (600–650 V) of the photomultipliers were adjusted to give similar anode currents in both channels. One microlight guide was subsequently moved to a pericentral region. 7-Ethoxycoumarin was infused during the time indicated by the *horizontal base* and *vertical arrows*

added sulfate (REINKE et al. 1981); in contrast, glucuronidation occurs with lower affinity but has a much higher capacity (THURMAN et al. 1981). When hepatotoxicants were used to destroy selected regions of the liver lobule, results indicated that glucuronosyltransferases and sulfotransferases are localized predominantly in periportal zones (JAMES et al. 1981). Studies with pharmacokinetic modeling also indicated that sulfation of acetaminophen generated from phenacetin by perfused liver was greater in periportal than in pericentral areas (PANG and TERRELL 1981). Although such information was useful, quantitative data on rates of conjugation in specific sublobular regions of the liver were still needed. Microlight guides and miniature O_2 electrode technology have been used to obtain these data (CONWAY et al. 1982).

Rates of conjugation of fluorescent 7-hydroxycoumarin to nonfluorescent sulfates and glucuronides in periportal and pericentral areas of the perfused liver were determined with microlight guides (CONWAY et al. 1982). When 7-hydroxycoumarin (up to $30\,\mu M$) was infused during perfusion in the anterograde direction, fluorescence of free 7-hydroxycoumarin was detected only in periportal areas; however, fluorescence was detected only in pericentral areas during perfusion in the retrograde direction. This study demonstrated that conjugates are formed in only one zone of the liver lobule with relatively low concentrations of substrate. To estimate rates of sulfation and glucuronidation in periportal and pericentral regions, conjugates of 7-hydroxycoumarin in the effluent perfusate were measured when perfusion was in the anterograde or retrograde direction. When less than 10 μM 7-hydroxycoumarin was infused in the anterograde direction, sulfation predominated over glucuronidation; in contrast, when 20–30 μM 7-hydroxycoumarin was infused, glucuronidation predominated (CONWAY et al. 1982). However, rates of glucuronidation and sulfation were similar when low concentrations of 7-hydroxycoumarin were infused in the retrograde direction, although glucuronidation still predominated at higher substrate concentrations. Thus, when low concentrations of 7-hydroxycoumarin were infused, sulfation was greater than glucuronidation in periportal zones but not in pericentral regions of the liver lobule. If sulfate-free perfusate were used, glucuronide was the major conjugate formed in both periportal and pericentral zones. Taken together, these data demonstrate that, at low substrate concentrations, sulfation competes successfully with glucuronidation for 7-hydroxycoumarin. Moreover, maximal rates of sulfation in periportal areas were double values obtained in pericentral regions (CONWAY et al. 1982). The variation in rates of sulfation across the liver lobule can result from differences in sulfotransferase and sulfatase activity as well as the supply of 3′-phosphoadenosine 5′-phosphosulfate.

2. Glucuronidation

Studies described above measured rates of glucuronidation of 7-hydroxycoumarin in specific regions of the liver lobule with low substrate concentrations (<20 μM) (CONWAY et al. 1982). Glucuronosyltransferases, however, have a relatively high K_m for substrate (>50 μM), and therefore glucuronidation was studied under conditions where substrate was not rate-limiting. For these experiments, a method employing microlight guides was designed to determine rates of glucuronidation of 7-hydroxycoumarin in specific regions of the liver lobule with 7-hydroxycoumarin in specific regions of the liver lobule with 7-hydroxycoumarin concentrations above the K_m. In these studies, livers were perfused under normoxic conditions with sulfate-free buffer, and fluorescence of free 7-hydroxycoumarin was measured from the surface of the liver (CONWAY et al. 1987). Nitrogen-saturated perfusate containing 20 mM ethanol was subsequently used to inhibit completely formation of nonfluorescent 7-hydroxycoumarin glucuronide (Fig. 3). Under these conditions, fluorescence recorded from the surface and the concentration of substrate infused were directly proportional (CONWAY et al. 1987). Thus, glucuronidation was responsible for differences in 7-hydroxycoumarin fluorescence observed between livers perfused with nitrogen+ethanol and

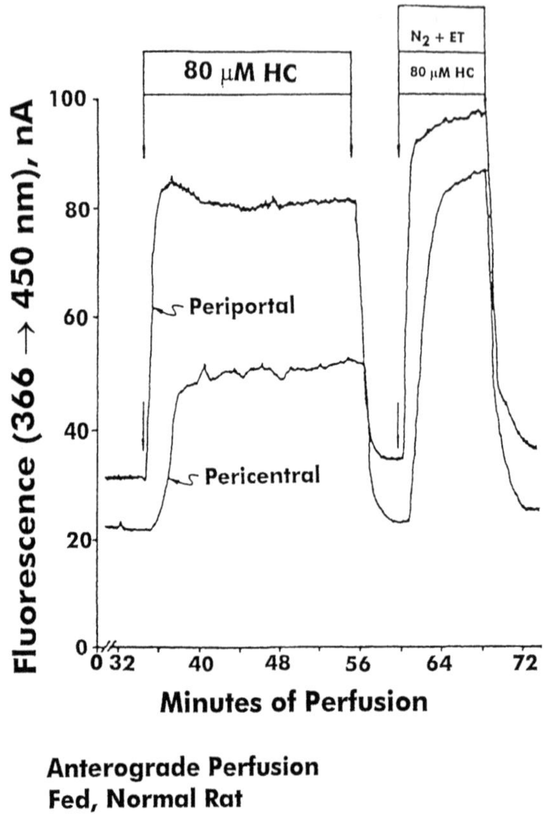

Fig. 3. Fluorescence increase due to 7-hydroxycoumarin (*HC*) and nitrogen-saturated perfusate containing ethanol (N_2 + *ET*) in periportal and pericentral zones of a liver from an untreated rat. Two microlight guides were placed on periportal and pericentral areas 1–3 mm apart. 7-Hydroxycoumarin (80 μM) and nitrogen-saturated perfusate containing ethanol (2 m*M*) were infused as indicated by the *horizontal bars* and *arrows*

normoxic medium. When livers from untreated rats were perfused with 80 μM 7-hydroxycoumarin, glucuronidation was similar in periportal and pericentral areas (Fig. 3). With this new method, maximal rates of glucuronidation in periportal and pericentral zones of the liver lobule were determined to be about 12–13 μmol/g per hour, and were half-maximal with 10–20 μM 7-hydroxycoumarin in both areas.

The activity of β-glucuronidase or glucuronosyltransferases and the supply of the cofactor uridine diphosphoglucuronic acid (UDPGA) are important factors in regulation of rates of glucuronide formation. β-Glucuronidase activity is distributed evenly in both zones of the liver louble (EL-MOUEHLI and KAUFFMAN 1986), and glucuronosyltransferase activity measured in microdissected, freeze-dried tissue samples in vitro (CONWAY et al. 1987) was two- to threefold greater in pericentral than in periportal regions. Thus, the maximal capacity of the glucuronidation system determined in vitro was about threefold greater in pericentral than in periportal areas even though rates of glucuronidation were similar in both regions of perfused livers. When epinephrine was infused, rates of glucuronidation were elevated by about 35%, probably due to increased supply of UDPGA through enhanced breakdown of glycogen. Therefore, UDPGA supply is an important rate-limiting factor for glucuronidation in livers from untreated rats.

III. Oxygen as a Determinant of Zone-Specific Hepatotoxicity

Study of the mechanisms of zone-specific hepatotoxicity due to allyl alcohol have also employed the isolated perfused liver (BELINSKY et al. 1984c). When allyl alcohol was infused for 60 min into livers from fed rats perfused in the anterograde direction, virtually all cells in periportal areas of the liver lobule were damaged as indexed by trypan blue uptake. In livers perfused in the absence of allyl alcohol, hepatocytes excluded trypan blue. Half-maximal uptake of dye occurred at 38 min (BADR et al. 1986). Under these conditions, oxygen uptake was inhibited only in periportal areas of the liver lobule. However, when the time of infusion of allyl alcohol was increased to 90 min, trypan blue was taken up by virtually all cells across the liver lobule, with half-maximal staining in pericentral zones occurring at 70 min. These results indicated that hepatocytes in pericentral regions were not immune to damage by allyl alcohol. Following 60 min of infusion of allyl alcohol during perfusion in the retrograde direction (i.e., the oxygen gradient was reversed), trypan blue was taken up by cells in pericentral but not periportal regions. Concomitantly, oxygen uptake was diminished only in pericentral areas. During perfusion in either direction, infusion of allyl alcohol in oxygen-saturated buffer resulted in release of lactate dehydrogenase and malondialdehyde (BADR et al. 1986). However, malondialdehyde release and trypan blue uptake were reduced markedly when oxygen tension was decreased by lowering the flow rate or perfusing with air-saturated buffer. Based on these data, it is concluded that local O_2 tension is a major determinant of zone-specific hepatotoxicity due to allyl alcohol. In addition, the generation of reactive oxygen species appears to play a role in the hepatotoxicity of allyl alcohol. Desferrioxamine, an iron-trapping agent, allopurinol, an inhibitor of xanthine oxidase, and (+)-cyanidanol-3, an oxygen radical scavenger, each prevented allyl alcohol-induced injury (BADR et al. 1986). Moreover, hepatic macrophages are involved, since injury was blocked only in vivo by a Kupffer cells toxicant, $GdCl_3$ (PRZYBOCKI et al. 1992). Thus, an oxygen-dependent mechanism involving the generation of reactive species participates in allyl alcohol-induced damage to regions of high oxygen tension.

Results from experiments with allyl alcohol outlined above raised the possibility that hepatotoxicity due to other agents generating free radicals may also be oxygen dependent. Chemicals containing a quinone nucleus undergo redox cycling in which the quinone is reduced to a semiquinone free radical, which in turn reacts with molecular oxygen to produce superoxide anion and

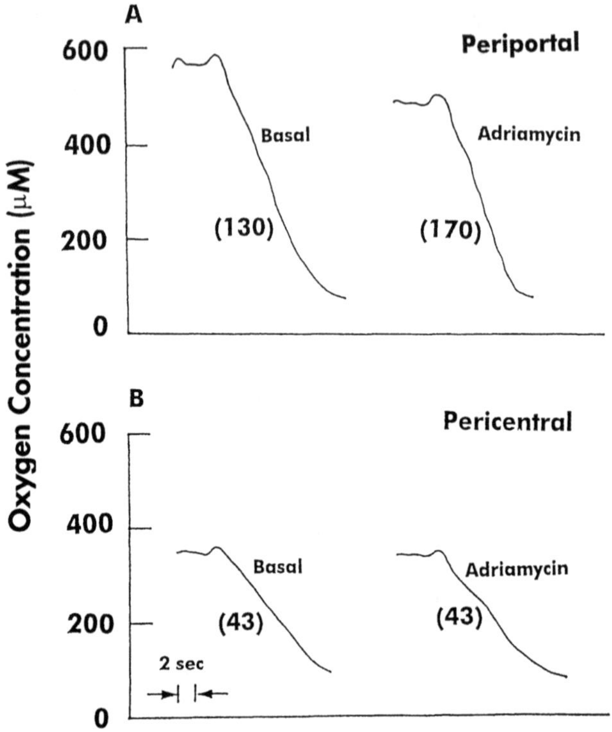

Fig. 4A,B. Oxygen uptake in periportal and pericentral areas of the livers perfused with Adriamycin. Livers from fasted, phenobarbital-treated rats were perfused with Krebs-Henseleit buffer containing 40% albumin for 20 min. Subsequently, livers were perfused with Adriamycin (300 μM). Local oxygen concentrations were measured using a miniature oxygen electrode placed sequentially on periportal (*light*) and pericentral (*dark*) regions of the liver lobule. Inflow and outflow were halted simultaneously, and local oxygen concentration decreased linearly. Basal values were determined during the first 20 min of perfusion before addition of Adriamycin. A driamycin values were determined 5–20 min later. **A** Periportal; **B** Pericentral. *Numbers in parentheses* represent corresponding rates of oxygen uptake in micromoles per grams per hour

regenerate the quinone. The superoxide anion then may enter into a series of reactions which ultimately result in cell damage. For example, menadione and doxorubicin (Adriamycin), which undergo redox cycling, both specifically injure oxygen-rich, periportal regions of the perfused liver lobule (BADR et al. 1987; GANEY et al. 1988). Hepatotoxicity due to doxorubicin was preceded by elevation in oxygen uptake due to redox cycling, which occurred exclusively in periportal areas of the lobule as determined by miniature oxygen electrodes (Fig. 4) In the presence of doxorubicin (300 μM), rates of oxygen uptake in periportal zones increased from 123 μmol/g per hour under basal conditions to 180 μmol/g per hour. Rates of oxygen uptake in pericentral areas were 42–43 μmol/g per hour in both the absence and presence of doxorubicin. Thus, redox cycling as well as toxicity due to doxorubicin was limited to areas of high oxygen tension. Further, doxorubicin toxicity was abolished when inflow oxygen tension was lowered (Ganey et al. 1988). Local oxygen tension may therefore be a major determinant of the hepatotoxicity of many compounds which undergo redox cycling.

D. Conclusions

The isolated perfused liver offers many advantages as an in vitro model for studying hepatotoxicity, particularly evaluating events that occur in periportal and pericentral regions of the liver lobule. The zone-specific nature of responses to chemicals is an important factor in understanding mechanisms of hepatotoxicity and providing insight into methods of therapy and prevention of toxicity. The types of studies involving the perfused liver presented in this chapter could be adapted to investigation of the bioactivation or metabolic inactivation of other drugs and chemicals. Recently, the perfused liver has been employed in evaluating the role of oxygen tension in hepatotoxicity of a number of chemicals, and this model is proving to be useful in studies of free radical-mediated toxicity. One as yet poorly explored use for the perfused liver is in investigation of the interaction among different cell types in hepatotoxic responses to xenobiotics. Since the lobular architecture is preserved, the perfused liver is ideal for studying hepatotoxicants that primarily affect nonparenchymal cells or that invoke interaction between different cell types, such as parenchymal and Kupffer cells, to produce toxicity. This has proven important in recent studies from our laboratory with CCl_4 (Edwards et al. 1993). In addition, blood elements can easily be introduced to the liver through the perfusate. Thus, the role of neutrophils, lymphocytes, platelets, or erythrocytes in hepatotoxicity could be evaluated using the perfused liver. Therefore, the perfused liver is an excellent model for the study of hepatotoxicity.

Acknowledgements. We gratefully acknowledge John J. Lemasters and Sungchul Ji for their contributions to the development of methods described here. This work was supported by NIH grant Nos. AA-03624, ES-04325, and AA-09156. P.E.G. was supported by T32-ES01726, F32-ES05431, and a Postdoctoral Fellowship from the American Liver Foundation.

References

Anundi I, Kauffman FC, El-Mouelhi M, Thurman RG (1986) Hydrolysis of organic sulfates in periportal and pericentral regions of the liver lobule: studies with 4-methylumbelliferyl sulfate in the perfused rat liver. Mol Pharmacol 29:599–605

Badr MZ, Belinsky SA, Kauffman FC, Thurman RG (1986) Mechanism of hepatoxicity in periportal regions of the liver lobule due to allyl alcohol: role of oxygen and lipid peroxidation. J Pharmacol Exp Ther 238:1138–1142

Badr MZ, Yoshihara H, Kauffman FC, Thurman RG (1987) Menadione causes selective toxicity to periportal regions of the liver lobule. Toxicol Lett 35:241–246

Baron J, Reddick JA, Greenspan P, Taira Y (1978) Immunohistochemical localization of NADPH-cytochrome c reductase in rat liver. Life Sci 22:1097–1102
Bartosek I, Guaitani A, Garattini S (1973) Prolonged perfusion of isolated rat liver. In: Bartosek I, Guaitani A, Miller LL (eds) Isolated liver perfusion and its application. Raven, New York, pp 63–72
Belinsky SA, Reinke LA, Kauffman FC, Thurman RG (1980) Inhibition of mixed-function oxidation of p-nitroanisole in perfused rat liver by 2,4-dinitrophenol. Arch Biochem Biophys 204:207–213
Belinsky SA, Kauffman FC, Ji S, Lemasters JJ, Thurman RG (1983) Stimulation of mixed-function oxidation of 7-ethoxycoumarin in periportal and pericentral regions of the perfused rat liver by xylitol. Eur J Biochem 137:1–6
Belinsky SA, Kauffman FC, Thurman RG (1984a) Reducing equivalents for mixed-function oxidation in periportal and pericentral regions of the liver lobule in perfused livers from normal and phenobarbital treated rats. Mol Pharmacol 26:574–581
Belinsky SA, Matsumura T, Kauffman FC, Thurman RG (1984b) Rates of allyl alcohol metabolism in periportal and pericentral regions of the liver lobule. Mol Pharmacol 25:158–164
Belinsky SA, Popp JA, Kauffman FC, Thurman RG (1984c) Trypan blue uptake as a new method to investigate hepatotoxicity in periportal and pericentral regions of the liver lobule. Studies with allyl alcohol in the perfused liver. J Pharmacol Exp Ther 230:755–760
Belinsky SA, Badr MZ, Kauffman FC, Thurman RG (1986) Mechanism of hepatotoxicity in periportal regions of the liver lobule due to allyl alcohol: studies on thiols and energy status. J Pharmacol Exp Ther 238:1132–1137
Bend JR, Smith BR, Van Anda J, Ryan AJ, Fouts JR (1978) Biotransformation of styrene oxide by the isolated perfused rat liver and by subtractions of homogenized liver cells. In: Fouts JR, Gut I (eds) Industrial and environmental xenobiotics: in vitro versus in vivo biotransformation and toxicity. Excerpta Medica, Amsterdam, pp 62–70
Bickel MH, Minder R (1970) Metabolism and biliary excretion of the lipophilic drug molecules, imipramine and desmethylimipramine in the rat. I. Experiments in vivo and with isolated perfused livers. Biochem Pharmacol 19:2425–2435
Bombeck CT, Biava C, London RE, Rybus LM (1968) Parameters of normal liver functions with the isolated perfused bovine liver. In: Norman JC (ed) Organ perfusion and preservation. Appleton-Century Crofts, New York, pp 573–608
Bradford BU, Marotto ME, Lemasters JJ, Thurman RG (1985) New, simple models to evaluate zone-specific damage due to hypoxia in the perfused rat liver: time course and effect of nutritional state, J Pharmacol Exp Ther 236:263–268
Brauer RW, Pessotti RL, Pizzolato P (1951) Isolated rat liver preparation. Bile production and other basic properties. Proc Soc Exp Biol Med 78:174–181
Brauser B, Bücher T, Sies H, Versmold H (1972) Control of mitochondrial activity by metabolites in the hemoglobin-free perfused liver. In: Gaede K, Horecker BL, Whelan WJ (eds) Molecular basis of biological activity. Academic, New York, pp 197–210
Chance B, Theorell B (1959) Localization and kinetics of reduced pyridine nucleotide in living cells by microflurometry. J Biol Chem 234:3044–3050
Chance B, Mayevsky A, Goodwin C, Mela L (1974) Factors in oxygen delivery to tissue. Microvasc Res 8:276–282
Chance B, Legallais V, Sorge J, Graham N (1975) A versatile time-sharing multichannel spectrophotometer, reflectometer, and fluorometer. Anal Biochem 66:498–514
Conway JG, Kauffman FC, Ji S, Thurman RG (1982) Rates of sulfation and glucuronidation of 7-hydroxycoumarin in periportal and pericentral regions of the liver lobule. Mol Pharmacol 22:509–516
Conway JG, Kauffman FC, Tsukuda T, Thurman RG (1987) Glucuronidation of 7-hydroxycoumarin in periportal and pericentral regions of the liver lobule in livers from untreated and 3-methylcholanthrene-treated rats. Mol Pharmacol 33:111–119

Edwards MJ, Keller BJ, Kauffman FC, Thurman RG (1993) The involvement of Kupffer cells in carbon tetrachloride toxicity. Toxicol Appl Pharmacol 119:275–279

El-Mouelhi M, Kauffman FC (1986) Sublobular distribution of transferases and hydrolases associated with glucuronide, sulfate and glutathione conjugation in human liver. Hepatology 6:450–456

Ganey PE, Kauffman FC, Thurman RG (1988) Oxygen-dependent hepatotoxicity due to doxorubicin: role of reducing equivalent supply in perfused rat liver. Mol Pharmacol 134:695–701

Garattini S, Guaitani A, Bartosek I (1973) Use of isolated perfused liver in the study of drug metabolism. In: Bartosek I, Guaitani A, Miller LL (eds) Isolated liver perfusion and its applications. Raven, New York, pp 225–234

Gooding PE, Chayen J, Sawyer B, Slater TF (1978) Cytochrome P-450 distribution in rat liver and the effect of sodium phenobarbitone administration. Chem Biol Interact 20:299–310

Goodman MN, Parrilla R, Toews CJ (1973) Influence of fluorocarbon emulsions on hepatic metabolism in perfused rat liver. Am J Physiol 225:1384–1388

Handler JA, Bradford BU, Glassman EB, Ladine JK, Thurman RG (1986) Catalase-dependent ethanol metabolism in vivo in deermice lacking alcohol dehydrogenase. Biochem Pharmacol 35:4487–4492

Hems R, Ross BD, Berry MN, Krebs HA (1966) Gluconeogenesis in the perfused rat liver. Biochem J 101:284–292

James R, Desmond P, Kupfer A, Schenker S, Branch RA (1981) The differential localization of various drug metabolizing systems within the rat liver lobule as determined by the hepatotoxins allyl alcohol, carbon tetrachloride, bromobenzene. J Pharmacol Exp Ther 217:127–132

Ji S, Chance B, Nishiki K, Smith T, Rich T (1979) Micro-light guides: a new method for measuring tissue fluorescence and reflectance. Am J Physiol 236:C144–C156

Ji S, Lemasters JJ, Thurman RG (1981) A fluorometric method to measure sublobular rates of mixed-function oxidation in the hemoglobin-free perfused rat liver. Mol Pharmacol 19:513–516

Ji S, Lemasters JJ, Thurman RG (1982) Intralobular hepatic pyridine nucleotide fluorescence: evaluation of the hypothesis that chronic treatment with ethanol produces pericentral hypoxia. Proc Natl Acad Sci USA 80:5415–5419

John DW, Miller LL (1969) Effect of aflatoxin B1 on net synthesis of albumin, fibrinogen, and al-acid glycoprotein by the isolated perfused rat liver. Biochem Pharmacol 18:1135–1146

Kauffman FC, Matschinsky FM (1986) Quantitative histochemical measurements within sublobular zones of the liver lobule. In: Thurman RG, Kauffman FC, Jungermann K (eds) Regulation of hepatic metabolism: intra- and intercellular compartmentation. Plenum, New York, pp 119–136

Kauffman FC, Evans RK, Thurman RG (1977) Alterations in nicotinamide and adenine nucleotide systems during mixed-function oxidation of p-nitroanisole in perfused livers from normal and phenobarbital-treated rats. Biochem J 166:583–592

Kruse PF, Patterson MK (1973) Tissue culture methods and application. Academic, New York

Lemasters JJ, Ji S, Thurman RG (1986) New micromethods for studying sublobular structure and function in the isolated, perfused rat liver. In: Thurman RG, Kauffman FC, Jungermann K (eds) Regulation of hepatic metabolism. Plenum, New York, pp 159–184

Lowry OH (1953) The quantitative histochemistry of the brain: histological sampling. J Exp Biol 1:20–428

Lowry OH (1973) An unlimited microanalytical system. Acc Chem Res 6:289–293

Lübbers DW, Kessler M, Scholz R, Bücher T (1965) Cytochrome reflection spectra and fluorescence of the isolated, perfused, hemoglobin-free rat liver during a cycle of anoxia. Biochem Z 341:346–350

Magee PN (1966) Toxic liver necrosis. Lab Invest 15:111–120
Matsumura T, Thurman RG (1983) Measuring rates of O_2 uptake in periportal and pericentral regions of liver lobule: stop-flow experiments with perfused liver. Am J Physiol 244:G656–G659
Mayevsky A, Chance B (1974) A new long-term method for the measurement of NADH fluorescence in intact rat brain with chronically implanted cannula. In: Bicher HI, Bruly DF (eds) Oxygen transport to tissue. Plenum, New York, pp 239–244
Miller JA (1970) Carcinogenesis by chemicals: an overview. Cancer Res 30:559–576
Miller LL (1973a) History of isolated liver perfusion and some still unsolved problems. In: Bartosek I, Guaitani A, Miller LL (eds) Isolated liver perfusion and its applications. Raven, New York, pp 1–9
Miller LL (1973b) Technique of isolated rat liver perfusion. In: Bartosek I, Guaitani A, Miller LL (eds) Isolated liver perfusion and its applications. Raven, New York, pp 10–52
Miller LL, Bly CG, Watson ML, Bale WF (1951) The dominant role of the liver in plasma protein synthesis. A direct study of the isolated perfused rat liver with the aid of lysine-5-C14. J Exp Med 94:431–453
Mitchell JR, Jollow DJ (1973) Metabolic activation of drugs to toxic substances. Gastroenterology 68:392–402
Mitchell JR, Jollow DJ, Gillette JR, Brodie BB (1973) Drug metabolism as a cause of drug toxicity. Drug Metab Dispos 1:418–438
Moldéus PW, Grundin R, Vadi H, Orrenius S (1974) A study of drug metabolism linked to cytochrome P-450 in isolated rat-liver cells. Eur J Biochem 46:351–360
Pang KS, Terrell JA (1981) Retrograde perfusion to probe the heterogeneous distribution of hepatic drug metabolizing enzymes in the rat. J Pharmacol Exp Ther 216:339–346
Przybocki JM, Reuhl KR, Thurman RG, Kauffman FC (1992) Involvement of nonparenchymal cells in oxygen-dependent hepatic injury by allyl alcohol. Toxicol Appl Pharmacol 115:57–63
Recknagel RO, Glende J (1973) Carbon tetrachloride hepatotoxicity: an example of lethal cleavage. CRC Crit Rev Toxicol 2:263–297
Rees KR, Tarlow MJ (1967) The hepatotoxic action of allyl formate. Biochem J 104:757–761
Reinke LA, Belinsky SA, Evans RK, Kauffman FC, Thurman RG (1981) Conjugation of p-nitrophenol in the perfused rat liver: the effect of substrate concentration and carbohydrate reserves. J Pharmacol Exp Ther 217:863–870
Schmassek H, Walli AK, Ferraudi M, Jost U (1973) Relationship of different techniques for studying liver metabolism. In: Lundquist F, Tygstrup N (eds) Regulation of hepatic metabolism. Academic, New York, pp 715–725
Schmucker DL, Jones AL, Michielsen CE (1975) An improved system for hemoglobin-free perfusion of isolated rat livers. Lab Invest 33:168–179
Scholz R, Thurman RG, Williamson JR, Chance B, Bücher T (1969) Flavin and pyridine nucleotide redox state in the hemoglobin-free perfused rat liver. Anoxia and subcellular localization of fluorescent falvins. J Biol Chem 244:2317–2324
Scrutton MC, Utter MF (1968) The regulation of glycolysis and gluconeogenesis in animal tissues. Annu Rev Biochem 37:249–302
Sies H, Brauser B (1970) Interaction of mixed function oxidase with its surface and associated redox transitions of cytochrome P-450 and pyridine nucleotides in perfused rat liver. Eur J Biochem 15:531–540
Sies H, Chance B (1970) The steady state level of catalase compound I in isolated hemoglobin-free perfused rat liver. FEBS Lett 11:172–176
Smith MT, Loveridge N, Wills E (1979) The distribution of glutathione in the rat liver lobule. Biochem J 182:103–108
Teutsch HF (1981) Chemomorphology of liver parenchyma. Prog Histochem Cytochem 14:1–92

Teutsch HF, Reider R (1979) NADP-dependent dehydrogenases in rat liver parenchyma. Histochemistry 60:43–52

Theorell H, Chance B, Yonetani T, Oshino N (1972) The combustion of alcohol and its inhibition by 4-methylpyrazole in perfused rat livers. Arch Biochem Biophys 151:434–444

Thurman RG, Kauffman FC (1980) Factors regulating drug metabolism in intact hepatocytes. Pharmacol Rev 31:229–251

Thurman RG, Kauffman FC (1985) SCOPE: metabolic fluxes in periportal and pericentral regions of the liver lobule. Hepatology 5:144–151

Thurman RG, Scholz R (1969) Mixed function oxidation in perfused rat liver. Oxygen uptake following aminopyrine addition. Eur J Biochem 10:459–467

Thurman RG, McKenna WR, Brentzel HJ, Hesse S (1975) Significant pathways of hepatic ethanol metabolism. Fed Proc 34:2075–2081

Thurman RG, Marazzo DP, Jones LS, Kauffman FC (1977) The continuous kinetic determination of p-nitroanisole O-demethylation in hemoglobin-free perfused rat liver. J Pharmacol Exp Ther 201:498–506

Thurman RG, Reinke LA, Belinsky SA, Evans RK, Kauffman FC (1981) Co-regulation of the mixed-function oxidation of p-nitroanisole and glucuronidation of p-nitrophenol in the perfused rat liver by carbohydrate reserves. Arch Biochem Biophys 209:137–142

von Bahr C, Alexanderson B, Azarnoff DL, Sjöqvist F, Orrenius S (1970a) A comparative study of drug metabolism in the isolated perfused liver and in vivo in rats. Eur J Pharmacol 9:99–105

von Bahr C, Sjöqvist F, Oreenius S (1970b) The inhibitory effects of hydrocortisone and testosterone on the plasma disappearance of nortriptyline in the dog and the perfused rat liver. Eur J Pharmacol 9:106–110

Williamson DH, Ellington EV, Ilic V, Saal J (1974) Hepatic effects of saturated and unsaturated short-chain fatty acids and the control of ketogenesis in vivo. In: Lundquist F, Tygstrup N (eds) Regulation of hepatic metabolism. Academic, New York, pp 191–206

Wollenberger A, Ristau O, Schoffa G (1960) A simple technique for extremely rapid freezing of large pieces of tissue. Pflugers Arch 270:399–412

Yoshimura S, Komatsu N, Watanabe K (1977) Purification and immunohistochemical localization of rat liver glutathione peroxidase in micro-dissected periportal and perivenous rat liver tissue. FEBS Lett 83:272–276

CHAPTER 6

Cytochromes P450 and Liver Injury

J.S. LEEDER and A.B. OKEY

A. Drug Biotransformation, Cytochromes P450 and the Liver

I. Drug Biotransformation by the Liver

Most drugs that are administered to patients must possess some degree of fat solubility or lipophilicity in order to be absorbed from the gastrointestinal tract. Once absorbed, they circulate in blood bound to plasma proteins such as albumin, and are sequestered into fat with relative tissue:blood ratios determined by the degree of lipophilicity. For these reasons, lipophilic drugs are not readily excreted by the kidney into urine; therefore conversion to more water-soluble or hydrophilic products is required to facilitate drug elimination from the body. Almost all tissues and organs possess some ability to biotransform lipophilic compounds into water-soluble metabolites. However, the liver is quantitatively the most important organ involved in drug biotransformation for several reasons: (a) the oral absorption of most drugs involves passive diffusion into the portal circulation and delivery to the liver before the drug is distributed throughout the body and exerts its therapeutic effects, (b) transcellular pores or fenestrations in the endothelial cells lining the sinusoidal spaces are unique to the liver and are sufficiently large to permit most plasma proteins to diffuse into the space of Disse where the protein-bound drugs can come in contact with the hepatocyte plasma membrane and (c), following passive diffusion or active transport into the hepatocyte, drug molecules are converted into more hydrophilic metabolites which may be excreted back into the space of Disse and eventually into the systemic circulation for subsequent renal elimination. Alternatively, they may be sorted to the canalicular membrane and be excreted in bile.

II. General Drug Biotransformation Processes

There are several processes by which lipophilic compounds are biotransformed to more water-soluble products. The numerous biotransformation reactions are conventionally classified into two main types, phase I and phase II, which generally occur sequentially. Phase I reactions introduce or reveal (by oxidation, reduction or hydrolysis) a functional group within the substrate that serves as a site for a phase II conjugation reaction. Conjugation with endogenous agents such as sulfate, acetate, glucuronic acid, glutathione and glycine further increases polarity and water solubility, thus facilitating elimination. Associated increases in molecular weight also reduce specific tissue interactions (such as ligand-receptor interactions) which, when coupled with enhanced excretion, result in inactivation or detoxification of the parent compound.

III. Phase I Reactions

The enzymes involved in phase I metabolism differ widely in their complexity. Some enzymes catalyze reactions with compounds containing a specific functional group while other enzymes are extremely promiscuous in terms of acceptable substrates. Although some phase I enzymes are involved in biosynthesis or degradation of physiologically important molecules, most appear to exist solely for the purpose of metabolizing exogenous compounds.

Phase I enzymes are found in several subcellular compartments: *cytosolic enzymes* include alcohol and aldehyde dehydrogenases, aldehyde oxidase and sulfoxide reductase. Reductases, which metabolize quinone, nitro- and ketone functional groups, can be found in cytosolic and microsomal fractions; ketone reductases are also found in mitochondria. *Mitochondrial enzymes* involved in phase I metabolism also include monoamine oxidase and some forms of *N*-oxide reductase and aldehyde dehydrogenase which are distinct from the cytosolic enzymes. *Microsomal* monooxygenases such as flavin-containing monooxygenase and, more importantly, the cytochromes P450 are quantitatively the most important oxidative enzymes responsible for xenobiotic activation and detoxification (GUENGERICH 1993).

IV. Introduction to the Cytochromes P450

The cytochromes P450 (or more properly the heme-thiolate P450s) are a superfamily of heme-containing proteins that catalyze the metabolism of many lipophilic endogenous substances (steroids, fatty acids, fat-soluble vitamins, prostaglandins, leukotrienes and thromboxanes) and exogenous compounds. It is estimated that an ancestral P450 gene existed more than 3.5 billion years ago: NEBERT (1991, 1994) has proposed that the function of P450s (and other "drug-metabolizing" enzymes) is to regulate the steady-state concentrations of endogenous ligands responsible for ligand-modulated transcription of genes involved in growth, differentiation and maintaining homeostasis. Subsequent events, such as the combustion of organic matter, adaptation to a relatively oxygen-rich environment and animal-plant interactions, are thought to be responsible for the emergence of the multiple P450 species now observed throughout the phylogenetic tree. The most recent update lists 221 P450 genes

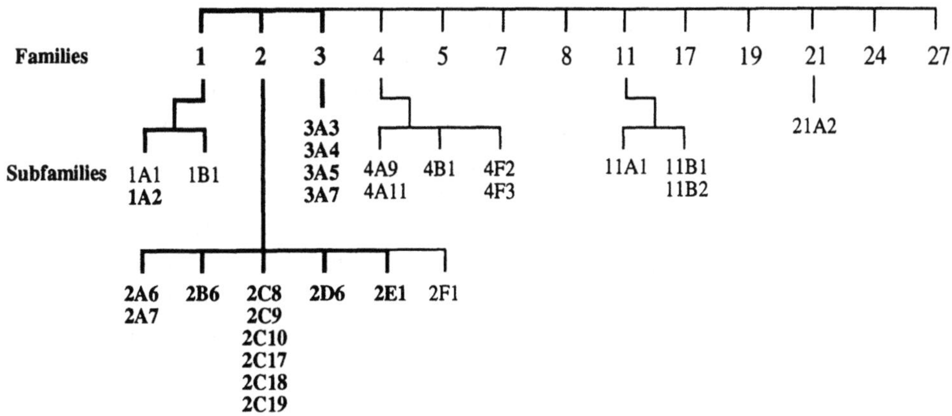

Fig. 1. The human cytochromes P450. P450s that share at least 40% homology are grouped into families *denoted by an Arabic number following the CYP root.* Subfamilies, *designated by a letter*, appear to represent clusters of highly related genes. Individual P450s in a subfamily are numbered sequentially. Hepatic P450s commonly involved in drug metabolism are shown in *bold type*

and 12 putative pseudogenes described in 31 eukaryotic species and 11 prokaryotic species (NELSON et al. 1993).

In humans, 32 genes and 5 putative pseudogenes have been described to date (NELSON et al. 1993). These can be functionally divided into two distinct classes: (a) the steroidogenic enzymes expressed in specialized tissues such as the adrenal glands, gonads and placenta, and (b) the P450s involved in the metabolism of drugs, pesticides and environmental contaminants. To unify (and simplify) P450 nomenclature, a convention based on evolutionary considerations was adopted in 1987 (NEBERT et al. 1987) and subsequently updated (NEBERT et al. 1989, 1991; NELSON et al. 1993). This system uses the root symbol "CYP," representing *cy*tochrome *P*450. P450s that share at least 40% homology are grouped into families denoted by an Arabic number following the CYP root. Subfamilies, designated by a letter, appear to represent clusters of highly related genes. Members of the human CYP2 family, for example, have greater than 67% amino acid sequence homology. Individual P450s in a subfamily are numbered sequentially, i.e., CYP3A3, CYP3A4, CYP3A5. Figure 1 lists known human cytochromes P450. Those that have been identified as being important in human drug metabolism are predominantly found in the CYP1, CYP2 and CYP3 gene families.

B. Cytochromes P450 and Drug Biotransformation

I. Human Hepatic Cytochromes P450

Historically, P450s have been associated with "broad and overlapping substrate specificities." It is now apparent that this broad substrate specificity can be attributed both to multiple forms of P450 in the liver, and to enzyme kinetics that, with substrate concentrations found under physiological conditions, favor a single form of P450 being the primary catalyst of metabolism. Technical developments over the past 10 years have permitted a better definition of the role of individual P450s in human drug biotransformation, and it is now quite apparent that there is considerable interindividual variability in the hepatic expression of P450 enzymes (FORRESTER et al. 1992; SHIMADA et al. 1994). It is not surprising, then, that the pathway and rate of a given compound's metabolic clearance in an individual would be a function of that individual's unique phenotype with respect to the forms and amounts of P450 species expressed in the liver (see below) (WRIGHTON and STEVENS 1992).

CYP 1 Family. Only one member of the CYP1 family, CYP1A2, is expressed at appreciable levels in human liver. The expression of this isoform varies approximately 60-fold, and is approximately fourfold higher in smokers than in nonsmokers (SESARDIC et al. 1988). CYP1A1 mRNA is detectable in human liver, but the amount of CYP1A1 protein is low or absent (SCHWEIKL et al. 1993; HAKKOLA et al. 1994).

The CYP2 family contains the largest number of P450 isoforms; these have considerable diversity in their expression and substrate specificities.

CYP2A Subfamily. The CYP2A subfamily has not been extensively studied in humans. Available data suggest that CYP2A6 represents ≤4% of the total P450 present in human liver (SHIMADA et al. 1994) but may vary approximately 100-fold (YUN et al. 1991).

CYP2B Subfamily. The CYP2B subfamily or the "phenobarbital-inducible" P450s have been extensively studied in experimental animals but their role in human drug metabolism is poorly understood. Recent data indicate that immunochemically detectable CYP2B6 is present in only 24% of human livers and, even then, at levels that are ≤1% of the total P450 content (MIMURA et al. 1993; SHIMADA et al. 1994).

CYP2C Subfamily. Several members of the CYP2C subfamily are present in human liver. CYP2C8 is reported to be bimodally expressed, with 30% of human liver specimens showing higher activities than the rest (WRIGHTON et al. 1987). CYP2C9 and CYP2C10 differ by only two amino acids but are thought to be the products of two distinct genes (NELSON et al. 1993). The activity of these P450s towards substrates such as tolbutamide and (*S*)-warfarin varies approximately 30-fold (RELLING et al. 1990). The P450 responsible for the polymorphic expression of (*S*)-mephenytoin 4′-hydroxylation is also a member of the CYP2C subfamily and now has been identified as CYP2C19 (WRIGHTON et al. 1993a; GOLDSTEIN et al. 1994). The poor metabolizer phenotype is inherited as an autosomal recessive trait in 3%–5% of Caucasians, and approximately 20% of Orientals (WILKINSON et al. 1989; DE MORAIS et al. 1994) such that this enzyme activity is highly variable (>100-fold) in the population (FORRESTER et al. 1992).

CYP2D Subfamily. A similar broad range of activity is observed for CYP2D6, which also is polymorphically expressed (see below). Like CYP2C19, the inheritance of the poor metabolizer phenotype is autosomal recessive with clear ethnic differences in the frequency of this phenotype: 5%–10% in Caucasians compared to <1% in Orientals. Over 30 drugs in clinical use are metabolized by this P450 (MEYER 1990).

CYP2E Subfamily. CYP2E1 is very important from a toxicological perspective since it bioactivates several low molecular weight organic compounds, such as carbon tetrachloride, ethanol and acetaminophen, to reactive intermediates (GUENGERICH et al. 1991). The hepatic expression of CYP2E1 is also quite variable; increased levels have been reported in patients receiving alcohol and isoniazid (PERROT et al. 1989), both of which are known inducers of CYP2E1 in the rat. It also is likely that CYP2E1 expression will also be increased in physiologic states associated with increased levels of acetone or ketone bodies (diabetes mellitus, fasting, obesity) as is observed in rats.

CYP3A Subfamily. The CYP3A subfamily consists of four members in humans and catalyzes the oxidation of many different compounds with structures as diverse as dapsone and steroid molecules as well as more complex molecules like cyclosporine A. Significant correlations between the amounts of immunoreactive CYP3A3/4 and total hepatic P450 content suggest that these isozymes are the major P450 species in human liver.[1] However, while total P450 levels varied only two- to threefold in a sample of human liver microsomes, the amount of immunoreactive CYP3A3/4 varied approximately 60-fold, demonstrating that there are many cases in which CYP3A3/4s are not necessarily the most abundant P450s (FORRESTER et al. 1992). Some of this variability may be related to induction since CYP3A3/4-related catalytic activities are elevated in patients receiving barbiturates, phenytoin, rifampin and glucocorticoids (see following section) (WATKINS et al. 1985). CYP3A5 is polymorphically expressed, being present in approximately 25% of liver microsomal samples tested (WRIGHTON et al. 1989). CYP3A7 was originally thought to be expressed only in fetal liver, comprising 30%–50% of total fetal hepatic P450 (WRIGHTON and VANDENBRANDEN 1989). More recent data indicate that CYP3A7 also is expressed to a varying degree in adult liver (SCHEUTZ et al. 1994). Unfortunately, the role of CYP3A5 and CYP3A7 in drug biotransformation and bioactivation has not been investigated to any great extent.

Clinically relevant substrates, inhibitors and inducers of the CYP1, CYP2 and CYP3 families are summarized in Table 1. This is not meant to a comprehensive listing of P450-mediated drug biotransformation in human

[1] CYP3A3 and CYP3A4 are so highly related (97% homologous) that they cannot be distinguished by immunochemical methods or catalytic properties. For this reason, most investigators use the term "CYP3A3/4" to denote this fact (WRIGHTON and STEVENS 1992).

Table 1. Representative substrates, catalytic activities, inducers and inhibitors of human cytochromes P450

	Substrate and reaction catalyzed	Inducers	Inhibitors
CYP1A2	Caffeine 3-demethylation	Cigarette smoke	Ciprofloxacin
	Phenacetin *O*-deethylation	Charcoal-broiled foods	Enoxacin
	Theophylline 3-demethylation	Cruciferous vegetables	Perfloxacin
	Acetaminophen NAPQI formation	Omeprazole	Furaphylline
CYP2C9/10	Tolbutamide hydroxylation	Rifampin	Cimetidine
	Phenytoin 4-hydroxylation		Sulfaphenazole
	Warfarin (*S*)-7-hydroxylation		Sulfinpyrazone
			Fluconazole
CYP2C19	(*S*)-Mephenytoin 4′-hydroxylation	Rifampin	
	Diazepam *N*-demethylation		
	Propranolol side chain oxidation		
CYP2D6	Debrisoquine 4-hydroxylation		Quinidine
	Alprenolol aromatic hydroxylation		Fluoxetine
	Bufurolol 1′-hydroxylation		
	Metoprolol *O*-dealkylation; aliphatic hydroxylation		
	Propranolol 4-hydroxylation		
	Timolol *O*-dealkylation		
	Amiodarone hydroxylation		
	Encainide *O*-demethylation		
	Flecainide *O*-dealkylation		
	Propafenone 5-hydroxylation		
	Amitriptyline hydroxylation		
	Clomipramine hydroxylation		
	Desipramine *O*-demethylation		
	Imipramine 2-hydroxylation		
	Nortriptyline benzylic hydroxylation		
	Perphenazine		
	Thioridazine		
	Codeine *O*-demethylation		
	Dextromethorphan *O*-demethylation		
CYP2E1	Acetaminophen NAPQI formation	Ethanol	Disulfiram
	Benzene hydroxylation	Isoniazid	
	Chlorzoxazone 6-hydroxylation	Ketone bodies (diabetes)	
	Enflurane defluorination		
	Ethanol oxidation		
	Isoflurane defluorination		
	Organic solvents		
CYP3A3/4	Acetaminophen NAPQI formation	Carbamazepine	Ketoconazole
	Amiodaraone *N*-deethylation	Clotrimazole	Grapefruit juice
	Carbamazepine 10,11-epoxidation	Dexamethasone	Troleandomycin

Table 1. (*Contd.*)

	Substrate and reaction catalyzed	Inducers	Inhibitors
	Cortisol 6-β-hydroxylation	Phenobarbital	
	Cyclosporine *N*-demethylation	Phenytoin	
	Dapsone *N*-hydroxylation	Phenylbutazone	
	Diazepam 3-hydroxylation		
	Diltiazem		
	Ergot alkaloids		
	Erythromycin *N*-demethylation		
	Estrogens		
	FK506 *O*-demethylation		
	Imipramine *N*-demethylation		
	Ketoconazole		
	Lidocaine		
	Lovastatin		
	Methylprednisolone		
	Miconazole		
	Midazolam		
	Nifedipine		
	Progesterone 6-β-hydroxylation		
	Propafenone *N*-dealkylation		
	Quinidine		
	Rapamycin 41-*O*-demethylation		
	Taxol 3′-hydroxylation		
	Terfenadine *N*-dealkylation		
	Testosterone 6-β-hydroxylation		
	Theophylline 8-hydroxylation		
	Tienilic acid *S*-oxidation		
	Troleandomycin *N*-dealkylation		
	Triazolam		
	Verapamil *N*-dealkylation		

liver but rather is to provide an idea of which P450s are primarily responsible for the metabolism of commonly used agents. It should be noted that a given compound may be metabolized by more than one P450, often at a different site on the drug molecule; in the majority of cases, the P450 listed catalyzes the biotransformation pathway which is quantitatively most important.

II. Sources of Variability in P450 Expression and Activity

The level and activity of various members of the P450 superfamily obviously is a key factor in determining the rate at which different drug substrates will be biotransformed and in determining the chemical nature and reactivity of the products. Although there is some consistency in the pattern and activity of P450 enzymes across the human population, several factors alter the repertoire of P450 forms expressed at any given time in a given individual. Chief among these are: (a) the genetic background, (b) exposure to chemicals that induce P450 proteins, (c) exposure to chemicals that inhibit the activity of P450 enzymes and (d) tissue-specific expression. Thus, as with other biological traits, the level and activity of P450 enzymes is determined both by heredity and by environment.

There is an enormous and continually expanding literature on the genetics of P450 enzymes and on regulation of their expression in different tissues by endogenous and exogenous chemical signals. Here we will summarize only briefly some particular findings that may be of relevance to drug-induced hepatotoxicity.

1. P450 Genetics and Polymorphisms

Polymorphisms potentially may exist either in the gene for the P450 protein itself or in genes or noncoding regions that regulate expression of the P450 enzyme. The most extensively studied polymorphism in human P450s involves CYP2D6. About 5%–10% of Caucasians are "poor metabolizers" of drugs that are substrates for CYP2D6 whereas only about 1%–2% of Asian subjects exhibit the "poor metabolizer" phenotype. The "poor metabolizer" phenotype results from several different mutations in the *CYP2D6* gene which prevent synthesis of functional CYP2D6 protein (MEYER et al. 1992). Defective metabolism of drugs that are substrates for CYP2D6 may lead to plasma levels of the parent drug that exceed the expected therapeutic range and cause dose-related toxicity (EICHELBAUM and GROSS 1990). Since CYP2D6 is a primary biotransformation pathway for a wide range of therapeutic agents (see Table 1), the potential clinical impact of the CYP2D6 polymorphism is significant. However, at this time, decreased CYP2D6 activity in "poor metabolizers" has only been shown to be associated with hepatotoxicity with one drug, perhexilene (MORGAN et al. 1984). This implies that CYP2D6-mediated biotransformation of perhexilene to its mono- and dihydroxy metabolites represents a protective, detoxification pathway. Recently a few subjects have been identified who are "ultrarapid metabolizers" of CYP2D6 substrates due to amplification of the *CYP2D6* gene to as much as 12-fold the normal copy number (JOHANSSON et al. 1993); it remains to be seen if expression of "excessive" CYP2D6 will lead to any adverse drug reactions, including hepatotoxicity.

The other major P450 polymorphism originally was discovered as a defect in metabolism of *S*-mephenytoin. The incidence of "poor metabolizers" of *S*-mephenytoin is about 2%–5% in Caucasians and about 20% in Asian populations (WILKINSON et al. 1989). The major defect in *S*-mephenytoin metabolism has been shown to result from a mutation in the *CYP2C19* gene which creates an aberrant splice site, resulting in a truncated nonfunctional CYP2C19 protein (DE MORAIS et al. 1994). Although there are dose-related adverse effects associated with the *S*-mephenytoin "poor metabolizer" phenotype (WILKINSON et al. 1989), no overt increase in hepatotoxicity has been observed to result from the CYP2C19 defect per se. However, since CYP2C19 is apparently responsible for the *R-p*-hydroxylation of phenytoin, a minor biotransformation pathway in man (FRITZ et al. 1987), it will be of interest to determine if defective metabolism through the CYP2C19 pathway either increases or decreases the risk of hepatotoxicity in patients treated with anticonvulsants.

2. P450 Induction

Not all P450s in liver are inducible. However, for those P450 species that are inducible the level and activity of the enzyme may rise dramatically after exposure to specific drugs and environmental chemicals. Table 1 lists P450 species in human liver, including those that are inducible, along with the agents that induce these enzymes.

a) CYP1A Enzymes

The most widely studied inducible P450 subfamily is CYP1A. In laboratory animals and in many human tissues CYP1A1 is induced as much as 100-fold after exposure to polycyclic aromatic hydrocarbons such as 3-methylcholanthrene or halogenated aromatic hydrocarbons such as 2,3,7,8-tetrachlorodibenzo-*p*-dioxin (TCDD) (OKEY 1992). In rodents CYP1A1 induction is high in liver as well as in most nonhepatic tissues. In humans CYP1A1 can be induced in many nonhepatic cells and tissues (OKEY 1992). However, in human liver, CYP1A1 mRNA is expressed only at very low levels and CYP1A1 protein is virtually absent, even in subjects exposed to known inducing stimuli (SCHWEIKL et al. 1993; HAKKOLA et al. 1994). Therefore, in humans, CYP1A1 is unlikely to play a role in hepatotoxicity. Even though CYP1A1 may not be a significant factor in hepatotoxicity in humans, we present this discussion on CYP1A1 to emphasize that P450s may be regulated by mechanisms that lead to profound tissue-specific and species-specific expression patterns; hence extrapolation of toxicologic findings from one tissue to another or from one species to another should be undertaken with appropriate care. The expanding repertoire of methods for studying drug metabolism directly in human systems in vitro and in vivo may provide the best avenue for avoiding the pitfalls of misinterpretation due to species variation.

Whereas CYP1A1 is widely expressed in human nonhepatic tissues but not in human liver, expression of the other member of the CYP1A subfamily, CYP1A2, is just the opposite. CYP1A2 appears to be expressed only in liver in humans and not to any significant extent in nonhepatic tissues (WRIGHTON et al. 1993b; GONZALEZ and GELBOIN 1994). There is considerable variation among human subjects in the hepatic level of CYP1A2 mRNA and CYP1A2 protein; the highest levels tend to be found in cigarette smokers (SCHWEIKL et al. 1993). The fact that CYP1A2 in humans is confined to liver coupled with the fact that CYP1A2 is the primary pathway for caffeine metabolism has led to noninvasive tests for CYP1A2 activity based upon measurement of caffeine metabolites in urine. By the caffeine-phenotyping method KALOW and TANG (1991, 1993) showed that hepatic CYP1A2 activity in human subjects was induced in a manner that was correlated with the number of cigarettes smoked and with the level of the nicotine metabolite, cotinine, excreted in urine. Caffeine metabolism also can be induced in human hepatocyte cell lines derived from normal liver when these cells are exposed in culture to the smoke constituent, dibenz[*a,h*]anthracene; this increased caffeine metabolism may be due to induction of CYP1A2 (ROBERTS et al. 1994). In addition to smoking, the metabolism of caffeine and other selective CYP1A2 substrates such as phenacetin also is elevated in persons eating large amounts of charcoal-broiled foods or cruciferous vegetables and in subjects given the proton pump inhibitor omeprazole (reviewed in OKEY 1992; ROST et al. 1992). CYP1A2 is a major enzyme in the bioactivation of many chemical carcinogens (GUENGERICH and SHIMADA 1991); however, it has not yet been established whether the risk of hepatotoxicity is increased in humans following elevation of hepatic CYP1A2 by smoking or other chemical exposures.

The mechanism by which CYP1A1 and CYP1A2 are induced involves binding of the inducing agent to a soluble intracellular protein, the AH (aromatic hydrocarbon) receptor. The AH receptor mechanism was initially discovered in rodent liver (POLAND et al. 1976). Experiments over the past decade indicate that the induction mechanism is fundamentally the same in humans as in rodents (OKEY 1992; SWANSON and BRADFIELD 1993; QUATTROCHI 1994). The AH receptor has been demonstrated in many human cells and tissues including human liver (reviewed in OKEY et al. 1994a,b) as well as in human hepatoma cell lines in culture (LABRUZZO et al. 1989; ROBERTS et al. 1990, 1991).

Polymorphisms are not known in the coding regions of human *CYP1A1* or *CYP1A2* genes. The wide variation in *CYP1A* enzyme activities among human subjects may be related to polymorphisms in the regulatory mechanism, including the AH receptor (NEBERT et al. 1993; GONZALEZ and GELBOIN 1994) and the search for such regulatory polymorphisms is an active field of investigation.

b) *CYP2E1*

The levels and activity of CYP2E1 vary among livers from different humans and this variation may be dependent upon the degree of exposure to inducing agents (GONZALEZ and GELBOIN 1994). The most commonly encountered CYP2E1 inducer in humans is ethanol, but CYP2E1 also can be induced by a wide variety of volatile solvents. Elevation of CYP2E1 appears to be primarily via stabilization of the protein by the inducer rather than through increased transcription of the *CYP2E1* gene (GONZALEZ and GELBOIN 1994). CYP2E1 induction may be of considerable toxicologic importance because this enzyme activates many small molecules (see below).

c) *CYP3A Enzymes*

Enzymes in the CYP3A subfamily are the most abundant P450s in human liver and they are susceptible to induction by a wide variety of agents in laboratory animals and in humans (Table 1). One of the substrates bioactivated by *CYP3A* enzymes is the potent hepatocarcinogen, aflatoxin B_1 (GONZALEZ and GELBOIN 1994). *CYP3A* enzymes also can bioactivate acetaminophen (see below); hence induction of *CYP3A* enzymes has the potential to substantially alter activation or clearance of some important hepatotoxins.

This leads to the question of whether induction of P450 enzymes is beneficial to the host or detrimental. In laboratory animals it is possible to manipulate P450 levels, through induction, in such ways that toxicity is enhanced – for example, P450 induction by phenobarbital potentiates the hepatotoxicity of bromobenzene in rodents and also potentiates hepatotoxicity of the anticonvulsant drug valproic acid. On the other hand, it also is possible to reduce bromobenzene hepatotoxicity in rodents by inducing P450s with 3-methylcholanthrene (reviewed in OKEY 1992). Whether P450 induction is "good" or "bad" for the liver depends upon very particular circumstances including definition of the specific P450 induced, the chemical identity of the potential toxicant and the route of exposure to that toxicant. It is perhaps fortunate that induction of P450 enzymes (which may bioactivate drugs to toxic metabolites) often is accompanied by induction of phase II enzymes that can conjugate the reactive metabolites and facilitate excretion. From the viewpoint of the integrated organism, P450 induction in liver, in most instances, will be highly beneficial since it enhances first-pass clearance of potentially toxic xenobiotic chemicals and reduces the exposure of extrahepatic tissues to these agents.

3. P450 Inhibition

Given that those P450s which metabolize xenobiotic chemicals usually recognize a very large number of substrates, it would be expected that competitive inhibition will be common. Indeed, reciprocal inhibition studies are a very useful tool for determining if two or more different substrates share the same enzymatic pathway. Substrate overlap also means that very few inhibitors are specific to a single P450 species; at best the inhibitor may be selective rather than truly specific. Table 1 lists some P450 inhibitors that act on the P450s that are most prominent in human liver. One of the most interesting inhibitors to emerge in recent years is grapefruit juice, which has been shown to inhibit metabolism of substances such as felodipine and nifedipine (substrates for CYP3A3/4; BAILEY et al. 1994) and caffeine (a CYP1A2 substrate; FUHR et al. 1993). Part of the inhibition may be due to naringin, the chemical which gives grapefruit juice its distinctive flavor, but it appears that grapefruit juice also contains other unidentified P450 inhibitors.

The grapefruit juice story illustrates the fact that not all modulators of P450s are drugs and environmental chemicals; dietary constituents also are important. As was the case with P450 induction, there is no basis to state that P450 inhibition will be universally beneficial or universally detrimental. Inhibition of hepatic P450s might be beneficial to the liver itself, but could lead to an increased exposure of extrahepatic tissues to potential toxicants (YANG et al. 1994).

4. Liver Disease: Effects on Drug Biotransformation

As a final brief word on factors that alter P450 activity in liver, the very existence of liver disease itself can have a major impact on drug biotransformation and levels of P450 enzymes. Viral or bacterial infections in laboratory animals can significantly reduce the biotransformation and elimination of a wide variety of drugs (RENTON and KNICKLE 1990) and this may be associated with either an increase or a decrease in the capacity to bioactivate xenobiotic chemicals to toxic or carcinogenic products (CRIBB et al. 1994). Cytochrome P450 levels also generally are decreased in various hepatic disease states such as cirrhosis and chemical hepatitis and this impairs drug elimination (MURRAY 1992). Thus "faulty" metabolism of drugs can lead to liver disease and liver disease can lead to "faulty" metabolism of drugs.

II. Reaction Mechanism

P450s in the CYP1, CYP2 and CYP3 families are able to catalyze oxidation of many substrates that are quite diverse in size (for example, ethylene: M_r 28, and cyclosporine A: M_r 1201) and shape (planar polyaromatic hydrocarbons and large, "bulky" molecules such as cyclosporine A). Although known substrates for the entire P450 superfamily number in the thousands, the reactions catalyzed are much more limited, encompassing aliphatic oxidation, aromatic hydroxylation, heteroatom (nitrogen, sulfur) oxygenation and heteroatom dealkylation reactions. These reactions are characterized by the incorporation of one oxygen atom from molecular oxygen (O_2) into the substrate while the other oxygen atom combines with two hydrogen atoms (from NADPH) to form H_2O and share a common stoichiometry (Fig. 2):

$$RH + 2NADPH + O_2 \rightarrow ROH + 2NADP + H_2O$$

To facilitate this process, there are two features that are common to all P450s: a prosthetic heme group and a conserved active-site cysteine to which the heme iron is anchored. The heme iron has six potential ligand positions, four of which join the iron to the four pyrrole nitrogens of the heme ring. The fifth (thiolate) ligand is the sulfur atom of the conserved active-site cysteine while the sixth coordination site undergoes reversible, weak ligation to an oxygen-containing molecule. In the endoplasmic reticulum, P450s exist in an equilibrium between a hexacoordinate form or "low-spin" state in which the

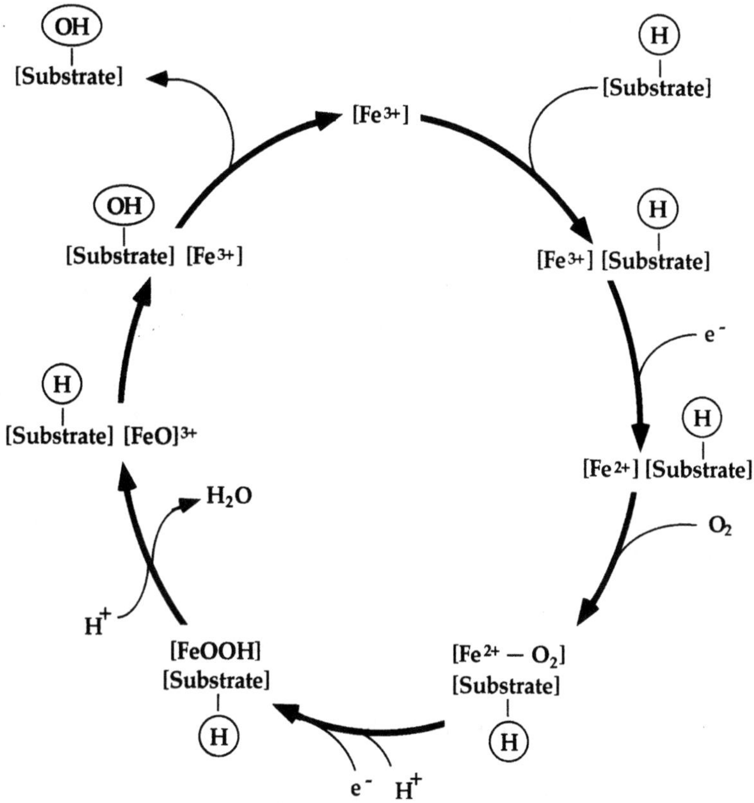

Fig. 2. Cytochrome P450 catalytic cycle. The process of P450-mediated oxidation is initiated by substrate binding to the ferric (Fe^{3+}) form of the enzyme. The substrate-induced conversion from the low-spin to the high-spin state facilitates transfer of the first electron from NADPH via NADPH-dependent cytochrome P450 reductase to the heme iron, resulting in its reduction to the ferrous (Fe^{2+}) state. The ferrous form of P450 then binds O_2 and, following the addition of a proton and a second electron (from either NADPH-reductase or cytochrome b_5), an FeOOH complex is formed. The release of H_2O leaves an $(FeO)^{3+}$ complex that directly oxidizes the substrate

heme iron is located in the plane of the tetra-pyrrole ring (one electron in the outer orbitals) and a pentacoordinate or "high-spin" form in which there is no sixth ligand, and the iron is skewed out of plane towards the thiolate ligand (five unpaired electrons in the outer orbitals).

The process of P450-mediated oxidation is initiated by substrate binding to the ferric (Fe^{3+}) form of the enzyme (Fig. 2). In the most common situation, the insertion of substrate into the substrate-binding site prevents the partial sixth ligation, thereby converting the P450 from the low-spin to the high-spin state. This substrate-induced spin-state conversion facilitates transfer of the first electron from NADPH via NADPH-dependent cytochrome P450 reductase to the heme iron, resulting in its reduction to the ferrous (Fe^{2+}) state. The ferrous form of P450 then binds O_2 and, following the addition of a proton and a second electron (from either NADPH reductase or cytochrome b_5), an FeOOH complex is formed. The release of H_2O leaves an $(FeO)^{3+}$ complex that directly oxidizes the substrate.

While the heme moiety is responsible for the common reaction mechanism among P450s, the substrate preference of an individual P450 is a function of the apoprotein component. Based on sequence alignment studies with members of the CYP2 family, GOTOH (1992) has identified six distinct, highly variable amino acid sequences distributed among the more conserved regions. He proposed that these hypervariable regions (or substrate recognition sequences) were responsible for the unique substrate recognition patterns of individual members of the CYP2 family. This has been confirmed by several studies comparing the structure-activity relationships between P450s within the same family or subfamily, allelic variants of the same P450 and P450s in which single amino acids have been altered by site-directed mutagenesis. In all cases, amino acids identified as critical for substrate specificity fall within or near these putative substrate recognition sequences (HALPERT and HE 1993; HSU et al. 1993; HE et al. 1994).

III. Drug Biotransformation and Drug Toxicity

1. Cytochrome P450 and Bioactivation

In most cases, P450-mediated oxidative metabolism gives rise to chemicaly stable metabolites which have (a) no pharmacological activity, (b) reduced or increased activity relative to the parent compound or (c) a qualitative change in pharmacological activity (i.e., imipramine demethylation to desipramine converts a serotonin uptake inhibitor to a norepinephrine uptake inhibitor). Structural modifications from P450 biotransformation may also result in bioactivation to reactive, electrophilic metabolites capable of interacting covalently with cellular macromolecules (Fig. 3). Modification of protein targets can result in end organ toxicities (liver necrosis, nephrotoxicity), hypersensitivity reactions or teratogenicity. Alterations in nucleic acids can lead to mutagenesis and carcinogenesis. Examples of potentially hepatotoxic drugs and other xenobiotics that are bioactivated by cytochromes P450 to reactive metabolites are listed in Table 2.

2. Activation/Detoxification Balance

Biotransformation of xenobiotic chemicals into excretable products is essential to survival for organisms living in a "chemically hostile" world. P450 enzymes are indispensable to biotransformation and elimination of lipophilic drugs and environmental chemicals. Yet P450s also bioactivate many xenobiotics into toxic reactive metabolites, an activity, per se, that clearly is deleterious to the host.

From an evolutionary perspective, the beneficial actions of P450s, in concert with other phase I and phase II enzymes, outweigh the risks associated

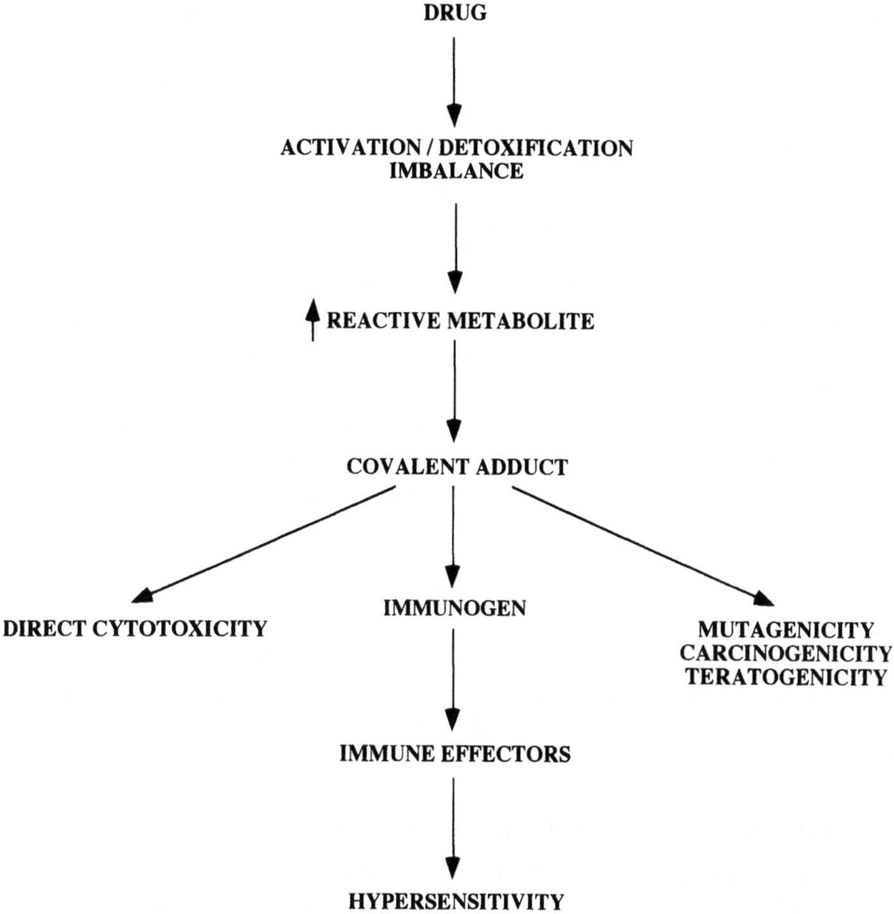

Fig. 3. Role of reactive metabolites in drug toxicity

Table 2. Potentially hepatotoxic drugs and other xenobiotics bioactivated to reactive intermediates by cytochromes P450. (Adapted from GUENGERICH and SHIMADA 1991; BOELSTERLI 1993; PESSAYRE 1993)

Drug	Reference
Acetaminophen	PATTEN et al. 1993
Amineptine	GENÈVE et al. 1987; LARREY et al. 1989
Amitriptyline	RILEY et al. 1990
Carbamazepine	PIRMOHAMED et al. 1992a,b
Carbon tetrachloride	DAVIES et al. 1986
Cocaine	PELLINEN et al. 1994
Diclofenac	KRETZ-ROMMEL and BOELSTERLI 1993
Erythromycin	DANAN et al. 1981
Ethanol	RYAN et al. 1985
Halothane	GANDOLFI et al. 1980
Isoniazid	TIMBRELL et al. 1980
Phenytoin	RILEY et al. 1990
Tienilic acid	LÓPEZ-GARCIA et al. 1993, 1994
Trichlorethylene	ALLEMAND et al. 1978
Valproic acid	RETTIE et al. 1987

with bioactivation to reactive metabolites. The current human repertoire of phase I and phase II enzymes may not always act in an ideal way to preserve the integrity of the host. However, in most instances the bulk of the myriad of ingested lipophilic xenobiotics compounds is excreted, as innocuous metabolites, without adverse effects on the host. Those instances in which overt toxicity is produced in the host typically result either from the detoxification pathways being overwhelmed by reactive metabolites (as in the case of acetaminophen overdose) or from a rare combination of failures in the host biotransformation defense mechanisms coupled with an "idiosyncratic" sensitivity to the products of drug biotransformation. The biochemical and immunologic mixture of factors that leads to "idiosyncratic" susceptibility may not be the same for all individuals. The elucidation of factors underlying idiosyncratic reactions remains a major challenge in drug-induced hepatotoxicity.

The role of biotransformation reactions in mediating drug activation and detoxification (and, by extension, possible toxicity) is a complex interplay of many variables. Knowledge of the human P450s and other enzymes responsible for generating specific reactive intermediates or nontoxic metabolites is critical for developing models of individual susceptibility to hepatotoxic events and for determining the propensity of a given compound to produce a hepatotoxic response.

3. "Probe Drugs" for Determining P450 Activities in Humans In Vivo

For purposes of both research and clinical management it would be of great value to be able to determine the level and activity of specific P450 enzymes in human subjects without needing to rely upon invasive tests such as liver biopsies. Properties of an ideal probe drug include: (a) that it can be

Table 3. Potential noninvasive assays to determine activity of individual P450 enzymes in human subjects. (From GUENGERICH and SHIMADA 1991)

P450 species	Diagnostic catalytic activity
CYP1A2	Phenacetin *O*-deethylation
	Caffeine demethylation
CYP2A6	Coumarin 7-hydroxylation
CYP2C9	Tolbutamide hydroxylation
CYP2D6	Debrisoquine 4-hydroxylation
	Sparteine δ-2 and δ-4 oxidation
	Dextromethorphan *O*-demethylation
CYP2E1	Chlorzoxazone 6-hydroxylation
CYP3A4	Nifedipine oxidation
	Erythromycin *N*-demethylation
	Dapsone *N*-hydroxylation
	Lidocaine *N*-deethylation
	Cortisol 6β-hydroxylation

harmlessly administered to a broad range of healthy subjects or patients, (b) that its metabolites be excreted in urine, saliva or breath at levels easily measured by standard chemical methods and (c) that it be metabolized exclusively by a single species of P450. For many forms of P450, probe drugs specific to the P450 have not yet been developed. The very fact that there is extensive overlap in substrate recognition among many members of the P450 superfamily makes it difficult to identify chemical probes whose metabolic products are solely produced by a single P450. Nevertheless, in recent years several probe drugs have proven very useful in phenotyping human subjects for certain P450 pathways; these are listed in Table 3.

C. Mechanisms of P450-Mediated Liver Injury

Drugs implicated in the development of hepatic injury mumber in the hundreds (BIOUR et al. 1994) and are classified for mechanistic purposes as "intrinsic" or "idiosyncratic" hepatotoxins (ZIMMERMAN 1990). Intrinsic hepatotoxity refers to events that are dose dependent and largely predictable from animal studies, for example, acetaminophen- and carbon tetrachloride-induced hepatotoxicity. In contrast, idiosyncratic hepatotoxicity is unpredictable from animal studies, is independent of the dose administered and is determined by (as yet) poorly understood characteristics unique to susceptible individuals. The idiosyncrasy may be either metabolic or immunologic, with the latter being more common. Regardless of whether the mechanism is intrinsic or idiosyncratic, it appears that reactive drug metabolites, rather than the parent compound, are responsible for the toxic effects.

I. Reactive Metabolites

The "reactivity" of metabolites is best understood in terms of a continuum ranging from stable metabolites that exit the organ where they are formed and are excreted, to ultra-short-lived reactive metabolites that form covalent adducts at their site of generation, thereby inactivating the enzyme (GUENGERICH and LIEBLER 1985). In between are reactive intermediates that can leave the tissue of origin (long lived), those that are sufficiently stable to leave the cells of origin but not the tissue (intermediate lived) and those that diffuse away from the enzyme of origin but are inactivated before they can leave the cell (short lived).

Cytochrome P450-mediated bioactivation can result in several different "reactive" species including free radical compounds and other electrophilic metabolites such as aromatic and aliphatic epoxides, quinoneimines and acyl halides (Fig. 4). The potentially harmful sequelae of these reactive metabolites are dependent on the chemical reactivity of the metabolite and the nature of the cellular target. Cellular damage may result from covalent modification of cellular macromolecules (proteins) or by noncovalent interactions such as oxidative stress. Some toxic species, such as quinones and related compounds,

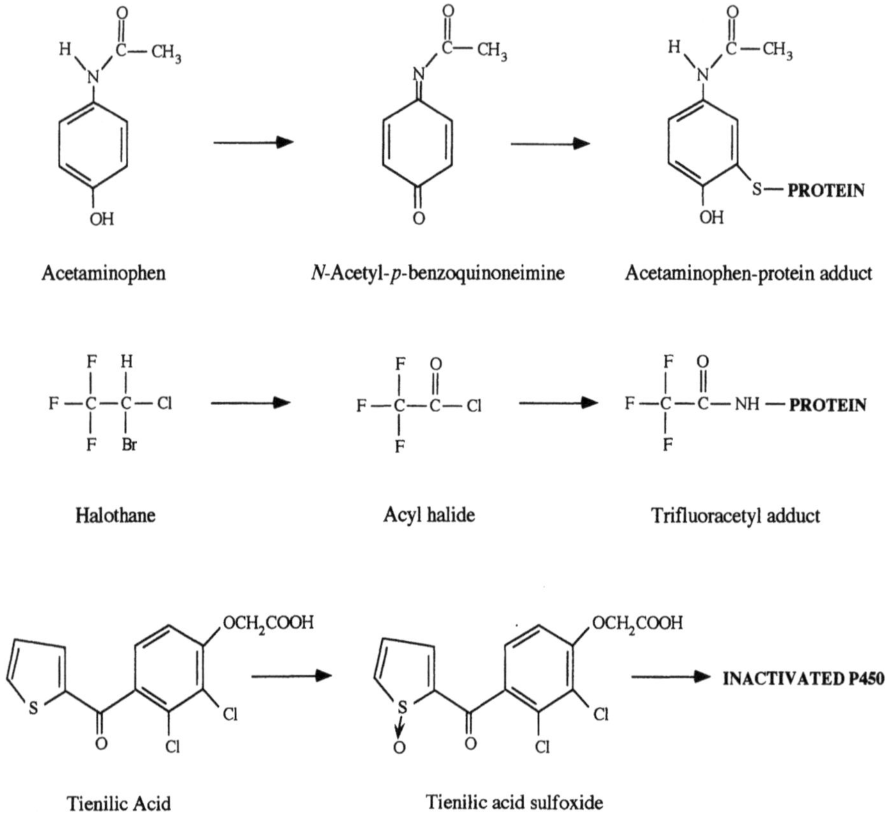

Fig. 4. Examples of hepatotoxic drugs and associated reactive intermediates

interact with biological systems by both covalent and noncovalent mechanisms such that it can be difficult to determine the relative contribution of each pathway to the overall toxic event.

1. Noncovalent Interactions

Noncovalent modification of proteins may occur as a consequence of interactions between rective oxygen metabolites and cellular constituents. Termed "oxidative stress," the toxic effects may manifest as glutathione depletion, alteration in redox balance or lipid peroxidation. The reactive oxygen species superoxide, hydrogen peroxide and hydroxyl radical are interrelated oxidizing agents. For example, superoxide can dismutate, either enzymatically or nonenzymatically, to form hydrogen peroxide and oxygen. The extremely reactive hydroxyl radical can be formed from either hydrogen peroxide or superoxide. Reactive oxygen species may be formed by redox cycling, a process in which a compound such as nitrofurantoin is reduced by an intracellular reductant (NADPH) to an intermediate (free radical) that is subsequently oxidized by molecular oxygen producing superoxide and regenerating the parent compound. The parent compound can then undergo another cycle of reduction and oxidation; this futile recycling will eventually lead to depletion of intracellular reducing equivalents, and cellular defense mechanisms such as glutathione stores and glutathione peroxidase will be compromised. Likewise, enzymatic bioactivation may result in a metabolite capable of undergoing redox cycling. Subsequent oxidation of cellular proteins may result in functional inactivation which could lead to cell death.

2. Covalent Adduct Formation

Covalent adduct formation refers to the irreversible binding of a drug or drug metabolite to a cellular macromolecule which, for the purposes of this review, is the chemical interaction between a reactive metabolite and relatively electron rich or nucleophilic amino acids in the target protein. Irreversible binding in this context is defined as the retention of radiolabeled drug after exhaustive washings with polar and organic solvents until no further radiolabel is detected in the washes. Thus, a covalent interaction is inferred from irreversible binding data rather than being formally elucidated at a structural level.

Several drugs implicated in hepatotoxic reactions form covalent adducts with hepatic proteins which in most, but not all, cases is due to bioactivation by a cytochrome P450 enzyme. There are two general mechanisms by which covalent drug-protein interactions are thought to result in end organ toxicity. First, covalent interaction may interfere with the normal functioning of the target macromolecule. If this function is critical for cell viability – for example, energy production or ion homeostasis – the reactive metabolite may be directly cytotoxic. A role for covalent binding in mediating direct toxicity is largely inferred from findings that the degree of hepatocellular damage parallels the extent of covalent binding. However, a causal relationship between covalent binding of drug or metabolite to a cellular protein and the observed hepatotoxicity has been difficult to demonstrate. It is now apparent that the ability of a drug or metabolite to form a covalent adduct is of less importance than understanding the particular protein target(s) of the reactive metabolite and the functional role of those proteins in the cell.

The second general mechanism accounts for the apparent immune involvement in idiosyncratic hepatotoxicity. It has been proposed that covalent adduct formation produces a drug-modified protein that is potentially immunogenic, that is, capable of initiating an immune response. Most organic compounds are generally assumed to be too small (less than 1000 daltons) to be immunogenic themselves (Park et al. 1987). Although compounds such as penicillin, penicillamine and captopril are chemically reactive, most drugs associated with hepatotoxicity and other hypersensitivity reactions are not. Hence, bioactivation of the small drug molecule (hapten) is required to form a drug-carrier complex that can elicit the formation of specific immune effectors such as antibodies, T cells or both. The targets of the immune responses or antigenic determinants (epitopes) may include the free hapten or the bound derivative of the drug. New antigenic determinants might also arise from conformation changes created by hapten binding or from native carrier epitopes that, as a consequence of covalent adduct formation, are no longer perceived as self and bypass self tolerance (POHL et al. 1988; POHL 1990). Immune involvement in drug hepatotoxicity is not unreasonable given the liver's inherent capacity to generate covalent adducts and thus potentially antigenic species.

Much of our current understanding of the role of drug bioactivation and covalent adduct formation in direct or immunologically mediated drug toxicity has been derived from work with model compounds such as acetaminophen and halothane. These are discussed in more detail below, focusing, when known, on the role of specific human cytochromes P450 in generating reactive metabolites, on the cellular targets of those metabolites and on the toxic consequences of the interactions.

II. P450s as Targets of Immune Effectors

Hepatic damage involving the cytochromes P450 may occur independent of their role in drug bioactivation. In 1973, an autoantibody with a characteristic immunofluorescence pattern was reported in patients with hepatitis B surface antigen-negative liver disease (RIZZETTO et al. 1973). This antibody was termed anti-liver/kidney microsomal (anti-LKM) antibody because its binding to antigens in hepatocyte cytoplasm and the distal third of the proximal renal tubule could be removed by preadsorption with liver microsomes (SMITH et al. 1974). With the discovery of two additional, different antimicrosomal antibodies, LKM antibodies were renamed LKM_1. Patients with anti-LKM_1 rarely possess antinuclear or anti-smooth muscle antibodies, and it was proposed that the autoimmune hepatitis associated with anti-LKM_1 antibodies be called autoimune hepatitis type II (HOMBERG et al. 1987). The microsomal antigen was determined to be a 50-kDa protein (ALVAREZ et al. 1985) that was subsequently identified as the polymorphically expressed debrisoquine hydroxylase, CYP2D6 (GUEGUEN et al. 1988; KIFFEL et al. 1989; MANNS et al. 1989).

A second type of antimicrosomal antibody, anti-LKM_2, can be distinguished from anti-LKM_1 by its reactivity with the initial third of the proximal renal tubule. This has been observed in patients with tienilic acid-induced hepatitis (HOMBERG et al. 1984). Antimicrosomal antibodies of the third type do not react with renal tissue at all and are called anti-liver microsomal (anti-LM) antibodies. This particular fluorescent pattern was first observed in hepatitis associated with the antihypertensive agent dihydralazine (NATAF et al. 1986), but has also been observed in one child with autoimmune hepatitis (MANNS et al. 1990). The two human autoantigens have been identified as CYP2C9 for anti-LKM_2 (LECOEUR et al. 1994) and CYP1A2 for anti-LM (BOURDI et al. 1990; MANNS et al. 1990). Tienilic acid- and dihydralazine-induced hepatitis are discussed in more detail later.

The appearance of anti-cytochrome P450 antibodies in non-drug-related hepatotoxicity is particularly intriguing. One possibility is that dietary components are metabolized by P450s to reactive intermediates that modify the P450 structure, resulting in an immunogenic species (WATKINS 1991). Another possibility arises from studies investigating the region of the P450 autoantigens recognized by patient antibodies. Three groups have mapped independently the epitope recognized by anti-LKM_1 (anti-CYP2D6) antibodies to a linear segment centering around the consensus sequence DPAQPPRD (Asp-Pro-Ala-Gln-Pro-Pro-Arg-Asp). Homologies have been found between the mapped amino acid segments and herpes simplex virus type 1 and hepatitis C virus (HCV) proteins, suggesting that mimicry between CYP2D6 and viral antigens may occur (GUEGUEN et al. 1991; MANNS et al. 1991; YAMAMOTO et al. 1993a). The relationship between HCV infection and type II autoimmune hepatitis has been of particular interest to several groups and there now appear to be two distinct populations of patients with anti-CYP2D6 antibodies: (a) LKM_1-positive patients without HCV markers who tend to be young females with other associated autoimmune disorders or a family history of autoimmune hepatitis who respond to immunosuppressive therapy and (b) LKM_1-positive patients with HCV markers who are more likely to be older males without other autoimmune manifestations and who may respond better to antiviral therapy. Recent data suggest that anti-LKM_1 antibodies from patients with autoimmune hepatitis type II recognize a linear epitope while those from HCV-positive patients recognize a conformational epitop(s) (YAMAMOTO et al. 1993b). Clearly, much remains to be elucidated concerning the link between anti-LKM_1 antibodies and HCV. A more complete discussion of the issues and controversies can be found elsewhere (VERGANI and MIELI-VERGANI 1993a).

D. Specific Drugs/P450s and Liver Injury

Several drugs associated with hepatotoxicity, whether "intrinsic" or "idiosyncratic," covalently interact with hepatic proteins. In many cases, the specific target protein modified by the reactive metabolite has been identified (BOELSTERLI 1993). It must be reiterated, however, that the functional consequences of covalent or noncovalent interactions are less clear. Some specific examples that illustrate the complexities of these processes are presented in the following section with an emphasis on the role played by cytochrome P450-mediated bioactivation.

I. Acetaminophen

A correlation between acetaminophen covalent binding to hepatic proteins and the incidence and severity of hepatic necrosis in mice was established more than 20 years ago (MITCHELL et al. 1973). Cytochrome P450 was implicated in the bioactivation process by studies using classical P450 inhibitors such as piperonyl butoxide and cobaltous chloride. It is now apparent that acetaminophen is metabolized by P450 enzymes directly to the reactive metabolite *N*-acetyl-*p*-benzoquinone imine (DAHLIN et al. 1984). After therapeutic doses, the small amount of reactive metabolite formed is promptly detoxified by cellular glutathione to form 3-(glutathione-*S*-yl)acetaminophen. After toxic doses, glutathione is depleted and the reactive metabolite binds to proteins that, when released following lysis of hepatocytes, can be detected by immunological reagents specific for 3-(cystein-*S*-yl)acetaminophen derivatives (ROBERTS et al. 1987).

The fact that there is a correlation between the degree of P450-mediated bioactivation of acetaminophen to 3-(cystein-*S*-yl)acetaminophen adducts and the severity of hepatic necrosis does not necessarily imply a causal relationship. Two dimethylated acetaminophen analogues – 3,5-dimethyl acetaminophen and 2,6-dimethyl acetaminophen – are also bioactivated to the corresponding quinone imine metabolites by cytochrome P450. However, the relative propensity of acetaminophen and these two analogues to produce hepatotoxicity does not correlate with their ability to form covalent adducts (BIRGE et al. 1988). Mechanistic studies have demonstrated that the toxic consequences of bioactivation differ for each compound despite the structural similarity of the reactive metabolites. For example, alkylation of critical protein thiols appears to predominate for acetaminophen. Despite identification of a 56-kDa selenium-binding protein (PUMFORD et al. 1990, 1992) and a 44-kDa microsomal protein (BARTOLONE et al. 1987) as the primary cellular targets of intracellularly generated *N*-acetyl-*p*-benzoquinone imine, a causal relationship with cellular toxicity remains to be established. In contrast, for 3,5-dimethyl acetaminophen-dependent toxicity, oxidation of protein thiol groups is important while 2,6-dimethyl acetaminophen toxicity is dependent on a combination of covalent adduct formation and lipid peroxidation (PORUBEC et al. 1987). Thus, bioactivation of acetaminophen or its dimethyl analogues by cytochrome(s) P450 appears to be essential for manifestation of toxicity whereas the ultimate mechanism of toxicity is dependent on the specific chemical properties of the reactive metabolite.

The formation of acetaminophen-glutathione adducts has been exploited for studies investigating the abilities of individual human P450s to generate the reactive *N*-acetyl-*p*-benzoquinone imine. Studies using various experimental approaches have revealed a role for CYP1A2, CYP2E1 and CYP3A4 in bioactivating acetaminophen to reactive species detected as glutathione conjugates (RAUCY et al. 1989; PATTEN et al. 1993; THUMMEL et al. 1993b). Acetaminophen has the highest affinity for CYP3A4 ($150 \mu M$) and this P450 contributes appreciably to *N*-acetyl-*p*-benzoquinone imine formation at therapeutically relevant drug concentrations (THUMMEL et al. 1993b). At higher acetaminophen concentrations, the importance of CYP3A4 declines such that in overdose situations (plasma concentrations exceeding $2 mM$) bioactivation by CYP2E1 and CYP1A2 predominates (RAUCY et al. 1989; PATTEN et al. 1993). Of these, CYP2E1 appears to be quantitatively more important based on a threefold higher affinity and approximately fivefold greater product formation compared to CYP1A2 (PATTEN et al. 1993). These results suggest that concomitant administration of inducers of CYP3A4 or CYP2E1 inducers could predispose patients to acetaminophen hepatotoxicity at lower than conventional "toxic" doses. This appears to be the case since both chronic anticonvulsant therapy (leading to CYP3A induction) and isoniazid treatment (CYP2E1 induction) have been reported to potentiate acetaminophen hepatotoxicity (MURPHY et al. 1990; BRAY et al. 1992). It has also been suggested that chronic alcoholics (associated with CYP2E1 induction) are at increased risk (GOLDFINGER et al. 1978). Therefore, susceptibility to acetaminophen hepatotoxicity is a function of an individual's particular P450 profile, at least in terms of the relative amounts of CYP3A4, CYP2E1 and CYP1A2, and their exposure to drugs and other agents known to modulate cytochrome P450 expression (see Table 1).

II. Halothane

Fulminant liver necrosis is a rare, idiosyncratic response to the inhalational anesthetic halothane. This halothane hepatitis has an estimated incidence of 1:30000 exposure, and is approximately ten fold more frequent following repeated exposure (POHL et al. 1988). An immunologic etiology has been proposed based on the identification of specific IgG antibodies directed against hepatic proteins that have been modified by a trifluoroacetyl group derived from halothane. These neoantigens are primarily associated with the lumen of the endoplasmic reticulum (KENNA et al. 1992), and may be involved with cellular calcium homeostasis and protein stability (POHL 1990). A 100-kDa trifluoroacetylated protein has been identified as ERp99 (endoplasmin; 94-kDa glucose-regulated protein) which is a calcium-binding protein and also binds malfolded proteins (THOMASSEN et al. 1990). Trifluoroacetyl conjugates of calreticulin (BUTLER et al. 1992), protein disulfide isomerase (MARTIN et al. 1993), a microsomal carboxylesterase (SATOH et al. 1989) and a 72-kDa heat shock protein (PUMFORD et al. 1993a) have all been isolated and found to be recognized to varying extents by antibodies from patients with halothane hepatitis. Current evidence indicates that all individuals exposed to halothane probably produce trifluoroacetylated proteins when exposed to halothane, but that only those individuals who develop the drug-induced disease present with antibodies against the modified proteins (KENNA et al. 1988a). Recent data indicate that the antitrifluoroacetyl antibodies found in halothane hepatitis also recognize lipoic acid-containing epitopes on the E2 subunit of pyruvate dehydrogenase (CHRISTEN et al. 1994). These data imply that the E2 subunit is an autoantigen in halothane hepatitis and that molecular mimicry between the structures of the trifluoroacetyl reactive metabolite of halothane and lipoic acid may be important in the pathogenesis of halothane hepatitis.

Halothane may be biotransformed by both reductive (AHR et al. 1982) and oxidative (GANDOLFI et al. 1980) P450-dependent pathways to potentially reactive metabolites. Studies with deuterated halothane indicate that the rate-limiting step in neoantigen formation is the breaking of the carbon–hydrogen bond. In addition, in vitro microsomal incubations with halothane led to neoantigens only under aerobic conditions, indicating that the oxidative trifluoroacetyl halide CF_3COCl (Fig. 4) rather than the reductive free radical $CF_3CHCl\bullet$ is responsible for neoantigen formation. Acylation of nucleophilic amino acids on target proteins, particularly the ε-amino group of lysine, produces the trifluoroacetyl-lysine-protein adducts recognized by patient antibodies (KENNA et al. 1988b).

Halothane bioactivation clearly appears to be a P450-dependent process, and available data implicate CYP2E1 in this process. In rats, the phenobarbital-inducible CYP2B can mediate trifluoroacetyl halide production and covalent adduct formation at high substrate concentrations (SATOH et al. 1985), whereas CYP2E1 is primarily responsible for this activity at lower concentrations (GRUENKE et al. 1988). In humans, CYP2E1 mediates the metabolism (defluorination) of other halogenated inhalational anesthetics such as enflurane (THUMMEL et al. 1993a), sevoflurane, isoflurane and methoxyflurane (KHARASCH and THUMMEL 1993). Structurally related compounds such as trichloroethylene, ethylene dichloride and 1,2-dichloropropane, among others, are bioactivated by CYP2E1 (GUENGERICH et al. 1991). Recent data indicate that human liver microsomal biotransformation of halothane (and the structurally related chlorofluorocarbon substitute 1,1-dichloro-2,2,2-trifluoroethane) to trifluoroacetic acid (via a reactive trifluoroacetyl halide) correlates with CYP2E1 content (URBAN et al. 1994). Thus, on the basis of available data, CYP2E1 appears responsible for halothane bioactivation in humans as well.

III. Tienilic Acid

Tienilic acid (also known as ticrynafen) was a uricosuric diuretic used in the management of hypertension until its withdrawal from sale in the United States in 1980 due to hepatic toxicity resembling viral hepatitis (ZIMMERMAN et al. 1984). An immunologic etiology is implied by the presence of fever, eosinophilic aggregates in the liver, prompt recurrence of clinical and serological features on rechallenge and the presence of unique antimicrosomal autoantibodies, termed anti-LKM-2, that decline with time after discontinuation of the drug (BEAUNE et al. 1987). LKM_2 autoantibodies can be distinguished from other antimicrosomal antibodies by their characteristic binding to the initial third of the proximal renal tubules. These autoantibodies are highly specific, recognizing CYP2C9 but not other members of the human CYP2C subfamily such as CYP2C8 or CYP2C18. CYP2C9 has special significance since it has been identified as the P450 responsible for tienilic acid bioactivation to a reactive metabolite that covalently binds to human liver microsomal proteins, possibly a thiophene *S*-oxide derivative (LÓPEZ-GARCIA et al. 1993, 1994). Moreover, the CYP2C9 protein is the target of the reactive metabolite; CYP2C9 oxidation of tienilic acid results in the formation of a reactive metabolite that binds in or near the active site of the P450 generating it (LECOEUR et al. 1994), ultimately resulting in inactivation of the enzyme (LÓPEZ-GARCIA et al. 1994). The anti-LKM-2 antibodies from patients inhibit CYP2C9 catalytic activity and appear to be true autoantibodies in that they recognize CYP2C9 without there being a strict requirement for drug to form part of the epitope.

This represents one of the few cases where there is a clear relationship between the cytochrome P450 responsible for drug bioactivation, the target of the reactive metabolite generated and the production of antibodies specific for the P450 that both produces and serves as the target of a reactive metabolite. However, several factors remain unresolved and are the subjects of ongoing research in this area. These include an understanding of how these drug-modified proteins are processed and presented to the immune system, and identification of the immune effectors responsible for the hepatotoxicity. It has been proposed that small amounts of CYPs 1A2, 2C, 2D6, 2E1 and 3A4 are present on hepatocyte plasma membranes and thus could be targets of immune effectors (LOEPER et al. 1993). However, while plasma membrane localization of P450s is generally accepted, there is some controversy as to whether the orientation (and thus accessibility to immune effectors) is cytosolic, corresponding to their orientation in the endoplasmic reticulum, or extracellular (VERGANI and MIELI-VERGANI 1993b; YAMAMOTO et al. 1993c).

IV. Dihydralazine

Like tienilic acid hepatitis, patients with dihydralazine-induced hepatitis have circulating antibodies which recognize a liver microsomal antigen. The different immunofluorescent staining pattern for these anti-LM antibodies implies that the autoantigen is distinct from either CYP2D6 or CYP2C9. Indeed, CYP1A2, has been identified as the human autoantigen in this case (BOURDI et al. 1990). The anti-CYP1A2 antibodies are quite specific since they do not recognize CYP1A1 despite its >80% homology with CYP1A2 (BOURDI et al. 1992).

A series of events analogous to those elucidated for tienilic acid has been proposed for dihydralazine: dihydralazine is bioactivated to a reactive metabolite that binds at or near the active site of the enzyme responsible for its bioactivation, in this case CYP1A2. The modified CYP1A2 then serves as an immunogen, leading to autoantibody formation. Direct reactive metabolite and covalent binding data in support of this model are limited. However, indirect data are consistent with the basic premise that CYP1A2 is involved in dihydralazine biotransformation; catalytic activities characteristic of CYP1A2 are inhibited in the presence of anti-LM-positive serum and are also inhibited by dihydralazine in a competitive manner (BOURDI et al. 1990). Moreover, addition of dihydralazine to human hepatocytes in culture is associated with a twofold increase in CYP1A-supported catalytic activities (BOURDI et al. 1992).

Although these data indicate that there is a relationship between dihydralazine and the CYP1A subfamily, the specific relationship between CYP1A2 and dihydralazine bioactivation remains to be determined.

V. Diclofenac

The nonsteroidal anti-inflammatory drug diclofenac has been associated with minor elevations of serum aminotransferase activity in approximately 15% of patients, and with rare cases of fulminant hepatic failure. Both direct cytotoxic and immunoallergic etiologies have been proposed for the severe toxic events (OULLETTE et al. 1991; PURCELL et al. 1991), but, to date, no drug- or organelle-specific antibodies have been identified in patient sera.

Diclofenac 4′-hydroxylation has been reported to be highly correlated with tolbutamide hydroxylation in human subjects, a reaction that is catalyzed by CYP2C9 and CYP2C10 (LEEMANN et al. 1993). In vitro studies with isolated rat hepatocytes suggest that the covalent binding of diclofenac to cellular proteins can be dissociated from the direct cytotoxic effects of the drug. Members of the rat CYP2C subfamily bioactivate diclofenac to a reactive intermediate that leads to acute lethal injury. In contrast, UDP-glucuronosyl transferases apparently bioactivate diclofenac to an acyl glucuronide intermediate that covalently modifies cellular proteins but that is not involved in the acute cytotoxicity (KRETZ-ROMMEL and BOELSTERLI 1993). Both radiochemical and immunochemical approaches have demonstrated that at least four proteins with apparent molecular masses between 50kDa and approximately 140kDa are selectively modified by diclofenac-reactive metabolites, primarily acyl glucuronides (PUMFORD et al. 1993b; KRETZ-ROMMEL and BOELSTERLI 1994). However, a recent report suggests that while the 70-, 110- and 140-kDa antigens are derived from diclofenac acyl glucuronide and are localized in the plasma membrane, the 50-kDa antigen is P450 dependent and microsomal in origin (HARGUS et al. 1994), possibly corresponding to a member of the rat CYP2C subfamily. Although similar studies have not been conducted with human hepatocytes, the cytotoxic and hypersensitivity features of reported cases of diclofenac hepatotoxicity may be a consequence of the relative production of directly cytotoxic CYP2C-generated metabolites and immunogenic acyl glucuronide adducts in susceptible individuals.

E. Conclusions

Many examples cited in this chapter establish that cytochromes P450 play at least three critical roles in drug-induced hepatotoxicity: (a) P450s are major pathways for bioactivation of parent drugs into reactive metabolites; (b) P450s frequently are cellular targets for reactive metabolites and (c), less frequently, P450s may be targets of immune effectors.

The dramatic improvement, especially over the last decade, in methods for detecting, identifying and characterizing individual forms of P450 has led to a much clearer understanding of which P450s are the primary activators and/or targets for specific drugs and environmental chemicals. Since it now is possible to genotype human subjects for several P450 polymorphisms and since it is becoming increasingly feasible to phenotype individuals for the actual level of expressed activity for many P450s, in principle we are much closer to being able to predict which patients might have increased risk of drug-induced hepatotoxicity from specific therapeutic agents. However, the quantitative importance of an individual P450 in bioactivation processes is likely dependent upon the repertoire of alternative biotransformation pathways, both phase I and phase II. Therefore, the practicality of implementing genotyping/phenotyping as routine pre-screening measures in the general population may be low. Nonetheless, in cases where there has been a family history of adverse reactions to certain drug categories or in cases where the individual patient previously has experienced an idiosyncratic reaction to any drug, it may eventually be both economically feasible and medically prudent to conduct genotyping/phenotyping tests before the first course of therapy. It must be kept in mind that, when there is a significant immune component to the hepatotoxic reaction, idiosyncrasy in the immune response is likely to be a more critical determinant of susceptibility than the genotype/phenotype of the particular cytochrome P450 involved.

The central challenge that persists is to determine the specific molecular, biochemical and cellular events that entrain from bioactivation and eventually manifest as hepatotoxicity. Although we have many clues as to relevant pathways, much of the link between bioactivation and ultimate toxic outcomes remains a black box. There are some common themes among the pathways for different drugs but it already is apparent that no single unifying scheme can be applied that will satisfactorily explain hepatotoxicity across all drug classes. However, recent developments in P450 research now make it feasible to identify the human P450(s) which are responsible for bioactivation. Similar advances will provide the key to tracking the fate of reactive metabolites and their cellular targets, and to elucidating the mechanisms of drug hepatotoxicity. The ultimate goals are to predict and prevent such adverse drug reactions.

References

Ahr HJ, King LJ, Nastainczyk W, Ullrich V (1982) The mechanism of reductive dehalogenation of halothane by liver cytochrome P-450. Biochem Pharmacol 31:383–390

Allemand H, Pessayre D, Descatoire V, Degott C, Feldmann G, Benhamou J-P (1978) Metabolic activation of trichlorethylene into a chemically reactive metabolite toxic to the liver. J Pharmacol Exp Ther 204:714–723

Alvarez F, Bernard O, Homberg JC, Kreibich G (1985) Anti-liver-kidney microsome antibody recognizes a 50000 molecular weight protein of the endoplasmic reticulum. J Exp Med 161:1231–1236

Bailey DG, Arnold JMO, Spence JD (1994) Grapefruit juice and drugs: how significant is the interaction? Clin Pharmacokinet 26:91–98

Bartolone JB, Sparks K, Cohen SD, Khairallah EA (1987) Immunochemical detection of acetaminophen-bound liver proteins. Biochem Pharmacol 36:1193–1196
Beaune P, Dansette PM, Mansuy D, Kiffel L, Finck M, Amar C, Leroux JP, Homberg JC (1987) Human anti-endoplasmic reticulum autoantibodies appearing in a drug-induced hepatitis are directed against a human liver cytochrome P-450 that hydroxylates the drug. Proc Natl Acad Sci USA 84:551–555
Biour M, Poupon R, Grangé J-D, Chazouillères O, Levy V-G, Bodin F, Cheymol G (1994) Hépatotoxicité des médicaments. 7e mise à jour du fichier bibliographique des atteintes hépatiques et des médicaments responsables. Gastroenterol Clin Biol 18:574–606
Birge RB, Bartolone JB, Nishanian EV, Bruno MK, Mangold JB, Cohen SD, Khairallah EA (1988) Dissociation of covalent binding from the oxidative effects of acetaminophen. Biochem Pharmacol 37:3383–3393
Boelsterli UA (1993) Specific targets of covalent drug-protein interactions in hepatocytes and their toxicological significance in drug-induced liver injury. Drug Metab Rev 25:395–451
Bourdi M, Larrey D, Nataf J, Bernuau J, Pessayre D, Iwasaki M, Guengerich FP, Beaune PH (1990) Anti-liver endoplasmic reticulum autoantibodies are directed against human cytochrome P-450IA2. J Clin Invest 85:1967–1973
Bourdi M, Gautier JC, Mircheva J, Larrey D, Guillouzo A, Andre C, Belloc C, Beaune PH (1992) Anti-liver microsomes autoantibodies and dihydralazine-induced hepatitis: specificity of autoantibodies and inductive capacity of the drug. Mol Pharmacol 42:280–285
Bray GP, Harrison PM, O'Grady JG, Tredger JM, Williams R (1992) Long term anticonvulsant therapy worsens outcome in paracetamol-induced fulminant hepatic failure. Hum Exp Toxicol 11:265–270
Butler LE, Thomassen D, Martin JL, Martin BM, Kenna JG, Pohl LR (1992) The calcium-binding protein calreticulin is covalently modified in rat liver by a reactive metabolite of the inhalation anesthetic halothane. Chem Res Toxicol 5:406–410
Christen U, Quinn J, Yeaman SJ, Kenna JG, Clarke JB, Gandolfi AJ, Gut J (1994) Identification of the dihydrolipoamide acetyltransferase subunit of the human pyruvate dehydrogenase complex as an autoantigen in halothane hepatitis. Eur J Biochem 223:1035–1047
Cribb AE, Delaporte E, Kim SG, Novak RF, Renton KW (1994) Regulation of cytochrome P-4501A and cytochrome P-4502E induction in the rat during the production of interferon α/β. J Pharmacol Exp Ther 268:487–494
Dahlin DC, Miwa GT, Lu AYH, Nelson SD (1984) N-Acetyl-p-benzoquinone imine: a cytochrome P-450-mediated oxidation product of acetaminophen. Proc Natl Acad Sci USA 81:1327–1331
Danan G, Descatoire V, Pessayre D (1981) Self-induction by erythromycin of its own transformation into a metabolite forming an inactive complex with reduced cytochrome P-450. J Pharmacol Exp Ther 218:509–514
Davies HW, Britt SG, Pohl LR (1986) Carbon tetrachloride and 2-isopropyl-4-pentenamide-induced inactivation of cytochrome P-450 leads to heme-derived protein adducts. Arch Biochem Biophys 244:387–392
de Morais SMF, Wilkinson GR, Blaisdell J, Nakamura K, Meyer UA, Goldstein JA (1994) The major genetic defect responsible for the polymorphism of *S*-mephenytoin metabolism in humans. J Biol Chem 269:15419–15422
Eichelbaum M, Gross AS (1990) The genetic polymorphism of debrisoquine/sparteine metabolism – clinical aspects. Pharmacol Ther 46:377–394
Forrester LM, Henderson CJ, Glancy MJ, Back DJ, Park BK, Ball SE, Kitteringham NR, McLaren AW, Miles JS, Skett P, Wolf CR (1992) Relative expression of cytochrome P450 isoenzymes in human liver and association with the metabolism of drugs and xenobiotics. Biochem J 281:359–368
Fritz S, Lindner W, Roots I, Frey BM, Küpfer A (1987) Stereochemistry of aromatic phenytoin hydroxylation in various drug hydroxylation phenotypes in humans. J Pharmacol Exp Ther 241:615–622

Fuhr U, Klittich K, Staib AH (1993) Inhibitory effect of grapefruit juice and its bitter principal, naringenin, on CYP1A2 dependent metabolism of caffeine in man. Br J Clin Pharmacol 35:431–436

Gandolfi AJ, White RD, Sipes IG, Pohl LR (1980) Bioactivation and covalent binding of halothane in vitro. Studies with [^{3}H]-and [^{14}C]-halothane. J Pharmacol Exp Ther 214:721–725

Genève J, Larrey D, Lettéron P, Descatoire V, Tinel M, Amouyal G, Pessayre D (1987) Metabolic activation of the tricyclic antidepressant amineptine. I. Cytochrome P-450-mediated in vitro covalent binding. Biochem Pharmacol 36:323–329

Goldfinger R, Ahmed KS, Pitchumoni CS, Wesely SA (1978) Concomitant alcohol and drug abuse enhancing acetaminophen toxicity. Am J Gastroenterol 70:385–388

Goldstein JA, Faletto MB, Romkes-Sparks M, Sullivan T, Kitareewan S, Raucy JL, Lasker JM, Ghanayem BI (1994) Evidence that CYP2C19 is the major (*S*)-mephenytoin 4′-hydroxylase in humans. Biochemistry 33:1743–1752

Gonzalez FJ, Gelboin HV (1994) Role of human cytochromes P450 in the metabolic activation of chemical carcinogens and toxins. Drug Metab Rev 26:165–183

Gotoh O (1992) Substrate recognition sites in cytochrome P450 family 2 (CYP2) proteins inferred from comparative analyses of amino acid and coding nucleotide sequences. J Biol Chem 267:83–90

Gruenke LD, Konopka K, Koop DR, Waskell LA (1988) Characterization of halothane oxidation by hepatic microsomes and purified cytochromes P-450 using a gas chromatografic mass spectrometric assay. J Pharmacol Exp Ther 246: 454–459

Gueguen M, Meunier-Rotival M, Bernard O, Alvarez F (1988) Anti-liver kidney microsome antibody recognizes a cytochrome P450 from the IID family. J Exp Med 168:801–806

Gueguen M, Boniface O, Bernard O, Clerc F, Cartwright T, Alvarez F (1991) Identification of the main epitope on human cytochrome P450 IID6 recognized by anti-liver kidney microsome antibody. J Autoimmun 4:607–615

Guengerich FP (1993) Cytochrome P450 enzymes. Am Sci 81:440–447

Guengerich FP, Liebler DC (1985) Enzymatic activation of chemicals to toxic metabolites. CRC Crit Rev Toxicol 14:259–307

Guengerich FP, Shimada T (1991) Oxidation of toxic and carcinogenic chemicals by human cytochrome P-450 enzymes. Chem Res Toxicol 4:391–407

Guengerich FP, Kim D-H, Iwasaki M (1991) Role of human cytochrome P-450 IIE1 in the oxidation of many low molecular weight cancer suspects. Chem Res Toxicol 4:168–179

Hakkola J, Pasanen M, Purkunen R, Saarikoski S, Pelkonen O, Mäenpää J, Rane A, Raunio H (1994) Expression of xenobiotic-metabolizing cytochrome P450 forms in human adult and fetal liver. Biochem Pharmacol 48:59–64

Halopert JR, He Y (1993) Engineering of cytochrome P450 2B1 specificity. Conversion of an androgen 16β-hydroxylase to a 15α-hydroxylase. J Biol Chem 268: 4453–4457

Hargus SJ, Amouzedeh HR, Pumford NR, Myers TG, McCoy SC, Pohl LR (1994) Metabolic activation and immunochemical localization of liver protein adducts of the nonsteroidal anti-inflammatory drug diclofenac. Chem Res Toxicol 7:575–582

He Y, Luo Z, Klekotka PA, Burnett VL, Halpert JR (1994) Structural determinants of cytochrome P450 2B1 specificity: evidence for five substrate recognition sites. Biochemistry 33:4419–4424

Homberg J, Abuaf N, Bernard O, Islam S, Alvarez F, Khalil SH, Poupon R, Darnis F, Lévy V-G, Grippon P, Opolon P, Bernuan J, Benhamou J-P, Alaqille D (1987) Chronic active hepatitis associated with anti-liver/kidney microsome antibody type I: a second type of "autoimmune" hepatitis. Hepatology 7:1333–1339

Homberg JC, André C, Abuaf N (1984) A new anti-liver-kidney microsome antibody (anti-LKM2) in tienilic acid-induced hepatitis. Clin Exp Immunol 55:561–570

Hsu M-H, Griffin KJ, Wang Y, Kemper B, Johnson EF (1993) A single amino acid substitution confers progesterone 6β-hydroxylase activity to rabbit cytochrome P450 2C3. J Biol Chem 268:6939–6944

Johansson I, Lundqvist E, Bertilsson L, Dahl M-L, Sjöqvist F, Ingelman-Sundberg M (1993) Inherited amplification of an active gene in the cytochrome P450 CYP2D locus as a cause of ultrarapid metabolism of debrisoquine. Proc Natl Acad Sci USA 90:11825–11829

Kalow W, Tang BK (1991) Caffeine as a metabolic probe: exploration of the enzyme-inducing effect of cigarette smoking. Clin Pharmacol Ther 49:44–48

Kalow W, Tang BK (1993) The use of caffeine for enzyme assays: a critical appraisal. Clin Pharmacol Ther 53:503–514

Kenna JG, Neuberger J, Williams R (1988a) Evidence for expression in human liver of halothane-induced neoantigens recognized by antibodies in sera from patients with halothane hepatitis. Hepatology 8:1635–1641

Kenna JG, Satoh H, Christ DD, Pohl LR (1988b) Metabolic basis for a drug hypersensitivity: antibodies in sera from patients with halothane hepatitis recognize liver neoantigens that contain the trifluoroacetyl group derived from halothane. J Pharmacol Exp Ther 245:1103–1109

Kenna JG, Martin JL, Pohl LR (1992) The topography of trifluoroacetylated protein antigens in liver microsomal fractions from halothane treated rats. Biochem Pharmacol 44:621–629

Kharasch ED, Thummel KE (1993) Identification of cytochrome P450 2E1 as the predominant enzyme catalyzing human liver microsomal defluorination of sevoflurane, isoflurane, and methoxyflurane. Anesthesiology 79:795–807

Kiffel L, Loeper J, Homberg JC, Leroux JP (1989) A human cytochrome P-450 is recognized by anti-liver/kidney microsome antibodies in autoimmune chronic hepatitis. Biochem Biophys Res Commun 159:283–289

Kretz-Rommel A, Boelsterli UA (1993) Diclofenac covalent protein binding is dependent on acyl glucuronide formation and is inversely related to P450-mediated acute cell injury in cultured rat hepatocytes. Toxicol Appl Pharmacol 120:155–161

Kretz-Rommel A, Boelsterli UA (1994) Selective protein adducts to membrane proteins in cultured rat hepatocytes exposed to diclofenac: radiochemical and immunochemical analysis. Mol Pharmacol 45:237–244

Labruzzo P, Yu XF, Dufresne MJ (1989) Induction of aryl hydrocarbon hydroxylase and demonstration of a specific nuclear receptor for 2,3,7,8-tetrachlorodibenzo-p-dioxin in two human hepatoma cell lines. Biochem Pharmacol 38:2339–2348

Larrey D, Berson A, Habersetzer F, Tinel M, Castot A, Babany G, Lettéron P, Freneaux E, Loeper J, Dansette P, Pessayre D (1989) Genetic predisposition to drug hepatotoxicity: role in hepatitis caused by amineptine, a tricyclic antidepressant. Hepatology 10:168–173

Lecoeur S, Bonierbale E, Challine D, Gautier JC, Valadon P, Dansette PM, Catinot R, Ballet F, Mansuy D, Beaune P (1994) Specificity of in vitro covalent binding of tienilic acid metabolites to human liver microsomes in relationship to the type of hepatotoxicity: comparison with two directly hepatotoxic drugs. Chem Res Toxicol 7:434–442

Leemann TD, Transon C, Bonnabry P, Dayer P (1993) A major role for cytochrome P450TB (CYP2C subfamily) in the actions of non-steroidal antiinflammatory drugs. Drugs Exp Clin Res 19:189–195

Loeper J, Descatoire V, Maurice M, Beaune P, Belghiti J, Houssin D, Ballet F, Feldman G, Guengerich FP, Pessayre D (1993) Cytochromes P-450 in human hepatocyte plasma membrane: recognition by several autoantibodies. Gastroenterology 104:203–216

López-Garcia MP, Dansette PM, Valadon PCA, Beaune PH, Guengerich FP, Mansuy D (1993) Human liver cytochromes P-450 expressed in yeast as tools for reactive-metabolite formation studies. Oxidative activation of tienilic acid by cytochromes P-450 2C9 and 2C10. Eur J Biochem 213:223–232

López-Garcia MP, Dansette PM, Mansuy D (1994) Thiophene derivatives as new mechanism-based inhibitors of cytochromes P-450: inactivation of yeast-expressed human liver cytochrome P-450 2C9 by tienilic acid. Biochemistry 33:166–175

Manns MP, Johnson EF, Griffin KJ, Tan EM, Sullivan KF (1989) Major antigen of liver kidney microsomal autoantibodies in idiopathic autoimmune hepatitis is cytochrome P450db1. J Clin Invest 83:1066–1072

Manns MP, Griffin KJ, Quattrochi LC, Sacher M, Thaler H, Tukey RH, Johnson EF (1990) Identification of cytochrome P450IA2 as a human autoantigen. Arch Biochem Biophys 280:229–232

Manns MP, Griffen KJ, Sullivan KF, Johnson EF (1991) LKM-1 autoantibodies recognize a short linear sequence in P450IID6, a cytochrome P450 monooxygenase. J Clin Invest 88:1370–1378

Martin JL, Kenna JG, Martin BM, Thomassen D, Reed GF, Pohl LR (1993) Halothane hepatitis patients have serum antibodies that react with protein disulfide isomerase. Hepatology 18:858–863

Meyer U, Skoda RC, Zanger UM, Heim M, Broly F (1992) The genetic polymorphism of debrisoquine/sparteine metabolism – molecular mechanisms. In: Kalow W (ed) Pharmacogenetics of drug metabolism. Pergamon, New York, pp 609–623

Meyer UA (1990) Genetic polymorphisms of drug metabolism. Fund Clin Pharmacol 4:595–615

Mimura M, Baba T, Yamazaki H, Ohmori S, Inui Y, Gonzalez FJ, Guengerich FP, Shimada T (1993) Characterization of cytochrome P-450 2B6 in human liver microsomes. Drug Metab Dispos 21:1048–1056

Mitchell JR, Jollow DJ, Potter WZ, Davis DC, Gillette JR, Brodie BB (1973) Acetaminophen-induced hepatic necrosis. I. Role of drug metabolism. J Pharmacol Exp Ther 187:185–194

Morgan MY, Reshef R, Shah RR, Oates NS, Smith RL, Sherlock S (1984) Impaired oxidation of debrisoquine in patients with perhexilene liver injury. Gut 25:1057–1064

Murphy R, Scartz R, Watkins PB (1990) Severe acetaminophen toxicity in a patient receiving acetaminophen. Ann Intern Med 113:799–800

Murray M (1992) P450 enzymes: inhibition mechanisms, genetic regulation and effects of liver disease. Clin Pharmacokinet 23:132–146

Nataf J, Bernuau J, Larrey D, Guillin MC, Rueff B, Benhamou JP (1986) A new anti-liver microsome antibody: a specific marker of dihydralazine hepatitis? Gastroenterology 90:1751

Nebert DW (1991) Proposed role of drug-metabolizing enzymes: regulation of steady state levels of the ligands that effect growth, homeostasis, differentiation, and neuroendocrine functions. Mol Endocrinol 5:1203–1214

Nebert DW (1994) Drug-metabolizing enzymes in ligand-modulated transcription. Biochem Pharmacol 47:25–37

Nebert DW, Adesnik M, Coon MJ, Estabrook RW, Gonzalez FJ, Guengerich FP, Gunsalus IC, Johnson EF, Kemper B, Levin W, Phillips IR, Sato R, Waterman MR (1987) The P450 gene superfamily: recommended nomenclature. DNA 6:1–11

Nebert DW, Nelson DR, Adesnik M, Coon MJ, Estabrook RW, Conzalez FJ, Guengerich FP, Gunsalus IC, Johnson EF, Kemper B, Levin W, Phillips IR, Sato R, Waterman MR (1989) The P450 superfamily: updated listing of all genes and recommended nomenclature for the chromosomal loci. DNA 8:1–13

Nebert DW, Nelson DR, Coon MJ, Estabrook RW, Feyereisen R, Fujii-Kuriyama Y, Gonzalez FJ, Guengerich FP, Gunsulas IC, Johnson EF, Loper JC, Sato R, Waterman MR, Waxman DJ (1991) The P450 superfamily: update on new sequences, gene mapping, and recommended nomenclature. DNA Cell Biol 10: 1–14

Nebert DW, Puga A, Vasilou V (1993) Role of the Ah receptor and the dioxin-inducible [Ah] gene battery in toxicity, cancer, and signal transduction. Ann NY Acad Sci 685:624–640

Nelson DR, Kamataki T, Waxman DJ, Guengerich FP, Estabrook RW, Feyereisen R, Gonzalez FJ, Coon MJ, Gunsalus IC, Gotoh O, Okuda K, Nebert DW (1993) The P450 superfamily: update on new sequences, gene mapping, accession numbers, early trivial names of enzymes, and nomenclature. DNA Cell Biol 12:1–51

Okey AB (1992) Enzyme induction in the cytochrome P-450 system. In: Kalow W (ed) Pharmacogenetics of drug metabolism. Pergamon, New York, pp 549–608

Okey AB, Riddick DS, Harper PA (1994a) The Ah receptor: mediator of the toxicity of 2,3,7,8-tetrachlorodibenzo-p-dioxin (TCDD) and related compounds. Toxicol Lett 70:1–22

Okey AB, Riddick DS, Harper PA (1994b) Molecular biology of the aromatic hydrocarbon (dioxin) receptor. Trends Pharmacol Sci 15:226–232

Oullette GS, Slitzky BE, Gates JA, Lagarde S, West AB (1991) Reversible hepatitis associated with diclofenac. J Clin Gastroenterol 13:205–210

Park BK, Coleman JW, Kitteringham NR (1987) Drug disposition and drug hypersensitivity. Biochem Pharmacol 36:581–590

Patten CJ, Thomas PE, Guy RL, Lee M, Gonzalez FJ, Guengerich FP, Yang CS (1993) Cytochrome P450 enzymes involved in acetaminophen activation by rat and human liver microsomes and their kinetics. Chem Res Toxicol 6:511–518

Pellinen P, Honkakoski P, Stenbäck F, Niemitz M, Alhava E, Pelkonen O, Lang MA, Pasanen M (1994) Cocaine N-demethylation and the metabolism-related hepatotoxicity can be prevented by cytochrome P450 3A inhibitors. Eur J Pharmacol Environ Toxicol Pharmacol 270:35–43

Perrot N, Nalpas B, Yang CS, Beaune PH (1989) Modulation of cytochrome P450 isozymes in human liver, by ethanol and drug intake. Eur J Clin Invest 19:549–555

Pessayre D (1993) Physiopathologie des hépatopathies médicamenteuses. Gastroenterol Clin Biol 17:H3–H17

Pirmohamed M, Kitteringham NR, Breckenridge AM, Park BK (1992a) The effect of enzyme induction on the cytochrome P450-mediated bioactivation of carbamazepine by mouse liver microsomes. Biochem Pharmacol 44:2307–2314

Pirmohamed M, Kitteringham NR, Guenthner TM, Breckenridge AM, Park BK (1992b) An investigation of the formation of cytotoxic, protein-reactive and stable metabolites from carbamazepine in vitro. Biochem Pharmacol 43:1675–1682

Pohl LR (1990) Drug-induced allergic hepatitis. Semin Liver Dis 10:305–315

Pohl LR, Satoh H, Christ DD, Kenna JG (1988) The immunologic and metabolic basis of drug hypersensitivities. Annu Rev Pharmacol 28:367–387

Poland A, Glover E, Kende AS (1976) Stereospecific high affinity binding of 2,3,7,8-tetrachloro-p-dioxin by hepatic cytosols: evidence that the binding species is a receptor for induction of aryl hydrocarbon hydroxylase. J Biol Chem 251:4936–4946

Porubec DJ, Rundgren M, Harvison PJ, Nelson SD, Moldéus P (1987) Investigation of mechanisms of acetaminophen toxicity in isolated rat hepatocytes with the acetaminophen analogues 3,5-dimethylacetaminophen and 2,6-dimethylacetaminophen. Mol Pharmacol 31:647–653

Pumford NR, Hinson JA, Benson RW, Roberts DW (1990) Immunoblot analysis of protein containing 3-(cystein-s-yl)acetaminophen adducts in serum and subcellular liver fractions from acetaminophen-treated mice. Toxicol Appl Pharmacol 104:521–532

Pumford NR, Martin BM, Hinson JA (1992) A metabolite of acetaminophen covalently binds to the 56 kDa selenium binding protein. Bichem Biophys Res Commun 182:1348–1355

Pumford NR, Martin BM, Thomassen D, Burris JA, Kenna JG, Martin JL, Pohl LR (1993a) Serum antibodies from halothane hepatitis patients react with the rat endoplasmic reticulum protein ERp72. Chem Res Toxicol 6:609–615

Pumford NR, Myers TM, Davila JC, Highet RJ, Pohl LR (1993b) Immunochemical detection of liver protein adducts of the nonsteroidal antiinflammatory drug diclofenac. Chem Res Toxicol 6:147–150

Purcell P, Henry D, Melville G (1991) Diclofenac hepatitis. Gut 32:1381–1385
Quattrochi L (1994) The human CYP1A2 gene and induction by 3-methylcholanthrene: a region of DNA that supports AH-receptor binding and promoter-specific induction. J Biol Chem 269:6949–6954
Raucy JL, Lasker JM, Lieber CS, Black M (1989) Acetaminophen activation by human liver cytochromes P450IIE1 and P450IA2. Arch Biochem Biophys 271:270–283
Relling MV, Aoyama T, Gonzalez FJ, Meyer UA (1990) Tolbutamide and mephenytoin hydroxylation by human cytochrome P450s in the CYP2C subfamily. J Pharmacol Exp Ther 252:442–447
Renton KW, Knickle LC (1990) Regulation of cytochrome P-450 during infectious disease. Can J Pharmacol Physiol 68:777–781
Rettie AE, Rettenmeier AW, Howald WN, Baillie TA (1987) Cytochrome P-450-catalyzed formation of Δ^4-VPA, a toxic metabolite of valproic acid. Science 235:890–893
Riley RJ, Roberts P, Kitteringham NR, Park BK (1990) Formation of cytotoxic metabolites from phenytoin, imipramine, desipramine, amitriptyline and mianserin by mouse and human hepatic microsomes. Biochem Pharmacol 39:1951–1958
Rizzetto M, Swana G, Doniach D (1973) Microsomal antibodies in active chronic hepatitis and other disorders. Clin Exp Immunol 15:331–344
Roberts DW, Pumford NR, Potter DW, Benson RW, Hinson JA (1987) A sensitive immunochemical assay for acetaminophen-protein adducts. J Pharmacol Exp Ther 241:527–533
Roberts EA, Johnson KC, Harper PA, Okey AB (1990) Characterization of the Ah receptor mediating aryl hydrocarbon hydroxylase induction in the human liver cell line Hep G2. Arch Biochem Biophys 276:442–450
Roberts EA, Johnson KC, Dippold WG (1991) Ah receptor mediating induction of cytochrome P450IA1 in a novel continuous human liver cell line (Mz-Hep-1): detection by binding with [^{3}H]2,3,7,8-tetrachlorodibenzo-p-dioxin and relationship to the activity of aryl hydrocarbon hydroxylase. Biochem Pharmacol 42:521–528
Roberts EA, Furuya KN, Tang BK, Kalow W (1994) Caffeine biotransformation in human hepatocyte cell lines derived from normal tissue. Biochem Biophys Res Commun 201:559–566
Rost KL, Brösicke H, Brockmöller J, Scheffler M, Helge H, Roots I (1992) Increase of cytochrome P450IA2 activity by omeprazole: evidence by the ^{13}C-[N-3-methyl]-caffeine breath test in poor and extensive metabolizers of mephenytoin. Clin Pharmacol Ther 52:170–180
Ryan DE, Ramanathan L, Iida S, Thomas PE, Haniu M, Shively JE, Lieber CS, Levin W (1985) Characterization of a major form of rat hepatic microsomal cytochrome P-450 induced by isoniazid. J Biol Chem 260:6385–6393
Satoh H, Gillette JR, Davies HW, Schulik RD, Pohl LR (1985) Immunochemical evidence of trifluoroacetylated cytochrome P-450 in the liver of halothane-treated rats. Mol Pharmacol 28:468–474
Satoh H, Martin BM, Schulik AH, Christ DD, Kenna JG, Pohl LR (1989) Human anti-endoplasmic reticulum antibodies in sera of patients with halothane-induced hepatitis are directed against a trifluoroacetylated carboxylesterase. Proc Natl Acad Sci USA 86:322–326
Scheutz JD, Beach DL, Guzelian PS (1994) Selective expression of cytochrome P450 CYP3A mRNAs in embryonic and adult human liver. Pharmacogenetics 4:11–20
Schweikl H, Taylor JA, Kitareewan S, Linko P, Nagorney D, Goldstein JA (1993) Expression of CYP1A1 and CYP1A2 genes in human liver. Pharmacogenetics 3:239–249
Sesardic D, Boobis AR, Edwards RJ, Davies DS (1988) A form of cytochrome P450 in man, orthologous to form d in the rat, catalyses the O-deethylation of phenacetin and is inducible by cigarette smoking. Br J Clin Pharmacol 26:363–372

Shimada T, Yamazaki H, Mimura M, Inui Y, Guengerich FP (1994) Interindividual variations in huamn liver cytochrome P-450 enzymes involved in the oxidation of drugs, carcinogens and toxic chemicals: studies with liver microsomes of 30 Japanese and 30 Caucasians. J Pharmacol Exp Ther 270:414–423

Smith MGM, Williams R, Walker G, Rizzetto M, Doniach D (1974) Hepatic disorders associated with liver/kidney microsomal antibodies. Br Med J 2:80–84

Swanson HI, Bradfield CA (1993) The AH-receptor: genetics, structure and function. Pharmacogenetics 3:213–230

Thomassen D, Martin BM, Martin JL, Pumford NR, Pohl LR (1990) The role of a stress protein in the development of a drug-induced allergic response. Eur J Pharmacol 183:1138–1139

Thummel KE, Kharasch ED, Podoll T, Kunze KL (1993a) Human liver microsomal enflurane defluorination catalyzed by cytochrome P-450 2E1. Drug Metab Dispos 21:350–357

Thummel KE, Lee CA, Kunze KL, Nelson SD, Slattery JT (1993b) Oxidation of acetaminophen to N-acetyl-p-aminobenzoquinone imine by human CYP3A4. Biochem Pharmacol 45:1563–1569

Timbrell JA, Mitchell JR, Snodgrass WR, Nelson SD (1980) Isoniazid hepatotoxicity: the relationship between covalent binding and metabolism in vivo. J Pharmacol Exp Ther 213:364–369

Urban G, Speerschneider P, Dekant W (1994) Metabolism of the chlorofluorocarbon substitute 1,1-dichloro-2,2,2-trifluoroethane by rat and human liver microsomes: the role of cytochrome P450 2E1. Chem Res Toxicol 7:170–176

Vergani D, Mieli-Vergani G (1993a) Type II autoimmune hepatitis. What is the role of the hepatitis C virus. Gastroenterology 104:1870–1873

Vergani D, Mieli-Vergani G (1993b) Type II autoimmune hepatitis: the conundrum of cytochrome P450IID6. Clin Exp Immunol 92:367–368

Watkins PB (1991) Antimicrosomal antibodies: what are they telling us. Hepatology 13:385–387

Watkins PB, Wrighton SA, Maurel P, Schuetz EG, Mendez-Picon G, Parker GA, Guzelian PS (1985) Identification of an inducible form of cytochrome P-450 in human liver. Proc Natl Acad Sci USA 82:6310–6314

Wilkinson GR, Guengerich FP, Branch RA (1989) Genetic polymorphism of S-mephenytoin hydroxylation. Pharmacol Ther 43:53–76

Wrighton SA, Stevens JC (1992) The human hepatic cytochromes P450 involved in drug metabolism. CRC Crit Rev Toxicol 22:1–21

Wrighton SA, VandenBranden M (1989) Isolation and characterization of human fetal liver cytochrome P450HLp2: a third member of the P450III gene family. Arch Biochem Biophys 268:144–151

Wrighton SA, Thomas PE, Willis P, Maines SL, Watkins PB, Levin W, Guzelian PS (1987) Purification of a human liver cytochrome P-450 immunochemically related to several cytochromes P-450 purified from untreated rats. J Clin Invest 80:1017–1022

Wrighton SA, Ring BJ, Watkins PB, Vandenbranden M (1989) Identification of a polymorphically expressed member of the human cytochrome P-450III family. Mol Pharmacol 36:97–105

Wrighton SA, Stevens JC, Becker GW, Vandenbranden M (1993a) Isolation and characterization of human liver cytochrome P450 2C19 – correlation between 2C19 and S-mephenytoin-4′-hydroxylation. Arch Biochem Biophys 306:240–245

Wrighton SA, VandenBranden M, Stevens JC, Shipley LA, Ring BJ (1993b) In vitro methods for assessing human hepatic drug metabolism: their use in drug development. Drug Metab Rev 25:453–484

Yamamoto AM, Cresteil D, Boniface O, Clerc FF, Alvarez F (1993a) Identification and analysis of cytochrome P450IID6 antigenic sites recognized by anti-liver-kidney microsome type-1 antibodies (LKM1). Eur J Immunol 23:1105–1111

Yamamoto AM, Cresteil D, Homberg JC, Alvarez F (1993b) Characterization of anti-liver-kidney microsome antibody (anti-LKM1) from hepatitis C virus-positive and -negative sera. Gastroenterology 104:1762–1767

Yamamoto AM, Mura C, de Lemos-Chiarnadini C, Krishnamoorthy R (1993c) Cytochrome P450IID6 recognized by LKM1 antibody is not exposed on the surface of hepatocytes. Clin Exp Immunol 92:381–390

Yang CS, Smith TJ, Hong J-Y (1994) Cytochrome P-450 enzymes as targets for chemoprevention against chemical carcinogenesis and toxicity: opportunities and limitations. Cancer Res 54:1982s–1986s

Yun C-H, Shimada T, Guengerich FP (1991) Purification and characterization of human liver microsomal cytochrome P-450 2A6. Mol Pharmacol 40:679–685

Zimmerman HJ (1990) Update of hepatotoxicity due to classes of drugs in common clinical use: non-steroidal drugs, anti-inflammatory drugs, antibiotics, antihypertensives, and cardiac and psychotropic agents. Semin Liver Dis 10:322–338

Zimmerman HJ, Lewis JH, Ishak KG, Maddrey WC (1984) Ticrynafen-associated hepatic injury: analysis of 340 cases. Hepatology 4:315–323

CHAPTER 7

Mechanisms of Drug-Induced Cholestasis

J.B. WATKINS III and C.D. KLAASSEN

A. Definition of Cholestasis

Cholestasis means stagnation of bile, and includes biochemical, morphological, and physiological features. Clinically determined signs and symptoms result from accumulation in blood of compounds normally excreted in bile, such as bilirubin, bile acids, cholesterol, alkaline phosphatase, 5′-nucleotidase, γ-glutamyltranspeptidase, leucine aminopeptidase, lipoprotein X, and immunoglobulin A. The response of these compounds and the time course for elevation in serum varies after bile duct ligation (KAPLAN et al. 1979; FREDERIKS et al. 1990) and after different cholestatic toxins (KEEFFE et al. 1979). Hyperbilirubinemia in combination with elevated serum alkaline phosphatase is typically a reliable laboratory parameter, and determination of serum bile acid concentration has been proposed as a semiquantitative measure of cholestasis (BERRY and REICHEN 1983). Cholestasis may be defined morphologically as visible accumulation of bile pigments in the canaliculi and hepatocytes, dilation of the canalicular space with a reduction of microvilli, feathery degeneration, accumulation of copper, and Mallory body-like cytoplasmic inclusions. Finally, the simplest functional definition of cholestasis is a decrease in bile flow. Cholestasis can be due to either a failure to secrete bile (intrahepatic) or to a mechanical obstruction (extrahepatic cholestasis) of the bile ducts. Laboratory tests may reflect the severity of cholestasis, but they do not identify the etiology of the disorder or distinguish between extra- and intrahepatic forms. Additional information on cholestasis may be found elsewhere (ZYSSET and REICHEN 1988; REICHEN and SIMON 1988; KING and BLITZER 1990; VORE 1991; FEUER and DIFONZO 1992; FALLON et al. 1993). Numerous other drugs are capable of inducing cholestasis, and interested readers should consult other comprehensive reviews (ZIMMERMAN and LEWIS 1987; HORSMANS and HARVENGT 1991). A recent issue of *Seminars in Liver Diseases* was devoted exclusively to cholestasis (LESTER 1993). This chapter will present potential mechanisms by which chemicals can induce cholestasis and ten overview several known cholestatic agents. one problem with each of the mechanisms discussed is that it is not known whether any of these changes is a primary mechanism or a secondary consequence of cholestasis.

B. Mechanisms of Canalicular Bile Formation

An understanding of bile formation is needed to fully appreciate the mechanisms by which drugs can induce cholestasis. Although some detail is included here, more information on bile formation, hepatic uptake and biliary excretion may be obtained elsewhere (KLAASSEN and WATKINS 1984; HOFMANN 1990; ANWER 1991; SIEGERS and WATKINS 1991; COLEMAN and RAHMAN 1992; ARIAS et al. 1993; ERLINGER 1993).

Hepatic parenchymal cells function as a polarized epithelium actively transporting bile acids, other organic chemicals and inorganic solutes from the hepatic sinusoid across the basolateral membrane through the cell and finally across the canalicular membrane into bile. Water and cations like Na^+ contribute to bile formation by crossing the canalicular membrane and tight junctions in response to osmotic and electrochemical gradients generated by the transport of impermeant anions. Besides the transcellular route across sinusoidal and basolateral membranes, water and solutes can enter bile via the paracellular pathway across the tight junctions, or by combination of the transcellular and paracellular routes.

I. Transport of Bile Acids

Bile acid secretion into bile provides the major osmotic driving force for bile formation. Bile acid secretion depends on bile salt delivery from the intestine, hepatic uptake, and biliary excretion. Intestinal absorption and the portal circulation provide 90% of biliary bile acids. It is now clear that the basolateral membrane contains at least two carriers, a 48-kDa sodium-dependent protein highly specific for bile acids (FRIMMER and ZIEGLER 1988; MEIER 1989) and a 54-kDa multispecific anion/hydroxyl exchanger (HUGENTOBLER and MEIER 1986; FRIMMER and ZIEGLER 1988), capable of moving bile acids into the cell against a concentration gradient. These transporters are driven by an inwardly directed Na^+ gradient maintained by Na^+-K^+-ATPase (BLITZER and BOYER 1978; DUFFY et al. 1983). The in-to-out OH^- gradient is thought to be generated by Na^+/H^+ exchange driven by the out-to-in Na^+ (coupled with HCO_3^-) gradient produced by the Na^+-K^+-ATPase pump (HUGENTOBLER and MEIER 1986).

Bile acids are then transported to the canalicular membrane by at least two mechanisms. First, the bile acids move by rapid diffusion after coupling to a class of cytosolic proteins (STOLZ et al. 1989). Second, transcytotic vesicles may move bile acids across the cell more slowly via the microtubules once bile acid concentrations rise above physiologic levels (CRAWFORD et al. 1988; SAKISAKA et al. 1988).

Secretion of bile acids across the canalicular membrane is mediated by a 110-kDa integral membrane transporter (MEIER et al. 1984, 1985, 1987; REUTZ et al. 1988; SIPPEL et al. 1990). Bile acid excretion is driven by the negative intracellular potential (INOUE et al. 1983, 1984; MEIER et al. 1984; WEINMAN et al. 1989). ATP-dependent transport of bile acids may also occur (NISHADA et al. 1991). The predominant P-glycoprotein in canalicular membrane is the product of the multidrug resistance-2 gene, but the natural substrate has yet to be identified (BUSHMAN et al. 1992). Substrates for ATP-dependent transport by the multidrug resistance-3 gene product include colchicine, vinblastine, calcium channel blockers, and cyclosporine A (KAMIMOTO et al. 1989). Although much is known about canalicular secretion (ARIAS et al. 1993; ERLINGER 1993; FALLON et al. 1993; ZIMNIAK et al. 1992; ZIMNIAK and AWASTHI 1993), knowledge of canalicular ATP-dependent transporters is currently an active area of intense research.

II. Transport of Inorganic Ions and Glutathione

The bile acid-independent fraction of bile formation is due to transport of other organic and inorganic anions. Biliary secretion is clearly affected by glutathione depletion (AKERBOOM et al. 1984): glutathione undergoes carrier-mediated translocation across the canalicular membrane (BALLATORI and TRUONG 1990) with passive water movement to maintain osmotic pressure. In addition, a Cl^-/HCO_3^- exchanger (MEIER et al. 1985) contributes to bicarbonate-induced bile flow. Moreover, organic anions like bilirubin and sulfobromophthalein share an ATP-dependent multiple organic anion carrier that is distinct from the canalicular bile acid transporter (ISHIKAWA et al. 1990; KITAMURA et al. 1990), and secretion of these anions may also contribute to bile formation.

III. Other Mechanisms

Microfilaments and microtubules help to maintain cell shape and to secrete various substances, including lipoproteins, proteins and bile acids into bile. The pericanalicular ectoplasm contains a web of thick (10 nm) and thin (5 nm) microfilaments that surround the canaliculus, inserting into the junctional complex and extending into the canalicular microvilli (FRENCH and DAVIES 1975). The microfilaments form the contractile system which provides "tone" to the canaliculus and facilitates canalicular bile flow by means of active contractions of the canalicular walls of adjacent hepatocytes (PHILLIPS et al. 1978, 1986). An intact microtubular system is needed for transcytotic vesicular secretion of bile acids (COLEMAN 1987; HAYAKAWA et al. 1990). In addition, the microtubular system is involved in vesicular transport of bulk fluid into bile by exocytosis in sucrose-loaded rats (LESAGE et al. 1990). Moreover, tight junction permeability may be influenced by contraction of actin and myosin associated with the plasma membrane in the perijunctional area (ELIAS et al. 1980; YAMAGUCHI et al. 1991).

C. Mechanisms of Cholestasis

I. Alterations is Basolateral Membrane Function

Long considered a disease of the canalicular membrane (SIMON and ARIAS 1973), cholestasis may occur at the sinusoidal membrane as well (BERR et al. 1984). Monohydroxy bile acids produce both competitive (HARDISON et al. 1984) and noncompetitive (SCHWENK et al. 1977) inhibition of bile acid uptake in the elevated concentrations found in cholestasis. Decreased uptake of taurocholate into hepatocytes isolated from ethinyl estradiol-treated rats (BERR et al. 1984) may result from altered lipid structure of the membrane (DAVIS et al. 1978), because the number of carriers is not affected (SIMON et al. 1980). Other forms of cholestasis where impaired bile acid transport has been demonstrated include those induced by bile duct ligation (ACCATINO et al. 1981), androgenic steroids (SCHWARZ et al. 1977), chlorpromazine (ROS et al. 1979), and taurolithocholate (SCHWENK et al. 1977). Although hepatic lithocholate uptake occurs by diffusion, uptake of the glucuronide and sulfate conjugates is mediated by a Na^+-independent carrier (TAKIKAWA et al. 1991). Finally, elevation of monohydroxy bile acids has also been implicated in cholestasis associated with total parenteral nutrition (FOUIN-FORTUNET et al. 1982). Future studies will need to conclusively elucidate the mechanisms by which bile acids alter uptake. Theoretical possibilities include: (1) a decreased number of bile acid carriers; (2) an alteration in the driving forces for solute transport; (3) an alteration in the membrane characteristics; or (4) some other intracellular event.

II. Alterations in Canalicular Membrane Function

Ethinyl estradiol decreases the biliary transport maximum for taurocholate in vivo (GUMUCIO and VALDIVIESO 1971) and the efflux of taurocholate from isolated hepatocytes (TARAO et al. 1982). The canalicular membrane likely participates in the lipid alterations induced by ethinyl estradiol because secretory maximum and lipid fluidity correlate (DAVIS et al. 1978; SIMON et al. 1980). Biliary excretion of bilirubin and sulfobromophthalein is diminished by anabolic steroids (ARIAS 1963) and estrogens (DAHL et al. 1978; REYES et al. 1981). Low doses of estradiol minimally effect bile flow; but significantly decrease transport of morphine glucuronide (AUANSAKUL and VORE 1982). Also, bicarbonate deprivation abolishes part of the bile acid-independent fraction of bile flow (MIYAI and HARDISON 1982). Moreover, inhibition of glutathione transport may be the mechanism for sulfobromophthalein-induced cholestasis (SCHULZE and CZOK 1975). α-Naphthylisothiocyanate reduces cellular glutathione concentrations through a reversible conjugation process in freshly isolated rat hepatocytes (CARPENTER et al. 1991; DAHM and ROTH 1991). How cholestatic agents affect the bicarbonate/chloride exchanger (MEIER et al. 1985), the putative chloride channel (BEAR et al. 1985), and the carriers for glutamate (BALLATORI et al. 1986) and other unidentified anions (KLOS et al. 1979) has yet to be completely defined. However, these studies indicate that altered canalicular excretion of organic anions and electrolytes may be involved in the etiology of cholestasis.

III. Alterations in Intracellular Events

1. Binding to Intracellular Proteins and Conjugation Enzymes

Ethinyl estradiol decreases ligandin concentration in liver, thereby increasing sulfobromophthalein efflux and diminishing net transport (REYES et al. 1972). Alterations of intrahepatic binding proteins are probably not important in the pathogenesis of cholestasis, but these changes could exacerbate cholestasis through an increase in intracellular concentration of cytotoxic substances such as monohydroxy bile acids and possible impairment of organic anion transport.

Sulfation and glucuronidation of bile acids, which are minor pathways under physiological conditions, are increased in cholestasis (BACK 1976). Sulfotransferases are under hormonal control, and estrogens are a potent stimulus (KANE et al. 1984). Cholestatic doses of ethinyl estradiol markedly induce hepatic glycolithocholate sulfotransferase (KIRKPATRICK and KILLENBERG 1980). However, sulfation is not induced by lithocholate treatment (BALISTERI et al. 1984), and sulfotransferase activity is typically normal in cholestatic liver (LOOF and WENGLE 1982). Sulfation and glucuronidation provide an alternate pathway for elimination of toxic bile acids (GALEAZZI and JAVITT 1977), thereby protecting against cholestatic sulfate and glucuronide conjugates of cholestatic bile acids (YOUSEF et al. 1981; MATHIS et al. 1983; OELBERG et al. 1984).

Intracellular translocation of bile acids is decreased in calcium deprivation-induced cholestasis (REICHEN et al. 1985). Similarly, ethinyl estradiol inhibits translocation of cholylglycylhistamine, a bile acid analog (SHEPHERD et al. 1984). The vesicular translocation of horseradish peroxidase is not affected by ethinyl estradiol (GOLDSMITH et al. 1983), but chlorpromazine is inhibitory on both sinusoidal uptake and translocation of the peroxidase (OKANUE et al. 1984). Increased biliary resistance decreases biliary immunoglobulin A excretion (RANK and WILSON 1983), but it is unknown whether this is due to a translocation defect.

2. Cytoskeleton

Altered function of different components of the cytoskeleton could lead to cholestasis by interference with tight junctional permeability, transcellular transport processes, contraction of canaliculi (OSHIO and PHILLIPS 1981), or carrier proteins (REICHEN et al. 1981). Two microfilament inhibitors, cytochalasin B and phalloidin, have been of value in determining the effects of microfilaments in bile formation. Cytochalasin B prevents the polymerization of actin (MCLEAN-FLETCHER and POLLARD 1980), causes detachment of microfilaments from the plasma membrane (ODA and PHILLIPS 1977), and provokes a reversible inhibition of canalicular contractions in isolated hepatocyte couplets (PHILLIPS et al. 1983). Chronic low-dose administration of cytochalasin causes cholestasis with dilatation of canaliculi and loss of canalicular microvilli (PHILLIPS et al. 1975), interferes with canalicular contractions in cell culture (PHILLIPS et al. 1983), inhibits taurocholate transport (REICHEN et al. 1981; KACICH et al. 1983), interferes with the translocation of immunoglobulin A across the hepatocyte (GEBHARDT 1984), and, in other epithelia, interferes with glucose uptake and formation of tight junctions.

Chronic administration of phalloidin leads to lesions characterized by an increase in filamentous actin around the canaliculi and the tight junction (MONTESANO et al. 1976; DUBIN et al. 1980). A motility disorder of the canaliculi may occur in phalloidin-induced cholestasis (WATANABE et al. 1983). Similar changes have been described in chlorpromazine-(ELIAS and BOYER 1979) and norethindrone- (PHILLIPS et al. 1978) produced cholestasis, and in vinblastine-treated cultured rat hepatocytes (ROBENEK and GEBHARDT 1983). Phalloidin undergoes uptake by the bile acid transport system and is concentrated by hepatocytes (KRAMER et al. 1982; PETZINGER and FRIMMER 1980; WIELAND et al. 1984). Low doses of phalloidin to rats cause marked accumulation of actin microfilaments in the pericanalicular region of the hepatocyte and a parallel decrease in bile flow (DUBIN et al. 1978; PHILLIPS et al. 1975; TUCHWEBER and GABBIANI 1976), as well as a decreased bile flow and bile acid secretion and an increased bile-to-plasma ratio of [^{3}H]inulin and [^{14}C]sucrose (ELIAS et al. 1980). In the isolated hepatocyte couplet model, phalloidin decreases the number of canalicular contractions and causes a spastic type of contraction (WATANABE et al. 1983). Phalloidin alters the permeability of tight junctions such that bile constituents can reflux from the canaliculus into the intercellular space. Because bile acid concentration in bile was not decreased in phalloidin-treated animals, the selective permeability changes resulted in an increased penetration of sucrose and inulin from plasma into bile, but not in the regurgitation of bile acids from bile to plasma (ELIAS et al. 1980).

Colchicine, an inhibitor of tubulin polymerization, does not affect basal bile flow but decreases bile acid excretion, and, when administered together with phalloidin, it decreases bile flow synergistically (DUBIN et al. 1980). Colchicine also inhibits bile acid uptake (REICHEN et al. 1981), and influences nonspecific protein secretion (KACICH et al. 1983; BARNWELL et al. 1984) as well as the receptor-mediated pathways for immunoglobulin A (GEBHARDT 1984) and lysosomal contents (SEWELL et al. 1984). In addition, colchicine markedly inhibits excretion of a physiologic load of taurocholate in bile acid depleted rats (CRAWFORD et al. 1988).

IV. Permeability Changes in the Biliary Tree

The regurgitation theory, proposed for estrone-induced cholestasis in rats (FORKER 1969), assumes that increased permeability of the biliary tree can be assessed indirectly by determining the clearance of inert solutes, such as inulin or sucrose (FORKER 1969). Measurement of the biliary recovery of retrogradely injected marker substances (OLSON and FUJIMOTO 1980) and electron microscopic demonstration of peroxidase penetrating into the canaliculus (METZ et al. 1977) both fail to identify the level at which permeability changes occur or permit quantitation. However, dual clearance (BRADLEY and HERZ 1978) and biliary multiple indicator dilution (REICHEN et al. 1985) techniques may differentiate between alterations in transcellular and paracellular permeability (REICHEN and LE 1985).

1. Altered Permeability of the Junctional Complex

The paracellular pathway for fluid transport goes through tight junctions, which are characterized morphologically (LAYDEN et al. 1978) as three to five parallel strands with an average depth of 0.15 μm (LAGARDE et al. 1981). Electrophysiologically, the hepatocyte tight junction is leaky (GRAF et al. 1984). Increased biliary permeability can occur at the level of the tight junction (ELIAS et al. 1980) and morphologic evidence of alterations of tight junctional organization has been described (ROBENEK et al. 1980, 1982). Circumstantial evidence for altered function of the tight junction is provided by a decrease in the number of strands, strand disruption, and a loss of parallel strand orientation observed after bile duct ligation (METZ et al. 1977) and cholestasis induced by phalloidin (MONTESANO et al. 1976; DUBIN et al. 1978; ELIAS et al. 1980, estrogen (DE VOS and DESMET 1981; ELIAS and IQBAL 1983), and taurolithocholate (JUNG et al. 1982). Increased permeability to inert solutes also occurs in cholestasis induced by taurocholate (REICHEN and LE 1983), α-naphthylisothiocyanate (KRELL et al. 1982), calcium deprivation (REICHEN et al. 1985), and microfilament inhibition (MONTESANO et al. 1976; ELIAS et al. 1980; DUBIN et al. 1980). The finding that the morphology of the tight junction is disrupted in parallel with increased permeability to inert solutes suggests that its integrity is required for normal bile formation. Furthermore, vasopression and epinephrine modulate hepatocyte tight junctional permeability, permitting biliary glutathione to reflux from bile to plasma (BALLATORI and TRUONG 1990). Whether altered permeability of the paracellular pathway is a primary pathogenetic event or a universal sequelae of cholestasis remains to be established.

2. Altered Permeability of the Canalicular Membrane

Altered canalicular permeability has been demonstrated in cholestasis induced by estrone (FORKER 1969), taurolithocholate (REICHEN et al. 1985), ethinyl estradiol (PETERSON and FUJIMOTO 1977), estradiol glucuronide (ADINOLFI et al. 1984), and α-naphthylisothiocyanate (JAESCHKE et al. 1983). Increased permeability after ethinyl estradiol administration is observed by the retrograde infusion method (PETERSON and FUJIMOTO 1977; IQBAL et al. 1985), but not by the steady-state clearance technique (JAESCHKE et al. 1983). Colchicine inhibition of vesicular transport and increased permeability to retrogradely injected sucrose and mannitol may result from increased permeability of the canalicular membrane (BAJWA and FUJIMOTO 1983). However, disruption of junctional complexes may be a response to cholestatic injury rather than its cause, and quantification of the number of strands may be a better morphologic expression of permeability (EASTER et al. 1983). Studies in canalicular vesicles and hepatocyte couplets are needed to pinpoint more accurately the site of increased permeability.

The multiple biliary indicator dilution technique provides evidence that transcellular rather than paracellular permeability may be altered in taurolithocholate-produced cholestasis (REICHEN and LE 1985). Administration of taurocholate with taurolithocholate prevents increased permeability to inulin and membrane alterations produced by taurolithocholate (LAYDEN and BOYER 1977). Ethinyl estradiol-produced cholestasis is characterized by an increased cholesterol ester content of the plasma membrane (DAVIS et al. 1978), which can be reversed by Triton WR 1339 administration (SIMON et al. 1980). Increased canalicular membrane permeability may be involved in manganese/bilirubin-induced cholestasis (AYOTTE and PLAA 1986).

3. Alterations in Membrane Proteins

Na^+-K^+-ATPase couples the hydrolysis of ATP to active transport of Na^+ and K^+ across the plasma membrane. Na^+-K^+-ATPase is a hydrophobic transmembrane protein, and the α subunit, molecular weight approximately 100 kDa, binds ATP on the inside of the cell and probably has eight membrane-spanning domains (CANTLEY 1981; HUBERT et al. 1986). Histochemical studies have localized functional units to the hepatic sinusoidal surface (BLITZER and BOYER 1978), but immunohistochemical studies have found immunoreactive proteins on the canalicular surface as well (LEFFERT et al. 1985). Na^+-K^+-ATPase activity depends on optimal membrane fluidity for required conformational changes (CANTLEY 1981). Thus, the protein is conceivably localized on both surfaces, but functionally inactive on canalicular membrane because of its viscous lipid environment. Rapid changes in canalicular membrane fluidity or redistribution of enzyme units from inactive canalicular sites to the sinusoidal surface have been proposed as regulators of its function (SCHARSCHMIDT et al. 1981; SCHENK et al. 1984). Na^+-K^+-ATPase largely controls the membrane potential in hepatocytes, thereby affecting internal pH, intracellular free calcium, cytoskeletal function, and secondary active transporters, which in turn may regulate both bile acid transport and bile acid-independent flow. Thus, short- as well as long-term regulation of Na^+-K^+-ATPase functional units may be integral to understanding cholestasis.

Decreased activity of Na^+-K^+-ATPase in hepatocellular plasma membrane fractions has been described in cholestasis induced by ethinyl estradiol (REICHEN and PAUMGARTNER 1977; DAVIS et al. 1978), chlorpromazine (SAMUELS and CAREY 1978; KEEFE et al. 1980), monohydroxy bile salts (KAKIS and YOUSEF 1978; REICHEN and PAUMGARTNER 1979), taurolithocholate

(REICHEN and PAUMGARTNER 1979), bile duct obstruction (WANNAGAT et al. 1978), endotoxin (UTILI et al. 1977), rose bengal (LAPERCHE et al. 1972), and protoporphyrin (AVNER et al. 1983). A decrease in the number of protein units has not yet been demonstrated, while upregulation follows administration of thyroid and adrenal hormones (LAYDEN and BOYER 1976; MINER et al. 1980) and phenobarbital (SIMON et al. 1977). Ethinyl estradiol or estradiol treatment of rats decreases Na^+-K^+-ATPase activity in plasma membranes (DAVIS et al. 1978; REICHEN and PAUMGARTNER 1977), reduces uptake of bile acids and steroid glucuronides into isolated hepatocytes (BERR et al. 1984; BROCK and VORE 1984), and abolishes both Na^+-dependent uptake of taurocholate in basolateral membrane vesicles and voltage-dependent taurocholate efflux from canalicular membrane vesicles (FRICKER et al. 1988). Changes in maximal bile acid secretory rate may be due to modifications in basolateral (ROSARIO et al. 1988) and in canalicular (FRICKER et al. 1988) membranes. The differences observed in these two studies may result from variations in the quality of the membrane preparations, in ethinyl estradiol-induced cholestasis, a lower hepatocellular potassium concentration and rubidium uptake have been described (BERR et al. 1984), suggesting that in vitro changes truly reflect in vivo alterations of cation pumping. Another clue that enzyme activity reflects pumping activity is the finding that reversal of Na^+-K^+-ATPase inhibition is associated with restoration of bile flow (SIMON et al. 1980; BOELSTERLI et al. 1983). In addition, some cholestatic agents, such as indocyanine green (HORAK et al. 1973), preferentially affect electrolyte transport. The role of the Na^+/H^+-antiporter (ARIAS and FORGAC 1984) in different forms of cholestasis remains to be established. Future studies of the selective impairment and(or) a generalized decreased activity of these different ion pumps will help define a role for these mechanisms in cholestasis. Whether this decrease in Na^+-K^+-ATPase activity is primarily pathogenetic or a sequel of cholestasis is unknown. Although Na^+-K^+-ATPase inhibition is often noted in cholestasis, it is not a generalized phenomenon (KAKIS and YOUSEF 1978; KAKIS et al. 1980; TODA et al. 1978; MEIJER et al. 1978).

Mg^{2+}-ATPase is an operational term that sums both Mg^{2+}- and Ca^{2+}-dependent ATP-splitting activity that is localized predominantly at the canalicular surface of hepatocytes (BLITZER and BOYER 1978; EVANS et al. 1976; KEEFFE et al. 1979). Although microfilaments have Mg^{2+}-ATPase activity, it is not known to what extent the pericanalicular web and microfilaments attached to membrane preparations contribute to the Mg^{2+}-ATPase activity measured in membrane preparations. The effect of different models of cholestasis on Mg^{2+}-ATPase in plasma membrane fractions is controversial. All bile acids, except dehydrocholate, inhibit Mg^{2+}-ATPase in vitro (SCHARSCHMIDT et al. 1981; MEIJER et al. 1978). Although bile duct ligation increases enzyme activity (SIMON and ARIAS 1973), conflicting reports concerning chlorpromazine (SAMUELS and CAREY 1978; TAVALONI and BOYER 1980) and ethinyl estradiol (SIMON and ARIAS 1973; SIMON et al. 1980; REICHEN and PAUMGARTNER 1977) have appeared. Cytochalasin B induces a parallel loss of microfilaments and enzyme activity (ODA and PHILLIPS 1977), supporting a relationship between Mg^{2+}-ATPase and microfilaments.

Membrane-bound hepatocellular alkaline phosphatase is increased in cholestasis (SIMON and ARIAS 1973; TODA et al. 1980) and is likely to be derived from the basolateral membranes (DE BROE et al. 1985; KOMODA et al. 1984). The increase in hepatocellular alkaline phosphatase activity reaches its peak 24h after bile duct ligation, whereas ductular proliferation increases up to 7 days (KAPLAN et al. 1979). Moreover, distinct isoforms of alkaline phosphatase may be isolated from hepatocellular and ductular epithelial cells by their different electrophoretic properties (HATOFF et al. 1985). Elevated hepatic alkaline phosphatase following bile duct ligation in rats is due to increased synthesis (KAPLAN et al. 1983). However, mRNA content after bile duct ligation is unaltered, suggesting that increased alkaline phosphatase activity is translationally regulated (SEETHARAM et al. 1986). Bile acid-stimulated synthesis of alkaline phosphatase is cycloheximide sensitive (HATOFF and HARDISON 1979, 1981), raising the possibility that bile salt elevation in cholestasis may be the messenger.

4. Alterations in Membrane Composition and Function

Differences in lipid composition found between canalicular and sinusoidal domains are largely responsible for the measured fluidity differences in these membrane fractions (EVANS et al. 1976; SCHACHTER 1984). For example, acute but not chronic administration of cholic acid depletes total plasma membrane phospholipid content without changing specific phospholipid species (RAHMAN et al. 1986). Changes in membrane free cholesterol content in nonhepatic plasma membranes influence lipid fluidity, water permeability, enzyme function, and transport processes (SPECTOR and YOREK 1985; SANDERMANN 1978). Lithocholate and taurolithocholate administration reportedly increase free cholesterol content six- and twofold, respectively, in liver plasma membrane fractions (KAKIS and YOUSEF 1978). Ethinyl estradiol administration increases membrane content of cholesteryl esters (DAVIS et al. 1978). Contrasting results using lower doses of ethinyl estradiol indicate changes in bile flow, Na^+-K^+-ATPase activity, and membrane fluidity without increased cholesteryl ester accumulation (ROSARIO et al. 1988).

A key property in the regulation of transporter and ion carrier function is membrane fluidity and the ratio of cholesterol to phospholipid (SCHACHTER 1984). Other determinants include the ratio of sphingomyelin to phosphatidylcholine, and the length and degree of saturation of fatty acids (STUBBS 1983). Dietary factors influence membrane fluidity and may partially reverse ethinyl estradiol-induced cholestasis through changes in fatty acid composition (STORCH and SCHACHTER 1984). Liver plasma membrane fluidity was decreased in mixed membrane populations following administration of ethinyl estradiol (DAVIS et al. 1978) and chlorpromazine (KEEFFE et al. 1980), and after thyroidectomy (KEEFFE et al. 1979). Preliminary reports using specific plasma membrane domains showed that ethinyl estradiol selectively decreases sinusoidal fluidity, leaving the canalicular fractions unaltered (ROSARIO et al. 1988; ARIAS et al. 1986). Correlation of transport function data with lipid measurements in well-characterized plasma membrane vesicles is needed to completely describe how changes in lipid composition and fluidity are involved in many aspects of cholestasis and to conclude whether the described changes are real or result from a different mixture of surface membrane components.

D. Drugs and Other Chemicals Inducing Cholestasis

I. α-Naphthylisothiocyanate

α-Naphthylisothiocyanate (ANIT) induces a dose-dependent cholestasis following acute administration, and bile duct hyperplasia and biliary cirrhosis after chronic treatment (PLAA and PRIESTLEY 1976). Metabolism of ANIT is critical to its cholestatic activity. Potentiation or inhibition of oxidative desulfuration of [^{35}S]ANIT correlates with a corresponding potentiation or inhibition of ANIT cholestasis (TRAIGER et al. 1985). Moreover, pretreatment of rats with L-buthionine-*S,R*-sulfoximine protects against ANIT-induced cholestasis and hyperbilirubinemia, suggesting that a glutathione conjugate maybe involved (DAHM and ROTH 1991). Additional work indicates that ANIT depletes hepatocytes of glutathione through a reversible conjugation process (CARPENTER-DEYO et al. 1991).

ANIT is one of the few chemicals that induces cholestasis by disruption of the tight junctions, causing dilation of bile ducts, loss of microvilli from bile duct epithelial cells, and an apparent opening of the tight junctions between some bile duct epithelial cells that could be seen by electron microscopy within 4h of dosing rats with 300mg/kg ANIT (CONNOLLY et al. 1988). These changes were more pronounced after 6h and the majority of bile ducts were destroyed by 24h. Alterations in tight junctions between hepatocytes could be detected by electron microscopy as early as 6h, and evidence of parenchymal necrosis was first noted at 24h. In the isolated perfused liver preparation, 250mg ANIT/kg to rats decreased the permeability barrier between perfusate and bile for ^{14}C-sucrose, whereas taurocholate and sulfobromophthalein perfusate concentrations at equilibrium were increased about eightfold over that in control livers, with a comparable decrease in their biliary concentration (KRELL et al. 1982). Moreover, ANIT increased the rate of elimination of sucrose from bile in the fast phase via the paracellular pathway (JAESCHKE et al. 1987a), indicating a reflux of sucrose from the bile into the perfusate across the tight junctions. Thus, ANIT-induced cholestasis results from disruption of the tight junctions between hepatocytes and bile duct epithelial cells, with the subsequent diffusion of osmotically active solutes from bile into plasma. A decrease in the biliary concentration of solutes normally present in high concentrations is a critical feature of cholestasis due to an increased permeability of the tight junctions, and is not a common feature in most types of cholestasis. The molecular mechanism by which these tight junctions are disrupted and the identity of the active agent/metabolite is not known.

II. Androgenic and Estrogenic Steroids

Anabolic steroid medical use and misuse/abuse by athletes leads to several hepatic complications (ISHAK and ZIMMERMAN 1987). Methyl testosterone and norethandrolone impair sulfobromophthalein transport (DURHAM and VORE 1986). Several cholestatic steroids inhibit taurocholate uptake into isolated hepatocytes (SCHWARZ et al. 1977). Moreover, norethandrolone may alter hepatic microfilaments (PHILLIPS et al. 1978). In addition, D-ring glucuronides of testosterone and dihydrotestosterone are also cholestatic (VORE et al. 1989).

Estrogen-induced cholestasis was observed soon after introduction of oral contraceptives in 1960 in women who also developed intrahepatic cholestasis of pregnancy; ethinyl estradiol was the causative agent (KREEK 1987; REYES and SIMON 1993; VORE 1987). Transport of a number of organic anions is apparently inhibited even in normal human pregnancy. Plasma levels of bilirubin are at the upper limit of normal in many women during the later stages of pregnancy (REYES and SIMON 1993; VAN DYKE 1990). Bile acids also accumulate in plasma in normal pregnancy, although only rarely outside the normal range, so that levels at term are two- to threefold above those seen in early pregnancy (LUNZER et al. 1986; VAN DYKE 1990). These data indicate that estrogens decrease hepatic excretory function, and that, in some women, this inhibition is sufficient to precipitate pruritus and jaundice.

Several mechanisms have been proposed to explain estrogen-induced cholestasis. First, increased permeability of the biliary tree with diffusion of solutes from bile to plasma via the paracellular pathway may be the mechanism for the increased biliary clearance of sucrose and mannitol and the decreased biliary excretion of sulfobromophthalein induced by estrone (FORKER 1969). The increased bile: plasma ratio of sucrose and inulin could be due to decreased bile production, and the elevated bile acid concentration in bile argues against regurgitation of biliary contents into plasma (JAESCHKE et al. 1983). After 1 week of estradiol valerate (1 mg/kg per week), bile flow was decreased and biliary taurocholate concentration was increased (JAESCHKE et al. 1987b). After 3 weeks of treatment, bile flow remained depressed, but taurocholate concentration in bile had decreased and the sucrose and inulin permeability coefficients increased, consistent with increased permeability of the tight junction. These data indicate that increased permeability is not causing the decreased bile flow induced by estrogens, although it may be the consequence of the cholestasis.

Decreased fluidity of the plasma membrane may be responsible for estrogen-induced cholestasis (SIMON et al. 1980). For example, ethinyl estradiol induces hepatic low-density lipoprotein receptors and subsequently increases clearance of plasma lipoproteins (KOVANEN et al. 1979; CHAO et al. 1979).

Although the cholesterol ester content of liver homogenate and plasma membranes is increased, their membrane fluidity is decreased (DAVIS et al. 1978; KEEFFE et al. 1979; SIMON et al. 1980). Thus, decreased membrane fluidity of the basolateral domain that is induced with ethinyl estradiol does not correlate with increased cholesterol ester content (ROSARIO et al. 1988). Also, addition of *S*-adenosylmethionine to the vesicles in vitro restores taurocholate transport activity in both basolateral and canalicular membrane fractions (FRICKER et al. 1988). Similarly, *S*-adenosylmethionine treatment in rats increases plasma membrane fluidity and Na^+-K^+-ATPase activity and partly reverses ethinyl estradiol-induced cholestasis (STRAMENTINOLI et al. 1981; BOELSTERLI et al. 1983). Moreover, intrahepatic cholestasis of pregnancy improves after *S*-adenosylmethionine treatment (FREZZA et al. 1984).

A third mechanism for estrogen-induced cholestasis involves biotransformation of estrogens to cholestatic glucuronide metabolites. In particular, glucuronide conjugates of the D-ring of estradiol, estriol, and ethinyl estradiol cause an immediate, profound, dose-dependent and reversible cholestasis following their intravenous administration to rats (MEYERS et al. 1980, 1981; VORE et al. 1983; VORE and SLIKKER 1985). Glucuronide conjugates of the A-ring administered under identical experimental conditions induce choleresis. The cholestatic glucuronides decrease both bile acid-dependent and bile acid-independent components of bile flow (MEYERS et al. 1981). Administration of estradiol-17β-D-glucuronide to the rhesus monkey (5.5–11 μmol/kg i.v.) significantly inhibited indocyanine green clearance, whereas estradiol-3-β-D-glucuronide had no effect (SLIKKER et al. 1983). These doses of estradiol-17β-D-glucuronide are similar to urinary levels of the cholestatic D-ring glucuronide, estriol-16α-glucuronide, of about 2 μmol/kg per day, seen in the third trimester of normal pregnancy (BAKER et al. 1979). These data suggest that retention of sulfobromophthalein in normal pregnancy may be due to high levels of D-ring glucuronides present at this time. How the cholestatic D-ring glucuronide conjugates of the estrogens induce cholestasis is not known. These agents probably interact at a specific site, based on the structure-activity relationships observed and the parallel dose-response curves seen for the induction of cholestasis by this group of compounds (VORE and SLIKKER 1985). The structural similarities between the cholestatic glucuronides and the bile acids suggest that this site may be a bile acid carrier. However, estradiol-17β-D-glucuronide does not inhibit Na^+-dependent taurocholate transport into isolated hepatocytes (BROUWER et al. 1987) or into hepatic basolateral membrane vesicles (ZIMMERLI et al. 1989). Taurocholate will protect against and reverse estradiol-17β-D-glucuronide-induced cholestasis in the isolated perfused liver (ADINOLFI et al. 1984; DURHAM and VORE 1986; UTILI et al. 1990); however, the interactions of estradiol-17β-D-glucuronide and taurocholate are not competitive in nature (DURHAM and VORE 1986). Paracellular permeability to horseradish peroxidase in the isolated perfused liver treated with estradiol-17β-D-glucuronide is increased about threefold under basal conditions, and about sixfold when taurodehydrocholate is infused to restore bile flow to initial levels (KAN et al. 1989). Although tight junctions are damaged by estradiol-17β-D-glucuronide, a causal relationship between increased paracellular permeability and estradiol-17β-D-glucuronide-induced cholestasis has not been determined (COLEMAN and KAN 1990; JAESCHKE 1990). Finally, future studies are needed to determine whether hepatic estrogen receptors mediate changes in the number or type of carriers involved in transport of osmotically active solutes into bile.

III. Bile Acids

Many bile acids are hepatotoxic and will induce cholestasis (RADOMINSKA et al. 1993). Monohydroxy bile acids are generally more toxic than dihydroxy bile acids, which are more toxic than trihydroxy bile acids (BILLINGTON et al. 1980; SCHOLMERLICH et al. 1984). The rank order of cholestatic potency of three bile acids following intravenous infusion in the rat was taurodeoxycholate > taurochenodeoxycholate > taurocholate > tauroursodeoxycholate (DREW and PRIESTLEY 1979; HARDISON et al. 1981).

Lithocholate treatment of rats causes cytoplasmic invaginations and bizarre lamellar transformations in the canalicular membrane (LAYDEN and BOYER 1975; MIYAI et al. 1975), increases cholesterol content of erythrocyte membranes (COOPER et al. 1972), and increases incorporation of cholesterol into hepatic plasma membranes (KAKIS and YOUSEF 1978). Electron microscopy studies failed to demonstrate a consistent relationship between the presence of lithocholate precipitates and cholestasis (MIYAI et al. 1977). Because cholesterol incorporation into membranes decreases membrane fluidity and permeability to water, small nonionic solutes, anions, and cations (OELBERG and LESTER 1986), lithocholate must induce cholestasis by decreasing fluidity and permeability of the canalicular membrane.

Conjugation of lithocholate with taurine or glycine and/or sulfate or glucuronic acid influences cholestatic potential. Sulfated glycolithocholic acid, the major metabolite of lithocholate in normal human bile (STIEHL et al. 1980), remains cholestatic, whereas sulfated taurolithocholate has minimal influence on bile flow rate in normal rats (YOUSEF et al. 1981; KUIPERS et al. 1988). Cholestatic lithocholate 3-*O*-β-glucuronide, found in serum and urine of patients with cholestatic liver disease, appears in rat bile as an opalescent lithocholic acid glucuronide-calcium complex (OELBERG et al. 1984). In pure aqueous solution, calcium and lithocholate glucuronide form stoichiometric insoluble complexes and the cholestatic bile salts, lithocholate sulfate, lithocholate glucuronide, and lithocholate, bind calcium with 10–60 times greater affinity than do the noncholestatic bile acids, taurocholate, glycocholate, and taurolithocholate sulfate (OELBERG et al. 1984).

There may be an association between disruption of hepatic Ca^{2+} homeostasis and bile acid-induced cholestasis (STORCH et al. 1983; OELBERG and LESER 1986; COMBETTES et al. 1988; ANWER et al. 1988; SPIVEY et al. 1993). However, 2,5-di(*tert*-butyl)-1,4-benzohydroquinone, a specific inhibitor of microsomal Ca^{2+} sequestration, causes a sustained (20 min) increase in cytosolic Ca^{2+}, release of the endoplasmic reticular Ca^{2+} pool, and an efflux of Ca^{2+} from liver cells without decreasing bile flow or inducing lactate dehydrogenase (LDH) release (FARRELL et al. 1990). In the isolated perfused rat liver system, lithocholate (25 μM) or taurolithocholate (5 μM) infusion for 10 or 30 min decreased bile flow by 80%-90% and caused significant lactate dehydrogenase release (FARRELL et al. 1990). However, glycochenodeoxycholate-induced cholestasis may result form ATP depletion followed by a subsequent rise in intracellular Ca^{2+}, producing an effect similar to that found in anoxia (SPIVEY et al. 1993). Lithocholate binding to plasma membranes and microsomes appears to correlate with the development of cholestasis in male rats, and glucuronidation of lithocholate contributes to the cholestasis (VU et al. 1992). Finally, rapid biliary secretion of sulfated glycolithocholate forms an insoluble complex with calcium in bile canaliculi, causing an obstructive cholestasis (KUIPERS et al. 1992). Thus, disruption of intracellular calcium homeostasis is probably not the mechanism for bile acid-induced cholestasis and liver injury.

Allo bile acids are structural analogues of natural bile acids in which the A and B rings of the steroid nucleus have a *trans* configuration and the hydrogen at C-5 is α-oriented rather than the A/B ring *cis* configuration and β-orientation of the C-5 hydrogen of natural bile acids. VONK et al. (1981) report that 3β-hydroxy-5α-cholanic acid is cholestatic in rats and is about four times more potent than the 5β analogue. When the cholestatic potency of a series of allobile acids, 3α-hydroxy-5α-cholanic acid, 3-keto-5α-cholanic acid, and 3β-hydroxy-5α-cholanic acid, was compared with that of their 5β analogues and with dihydrotestosterone glucuronide (DHTG), DHTG was two times more potent than 3-keto-5α-cholanic acid and five times more potent than lithocholate. Therefore, the glucuronic acid moiety and the A/B *trans* configuration contribute significantly but not essentially to the cholestatic activity of these bile acids (VORE et al. 1989).

A recent study indicates that significant interactions between bile acids and other chemicals may play a role in bile acid-induced cholestasis. For example, methyl isobutyl ketone treatment of rats for 3 days potentiates lithocholate-induced cholestasis by reducing the bile acid pool and by interfering with secretion of bile acids (JOSEPH et al. 1992). The hepatotoxic effects of the bile acids may also be due to their ability to damage membranes; however, the molecular mechanism(s) of these effects remain to be elucidated.

IV. Chlorpromazine and Other Phenothiazines

Chlorpromazine is a cationic detergent that binds membrane phospholipids and alters membrane fluidity and Na^+-K^+-ATPase activity (KEEFFE et al. 1980). Although some of the cholestatic response could be attributed to decreased hepatic perfusion (TAVOLONI and BOYER 1980), hydroxylated metabolites (7,8-dihydroxychlorpromazine) inhibit Na^+-K^+-ATPase in a dose-dependent manner (VAN DYKE and SCHARSCHMIDT 1987), whereas chlorpromazine sulfoxide is not cholestatic (SAMUELS and CAREY 1978). Chlorpromazine and estradiol-17β-D-glucuronide infusion into the isolated perfused liver induce fragmentation and loss of canalicular microvilli, dilation of canaliculi, and thickening of the pericanalicular ectoplasm, and these changes in ultrastructure parallel alterations in bile flow rate (ABERNATHY et al. 1992). Cholestatic jaundice is less frequently observed in patients taking other antipsychotic drugs.

V. Cyclosporine

Cyclosporine is a potent immunosuppressant with a very narrow therapeutic index used extensively in the management of transplant patients. Although nephrotoxicity is the primary adverse effect, cholestatic liver injury with hyperbilirubinemia (both total and direct) and elevated serum bile acids is also seen (SCHADE et al. 1983; ARIAS 1993). Cyclosporine can significantly decrease basal bile flow and bile acid secretory rates in rats without inducing histological lesions (LE THAI et al. 1988). Concomitant treatment with phenobarbital abolishes the cholestasis, suggesting that metabolism was a detoxication process. Cyclosporine decreases bile flow and bile salt secretion (ROTOLO et al. 1986; ROMAN et al. 1990) as well as biliary lipid secretion in rats (GALAN et al. 1992). Cyclosporine is a competitive inhibitor of taurocholate uptake in isolated hepatocytes (STACEY and KOTECKA 1988), but a noncompetitive inhibitor of Na^+-dependent taurocholate uptake in basolateral rat liver membrane vesicles (ZIMMERLI et al. 1989). In fact, cyclosporine A competitively inhibits Na^+-dependent uptake in both basolateral and canalicular membrane vesicles and inhibits Na^+-independent efflux of taurocholate from canalicular vesicles; two of its metabolites OL-17 and OL-21 were without significant effect in any of these systems (MOSELEY et al. 1990). Recent evidence in rat liver membrane vesicles indicated that cyclosporine A inhibited ATP-dependent carriers for both bile acids and cysteinyl leukotrienes (KADMON et al. 1993). Moreover, inhibition of bile acid-independent flow may be due to decreased glutathione secretion (ROMAN et al. 1990; FERNANDEZ et al. 1992). Further work is required to completely elucidate the mechanism of cyclosporine-induced cholestasis.

VI. Miscellaneous Cholestatic Agents

Combination of bilirubin and manganese sulfate induces dilation of canaliculi with swelling and loss of microvilli and decreased bilirubin transport (WITZLEBEN 1972). More recent studies have indicated that bile canalicular membranes from bilirubin-manganese-treated rats have higher levels of cholesterol and phospholipid, as well as incorporation of bilirubin and manganese (PLAA et al. 1982). Moreover, inhibition of the bile acid-independent fraction, but not the bile acid-dependent fraction, of bile flow is reduced (AYOTTE and PLAA 1988). Further studies are needed to identify the physical-chemical nature of any manganese-bilirubin complexes and the permeability of the paracellular pathway.

Cardiac glycosides at cholestatic doses probably alter the hemodynamic forces in bile formation (Tavoloni et al. 1978). Gram-negative bacterial sepsis releases an endotoxin capable of inducing cholestasis, perhaps via inhibition of Na^+-K^+-ATPase (Nolan 1981). In addition, the tricyclic antidepressants amitriptyline, imipramine, and amineptine are oxidized to metabolites that induce cholestasis in a small percentage of patients (Larrey et al. 1988, 1989). The antiarrhythmic propafenone has recently induced an acute cholestatic syndrome (Mondardini et al. 1993). Finally, erythromycins, especially estolate and ethylsuccinate derivatives, induce a cholestatic jaundice perhaps by inhibiting Na^+-K^+-ATPase and decreasing Na^+-dependent uptake of bile acid by hepatocytes (Gaeta et al. 1985; Zafrani et al. 1979; Diehl et al. 1984). Because erythromycin base can also induce rash, fever, and jaundice, a hypersensitivity reaction has been postulated as a mechanism for erythromycin liver disturbances (Shirin et al. 1992). Studies with an experimental immunological intrahepatic cholestasis model in guinea pigs indicate inhibition of bile acid uptake and secretion, decreased bile acid-independent flow, and unaltered tight junction permeability (Shin et al. 1992). Moreover, a biliary asialoglycoprotein stimulates T-cell proliferation in patients with primary biliary cirrhosis but not in drug-induced cholestasis (Onishi et al. 1991). In addition, a cholestatic factor identified immunocytochemically in patients with intrahepatic cholestasis in various liver diseases was localized to polysomes and filamentous structures around the canaliculus (Yamada et al. 1990). Moreover, a polyclonal antibody (anti-neutrophil serum) attenuates ANIT-induced cholestasis, indicating that polymorphonuclear leukocytes are involved by an as yet undetermined mechanism (Dahm et al. 1990). Future studies will need to asscertain the importance of the immune system in drug-induced cholestasis.

References

Abernathy CO, Zimmerman HJ, Ishak KG, Utili R, Gillespie J (1992) Drug-induced cholestasis in the perfused rat liver and its reversal by tauroursodeoxycholate: an ultrastructural study. Proc Soc Exp Biol Med 199:54–58

Accatino L, Contreras A, Berdichevksy E, Quintana C (1981) The effect of complete biliary obstruction on bile secretion. J Lab Clin Med 97:525–534

Adinolfi LE, Utili R, Gaeta GB, Abernathy CO, Zimmerman HJ (1984) Cholestasis induced by estradiol-17β-D-glucuronide: mechanisms and prevention by sodium taurocholate. Hepatology 4:30–37

Akerboom TP, Bilzer M, Sies H (1984) Relation between glutathione redox changes and biliary excretion of taurocholate in the perfused rat liver. J Biol Chem 259:5838–5843

Anwer MS (1991) Anatomy and physiology of bile formation. In: Siegers CP, Watkins JB III (eds) Progress in pharmacology and clinical pharmacology: biliary excretion of drugs and other chemicals. Fischer, Stuttgart, pp 3–23

Anwer MS, Engleking LR, Nolan K, Sullivan D, Zimniak P (1988) Hepatic activity of isolated rat hepatocytes. Hepatology 8:887–891

Arias IM (1963) Effects of a plant acid (icterogenin) and certain anabolic steroids on the hepatic metabolism of bilirubin and sulfobromophthalein (BSP). Ann NY Acad Sci 104:1014–1025

Arias IM (1993) Cyclosporin, the biology of the canaliculus, and cholestasis. Gastroenterology 104:1558–1560

Arias IM, Forgac M (1984) The sinusoidal domain of the plasma membrane of rat hepatocytes contains an amiloride-sensitive Na^{+}/H^{+} antiport. J Biol Chem 259:5406–5408

Arias IM, Adachi Y, Tran T (1986) Ethinylestradiol cholestasis: a disease of the sinusoidal domain of hepatocyte plasma membrane. Hepatology 3:872 (abstract)

Arias IM, Che M, Gatmaitman Z, Leveille C, Nishida T, St Pierre M (1993) The biology of the canaliculus, 1993. Hepatology 17:318–329

Avner DL, Larsen R, Berenson MM (1983) Inhibition of liver surface membrane Na^{+}, K^{+}-adenosine triphosphatase, Mg^{+2}-adenosine triphosphatase and 5′-nucleotidase activities by protoporphyrin. Observations in vitro and in the perfused rat liver. Gastroenterology 85:700–706

Auansakul AC, Vore M (1982) The effect of pregnancy and estradiol-17β treatment on the biliary transport maximum of dibromosulfophthalein, and the glucuronide conjugates of 5- isolated perfused rat liver. Drug Metab Dispos 10:344–349

Ayotte P, Plaa GL (1986) Modification of biliary tree permeability in rats treated with a manganese-bilirubin combination. Toxicol Appl Pharmacol 84:295–303

Ayotte P, Plaa GL (1988) Biliary excretion in Sprague-Dawley and Gunn rats during manganese-bilirubin-induced cholestasis. Hepatology 8:1069–1078

Back P (1976) Bile acid glucuronide I. Isolation and identification of a chenodeoxycholic acid glucuronide from human plasma in intrahepatic cholestasis. Z Physiol Chem 357:213–217

Bajwa RS, Fujimoto JM (1983) Effect of colchicine and S,S,S-tributyl phosphorotrithioate (DEF) on the biliary excretion of sucrose, mannitol and horseradish peroxidase in the rat. Biochem Pharmacol 32:85–90

Baker TS, Jennison KM, Kellie AE (1979) The direct radioimmunoassay of oestrogen glucuronides in human female urine. Biochem J 177:729–738

Balistreri WF, Zimmer L, Suchy FJ, Bove KE (1984) Bile salt sulfotransferase: alterations during maturation and non-inducibility during substrate ingestion. J Lipid Res 25:228–235

Ballatori N, Truong AT (1990) Cholestasis, altered junctional permeability, and inverse changes in sinusoidal and biliary glutathione release by vasopressin and epinephrine. Mol Pharmacol 38:64–71

Ballatori N, Jacob R, Boyer JL (1986) Intrabiliary glutathione hydrolysis. A source of glutamate in bile. J Biol Chem 261:7860–7865

Barnwell SG, Lowe PJ, Coleman R (1984) The effects of colchicine on secretion into bile of bile salts, phospholipids, cholesterol and plasma membrane enzymes: bile salts are secreted unaccompanied by phospholipids and cholesterol. Biochem J 220:723–731

Bear CE, Petrunka CN, Strasberg SM (1985) Evidence for a channel for the electrogenic transport of chloride ion in the rat hepatocyte. Hepatology 5:383–391

Berr F, Simon FR, Reichen J (1984) Ethinylestradiol impairs bile salt uptake and Na-K pump function of rat hepatocytes. Am J Physiol 247:G437–G443

Berry W, Reichen J (1983) Bile acid metabolism: its relation to clinical disease. Semin Liver Dis 3:330–340

Billington D, Evans CE, Godfrey PP (1980) Effects of bile salts on the plasma membranes of isolated rat hepatocytes. Biochem J 188:321–327

Blitzer BL, Boyer JL (1978) Cytochemical localization of Na,K-ATPase in the rat hepatocyte. J Clin Invest 62:1104–1108

Boelsterli UA, Rakhit G, Balazs T (1983) Modulation by S-adenosyl-L-methionine of hepatic Na,K-ATPase membrane fluidity, and bile flow in rats with ethinylestradiol-induced cholestasis. Hepatology 3:12–17

Bradley SE, Herz R (1978) Permselectivity of biliary canalicular membrane in rats – clearance probe analysis. Am J Physiol 235:E570–E576
Brock WJ, Vore M (1984) The effect of pregnancy and treatment with estradiol-17β on the transport of organic anions into isolated rat hepatocytes. Drug Metab Dispos 13:695–699
Brouwer KLR, Durham S, Vore M (1987) Multiple carriers for hepatocytes. Mol Pharmacol 32:519–523
Bushman E, Arceci RJ, Croop JM, Che M, Arias IM, Gousman DE, Gros P (1992) Mouse mdr2 encodes P-glycoprotein expressed in the bile canalicular membrane as determined by isoform specific antibodies. J Biol Chem 267:18093–18099
Cantley LC (1981) Structure and mechanism of the Na,K-ATPase. Curr Top Bioenerget 11:201–237
Carpenter-Deyo L, Marchand DH, Jean PA, Roth RA, Reed DJ (1991) Involvement of glutathione in α-naphthylisothiocyanate (ANIT) metabolism and toxicity to isolated hepatocytes. Biochem Pharmacol 42:2171–2180
Chao YS, Windler EE, Chen GC, Havel RJ (1979) Hepatic catabolism of rat and human lipoproteins in rats treated with 17α-ethinyl estradiol. J Biol Chem 254:11360–11366
Coleman R (1987) Biochemistry of bile secretion. Biochem J 244:249–261
Coleman R, Kan KS (1990) Oestradiol 17β-glucuronide and tight junctional permeability increase. Biochem J 266:622
Coleman R, Rahman K (1992) Lipid flow in bile formation. Biochim Biophys Acta 1125:113–133
Combettes L, Dumont M, Berthon B, Erlinger S, Claret M (1988) Release of calcium from the endoplasmic reticulum by bile acids in rat liver cells. J Biol Chem 263:2299–2303
Connolly AK, Price SC, Connelly JC, Hinton RH (1988) Early changes in bile duct lining cells and hepatocytes in rats treated with alpha-naphthylisothiocyanate. Toxicol Appl Pharmacol 93:208–219
Cooper RA, Garcia FA, Trey C (1972) The effect of lithocholic acid on red cell membranes in vivo. J Clin Invest 79:7–18
Crawford JM, Berken CA, Gollan JL (1988) Role of the hepatocyte microtubular system in the excretion of bile salts and biliary lipid: implications for intracellular vesicular transport. J Lipid Res 29:144–156
Dahl CR, Gonzalez MC, Simon FR (1978) Reversal of impaired sulfobromophthalein transport caused by ethinyl estradiol with Triton WR-1339 and phenobarbital. Gastroenterology 74:1023–1029
Dahm LJ, Roth RA (1991) Protection against alpha-naphthylisothiocyanate-induced liver injury by decreased hepatic non-protein sulfhydryl content. Biochem Pharmacol 42:1181–1188
Dahm LJ, Schultze AE, Roth RA (1990) An antibody to neutrophils attenuates alpha-naphthylisothiocyanate-induced liver injury. J Pharmacol Exp Ther 256:412–420
Davis RA, Kern F, Showalter R, Sutherland E, Sinensky M, Simon FR (1978) Alterations of hepatic Na^+,K^+-ATPase and bile flow by estrogen: effects on liver surface membrane structure and function. Proc Natl Acad Sci USA 75:4130–4134
De Broe ME, Roels F, Nouwen EJ, Claeys L, Wieme RJ (1985) Liver plasma membrane: the source of high molecular weight alkaline phosphatase in human serum. Hepatology 5:118–128
De Vos R, Desmet V (1981) Morphology of liver cell tight junctions in ethinyl estradiol induced cholestasis. Pathol Res Pract 171:381–388
Diehl AM, Latham P, Boitnott JK, Mann J, Maddrey WC (1984) Cholestatic hepatitis from erythromycin ethylsuccinate. Am J Med 76:931–934
Drew R, Priestly BG (1979) Choleretic and cholestatic effects of infused bile salts in the rat. Experientia 35:809–811
Dubin M, Maurice M, Feldman G, Erlinger S (1978) Phalloidin-induced cholestasis in the rat: relation to changes in microfilaments. Gastroenterology 75:450–455

Dubin M, Maurice M, Feldmann G, Erlinger S (1980) Influence of colchicine and phalloidin on bile secretion and hepatic ultrastructure in the rat: possible interaction between microtubules and microfilaments. Gastroenterology 79:646–654
Duffy MC, Blitzer BL, Boyer JL (1983) Direct determination of the driving forces for taurocholate uptake into rat liver plasma membrane vesicles. J Clin Invest 72:1470–1481
Durham S, Vore M (1986) Taurocholate and steroid glucuronides: mutual protection against cholestasis in the isolated perfused rat liver. J Pharmacol Exp Ther 237:490–495
Easter DW, Wade JB, Boyer JL (1983) Structural integrity of hepatocyte tight junctions. J Cell Biol 96:745–749
Elias E, Boyer JL (1979) Chlorpromazine and its metabolites alter polymerization and gelation of actin. Science 206:1404–1406
Elias E, Iqbal S (1983) Increased tight junction permeability: a possible mechanism of estrogen cholestasis. Eur J Clin Invest 13:383–390
Elias E, Hruban Z, Wade JB, Boyer JL (1980) Phalloidin-induced cholestasis: a microfilament-mediated change in junctional complex permeability. Proc Natl Acad Sci USA 77:2229–2233
Erlinger S (1993) Secretion of bile. In: Schiff L, Schiff ER (eds) Diseases of the liver, vol 1, 7th edn. Lippincott, Philadelphia, pp 85–107
Evans WH, Kremmer T, Culvenor JG (1976) Role of membranes in bile formation. comparison of the composition of bile and a liver bile-canalicular plasma membrane subfraction. Biochem J 154:589–595
Fallon MB, Anserson JM, Boyer JL (1993) Intrahepatic cholestasis. In: Shiff L, Schiff ER (eds) Diseases of the liver, vol 1, 7th edn. Lippincott, Philadelphia, pp 343–361
Farrell GC, Duddy SK, Kass GEN, Liopis J, Gahm A, Orrenius S (1990) Release of Ca^{2+} from the endoplasmic reticulum is not the mechanism for bile acid-induced cholestasis and hepatotoxicity in the intact rat liver. J Clin Invest 85:1255–1259
Fernandez E, Munoz ME, Roman ID, Galan AI, Gonzalez-Buitrago JM, Jimenez R (1992) Cyclosporin A-induced cholestasis in the rat. Beneficial effects of S-adenosyl-L-methionine. Drug Invest 4 [Suppl 4]:54–63
Feuer G, DiFonzo CJ (1992) Intrahepatic cholestasis: a review of biochemical-pathological mechanisms. Drug Metab Drug Interact 10:1–161
Forker EL (1969) The effect of estrogen on bile formation in the rat. J Clin Invest 48:654–663
Fouin-Fortunet H, LeQuernec L, Erlinger S, Loubours F, Colin R (1982) Hepatic alterations during total parenteral nutrition in patients with inflammatory bowel disease: a possible consequence of lithocholate toxicity. Gastroenterology 82:932–937
Frederiks WM, Van Noor Den CJF, Aronson DC, Marx F, Bosch KS, Jonges GN, Vogels IMC, James J (1990) Quantitative changes in acid phosphatase, alkaline phosphatase and 5′-nucleotidase activity in rat liver after experimentally induced cholestasis. Liver 10:158–166
French SW, Davies PL (1975) Ultrastructural localization of actin-like filaments in rat hepatocytes. Gastroenterology 68:765–774
Frezza MG, Pozzato G, Chiesa L, Stramentinoli G, DiPadova C (1984) Reversal of intrahepatic cholestasis of pregnancy in women after high doses of S-adenosyl-L-methionine. Hepatology 4:274–278
Fricker G, Landmann L, Meier PJ (1988) Ethinylestradiol (EE) induced structural and functional alterations of rat liver plasma membranes and their reversal by S-adenosylmethionine (SAMe) in vitro. Hepatology 8:1224 (abstract)
Frimmer M, Ziegler K (1988) The transport of bile acids in liver cells. Biochim Biophys Acta 947:75–99
Gaeta GB, Utili R, Adinolfi LE, Abernathy CO, Giusti G (1985) Characterization of the effects of erythromycin estolate and erythromycin base on the excretory function of the isolated rat liver. Toxicol Appl Pharmacol 80:185–192

Galan AI, Roman IS, Munoz ME, Cava F, Gonzalez-Buitrago JM, Jimenez R (1992) Inhibition of biliary lipid and protein secretion by cyclosporine A in the rat. Biochem Pharmacol 44:1105–1113

Galeazzi R, Javitt NB (1977) Bile acid excretion: the alternate pathway in the hamster. J Clin Invest 60:693–701

Gebhardt R (1984) Participation of microtubules and microfilaments in the transcellular biliary secretion of immunoglobulin A in primary cultures of rat hepatocytes. Experientia 40:269–271

Goldsmith MA, Huling S, Jones AL (1983) Hepatic handling of bile salts and protein in the rat during intrahepatic cholestasis. Gastroenterology 84:978–986

Graf J, Gautam A, Boyer JL (1984) Isolated rat hepatocyte couplets: a primary secretory unit for electrophysiologic studies of bile secretory function. Proc Natl Acad Sci USA 81:6516–6520

Gumucio JJ, Valdivieso VD (1971) Studies on the mechanism of ethinylestradiol impairment of bile flow and bile salt excretion in the rat. Gastroenterology 61:339–344

Hardison WGM, Hatoff DE, Miyai K, Weiner RG (1981) Nature of bile acid maximum secretory rate in the rat. Am J Physiol 241:G337–G343

Hardison WGM, Bellentani S, Heasley V, Shellhammer D (1984) Specificity of an Na^+-dependent taurocholate transport site in isolated rat hepatocytes. Am J Physiol 246:G477–G483

Hatoff DE, Hardison WGM (1979) Induced synthesis of alkaline phosphatase by bile acids in rat liver cell culture. Gastroenterology 77:1062–1067

Hatoff DE, Hardison WGM (1981) Bile acids modify alkaline phosphatase induction and bile secretion pressure after bile duct obstruction in the rat. Gastroenterology 80:666–672

Hatoff DE, Toyota N, Wong C, Miller AL, Takeya M, Miyai K (1985) Rat liver alkaline phosphatases. Evidence that hepatocyte and portal triad enzymes differ. Dig Dis Sci 30:564–572

Hayakawa T, Ng OC, Ma A, Boyer JL (1990) Taurocholate stimulates transcytotic vesicular pathways labelled by horseradish peroxidase in the isolated perfused rat liver. Gastroenterology 99:216–228

Hofmann AF (1990) Bile acid secretion, bile flow and biliary lipid secretion in humans. Hepatology 12:17S–25S

Horak W, Grabner G, Paumgartner G (1973) Inhibition of bile salt-independent bile formation by indocyanine green. Gastroenterology 64:1005–1012

Horsmans Y, Harvengt C (1991) Secondary drug-induced cholestasis with bile duct involvement. Acta Gastroenterol Belg 54:27–33

Hubert JJ, Schenk DB, Skelly H, Leffert HL (1986) Rat hepatic (Na^+,K^+)-ATPase: α-subunit isolation by immunoaffinity chromatography and structural analysis by peptide mapping. Biochemistry 25:4156–4163

Hugentobler G, Meier PJ (1986) Multispecific anion exchange in basolateral (sinusoidal) rat liver plasma membrane vesicles. Am J Physiol 251:G656–G664

Inoue M, Kinne R, Tran T, Biempica L, Arias IM (1983) Rat liver canalicular plasma membrane vesicles: isolation and topological characterization. J Biol Chem 258:5183–5188

Inoue M, Kinne R, Tran T, Arias IM (1984) Taurocholate transport by rat liver canalicular membrane vesicles. Evidence for the presence of an Na-independent transport system. J Clin Invest 73:659–663

Iqbal S, Mills CO, Elias E (1985) Biliary permeability during ethinyl estradiol-induced cholestasis studied by segmented retrograde intrabiliary injections in rats. J Hepatol 1:211–219

Ishak KG, Zimmermann HJ (1987) Hepatotoxic effects of the anabolic/androgenic steroids. Semin Liv Dis 7:230–236

Ishikawa T, Muller M, Klunemann C, Schaub T, Keppler D (1990) ATP-dependent primary active transport of cysteinyl leukotrienes across liver canalicular membrane. J Biol Chem 265:19279–19286

Jaeschke H (1990) The pathophysiological significance of increased tight-junctional permeability during oestrogen cholestasis. Biochem J 266:620–621

Jaeschke H, Krell H, Pfaff E (1983) No increase in biliary permeability in ethinylestradiol treated rats. Gastroenterology 85:808–814

Jaeschke H, Krell H, Pfaff E (1987a) Quantitative estimation of transcellular pathways of biliary sucrose in isolated perfused rat liver. Biochem J 241:635–640

Jaeschke H, Trummer E, Krell H (1987b) Increase in biliary permeability subsequent to intrahepatic cholestasis by estradiol valerate in rats. Gastroenterology 93:533–538

Joseph LD, Yousef IM, Plaa GL, Sharkawi M (1992) Potentiation of lithocholic-acid-induced cholestasis by methyl isobutyl ketone. Toxicol Lett 61:39–47

Jung W, Gebhardt T, Robenek H (1982) Primary cultures of rat hepatocytes as a model system for canalicular development, biliary secretion and intrahepatic cholestasis. II. Taurolithocholate-induced alterations of canalicular morphology and of the distribution of filipin-cholesterol complexes. Eur J Cell Biol 29:77–82

Kacich RL, Renston RH, Jones AL (1983) Effects of cytochalasin D and colchicine on the uptake, translocation and biliary secretion of horseradish peroxidase and [^{14}C]-taurocholate in the rat. Gastroenterology 85:385–394

Kadmon M, Kluenemann C, Boehme M, Ishikawa T, Gorgas K, Otto G, Herfarth C, Keppler D (1993) Inhibition by cyclosporin A of adenosine triphosphate-dependent transport from the hepatocyte into bile. Gastroenterology 104:1507–1514

Kakis G, Yousef IM (1978) Pathogenesis of lithocholate- and taurolithocholate-induced intrahepatic cholestasis in rats. Gastroenterology 75:595–607

Kakis G, Phillips MJ, Yousef IM (1980) The respective role of membrane cholesterol and of sodium potassium adenosine triphosphatase in the pathogenesis of lithocholate-induced cholestasis. Lab Invest 43:73–81

Kamimoto Y, Gatmaitman Z, Hsu J, Arias IM (1989) The function of Gp170, the multidrug resistance gene product, in rat liver canalicular membrane vesicles. J Biol Chem 264:11693–11698

Kan SK, Monte MJ, Parslow RA, Coleman R (1989) Oestradiol 17β-glucuronide increases tight-junctional permeability in rat liver. Biochem J 261:297–300

Kane RE, Chen LJ, Thaler MM (1984) Regulation of bile salt sulfotransferase isoenzymes by gonadal hormones. Hepatology 4:1195–1199

Kaplan MM, Kanel GC, Singer JA (1979) Enzyme changes and morphometric analysis of bile ducts in experimental bile duct obstruction. Clin Chim Acta 99:113–119

Kaplan MM, Ohkubo A, Quaroni EG, Sze-Tu D (1983) Increased synthesis of rat liver alkaline phosphatase by bile duct ligation. Hepatology 3:368–376

Keeffe EB, Scharschmidt BF, Blankenship NM, Ockner RK (1979) Studies of relationships among bile flow, liver plasma membrane Na,K-ATPase, and membrane microviscosity in the rat. J Clin Invest 64:1590–1598

Keeffe EB, Blankenship NM, Scharschmidt BF (1980) Alteration of rat liver plasma membrane fluidity and ATPase activity by chlorpromazine hydrochloride and its metabolites. Gastroenterology 79:222–231

King PD, Blitzer PL (1990) Drug-induced cholestasis: pathogenesis and clinical features. Semin Liver Dis 10:316–321

Kirkpatrick RB, Killenberg PG (1980) Effects of ethinylestradiol on enzymes catalyzing bile acid conjugation and sulfation. J Lipid Res 21:895–901

Kitamura T, Jansen P, Hardenbrook C, Kamimoto Y, Gatmaitan Z, Arias IM (1990) Defective ATP-dependent bile canalicular transport of organic anions in mutant (TR$^-$) rats with conjugated hyperbilirubinemia. Proc Natl Acad Sci USA 87:3557–3561

Klaassen CD, Watkins JB III (1984) Mechanisms of bile formation, hepatic uptake and biliary excretion. Pharmacol Rev 36:1–67

Klos C, Paumgartner G, Reichen J (1979) Cation-anion gap and choleretic properties of rat bile. Am J Physiol 236:E434–E440

Komoda T, Kumegawa M, Yajima T, Tamura G, Alpers DH (1984) Induction of rat hepatic and intestinal alkaline phosphatase activity produced by the bile from bile-duct ligated animals. Am J Physiol 246:G393–G400

Kovanen PT, Brown MS, Goldstein JL (1979) Increased binding of LDL to liver membranes from rats treated with 17-ethinylestradiol. J Biol Chem 254:11367–11373

Kramer W, Bickel U, Buscher HP, Gerok W, Kurz G (1982) Bile salt-binding polypeptides in plasma membranes of hepatocytes revealed by photoaffinity labelling. Eur J Biochem 129:13–24

Kreek MJ (1987) Female sex steroids and cholestasis. Semin Liver Dis 7:8–23

Krell H, Hoke H, Pfaff E (1982) Development of intrahepatic cholestasis by alpha-naphthylisothiocyanate in rats. Gastroenterology 82:507–514

Kuipers F, Enserink M, Havinga R, van der Steen ABM, Hardonk MJ, Fevery J, Vonk RJ (1988) Separate transport systems for biliary secretion of sulfated and unsulfated bile acids in the rat. J Clin Invest 81:1593–1599

Kuipers F, Hardonk MJ, Vonk RJ, Van der Meer R (1992) Bile secretion of sulfated glycolithocholic acid is required for its cholestatic action in rats. Am J Physiol 262:G267–G273

Lagarde S, Elias E, Wade JB, Boyer JL (1981) Structural heterogeneity of hepatocyte "tight" junctions: a quantitative analysis. Hepatology 1:193–203

Laperche Y, Launay A, Oudea P, Doulin A, Baraud J (1972) Effects of phenobarbital and rose bengal on the ATPases of plasma membranes of rat and rabbit liver. Gut 13:920–925

Larrey D, Amouyl G, Pessayre D, Degott C, Danne O, Machayekhi JP, Feldman G, Benhamon JP (1988) Amitriptyline-induced prolonged cholestasis. Gastroenterology 94:200–203

Larrey D, Berson A, Habersetzer F, Tinel M, Castot A, Babany G, Letteron P, Freneaux E, Loeper J, Dansette P, Pessayre D (1989) Genetic predisposition to drug hepatotoxicity: role in hepatitis caused by amineptine, a tricyclic antidepressant. Hepatology 10:168–173

Layden TJ, Boyer JL (1975) Scanning electron microscopy of the rat liver. Studies of the effect of taurolithocholate and other models of cholestasis. Gastroenterology 69:724–738

Layden TJ, Boyer JL (1976) The effect of thyroid hormone on bile salt-independent bile flow and Na^{+},K^{+}-ATPase activity in liver plasma membranes enriched in bile canaliculi. J Clin Invest 57:1009–1018

Layden TJ, Boyer JL (1977) Taurolithocholate-induced cholestasis: taurocholate but not dehydrocholate, reverses cholestasis and bile canalicular membrane injury. Gastroenterology 73:120–128

Layden TJ, Elias E, Boyer JL (1978) Bile formation in the rat. The role of the pericellular shunt pathway. J Clin Invest 62:1375–1385

Leffert HL, Schenk DB, Hubert JJ, Skelly H, Schumacher M, Ariyasu R, Ellisman M, Kock KS, Keller GA (1985) Hepatic Na,K-ATPase. A current view of its structure, function, and localization in rat liver as revealed by studies with monoclonal antibodies. Hepatology 5:501–507

LeSage GD, Robertson WE, Baumgart MA (1990) Demonstration of vesicular-dependent bile flow in the sucrose-loaded rat. Gastroenterology 99:478–487

Lester R (1993) Foreword. Semin Liver Dis 13:iii–vi

Le Thai B, Dumont M, Michel A, Erlinger S, Houssin D (1988) Cholestatic effect of cyclosporine in the rat. An inhibition of bile acid secretion. Transplantation 46:510–512

Loof L, Wengle B (1982) Enzymatic sulphation of bile salts in man. Bile salt sulfotransferase activity in percutaneous liver biopsy specimens from patients with liver disease. Scand J Gastroenterol 17:69–76

Lunzer M, Barnes P, Byth K, O'Halloran M (1986) Serum bile acid concentrations during pregnancy and their relationship to obstetric cholestasis. Gastroenterology 91:825–829

Mathis U, Karlaganis G, Preisig R (1983) Monohydroxy bile salt sulfates: tauro-3β-hydroxy-5-cholenoate-3-sulfate induces intrahepatic cholestasis in rats. Gastroenterology 85:674–681
McLean-Fletcher S, Pollard RD (1980) Mechanisms of action of cytochalasin B on actin. Cell 20:329–341
Meier PJ (1989) The bile salt secretory polarity of hepatocytes. J Hepatol 9:124–129
Meier PJ, Meier-Abt AS, Barrett C, Boyer JL (1984) Mechanisms of taurocholate transport in canalicular and basolateral rat liver plasma membrane vesicles. J Biol Chem 259:10614–10622
Meier PJ, Knickelbein R, Moseley RH, Dobbins JW, Boyer JL (1985) Evidence for carrier-mediated chloride/bicarbonate exchange in canalicular rat liver plasma membrane vesicles. J Clin Invest 75:1256–1263
Meier PJ, Meier-Abt AS, Boyer JL (1987) Properties of the canalicular bile acid transport system in rat liver. Biochem J 242:465–469
Meijer DKF, Vonk RJ, Weitering JG (1978) The influence of various bile salts and some cholephilic dyes on Na,K- and Mg-activated ATPase of rat liver in relation to cholestatic effects. Toxicol Appl Pharmacol 43:597–612
Metz J, Aoki M, Merlo M, Forssman WG (1977) Morphological alterations and functional changes of interhepatocellular junctions induced by bile duct ligation. Cell Tissue Res 182:299–310
Meyers M, Slikker W, Pascoe G, Vore M (1980) Characterization of cholestasis induced by estradiol-17B-D-glucuronide in the rat. J Pharmacol Exp Ther 214:87–93
Meyers M, Slikker W, Vore M (1981) Steroid D-ring glucuronides: characterization of a new class of cholestatic agents in the rat. J Pharmacol Exp Ther 218:63–73
Miner PB, Sutherland E, Simon FR (1980) Regulation of hepatic sodium plus potassium-activated adenosine triphosphatase activity by glucocorticoids in the rat. Gastroenterology 79:212–221
Miyai K, Hardison WGM (1982) Cholestasis induced by scillaren administration, bicarbonate deprivation, or reduced heptic blood flow. Exp Mol Pathol 36:333–346
Miyai K, Mayr WW, Richardson AL (1975) Acute cholestasis induced by lithocholic acid in the rat. A freeze-fracture replica and thin section study. Lab Invest 32:527–535
Miyai K, Richardson AL, Mayr WW, Javitt NB (1977) Subcellular pathology of rat liver in cholestasis and choleresis induced by bile salts. I. Effects of lithocholic, 3β-hydroxy-5-cholenoic, cholic and dehydrocholic acids. Lab Invest 36:249–258
Mondardini A, Pasquino P, Bernardi P, Aluffi E, Tartaglino B, Mazzucco G, Bonino F, Verne G, Negro F (1993) Propafenone-induced liver injury: report of a case and review of the literature. Gastroenterology 104:1524–1526
Montesano R, Gabbiani G, Perrelet A, Orci L (1976) In vivo induction of tight junction proliferation in rat liver. J Cell Biol 68:793–798
Moseley RH, Johnson TR, Morrissette JM (1990) Inhibition of bile acid transport by cyclosporine A in rat liver plasma membrane vesicles. J Pharmacol Exp Ther 253:974–980
Nishada T, Gatmaitan Z, Che M, Arias IM (1991) Rat liver canalicular membrane vesicles contain an ATP-dependent bile acid transport system. Proc Natl Acad Sci USA 88:6590–6594
Nolan JP (1981) Endotoxin, reticuloendothelial function and liver injury. Hepatology 1:458–465
Oda M, Phillips MJ (1977) Bile canalicular membrane pathology in cytochalasin B induced cholestasis. Lab Invest 37:350–356
Oelberg DG, Lester R (1986) Cellular mechanisms of cholestasis. Annu Rev Med 37:297–317
Oelberg DG, Dubinsky WP, Adcock EW, Lester R (1984) Calcium binding by lithocholic acid derivatives. Am J Physiol 247:G112–G115
Okanoue T, Kondo I, Ihrig TJ, French SW (1984) Effect of ethanol and chlorpromazine on transhepatic transport and biliary secretion of horseradish peroxidase. Hepatology 4:253–260

Olson JR, Fujimoto JM (1980) Evaluation of hepatobiliary function in the rat by the segmented retrograde intrabiliary injection technique. Biochem Pharmacol 29:205–211

Onishi S, Maeda T, Iwasaki S, Saibara T, Miyamoto T, Miyazaki M, Yamamoto Y, Enzan H (1991) A biliary protein identified by immunoblotting stimulates proliferation of peripheral blood T lymphocytes in primary biliary cirrhosis. Liver 11:321–328

Oshio C, Phillips MJ (1981) Contractility of bile canaliculi: implications for liver function. Science 212:1041–1042

Peterson RE, Fujimoto JM (1977) Increased biliary tree permeability produced in rats by hepatoactive agents. J Pharmacol Exp Ther 202:732–739

Petzinger E, Frimmer M (1980) Comparative studies on the rat liver cells. Arch Toxicol 44:127–135

Phillips MJ, Oda M, Mak E, Fisher MM, Jeejeebhoy KN (1975) Microfilament dysfunction as a possible cause of intrahepatic cholestasis. Gastroenterology 69:48–58

Phillips MJ, Oda M, Funatsu K (1978) Evidence for microfilament involvement in norethandrolone-induced intrahepatic cholestasis. Am J Pathol 93:729–744

Phillips MJ, Oshio C, Miyairi M, Smith CR (1983) Intrahepatic cholestasis as a canalicular motility disorder. Evidence using cytochalasin. Lab Invest 48:205–211

Phillips MJ, Poucell S, Oda M (1986) Biology of disease. Mechanisms of cholestasis. Lab Invest 54:593–608

Plaa GL, Priestly BG (1976) Intrahepatic cholestasis induced by drugs and chemicals. Pharmacol Rev 28:207–273

Plaa GL, De Lamirande E, Lewittes M, Yousef IM (1982) Liver cell plasma membrane lipids in manganese-bilirubin-induced intrahepatic cholestasis. Biochem Pharmacol 31:3698–3701

Radominska A, Treat S, Little J (1993) Bile acid metabolism and the pathophysiology of cholestasis. Semin Liver Dis 13:219–234

Rahman K, Hammond TG, Lowe PJ, Barnwell SG, Clark B, Coleman R (1986) Control of biliary phospholipid secretion. Effect of continuous and discontinuous infusion of taurocholate on biliary phospholipid secretion. Biochem J 234:421–427

Rank J, Wilson DI (1983) Changes in IgA following varying degrees of biliary obstruction in the rat. Hepatology 3:241–247

Reichen J, Le M (1983) Taurocholate, but not taurodehydrocholate, increases biliary permeability to sucrose. Am J Physiol 245:G651–G655

Reichen J, Le M (1985) Taurolithocholate induces cholestasis by altering transcellular but not pericellular biliary permeability. Clin Res 33:97A

Reichen J, Paumgartner G (1977) Relationship between bile flow and Na,K-adenosine triphosphatase in liver plasma membranes enriched in bile canaliculi. J Clin Invest 60:429–434

Reichen J, Paumgartner G (1979) Inhibition of hepatic Na,K-adenosine triphosphatase in taurolithocholate induced cholestasis in the rat. Experientia 35:1186–1188

Reichen J, Simon FR (1988) Cholestasis. In: Arias IM, Jakoby WB, Popper H, Schachter D, Shafritz DA (eds) The liver: biology and pathobiology. Raven, New York, pp 1105–1124

Reichen J, Berman MD, Berk PD (1981) The role of microfilaments and microtubules in taurocholate uptake by isolated rat liver cells. Biochim Biophys Acta 643:126–133

Reichen J, Berr F, Le M, Warren GH (1985) Characterization of calcium deprivation-induced cholestasis in the perfused rat liver. Am J Physiol 249:G48–G57

Reutz S, Hugentobler G, Meier PJ (1988) Functional reconstitution of hte canalicular bile transport system of rat liver. Proc Natl Acad Sci USA 85:6147–6151

Reyes H, Simon FR (1993) Intrahepatic cholestasis of pregnancy: an estrogen disease. Semin Liver Dis 13:289–301

Reyes H, Levi AJ, Gatmaitan Z, Arias IM (1972) Studies on Y and Z, two hepatic cytoplasmic organic anion-binding proteins: effect of drugs, chemicals, hormones and cholestasis. J Clin Invest 50:2242–2252

Reyes H, Ribalta J, Gonzalez MC, Segovia N, Oberhauser E (1981) Sulfobromophthalein clearance tests before and after ethinyl estradiol administration in women and men with familial history of intrahepatic cholestasis of pregnancy. Gastroenterology 81:226–231
Robenek H, Gebhardt R (1983) Primary cultures of rat hepatocytes as a model system of canalicular developments, biliary secretion and intrahepatic cholestasis. IV. Disintegration of bile canaliculi and disturbance of tight junction formation caused by vinblastine. Eur J Cell Biol 31:283–289
Robenek H, Herwig J, Themann H (1980) The morphologic characteristics of intercellular junctions between normal human liver cells and cells from patients with extrahepatic cholestasis. Am J Pathol 100:93–114
Robenek H, Rassat J, Grosser V, Themann H (1982) Ultrastructural study of cholestasis induced by long-term treatment with estradiol valerate. I. Tight junctional analysis and tracer experiments. Virchows Arch (Cell Pathol) 40:201–215
Roman ID, Monte MJ, Gonzalez-Buitrago JM, Esteller A, Jimenez R (1990) Inhibition of hepatocyte vesicular transport by cyclosporin A in the rat: relationship with cholestasis and hyperbilirubinemia. Hepatology 12:83–91
Ros E, Small DM, Carey MC (1979) Effects of chlorpromazine hydrochloride on bile salt synthesis, bile formation and biliary lipid secretion in the rhesus monkey: a model for chlorpromazine-induced cholestasis. Eur J Clin Invest 9:29–41
Rosario J, Sutherland E, Simon FR (1988) Ethinyl estradiol administration selectively alters liver sinusoidal membrane lipid fluidity and protein composition. Biochemistry 27:3939–3946
Rotolo FS, Branum GD, Bowers BA, Meyers WC (1986) Effect of cyclosporine on bile secretion in rats. Am J Surg 151:35–40
Ruetz S, Fricker G, Hugentobler G, Winterhalter K, Kurz G, Meier PJ (1987) Isolation and characterization of the putative canalicular bile salt transport system of rat liver. J Biol Chem 262:11324–11330
Sakisaka S, Ng OC, Boyer JL (1988) Tubulovesicular transcytotic pathway in isolated rat hepatocyte couplets in culture. Gastroenterology 95:793–804
Samuels AM, Carey MC (1978) Effects of chlorpromazine hydrochloride and its metabolites on Mg^{2+}- and Na,K-ATPase activities of canalicular enriched rat liver plasma membranes. Gastroenterology 74:1183–1190
Sandermann H (1978) Regulation of membrane enzymes by lipids. Biochim Biophys Acta 515:209–237
Schachter D (1984) Fluidity and function of hepatocyte plasma membranes. Hepatology 4:140–151
Schade RR, Guglielmi A, Van Thiel DH, Thompson ME, Warty V, Griffith B, Sanghvi A, Bahnson H, Hardesty R (1983) Cholestasis in heart transplant recipients treated with cyclosporine. Transplant Proc 25:2757–2760
Scharschmidt BF, Keeffe EB, Vessey DA, Blankenship MN, Ockner RK (1981) In vitro effects of bile salts on rat liver plasma membrane, lipid fluidity and ATPase activity. Hepatology 1:137–145
Schenk DB, Hubert JJ, Leffert HL (1984) Use of a monoclonal antibody to quantify (Na^+,K^+)-ATPase activity and sites in normal and regenerating rat liver. J Biol Chem 259:14941–14951
Scholmerlich J, Becher MS, Schmidt L, Schubert R, Kremer B, Feldhaus S, Gerok W (1984) Influence of hydroxylation and conjugation of bile salts on their membrane-damaging properties – studies on isolated hepatocytes and lipid membrane vesicles. Hepatology 4:661–666
Schulze PJ, Czok G (1975) Reduced bile flow in rats during sulfobromophthalein infusion. Toxicol Appl Pharmacol 32:213–224
Schwarz LR, Schwenk M, Pfaff E, Greim H (1977) Cholestatic steroid hormones inhibit taurocholate uptake into isolated rat hepatocytes. Biochem Pharmacol 26:2433–2437
Schwenk M, Schwarz LR, Greim H (1977) Taurolithocholate inhibits taurocholate uptake by isolated hepatocytes at low concentrations. Naunyn Schmiedebergs Arch Pharmacol 298:175–179

Seetharam S, Sussman NL, Komoda T, Alpers DH (1986) The mechanism of elevated alkaline phosphatase activity after bile duct ligation in the rat. Hepatology 6:374–380

Sewell RB, Barham SS, Zinsmeister AR, LaRusso NF (1984) Microtubule modulation of biliary excretion of endogenous and exogenous hepatic lysosomal constituents. Am J Physiol 246:G8–G15

Shepherd AN, Bedford GJ, Hill A, Bouchier IAD (1984) Primary biliary cirrhosis, dark adaptometry, electro-oculography and vitamin A state. Br Med J 289:1484–1485

Shin T, Mizoguchi Y, Kioka K, Kobayashi K, Morisawa S (1992) Study on the mechanism of an experimental immunological intrahepatic cholestasis model. Osaka City Medical J 38:111–125

Shirin H, Schapiro JM, Arber N, Pinkhas J, Sidi Y, Salomon F (1992) Erythromycin base-induced rash and liver function disturbances. Ann Pharmacother 26:1522–1523

Siegers CP, Watkins JB III (1991) Biliary excretion of drugs and other chemicals. Fischer, Stuttgart (Progress in pharmacology and clinical pharmacology, vol 8/4)

Simon FR, Arias IM (1973) Alteration of bile canalicular enzymes in cholestasis. A possible cause of bile secretory failure. J Clin Invest 52:765–775

Simon FR, Sutherland E, Accation L (1977) Stimulation of hepatic Na^+,K^+-ATPase activity by phenobarbital: its possible role in regulation of bile flow. J Clin Invest 59:849–861

Simon FR, Gonzalez M, Sutherland E, Accation L, Davis RA (1980) Reversal of ethinyl estradiol-induced bile secretory failure with Triton WR-1339. J Clin Invest 65:851–859

Sippel CJ, Ananthanarayanan M, Suchy FJ (1990) Isolation and characterization of the canalicular membrane bile acid transport protein. Am J Physiol 258:G729–G737

Slikker W, Vore M, Bailey JR, Meyers M, Montgomery C (1983) Hepatotoxic effects of estradiol-17β-D-glucuronide in the rat and monkey. J Pharmacol Exp Ther 225:138–43

Spector AA, Yorek MA (1985) Membrane lipid composition and cellular function. J Lipid Res 26:1015–1035

Spivey JR, Bronk SF, Gores GJ (1993) Glycochenodeoxycholate-induced lethal hepatocellular injury in rat hepatocytes: role of ATP depletion and cytosolic free calcium. J Clin Invest 92:17–24

Stacey NH, Kotecka B (1988) Inhibition of taurocholate and ouabain transport in isolated rat hepatocytes by cyclosporin A. Gastroenterology 95:780–786

Stiehl A, Becker M, Czygan P, Frohling W, Kommerell B, Rothauwe HW, Senn M (1980) Bile acids and their sulphated and glucuronidated derivatives in bile, plasma, and urine of children with intrahepatic cholestasis. effects of phenobarbital treatment. Eur J Clin Invest 10:307–316

Stolz A, Takikawa H, Ookhtens M, Kaplowitz N (1989) The role of cytoplasmic proteins in hepatic bile acid transport. Annu Rev Physiol 51:161–176

Storch J, Schachter D (1984) A dietary regimen alters hepatocyte plasma membrane fluidity and ameliorates ethinyl estradiol cholestasis in the rat. Biochim Biophys Acta 798:137–140

Storch J, Schachter D, Inoue M (1983) Lipid fluidity of hepatocyte plasma membrane subfractions and their differential regulation by calcium. Biochim Biophys Acta 727:209–212

Stubbs CD (1983) Membrane fluidity: structure and dynamics of membrane lipids. Essays Biochem 19:1–39

Stramentinoli G, DiPadova C, Gualano M, Rabagnati P, Galli-Kienle M (1981) Ethinylestradiol-induced impairment of bile secretion in the rat. Protective effects of S-adenosyl-l-methionine and its implication in estrogen metabolism. Gastroenterology 80:154–158

Takikawa H, Tomita J, Takemura T, Yamanaka M (1991) Cytotoxic effect and uptake mechanism by isolated rat hepatocytes of lithocholate and its glucuronide and sulfate. Biochim Biophys Acta 1091:173–178

Tarao K, Olinger EJ, Ostrow DJ, Balistreri WF (1982) Impaired bile acid efflux from hepatocytes isolated from the liver of rats with cholestasis. Am J Physiol 243:G253–G258
Tavaloni N, Boyer JL (1980) Relationship between hepatic metabolism of chlorpromazine and cholestatic effects in the isolated perfused rat liver. J Pharmacol Exp Ther 214:269–274
Tavolini N, Reed JS, Boyer JL (1978) Hemodynamic effects on determinants of bile secretion in isolated rat liver. Am J Physiol 234:E584–E592
Toda G, Kako M, Oka H, Oda T, Ikeda Y (1978) Uneven distribution of enzymatic alterations on the liver cell surface in experimental extrahepatic cholestasis of rat. Exp Mol Pathol 28:10–24
Toda G, Ikeda Y, Kako M, Oka H, Oda T (1980) Mechanism of elevation of serum alkaline phosphatase activity in biliary obstruction: an experimental study. Clin Chim Acta 107:85–96
Traiger GJ, Vyas KP, Hanzlik RP (1985) Effects of inhibitors of α-naphthylisothiocyanate induced hepatotoxicity on the in vivo metabolism of α-naphthylisothiocyanate. Chem Biol Interact 52:335–345
Tuchweber B, Gabbiani G (1976) Phalloidin-induced hyperplasia of actin microfilaments in rat hepatocytes. In: Preisig R, Bircher J, Paumgartner G (eds) The liver: quantitative aspects of structure and function. Karger, Basel pp 84–90
Utili R, Abernathy CO, Zimmermann HJ (1977) Studies on the effect of Escherichia coli endotoxin on canalicular bile formation in isolated perfused rat liver. J Lab Clin Med 89:471–482
Utili R, Tripodi MF, Adinolfi LD, Gaeta FB, Abernathy CO, Zimmerman HJ (1990) Estradiol-17β-D-glucuronide (E-17G) cholestasis in perfused rat liver: fate of E-17G and choleretic responses to bile salts. Hepatology 11:735–742
Van Dyke RW (1990) The liver in pregnancy. In: Zakim D, Boyer TD (eds) Hepatology. Saunders, New York, pp 1438–1459
Van Dyke RW, Scharschmidt BF (1987) Effect of chlorpromazine on Na^+-K^+-ATPase pumping and solute transport in rat hepatocytes. Am J Physiol 253:G613–G621
Vonk RJ, Tuchweber B, Masse D, Perea A, Audet M, Roy CC, Yousef IM (1981) Intrahepatic cholestasis induced by allo monohydroxy bile acid in rats. Gastroenterology 81:242–259
Vore M (1987) Estrogen cholestasis. Membranes, metabolites or receptors? Gastroenterology 93:643–649
Vore M (1991) Cholestasis. In: Siegers CP, Watkins JB III (eds) Progress in pharmacology and clinical pharmacology: biliary excretion of drugs and other chemicals. Fischer, Stuttgart, pp 455–474
Vore M, Slikker W (1985) Steroid D-ring glucuronides, a new class of cholestatic agents. Trends Pharmacol Sci 6:256–259
Vore M, Hadd H, Slikker W (1983) Ethinylestradiol-17β-D-ring glucuronide conjugates are potent cholestatic agents in the rat. Life Sci 32:2989–2993
Vore M, Montgomery C, Durham S, Schlarman D, Elliott WH (1989) Structure-activity relationship of the cholestatic activity of dihydrotestosterone glucuronide, allo bile acids and lithocholate. Life Sci 44:2033–2040
Vu DD, Tuchweber B, Plaa GL, Yousef IM (1992) Pathogenesis of lithocholate-induced intrahepatic cholestasis: role of glucuronidation and hydroxylation of lithocholate. Biochim Biophys Acta 1126:53–59
Wannagat FJ, Adler RD, Ockner RK (1978) Bile acid-induced increase in bile acid-independent flow and plasma membrane Na,K-ATPase activity in rat liver. J Clin Invest 61:297–307
Watanabe S, Miyairi M, Oshio C, Smith CR, Phillips MJ (1983) Phalloidin alters bile canalicular contractility in primary monolayer cultures of rat liver. Gastroenterology 85:245–253
Weinman SA, Graf J, Boyer JL (1989) Voltage-driven, taurocholate-dependent secretion in isolated hepatocyte couplets. Am J Physiol 256:G826–G832

Wieland LT, Nassal M, Kramer W, Fricker G, Bickel U, Kurz G (1984) Identity of hepatic membrane transport systems for bile salts, phalloidin, and antamanide by photoaffinity labeling. Proc Natl Acad Sci USA 81:5232–5236

Witzleben CL (1972) Physiologic and morphologic natural history of a model of intrahepatic cholestasis (manganese-bilirubin overload). Am J Pathol 65:577–588

Yamada S, Takehara K, Arai T, Takezawa J, Kobayashi S, Mizoguchi Y, Morisawa S, Yamamoto S, Nagura H (1990) Immunocytochemical studies on cholestatic factor in human liver with or without cholestasis. Liver 10:129–136

Yamaguchi Y, Dalle Molle E, Hardison WGM (1991) Vasopressin triggers myosin light chain phosphorylation in isolated rat hepatocytes. Am J Physiol 24:312–319

Yousef IM, Tuchweber R, Vonk RJ, Masse D, Audet M, Roy CC (1981) Lithocholate cholestasis-sulfated glycolithocholate-induced intrahepatic cholestasis in rats. Gastroenterology 80:233–241

Zafrani ES, Ishak KG, Rudzki C (1979) Cholestatic and hepatocellular injury associated with erythromycin esters. Report of nine cases. Dig Dis Sci 24:385–396

Zimmerli B, Valantinas J, Meier PJ (1989) Multispecificity (sinusoidal) rat liver plasma membrane vesicles. J Pharmacol Exp Ther 250:301–308

Zimmerman HJ, Lewis JH (1978) Drug-induced cholestasis. Med Toxicol 2:112–160

Zimniak P, Awasthi YC (1993) ATP-dependent transport systems for organic anions. Hepatology 17:330–339

Zimniak P, Ziller SA, Panfil I, Radominska A, Wolters H, Kuipers F, Sharma R, Saxena M, Moslen MT, Vore M, Vonk RJ, Awasthi YC, Lester R (1992) Identification of an anion-transport ATPase that catalyzes glutathione conjugate-dependent ATP hydrolysis in canalicular plasma membranes from normal rats and rats with conjugated hyperbilirubinemia (GY mutant). Arch Biochem Biophys 292:534–538

Zysset T, Reichen J (1988) Anticholestatic agents: experimental and clinical aspects. In: Testa B, Perrissoud D (eds) Liver drugs: from experimental pharmacology to therapeutic application. CRC Press, Boca Raton, pp 113–143

CHAPTER 8

Fatty Liver and Drugs

M.U. DIANZANI

A. General Mechanisms for Fatty Liver

Fatty infiltration of the liver is one of the most common responses of the liver to injury. The mechanisms, however, can differ according to the type of injury. To gain a good understanding of these mechanisms, the general scheme of triglyceride metabolism in the liver must be considered. Triglycerides (TGs), which are present in the hepatocytes, are synthesized locally from glycerol and fatty acids by TG synthetase. The liver uses TGs either to incorporate them in membranes, or to incorporate them in lipoproteins, which are "secreted" in the blood, or also, in restricted amounts, to hydrolyze them, usually within secondary lysosomes. The amount of TGs present inside a single hepatocyte therefore represents the balance between synthetic processes and removal.

In order to synthesize TGs, the hepatocyte needs glycerol and free fatty acids (FFAs). Whereas glycerol is easily synthesized within the hepatocytes, FFAs have a double origin. The most important part of them arrives preformed from the blood, and a minor portion is synthesized inside the hepatocytes, starting from acetyl-coenzyme A (acetyl-CoA). Only FFAs have access to the hepatocytes, whereas esterified fatty acids, as bound to chylomicrons or lipoproteins, need preliminary hydrolysis by lipoprotein lipase. Most of the FFAs present in the blood circulate bound to anionic proteins. From these they are released to hepatocytes. Inside these cells, they bind by specific transport proteins (especially ligandins, or proteins Y and protein Z). The level of circulating FFAs is modulated by the degree of activity of adipocyte lipase, which releases them from depot fat. The activity of lipase is strictly dependent upon the local concentration of cAMP, which is the balance between its production by adenylate cyclase and its destruction by the specific phosphodiesterase. Adenylate cyclase activity is stimulated by several hormones, such as epinephrine, norepinephrine, glucagon, adrenocorticotropic hormone (ACTH), glucocorticoids, and prostaglandins.

The synthesis of FFAs inside hepatocytes requires FFA activation to form acyl-coenzyme As (acyl-CoAs), and therefore energy in the form of ATP. It is favored by an increase in the local ratio between the reduced and oxidized forms of pyridine nucleotides. FFAs participating in the intrahepatocytic pool, independently of their origin, can be used by the cells in different ways. A certain portion can undergo oxidation either within mitochondria or within peroxisomes. Oxidation requires energy, as only acyl-CoAs are oxidized. Whereas inside the mitochondria oxidation is coupled to oxidative phosphorylation, thus producing much more energy than is consumed, oxidative phosphorylation is not present in peroxisomes. Therefore the oxidation in peroxisomes, which especially concerns long-chained fatty acids, is not energy producing.

Another portion of the FFAs is used by the hepatocytes for the synthesis of complex lipids. These may be either structural, i.e., they may contribute to the formation of membranes, or secretable, for instance lipoproteins. Secretable fats represent the most important portion; the bulk are represented by TG and by phospholipids. Lipoprotein secretion represents by far the most important pathway for the exit of TGs from their intracellular pool. A minor fraction, especially represented by TGs bound to membranes, is hydrolyzed inside cytolysosomes by a local acid lipase, after segregation of the membranes within autophagic vacuoles and their fusion with lysosomes.

Lipoproteins are formed by hydrophobic constituents (especially TGs and cholesterol esters), as well as by hydrophilic components (mainly proteins). Phospholipids (which contain both hydrophilic and hydrophobic portions) have the function of combining other components in a secretable micelle. The synthesis of the three main constituents of the lipoprotein molecule is done in the cytosol or in the endoplasmic reticulum, but their assembly occurs inside the Golgi apparatus. Here another important phenomenon occurs, i.e., the maturation of the micelles, by hexosylation (especially galactosylation), rendering them more easily secretable. The well-formed micelles migrate from the Golgi apparatus, as contained in the detached ends of the Golgi tubules, to the plasma membrane. The depolymerization of the main microtubular protein, i.e., tubulin, plays a role in this migration (see reviews by DIANZANI 1978, 1979a, 1992) (Fig. 1).

Accumulation of TGs inside the hepatocytes may occur either by increased production or by decreased release or destruction. Increased production requires an increased use of FFAs for this purpose, and this may depend either on an increase in the total FFA pool (depending either on an increased supply by the blood or on an increased local synthesis of new FFAs), or on a decrease in the portion of the pool used for other metabolic pathways (especially oxidation). Decreased TG destruction may occur either as a result of the

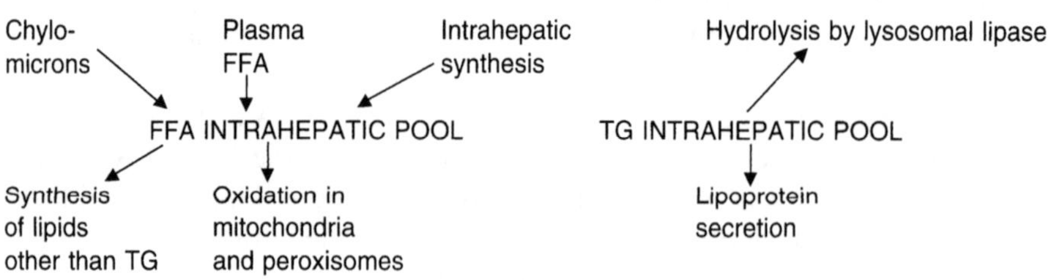

Fig. 1. The main pathways for FFA and TG metabolism in the hepatocyte

congenital deficiency of the lysosomal acid lipase (this is the cause of a very rare form of fatty liver, called Wolman's disease, where fat is segregated inside secondary lysosomes) or, much more frequently, as a result of an impairment of lipoprotein secretion.

This may be provoked by a block in the synthesis of the protein portion, by inhibition of the synthesis of the phospholipid portion, by defects in the assembly and maturation of the lipoprotein micelles in the Golgi apparatus, or by a defect in the migration of the well-formed micelles throughout the cytoplasm. Several drugs produce fatty liver. Each acts by one or more of these mechanisms.

B. Drugs Provoking Fatty Liver

I. Drugs Provoking Fatty Liver by Increasing FFA Supply to the Liver

Several drugs act in this way. Some increase FFAs in the blood by activating adipocyte adenylate cyclase. Others act by inhibiting adipocyte phosphodiesterase. Substances increasing adenylate cyclase activity are epinephrine, glucagon, ACTH, and glucocorticoids (see DIANZANI 1978, 1979a, 1992 for reviews). All these substances have been found capable of producing fatty liver.

Moreover, fatty liver is frequent during clinical stress, clearly as a consequence of the overproduction of some of these hormones. Stress can have several causes, including treatment with large enough amounts of poisons. Therefore, several toxic substances, for instance, ethanol or CCl_4, that produce fatty liver by direct action on the liver, act to increase TGs inside the liver also by this mechanism. It is important to mention here that as the amount of FFAs synthesized inside the liver cells is not high, arrival of FFAs from the blood is in any case necessary for the production of every type of fatty liver (HEIMBERG et al. 1964).

Other substances increase FFA supply to the liver by inhibiting adipocyte phosphodiesterase. The most powerful inhibitors of this enzyme so far known are methylxanthines, i.e., caffeine, theophylline, and theobromine. In the rat a single dose of 20 mg caffeine/100 g body wt. is sufficient to produce a fatty liver, which reaches a peak 24 h after treatment and is more sustained in adult than in young animals. Repeated treatments (five doses of 15 gm/100 g body wt., one/day) produce a much more intense fatty liver only in adult rats (DIANZANI et al. 1991). These doses are much higher than those usually taken by people consuming a moderate quantity of tea or coffee, but must be considered as possible causes of fatty liver in heavy drinkers.

In all these cases of fatty liver, the liver behaves as the innocent bystander of events occurring in other tissues. Liver function therefore remains normal, and no sign of clinical injury appears, with the only exception of a moderate increase in liver size. Cell damage may occur, however, in time, for several reasons, one of which is the fact that the increase in cell volume produces an increase in the mutual compression among the cells, and at the same time a compression on sinusoids. Therefore, some surface receptors may become obliterated, and the general blood supply restricted. This may be the cause of atrophy. Indeed, in long-term fatty livers, the cytoplasmic mass is generally reduced. Another reason for the damage may be the onset of lipid peroxidation (mostly due to the lack of balance present within cells between the peroxidizable substrate unsaturated fatty acids, or PUFAs) and the local level of antioxidants.

With the increased arrival of the FFAs, the PUFAs also increase, without a corresponding increase in vitamin E, the major lipid-soluble natural antioxidant. In caffeine-treated rats, a clear increase in lipid peroxidation occurs, whereas vitamin E decreases in whole hepatocytes and in the microsomes derived from them (DIANZANI et al. 1991). Lipid peroxidation may produce cell death.

II. Drugs Provoking Fatty Liver by Intrahepatic Mechanisms

Fatty livers related to intrahepatic causes are traditionally divided (see DIANZANI 1978, 1979a, 1992) into: (a) fatty livers due to increased local synthesis of FFAs, (b) fatty livers due to impairment in FFA oxidation, and (c) fatty livers due to decreased TG hydrolysis or release in the form of lipoproteins (LPs). Drugs are available to deal with each of these mechanisms.

1. Drugs Increasing Intrahepatic FFA Synthesis

Long-term treatment with barbiturates or related substances, as well as ethanol treatment, produces fatty liver by this mechanism. Treatment with phenobarbital (5 mg/100 g body wt.) three times a week produces fatty liver, more in female than in male rats (SALVADOR et al. 1970). It has been reported that the main reason is a stimulation of FFA synthesis from acetyl-CoA. This might be related to the increase in the NADPH/NADP ratio occurring during the oxidation of phenobarbital in the smooth endoplasmic reticulum (SER) of the liver cell. Moreover, phenobarbital is an inducer of the SER, whose mass increases, with the consequence that structural TGs also increase. Long-term barbiturate-induced fatty liver may cause lipoperoxidative damage (see DIANZANI 1992 for review), possibly due to the increase in the peroxidizable substrate. There is also the possibility, however, that the metabolism of barbiturates in the SER can produce a certain amount of oxygen free radicals, especially during the flavoprotein step of the chain. This may happen when the dehydrogenation of the substrate is faster than the oxidation of cytochrome P450. In this case, electrons can be released from $FADH_2$ to oxygen, so forming the superoxide anion $O_2^{-\bullet}$. This can accept hydrogen to form hydrogen peroxide, H_2O_2, which can produce the extremely reactive $OH^{\bullet}$ free radical in the presence of iron. Both $O_2^{-\bullet}$ and $OH^{\bullet}$ might be responsible for the onset of lipid peroxidation.

Ethanol treatment is an important cause of fatty liver. Two forms of ethanol-induced fatty liver do exist, i.e., the acute and the chronic forms. Acute fatty liver is a consequence of ethanol metabolism, which is usually oxidized to acetaldehyde by the cytosol NAD-dependent ethanol dehydrogenase. A small portion of the oxidation occurs, however, in the SER by the local monooxygenase chain, mainly by the isoform of cytochrome P450 IIE I, but also by H_2O_2 and by $OH^{\bullet}$ formed at the level of the flavoprotein. It is noteworthy that the ethanol-oxidizing activity of the SER increases after repeated treatments, as ethanol behaves as an inducer (see LIEBER and DE CARLI 1991 for review). Shortly after administration to rats of 6–8g ethanol/100g body wt., an increase in blood FFAs occurs; it precedes the onset of fatty liver, which usually occurs 6h after treatment and lasts for about 12h. For this reason, several authors have considered the toxic stress releasing FFAs from adipocytes as the most important cause of this type of fatty liver. This interpretation is substantiated by the fact that adrenalectomy or hypophysectomy, which abolish the stress-dependent release of FFA from adipocytes, prevent ethanol-induced fatty liver. POGGI and DI LUZIO (1964), however, stated that this mechanism was unimportant, as they found that stress did not provoke the release of ^{14}C-labeled palmitate from an implanted epididymal fat lobule containing this fatty acid. These authors claimed that the main reason for ethanol-induced fatty liver must be intrahepatic. This debate is now over. Undoubtedly, the release of FFAs from adipocytes permits this form of fatty liver, but the real damage is intrahepatic.

Many different intrahepatic causes have been considered as primary events. The most important remains the increased synthesis of FFAs from acetyl-CoA, which has been demonstrated both in vitro and in vivo (see LIEBER and DE CARLI 1991). The main reason for increased synthesis is considered to be the net increase in the ratio between the reduced and the oxidized forms of pyridine nucleotides occurring shortly after ethanol administration. However, this is still unclear.

The lack of fatty liver after administration of sorbitol, which is oxidized in the liver by an NAD-dependent sorbitol dehydrogenase and also provokes an increase in the ratio between reduced and oxidized forms of pyridine nucleotides, still awaits an explanation (SLATER et al. 1964).

Other authors have proposed that another cause for fat deposition is the decline in fatty acid oxidation, mostly related to mitochondrial damage, which has been well documented (see DIANZANI 1978, 1979a, 1992 for reviews). This decline may be a consequence of the decrease in availability of ATP due to uncoupling of oxidative phosphorylation (CUNNINGHAM et al. 1990). Uncoupling is, however, usually found after the onset in fat deposition, so it seems more probable that this factor may contribute to maintaining high levels of TG inside the liver as started by other mechanisms (see DIANZANI 1985, 1991a,b for reviews). It is noteworthy that peroxisomal oxidation does not seem to play an important role, at least in deer mice (INATOMI et al. 1989).

A block in lipoprotein secretion has also been discussed as the primary cause of ethanol-induced fatty liver, but negative results have been obtained by other authors (see DIANZANI 1978, 1979a and 1991 for reviews). Most authors taking a block in LP secretion to be the main cause of fat accumulation consider the inhibition in the protein part of the LP molecule as the primary event. No clear reason for this inhibition, however, has been produced, the only exception being the data reported by PERIN et al. (1974), who reported that relatively high concentrations of acetaldehyde, the main product of ethanol catabolism, increased the production of malonyldialdehyde. DIANZANI (1985) proposed a different kinetics of lipid peroxidation after ethanol, in comparison with that provoked by CCl_4. In the case of ethanol, an increased rate in the destruction of dienes might explain the apparently controversial results. Quite recently, SERGENT (1993) has shown that this is actually the case. Indeed, ethanol dehydrogenation by the NAD-dependent ethanol dehydrogenase produced an increase in the reduced forms of this pyridine nucleotide. NADH + H^+ has been found capable of releasing small amounts of free iron (Fe^{2+}) from heme, thus starting a free radical reaction characterized by the formation of the superoxide anion, hydrogen peroxide, and hydroxyl radical. This would start lipid peroxidation, and at the same time would increase the destruction of formed lipoperoxides, as well as of other substances displaying the diene conjugation absorption band. The experiments by SERGENT also allowed reconsideration of the problem of the intracellular sites for the formation of oxygen free radicals after ethanol. Until now, it has been considered that the microsomal ethanol-oxidizing system was the only site for the production of such radicals. The radicals were thought to be produced at the level of $FADH_2$, as well as at that of cytochrome P450 IIEI. SERGENT has shown that even the "innocent" ethanol dehydrogenase cytosolic pathway is producing free radicals. In any case, ethanol metabolism is responsible for the onset of lipid peroxidation, whose intensity appears to be dose dependent, and is much more intense after chronic than after acute treatment (see DIANZANI 1991a for review and also ANTONENKOV et al. 1989; KAMIMURA et al. 1992; NORDMANN et al. 1992). In chronic liver injury, the hepatic level of GSH has been found to be greatly decreased (see DIANZANI 1991a for review). Vitamin E is decreased both in plasma (KAWASE et al. 1989) and in the liver (BELL et al. 1992). Even the activity of the enzymes that represent a natural defense against free radicals, such as superoxide dismutase and glutathione peroxidase, show a decrease (ZIDENBERG-CHERR et al. 1991).

In addition to the oxygen and to the lipodienyl free radicals, ethanol treatment is characterized by the production of other radicals directly inhibiting protein synthesis in vitro. Even other aldehydes, and especially those produced from lipids undergoing lipid peroxidation, are able to block protein synthesis, but also at relatively high concentrations (DIANZANI 1979b, 1982, 1985). Therefore, it remains questionable whether such concentrations may be really reached in poisoned liver.

Another possible effect of the aldehydes, i.e., the block in tubulin depolymerization, that plays a role in the intracellular traffic of LP, is also difficult to accept as the main cause for fat accumulation, especially since it occurs again at relatively high aldehyde concentrations. BARAONA et al. (1977) indicated such an effect of acetaldehyde on tubulin in poisoned animals. BERMAN et al. (1983), however, found no morphological evidence for this effect. Colchicine, the most powerful drug affecting tubulin function, is capable of causing fat accumulation in isolated hepatocytes (POLI et al. 1979, 1987). Moreover, several authors (BARRY et al. 1987; XU et al. 1989) have demonstrated the formation of covalent bonds between acetaldehyde and the actin/microfilament system. Acetaldehyde binding has been demonstrated even with many other different proteins (DONAHUE et al. 1983; JUKKOLA and NIEMELÄ 1989; NIEMELÄ and ISRAEL 1992; WORRALL et al. 1991). It has been inferred that such adducts might be important in the initiation of an autoimmune reaction, which would play a role in the development of chronic hepatitis and fibrosis. In conclusion, the participation of aldehydes in blocking protein synthesis, as well as microtubule function, cannot be ruled out completely. It seems probable, however, that it can work only when particularly high concentrations of aldehydes are reached, i.e., in chronic ethanol poisoning.

Other authors have emphasized the role of lipid peroxidation in ethanol toxicity. The first approach to the problem was the demonstration by DI LUZIO and coworkers (DI LUZIO 1964) that the antioxidants display a protective action on ethanol-induced fatty liver. COMPORTI et al. (1967) found an increase in malonyl dialdehyde production both in vivo and in vitro after acute ethanol administration. HASHIMOTO and RECKNAGEL (1968), however, refuted the presence of lipid peroxidation, as they were unable to discover the appearance of the band of dienes in phospholipids isolated from microsomes of treated rats. This was confirmed by TORRIELLI et al. (1978), who confirmed a relationship to the ethanol molecule. ALBANO et al. (1987, 1988) have been able to detect the ethylhydroxy free radical by spin trapping. This free radical generates addition products with microsomal proteins (ALBANO et al. 1993a). The ethanol radical is formed especially at the level of cytochrome P450 IIEI, as antibodies against this isoform practically cancel the formation of the free radicals (ALBANO et al. 1993b; FRENCH et al. 1993); only a minor portion of them are formed after interaction with the oxygen free radicals produced in the first portion of the microsomal oxidizing chain, as shown by the inhibitory effects of the scavengers for $OH^{\bullet}$ (especially mannitol), and by desferroxiamine, sequestering iron that is needed for the formation of $OH^{\bullet}$ from $O_2^{\bullet}$ or H_2O_2 by a Haber-Weiss or a Fenton reaction. Another free radical is produced during the oxidation of acetaldehyde, but its nature is still controversial (Albano, personal communication). Undoubtedly, acetaldehyde oxidation by aldehyde oxidase or by xanthine oxidase gives rise to the superoxide anion (FRIDOVICH 1989; KERA et al. 1988; KATO et al. 1990). In this way, acetaldehyde contributes to stimulation of lipid peroxidation after ethanol (MÜLLER and SIES 1982).

In the acute ethanol treatment, lipid peroxidation probably plays a minor role, as also demonstrated by the absence of cell death; in contrast, after CCl_4 it is preventable by blocking lipid peroxidation by vitamin E preloading or promethazine pretreatment. The fact that antioxidants display a limited protection towards this type of fatty liver may indicate some participation of radical reactions in the fatty liver phenomenon, whereas other causes play a more important role.

Other alcohols, such as isopropanol, butanol, and pentanol, are also metabolized by the liver. They also give rise to the production of alcohol free radicals, which are generally more abundant than those following treatment with ethanol (ALBANO et al. 1987). It is possible that the higher toxicity of distilled heavy drinks, which contain more alcohols of this type than wine, is at least partially dependent upon their presence. An isopropanol-induced fatty liver has been described by NORDMANN et al. (1973). Its causes are probably similar to those occurring in ethanol poisoning.

2. Drugs Provoking Fatty Liver by Decreasing Fatty Acid Oxidation

A decrease in fatty acid oxidation occurs in the late stages of most toxic fatty livers. In the past, after the discovery of uncoupling of oxidative phosphorylation in mitochondria from fatty livers caused by CCl_4 or white phosphorus (DIANZANI 1954), this mechanism was thought to be the most important cause of fatty liver in such conditions. It was established, however, that the onset mechanisms were different, so the decline in oxidation remained only as a helper mechanism, contributing to the maintenance of high TG levels in the late stages of several poisonings. A primary involvement of this type of damage is, however, still possible for 4-pentenoic acid-induced fatty liver (THAYER 1984). This substance seems to interfere with the formation of CoA that is needed, together with ATP, for fatty acid activation, i.e., for the formation of acyl-CoAs, the only acid form suitable for oxidation in mitochondria. It is also possible that the block in oxidation plays a role even in arsenite-induced fatty liver. Arsenite is a poison for -SH groups, so even protein synthesis is precociously affected. The oxidative block occurs, however, at a very early stage (WEBB 1966).

3. Drugs Blocking Lipoprotein Secretion

The block of lipoprotein secretion represents by far the most important mechanism of toxic fatty liver. This block may occur either by inhibition of the synthesis of the phospholipid part of LPs, or also by inhibition of their protein part. Minor causes may be disturbances in the assembly or in the intracellular traffic of the LP micelles.

a) Drugs Affecting Phospholipid Synthesis

The prototype of this type of fatty liver is a nutritional one, i.e., fatty liver due to choline deficiency. Treatment with high doses of nicotinamide, which is frequently performed for therapeutic purposes can, however, produce a fatty liver by this mechanism. Indeed, nicotinamide is eliminated as *N*-methyl derivative, so that it acts as a depletor for methyl groups, thus preventing phospholipid synthesis. A mechanism related to a block in phospholipid synthesis has been proposed even for fatty livers following treatment with salts of the rare earths, such as lanthanium, cerium, praseodymium, neodymium, and samarium. GLENN et al. (1963) reported a decreased incorporation of palmitic acid into cardiolipin and phosphatidylinositol, thus suggesting such a mechanism for this type of fatty liver. Severe mitochondrial damage has been reported, however, even with this type of poisoning and the SER is also deeply affected (see DIANZANI 1978, 1979a, and 1992 for reviews). LOMBARDI and RECKNAGEL (1962) showed in any case that rare earths provoke a block in lipoprotein secretion.

b) Drugs Affecting Apolipoprotein Synthesis

Several drugs produce fatty liver by inhibiting protein synthesis. The block can occur at different steps of the complex mechanisms of protein synthesis. Several inhibitors act directly on the DNA template, so preventing the synthesis of mRNA. One of them is actinomycin D, which is, however, poorly steatogenic, probably due to the fact that the action of this drug affects protein synthesis even at the level of the adipocytes, so preventing the release of FFAs to the blood, permitting the development of fatty liver (DIANZANI and GRAVELA 1975). Aflatoxins, and especially aflatoxin B_1 toxic products of *Aspergillus flavus*, are, however, strongly steatogenic and cancerogenic when administered to rats. Their toxicity depends upon hydroxylation by the monooxygenase system of the SER (see DIANZANI 1992), the isoform of cytochrome P450 IIIA being the most effective (FORRESTER et al. 1990). The activation in the SER includes the formation of free radicals that have been detected by spin trapping (KODAMA et al. 1990). A protective effect of antioxidants, and especially of crocetin, a carotenoid, toward liver cell damage provoked by this mycotoxin has been reported (WANG et al. 1991a,b), thus suggesting participation of this free radical in toxicity. This depends upon the formation of adducts of hydroxylated aflatoxin with DNA, especially at the level of the guanine N7 position. Additional mechanisms for cell damage might be direct inhibition of RNA polymerase, or the formation of adducts with cytoplasmic RNA in addition to DNA (see DIANZANI 1978, 1979a, and 1992 for reviews).

An action at the level of template RNA is present even in the case of several alkylating substances, which, like aflatoxin, are at the same time steatogenic, necrogenic, and cancerogenic. Of such substances, including azodyes, ethionine, and alkylnitrosamines, especially ethionine, dimethylnitrosamine, and diethylnitrosamine have been the object of thorough study. The alkylation by such substances, however, is not restricted to DNA, but includes all the forms of cytoplasmic RNA. Moreover, ethionine is capable of trapping ATP to form the relatively stable adenosyl-*S*-ethionine, so depleting ATP in the liver cell. According to SHULL (1962), this is the main mechanism for the inhibition of protein synthesis displayed by ethionine. Without ATP, aminoacyl AMP and aminoacyl tRNA are not formed, so that protein synthesis is ineffective.

Dimethyl- and diethylnitrosamines provoke fatty liver in rats 5–6h after administration of a single dose of 30–50mg/kg body wt. Both substances are activated in the SER, possibly by a pathway including the formation of free radicals, diazomethane being one of the final products. The efficiency of the cytochrome P450 chain is required for toxicity. The onset of lipid peroxidation after dimethylnitrosamine has been reported (Slater 1972). Alkylation of mRNA, rRNA, and tRNA, in addition to DNA, has been observed (see Dianzani 1992 for review).

Other drugs affect protein synthesis by inhibiting mRNA formation. Amanitines, the most toxic poisons from the mushroom *Amanita phalloides*, specifically inhibit RNA polymerase II (see Dianzani 1992 for review). Fatty infiltration starts about 24h after poisoning. The penetration of the cyclopeptide across liver cell membrane requires the presence at its surface, especially in the sinusoidal face, of polypeptide receptors. Two of these, with molecular masses of 48 and 54kDa, respectively, have been characterized (Kroncke et al. 1986).

D-Galactosamine is another inhibitor of mRNA synthesis. Its action is related to the sequestration of intracellular UTP, which is trapped within uridine diphospho-D-galactosamine (see Dianzani 1992 for review). Galactosamination of plasma membranes would be responsible for the impairment in membrane function, and especially for the loss of the calcium pump, which has been considered as being responsible for cell death. Mourelle and Meza (1989) have found increased lipid peroxidation after D-galactosamine, as well as a protective effect of colchicine, probably related to its antioxidant properties.

Other steatogenic drugs act by blocking the fixation of aminoacyl tRNA to the large ribosomal subunit. Puromycin, a toxic antibiotic, acts in this way. Tetracyclines, which are steatogenic only at high dosage (800mg/kg body wt. in the rat, in the case of oleandomycin) specifically block the fixation on the 50S subunit of phenylalanyl tRNA (see Dianzani 1978, 1979a,b, and 1992 for reviews).

Cycloheximide, another toxic antibiotic, is an inhibitor of translation. When administered to rats, it "freezes" the polyribosomal profiles, as it prevents the movement of ribosomes along the messenger RNA. The same property is displayed by emetine, used for a long time in therapy as an antimalarial drug. Emetine is more steatogenic than cycloheximide, possibly due to their differential effect on FFA supply to the blood from adipocytes (see Dianzani 1978, 1979a, and 1992 for reviews). Other inhibitors of the translation provided with a modest steatogenic activity, possibly due to some extrahepatic effect, are diptheria toxin (Casu et al. 1966), ricin (Montanaro et al. 1973; Sperti et al. 1973), abrin (Olsnes and Pihl 1973), modeccin (a peptide from the African *Adenia digitata*) (Stirpe et al. 1978), volkensin (a peptide from

Adenia volkensi) (Barbieri et al. 1982) and viscumin (a protein from *Viscum album*) (Olsnes et al. 1982).

White phosphorus and halogenated hydrocarbons (especially CCl_4) are considered the most important poisons of the initiation reaction in vivo. The initiation reaction is needed to recycle ribosomal subunits which have escaped from the messenger RNA filament. It requires specific factors and -SH groups. Both white phosphorus and halogenoalkanes provoke the dissociation of polyribosomal profiles, as the detached subunits cannot cycle again. Therefore, the polyribosomal profiles are characterized by the sole presence of subunits, monomers, and some dimers, whereas polymers (i.e., a high number of ribosomes attached to the messenger filament) disappear. It is noteworthy that the previous treatment with cycloheximide or emetin, which block the translation, prevents the white phosphorus- or CCl_4-induced dissociation of the profiles. This proves that such poisons do not act on ribosomes still bound to mRNA, but are able to prevent the reattachment to it of the subunits (see Dianzani 1978, 1979, 1992 for reviews).

White phosphorus is the only poison whose toxicity is not dependent upon its chemical nature, but upon its physical structure. Indeed, the other allotropic forms of this element (black, red phosphorus), as well as P^{32}, are nontoxic (Dianzani 1972). The reasons for toxicity are still unknown, but some metabolic change is probably occurring in the SER since the destruction of the local drug-metabolizing system by SKF525A is protective (Torrielli et al. 1973). It has been reported that oxygenated derivatives of phosphorus, such as phosphonates and phosphinites, are able to inactivate cytochrome P450 (Dahl and Hodgson 1978). A radical involvement is suggested by the appearance of increased lipid peroxidation in treated rats (Ghoshal et al. 1971). Therefore, fatty liver is mostly due to a block in protein synthesis and of lipoprotein secretion (Recknagel et al. 1960, 1961; Lombardi and Recknagel 1962), but additional factors may collaborate, especially in the late phases of poisoning, where very heavy mitochondrial changes and uncoupling of oxidative phosphorylation are also present (Dianzani 1954, 1972).

Halogenated hydrocarbon toxicity is also dependent upon their metabolism in the drug-metabolizing system of the SER, the same isoform of cytochrome P450 being involved in ethanol metabolism, i.e., IIEI is the most important site for the production of $CCl_3^{\bullet}$ free radical, the primary metabolic product (Castillo et al. 1992). It is noteworthy that CCl_4 can be metabolized, at a slow rate, even in other intracellular sites, as nuclear membrane (Diaz Gomez and Castro 1980; Castro et al. 1990), plasma membrane (Wu and Cederbaum 1992), and mitochondria (Levy and Brabec 1984; Albano et al. 1985a; Tomasi et al. 1987). Toxicity is closely dependent upon the metabolism. Therefore, the most toxic haloalkanes are at the same time those which are more easily metabolized. Among the halomethanes, the most toxic is $CBrCl_3$, followed by CCl_4, $CHCl_3$, and CH_2Cl_2. Several haloalkanes or -alkenes are used in industry, e.g., 1,2-dibromoethane, which is a pesticide, CCl_4, chloroform and trieline, which are well-known solvents, halothane, which is used in anesthesia, and vinyl compounds, which are used in the industry of plastics. Free radicals of such compounds have been identified by spin trapping (TOMASI et al. 1985 for $CHCl_3$; TOMASI et al. 1985 for 1,2-dibromoethane; TOMASI et al. 1983a,b for halothane; and TOMASI et al. 1980 for CCl_4). The toxicity of such drugs, as well as the formation of free radicals, is increased by previous induction of hyperplasia of the SER by phenobarbital, or by other inducers. In contrast, the destruction of the drug-metabolizing system of SER by SKF525A, lead nitrate, methoxsalen, or small doses of CCl_4 itself (UGAZIO et al. 1973) strongly decreases toxicity. It is noteworthy that newborn rats, whose cytochrome P450-dependent chain is very low in activity, resist high doses of CCl_4 and that "regenerating" liver, where the chain is still poorly represented, also resists high doses of the poison (CHEESEMAN et al. 1986).

Even a protein-deficient diet, which decreases the activity of the metabolizing chain, decreases CCl_4 toxicity. The contemporary administration of drugs competing for the metabolic chain, for instance, aminopyrine or propylgallate, is also protective. (See DIANZANI 1978, 1979a and 1992 for reviews.) In contrast, a potentiation of toxicity occurs when CCl_4 is given together with 1,2-dibromoethane (DANNI et al. 1992) or with 1,2-dichloroethane (ARAGNO et al. 1992), the reason being that such haloethanes inactivate GSH transferase, so subtracting the metabolites of these substances from the interaction with GSH. Therefore, more haloethanes remain at the disposal of the free radical-producing microsomal chain (DANNI et al. 1991; CHIARPOTTO et al. 1993).

Trichloromethyl free radical is not the only free radical formed during CCl_4 metabolism. In the presence of oxygen, $CCl_3O_2^{\bullet}$ (trichloroperoxy) is formed. This is more short lived than $CCl_3^{\bullet}$ and reacts more easily with polyunsatured fatty acids, the interaction being prevented by promethazine (FORNI et al. 1983). In contrast, $CCl_3^{\bullet}$ reacts more easily with amino acids and proteins, its reactions not being prevented by promethazine. In vivo, CCl_4 produces two types of damage, i.e., covalent binding of the free radical to proteins, lipids, and nucleotides, and onset of lipid peroxidation (COMPORTI et al. 1965; RECKNAGEL and GHOSHAL 1966). It has been possible (DIANZANI and POLI 1985; POLI et al. 1987) to separate the covalent-binding-dependent damage from that dependent upon lipid peroxidation by pretreating the rats with promethazine, or also by preloading them with the natural antioxidant vitamin E. Promethazine and vitamin E cancel lipid peroxidation, as well as the reactions of $CCl_3^{\bullet}$.

Therefore, it seems evident that lipid peroxidation is provoked by $CCl_3O_2^{\bullet}$, whereas $CCl_3^{\bullet}$ is mostly responsible for covalent binding. A list of the enzymes and functions protected by promethazine and by vitamin E (and thus lipid peroxidation dependent) and of those not affected by such antioxidants (and thus mainly covalent binding dependent) is given in Table 1. It is noteworthy that the antioxidants cancel the acute cell death, without affecting fat deposition. Necrosis is thus dependent upon lipid peroxidation, at least in the acute phases of poisoning, whereas fatty liver is a consequence of covalent

Table 1. Protection by promethazine or by vitamin E preloading of different hepatocyte functions after administration of CCl_4. Results obtained both in vivo and in vitro on isolated hepatocytes

Function	CCl_4-induced inhibition (%)	Protection by promethazine or vitamin E
Microsomal glucose 6-phosphatase	35–40	Complete
Golgi galactosyl-transferase	35–40	Complete
Protein synthesis	40–50	Absent
Cytochrome P450 and related chain	30–35	Very low or absent
Ornithine decarboxylase	30–40	Very low or absent
Protein and lipoprotein secretion	65–80	Absent
Plasma membrane integrity	Time-dependent, usually cell death after 2–3 h	High or complete

Table 2. Time required for the appearance of fat infiltration after treatment with different drugs in the rat

Drug	Dose/100 g body wt.	Latency time (h)
CCl_4	0.26–2.6 m*M*	0.5–1
$CBrCl_3$	0.26 m*M*	0.5–1
CS_2 (males)	2.58 m*M*	12
CS_2 (females)	2.58 m*M*	6
White phosphorus	1.5 mg	6
Ethionine (females)	100 mg	6–7
Dimethylnitrosamine	20 mg	5–6
Diethylnitrosamine	20 mg	5–6
Cycloheximide	0.1 mg	5–6
Emetine	2 mg	3
Aflatoxin B_1	0.1 mg	6
α-Amanitine	0.5 μg	20–24

binding, like the inhibition in protein synthesis. Whereas with most inhibitors of protein synthesis the onset in fat accumulation occurs 5–6 h after poisoning, in the case of CCl_4 the onset time is only 1 h, and the block in protein synthesis does not seem sufficient to explain the early phase of fat deposition. Indeed, the real cause for this onset has been found to be the haloalkylation of apolipoproteins, which renders lipoproteins less easily secretable (POLI et al. 1983, 1987). Of course, other mechanisms (block in protein synthesis, decreased oxidation of fatty acids due to mitochondrial damage) may contribute to maintenance of the high fat levels in later stages of poisoning.

Moreover, lipoperoxidative degradation of fatty acids yields many toxic carbonyl compounds, about 30 of which have been identified so far (ESTERBAUER et al. 1982; POLI et al. 1985b, 1989). Of these, the most toxic products are the 4-hydroxy-2,3-transalkenal series, the most important members of which are 4-hydrox-hexenal, 4-hydroxy-octenal; 4-hydroxy-nonenal,4,5-dihidroxy-decenal, and 4-hydroxy-undecenal. The formation of such substances is strongly increased after CCl_4, which is also able to change the kinetics of lipid peroxidation (POLI et al. 1985b). These aldehydes can escape from still living cells, can form adducts with proteins, and can be found both in exudates and in blood plasma (CURZIO et al. 1986, 1987). Protein adducts can release free 4-hydroxy-nonenal when the concentration of this aldehyde in the medium is low. This may therefore represent a mechanism for exporting the effects of the aldehydes outside the liver in "distant" regions of the body. The formation of such aldehydes is prevented by pretreatment with promethazine (POLI et al. 1989). The aldehydes react either with -SH groups or with NH_2 groups. At high concentrations, which can be found in the liver of heavily poisoned rats, they produce a variety of enzymatic and functional damage. The effects of 4-hydroxynonenal at a concentration of 0.1 m*M* or higher are as follows:

1. Block of protein synthesis
2. Block in protein and lipoprotein secretion
3. Inhibition of ornithine decarboxylase
4. Block of tubulin function (GABRIEL et al. 1977)
5. Inhibition of mitochondrial oxidation
6. Partial impairment in the activity of lysosomal enzymes
7. Inhibition of glucose-6-phosphatase
8. Inhibition of galactosyl transferase

It is noteworthy that, at concentrations of 1 μM or lower, which exist in untreated tissues, 4-hydroxy-nonenal displays many other "physiological activities"; these are listed in Table 3. It is clear that 4-hydroxy-nonenal is able to

Table 3. Effects of 4-hydroxy-nonenal at a concentration of 1 μM or lower

1. Strong activation of plasma membrane adenylate cyclase (hepatocytes) (PARADISI et al. 1985; DIANZANI et al. 1989, 1990)
2. Strong activation of inositolphosphatide phospholipase C (hepatocytes, granulocytes) (ROSSI et al. 1988 a,b, 1990, 1991, 1993)
3. Stimulation of chemotaxis of rat granulocytes (CURZIO et al. 1982, 1983, 1985, 1986)
4. Stimulation of chemokinesis in human granulocytes (CURZIO et al. 1982, 1983, 1985, 1990)
5. Block of the expression of the oncogene c-*myc* in human erythroleukemic cells (line K562) and in promyelocytic human leukemic cells (line HL-60) (BARRERA et al. 1987, 1991; FAZIO et al. 1992, 1993)
6. Reexpression of the gene for gamma globulin in K562 cells (BARRERA et al. 1987) and maturation of chemiluminescent granules in HL-60 cells (BARRERA et al. 1991; FAZIO et al. 1992)
7. Inhibition of ornithine decarboxylase in HL-60 cells (FAZIO et al. 1993)
8. Inhibition of the expression of heat shock proteins in hepatocytes (CAJONE et al. 1989)
9. Inhibition of phospholipase D in NHI 3T3 cells (KISS et al. 1992)

affect cell proliferation and differentiation, as well as the movements of neutrophils.

It has been proposed that acute cell death is related to the block in the calcium pump. Experiments by ALBANO et al. (1985a, 1989a,b) suggest that the changes in Ca^{2+} content in hepatocytes occur in two phases: (a) the discharge of calcium from mitochondria and microsomes into the cytosol, with no change in total calcium content of the whole cell and (b) a second phase characterized by a real increase in intracellular Ca^{2+}. This phase is related to the impairment of the pump sited in plasmamembranes, possibly as consequence of the energetic loss of balance following mitochondrial damage.

The first phase is not directly responsible for cell death. Indeed, it cannot be prevented by pretreatment with promethazine or vitamin E, which are able to prevent cell death. It is probable that this phase is covalent binding dependent (see also SRIVASTAVA et al. 1990). The second phase seems to be more important for cell death, but it is still uncertain whether it is an epiphenomenon or the real cause itself. Incubation of hepatocytes with ATP produces a very strong increase in intracellular Ca^{2+}, without affecting cell viability (NAGELKERKE et al. 1989). Still unpublished experiments performed by CARINI et al. (1995) in this laboratory seem to support the conclusion that Na^{+} extrusion, more than Ca^{2+} extrusion, is responsible for the maintainance of cell life. Other substances provoking fatty liver, as well as a block in protein synthesis, act in less clear ways. Sporidesmin, a toxic product of the mushroom *Pytomyces chartarum*, blocks protein synthesis and lipoprotein secretion (see DIANZANI 1978, 1979, 1992 for reviews). Toxicity seems related to metabolism in the liver with production of superoxide anion (MUNDAY 1982).

Carbon disulfide produces centrilobular fatty infiltration 5–6h after administration (250 μl/100 g body wt.) to rats (BOND and DE MATTEIS 1967). Toxicity depends upon events occurring in the SER, as shown by the blocking of cytochrome P450 by CS_2, and by the increase in toxicity after phenobarbital induction. The intermediate formation of S-CO-S would be followed by its homolytic cleavage to S-CO$^{\bullet}$ and S$^{\bullet}$ free radicals.

Thioacetamide is also steatogenic, necrogenic, and cirrhogenic. When given acutely, it produces severe mitochondrial damage, resulting in a decrease in fatty acid oxidation (MÜLLER and DARGEL 1984). RNA (SMUCKLER and KOPLITZ 1974) and protein synthesis are inhibited. Moreover, an increase in lipid peroxidation occurs (MÜLLER and DARGEL 1990; CASCALES et al. 1991). Thioacetamide metabolism by the drug-metabolizing system seems to be involved in toxicity. Paracetamol at a high dosage is also strongly steatogenic and necrogenic. GSH levels decrease strongly in both the liver of rats treated in vivo and in isolated hepatocytes (ALBANO et al. 1983, 1985b).

Lipid peroxidation is strongly stimulated (see DIANZANI 1992 for reviews). Covalent binding of paracetamol derivatives to -SH-containing substances, such as G-SH or proteins, occurs. A free radical has been identified by spin trapping in vitro, when paracetamol is oxidized by hydrogen peroxide, but has not been found in vivo as yet. Its formation is, however, very probable, possibly at the level of the SER drug-metabolizing system. The chemical nature of the free radical has also clearly not been defined. It is very probably *N*-acetyl-semiquinone imine. This would react with G-SH, with the intermediate formation of thiol free radicals, which have been identified (Ross et al. 1984). Probably, this is the mechanism for G-SH depletion. Fatty liver seems to be a consequence of the block in protein synthesis, but mitochondrial damage is also important in the late stages of poisoning. Another important steatogenic and necrogenic substance is bromobenzene, which is especially active in mice (see COMPORTI 1985, 1989 for review).

This haloarene produces a big GSH depletion, as well as heavy mitochondrial damage (MAELLARO et al. 1990). Lipid peroxidation is much more intense than after CCl_4. It may be related to GSH depletion, but it seems probable that it depends upon the formation of free radicals due to the metabolism of the substance. Covalent binding of this free radical to GSH and to proteins occurs very quickly. It seems probable, however, that cell death even in this case is the consequence of lipid peroxidation. In fact, pretreatment with Trolox C (a soluble form of vitamin E) is protective against cell death. Fatty liver seems to depend, even in this case, on blocking the protein synthesis. It is not protected by Trolox C.

III. Drugs Decreasing Fat Infiltration in the Liver

Several drugs decrease the extent of fat infiltration, some of which act by decreasing TG hydrolysis in adipocytes, so decreasing FFA supply to hepatocytes, leading to every type of fatty liver. Other drugs act in different ways. Of these, one must consider first of all the specific inhibitors of the metabolism of steatogenic drugs, which is very often responsible for the development of fatty livers. Other drugs counteract not the primary event provoking the onset of fatty liver, but secondary events, mainly responsible for maintaining high intrahepatic levels of TG initiated by different mechanisms.

The use of epinephrine or norepinephrine receptor blockers results in a decrease in activation of adipocyte adenylate cyclase, and so in decreased activation of adipocyte lipase. FFA supply to the liver is therefore decreased and steatogenic substances cause a lower level of TG accumulation, if any (TORRIELLI et al. 1973). Adrenalectomy or hypophysectomy, as well as the transection of the spinal cord in the cervical region, also display a protective effect. Of course, the direct damage produced by the used poisons remains unaffected; only the hepatic level of TG is lower. In the case of cordectomy, however, there is some protection even from the intrahepatic damage, at least in the case of CCl_4. Indeed, the metabolism of CCl_4 producing the real toxic derivatives is decreased due to hypothermia. Treatment with adrenergic substances, in contrast, increases fat accumulation (TORRIELLI et al. 1973). Adenylate cyclase activation may be blocked even by inhibitors of the local protein synthesis, such as cycloheximide, actinomycin D, or emetine (DIANZANI 1992 for review).

Another method to decrease TG infiltration is the use of substances which increase fatty acid oxidation. Clofibrate, a substance provoking an increase in peroxisomes and of related enzymes, including fatty acid oxidase, has been reported to act in this way (SCHOFIELD et al. 1982). Due to its damaging effects, clofibrate has now been practically abandoned. WOOLES and WEYMOUTH (1968) used chlorcyclizine to increase fatty acid oxidation and reported a protective effect towards acute ethanol-induced fatty liver.

Ethanol-induced fatty liver is reported to be strongly negatively influenced by inhibiting ethanol oxidation by ethanol dehydrogenase. Pyrazol and related substances (especially 4-methylpyrazol) (LIEBER et al. 1970; see DIANZANI 1991a and 1992 for reviews), which inhibit ethanol dehydrogenase, have been reported to be protective towards ethanol-induced liver damage. Not all authors, however, have obtained positive results, and some have claimed toxicity for pyrazole. According to SERGENT (1993), pyrazole acts by preventing the increase in the ratio between reduced and oxidized forms of pyridine nucleotides, so preventing the release of free iron from heme. The latter phenomenon would be the real mechanism responsible for the onset of lipid peroxidation.

According to several authors, a better protection against ethanol toxicity, including fatty liver, would be achieved by prevention of ethanol metabolism by the drug-metabolizing system of the SER. 3-Amino-1,2,4-triazole, an inhibitor of catalase, which would be partially responsible for the production of the oxygen radicals in this chain, has been reported to be protective. Moreover, competition for the cytochrome P450 chain by other drugs (for instance, phenobarbital given simultaneously, or aspirin) decreases ethanol metabolism in this chain, as well as toxicity, and is protective toward fat accumulation. The same result is achieved by destruction of the chain by small doses of CCl_4. Substances such as propylgallate and diphenylphenylene diamine, which are antioxidants, act by competing for the cytochrome P450-dependent chain (TORRIELLI et al. 1978).

A last method for counteracting some of the damage produced by ethanol is the use of antioxidants. The first approach to this was made by the group of DI LUZIO (1964), who reported a lower TG content in the liver when antioxidants such as hexachromanol or vitamin E were given to rats together with ethanol, both in acute and in chronic tests. We have found, at least in the case of CCl_4, vitamin E preloading did not produce substantial protection toward fat accumulation. Some protective effect, even in the case of ethanol-induced fat accumulation, was seen after parenteral administration of GSH (DIANZANI 1981). One cannot exclude, however, that GSH administered in this way may demonstrate extrahepatic actions.

Fatty livers characterized by the presence of increased lipid peroxidation may receive some benefit from the administration of antioxidants. We have seen in Sect. B.II that in CCl_4-induced cell damage, fatty infiltration is poorly affected by vitamin E preloading or promethazine pretreatment, which, in contrast, practically abolish lipid peroxidation and related damage. Indeed, in this type of fatty liver, fat accumulation mostly depends upon trichloromethylation of apolipoproteins, i.e., upon an interaction that is not related to lipid peroxidation. Only in repeated cirrhogenic treatments with CCl_4 and vitamin E, which strongly reduce the fibrosis, is limited protection afforded against fat accumulation. This may mean that lipid peroxidation is involved in maintaining high levels of fat inside the liver in this type of treatment. Acute damage is, however, prevented by the administration of spin traps, such as phenylbutylnitrone or 2,5,5-trimethylpyrroline oxide (TOWNER et al. 1993). Such substances trap $CCl^{\bullet}_3$, so preventing both its covalent binding and the formation of $CCl_3O^{\bullet}_2$, which is responsible for the onset of lipid peroxidation. It is noteworthy that in chronic CCl_4 treatment, TGFβ_1, a monokine that is considered an inducer of the expression of the gene for procollagen α_1(I), is overproduced (ARMENDARIZ-BORUNDA et al. 1990; PAROLA et al. 1992a,b). Both the overproduction of TGFβ_1 and the overexpression of the gene for procollagen are prevented by vitamin E administration. In Ito cells (fat-storing cells) cultivated in vitro, ascorbate/iron induces both lipid peroxidation and the overexpression of procollagen gene, and 4-hydroxynonenal, the major toxic product of lipid peroxidation, displays a similar action (PAROLA et al. 1993).

Vitamin E and GSH display a protective effect on diethylmaleate (a GSH depletor poisoning), as well as on bromotrichloromethane poisoning (DILLARD et al. 1991). Parenteral treatment with cysteamine or with GSH affords some protection not only against CCl_4 poisoning, but even against paracetamol poisoning (CHU and BHAKHTAN 1978). It is clear, however, that antioxidants abolish only the lipid peroxidation-dependent damage, and not that related to covalent binding. The protective effect of GSH against paracetamol poisoning can be interpreted not only as being related to its antioxidant properties, but also as a substitutive therapy for the replacement of the intracellular GSH, which is depleted by covalent binding of paracetamol metabolites.

Substitutive therapy may even be considered the protectory effect displayed by adenosine (SHULL 1962) in ethionine poisoning, and that displayed by uridine in D-galactosamine poisoning (SHINOZUKA et al. 1973). Indeed, ethionine acts by trapping ATP, an adenosine compound, whereas D-galactosamine traps UTP.

References

Albano E, Poli G, Chiarpotto E, Biasi F, Dianzani MU (1983) Paracetamol-stimulated lipid peroxidation in isolated rat and mouse hepatocytes. Chem Biol Interact 47:249–263

Albano E, Bellomo G, Carini R, Biasi F, Poli G, Dianzani MU (1985a) Mechanisms responsible for carbon tetrachloride-induced perturbation of mitochondrial calcium homeostasis. FEBS 192:184–188

Albano E, Rundgren M, Harrison PJ, Nelson SD, Moldeus P (1985b) Mechanisms of N-acetyl-p-benzoquinone imine toxicity. Mol Pharmacol 28:306–311

Albano E, Tomasi A, Goria-Gatti L, Poli G, Vannini V, Dianzani MU (1987) Free radical metabolism of alcohols by rat liver microsomes. Free Rad Res Comms 3:243–249

Albano E, Tomasi A, Goria-Gatti L, Dianzani MU (1988) Spin trapping of free radical species produced during the microsomal metabolism of ethanol. Chem Biol Interact 65:223–236

Albano E, Carini R, Parola M, Bellomo G, Goria-Gatti L, Poli G, Dianzani MU (1989a) Effects of carbon tetrachloride in calcium homeostasis. A critical reconsideration. Biochem Pharmacol 38:2719–2725

Albano E, Carini R, Parola M, Bellomo G, Poli G, Dianzani MU (1989b) Increase in cytosolic free calcium and its role in the pathogenesis of hepatocyte injury induced by carbon tetrachloride. Adv Biosci 76:45–53

Albano E, Parola M, Comoglio A, Dianzani MU (1993a) Evidence for the covalent binding of hydroxyethyl radicals to rat liver microsomal proteins. Alcohol Alcohol 28:453–459

Albano E, Tomasi A, Persson JO, Terelius Y, Goria-Gatti L, Ingelman-Sundberg M, Dianzani MU (1993b) Role of ethanol-inducible cytochrome P450 II E I in catalyzing the free radical activation of aliphatic alcohols. Biochem Pharmacol 41:1895–1902

Antonenkov VD, Pirozhkov SV, Popova SV, Pachenko LF (1989) Effect of chronic ethanol treatment on lipid peroxidation in rat liver homogenate and subcellular fractions. Int J Biochem 21:1191–1195

Aragno M, Tamagno E, Danni O, Ugazio G (1992) In vivo studies in halogenocompound interactions. III. Effect of carbon tetrachloride plus 1,2-dichloroethane on liver necrosis and fat accumulation. Res Commun Chem Pathol Pharmacol 76:341–354

Armendariz-Borunda J, Seyer JM, Kang AH, Raghow (1990) Regulation of TGFβ_1 gene expression in rat liver intoxicated with carbon tetrachloride. FASEB J 4:215–221

Baraona E, Leo MA, Borowsky SA, Lieber CS (1977) Pathogenesis of alcohol-induced accumulation of proteins in the liver. J Clin Invest 60:546–554

Barbieri L, Falasca AI, Stirpe F (1982) Volkensin, the toxin of *Adenia volkensii* (Kiliambiti plant). FEBS 171:277–279

Barrera G, Martinotti S, Fazio V, Manzari V, Paradisi L, Parola M, Frati L, Dianzani MU (1987) Effect of 4-hydroxynonenal on c-myc expression. Toxicol Pathol 15:238–240

Barrera G, Di Mauro C, Muraca R, Ferrero D, Cavalli G, Fazio VM, Paradisi L, Dianzani MU (1991) Induction of differentiation in human HL-60 cells by 4-hydroxynonenal, a product of lipid peroxidation. Exp Cell Res 197:148–152

Barry RE, Williams AJK, McGwan JD (1987) The detection of acetaldehyde-liver plasma membrane protein adduct formed in vivo by alcohol feeding. Liver 7:364–368

Bell H, Bjørneboe A, Eidsvoll B, Norum KR, Rakherud N, Try K, Thomassen Y, Drevon CA (1992) Alcohol Alcohol 27:39–46

Berman WJ, Gil J, Jennett RB, Tuma D, Sorrell MF, Rubin E (1983) Ethanol, hepatocellular organelles and microtubules. A morphometric study in vivo and in vitro. Lab Invest 48:760–767

Bond EJ, De Matteis F (1967) Biochemical changes in rat liver after administration of carbon disulphide, with particular reference to microsomal changes. Biochem Pharmacol 18:2531–2549

Cajone F, Salina M, Bernelli Zazzera A (1989) 4-Hydroxynonenal induces a DNA-binding protein similar to heat shock factor. Biochem J 262:977–979

Carini R, Bellomo G, Dianzani MU, Albano E (1995) The operation of Na^+/Ca^{2+} exchanger prevents intracellular Ca^{2+} overload and hepatocyte killing following iron-induced lipid peroxidation. Biochem Biophys Res Comm 208:813–818

Cascales M, Martin-Sanz P, Craciunescu DG, Mayo I, Aguilar A, Roble-Chillidis EM, Cascales C (1991) Alteration in hepatic peroxidation mechanisms in thioacetamide-induced tumors in rats. Effect of a rhodium (III) complex. Carcinogenesis 12:233–240

Castillo T, Koop DR, Kamimura S, Triadafopoulos G, Tzukamoto H (1992) Role of cytochrome P-450 IIE I in ethanol, carbon tetrachloride and from dependent microsomal lipid peroxidation. Hepatology 16:992–996

Castro GD, Diaz Gomez MI, Castro JA (1990) Biotransformation of carbon tetrachloride and lipid peroxidation promotion by liver nuclear preparations from different animal species. Cancer Lett 53:9–15

Casu A, Monacelli R, Pala V (1966) Triglyceride behaviour in liver and serum of rabbits treated with dyphteria toxin. Experientia 22:544–545

Cheeseman KH, Collins M, Maddix J, Milia A, Proudfoot K, Slater TF, Burton GW, Webb A, Ingold KV (1986) Lipid peroxidation in regenerating rat liver. FEBS Lett 209:191–196

Chiarpotto E, Biasi F, Aragno M, Scavazza A, Danni O, Albano E, Poli G (1993) Change of liver metabolism of 1,2-dibromoethane during simultaneous treatment with carbon tetrachloride. Cell Biochem Funct II:71–75

Chu S, Bhakhtan NMG (1978) Experimental acetaminophen-induced hepatic necrosis. Biochemical and electron microscopic study cystamine protection. Lab Invest 39:193–203

Comporti M (1985) Biology of disease. Lipid peroxidation and cellular damage in toxic liver injury. Lab Invest 53:599–623

Comporti M (1989) Three models of free-radical-induced cell injury. Chem Biol Interact 72:1–56

Comporti M, Benedetti A (1972) Carbon tetrachloride induced peroxidation of liver lipids in vitamin E-pretreated rats. Biochem Pharmacol 21:418–420

Comporti M, Saccocci C, Dianzani MU (1965) Effect of CCl_4 in vitro and in vivo on lipid peroxidation of rat liver homogenates and subcellular fractions. Enzymologia 29:185–203

Comporti M, Harman AD, Luzio NR (1967) Effect of in vivo and in vitro ethanol administration on liver lipid peroxidation. Lab Invest 16:616–624

Cunningham CC, Coleman WB, Spach PI (1990) The effect of chronic ethanol consumption on hepatic mitochondrial energy metabolism. Alcohol Alcohol 25:127–136

Curzio M, Torrielli MV, Giroud J, Esterbauer H, Dianzani MU (1982) Neutrophil chemotactic responses to aldehydes. Res Comm Chem Pathol Pharmacol 36:463–467

Curzio M, Dianzani MU (1983) Effects of hydroxyalkenals on neutrophil migration. Atti Acc Scienze Torino 117:245–256

Curzio M, Esterbauer H, Dianzani MU (1985) Chemotactic activity of hydroxyalkenals on rat neutrophils. Int J Tissue React 7:137–142

Curzio M, Poli G, Esterbauer H, Biasi F, Di Mauro C, Dianzani MU (1986a) Detection of carbonyl products of lipid peroxidation in rat pleural exudate. IRCS Med Sci 14:98

Curzio M, Esterbauer H, Di Mauro C, Cecchini G, Dianzani MU (1986b) Chemotactic activity of lipid peroxidation product 4-hydroxynonenal and homologous hydroxyalkenals. Biol Chem Hoppe Seyler's 367:321–329

Curzio M, Di Mauro C, Esterbauer H, Dianzani MU (1987) Chemotactic activity of aldehydes. Structural requirements. Role in inflammatory process. Biomed Pharmacother 41:304–314

Curzio M, Esterbauer H, Di Mauro C, Dianzani MU (1990) Influence of the lipid peroxidation product 4-hydroxynonenal in human neutrophil migration. Intern J Immunother 6:13–18

Dahl HL, Hodgson E (1978) Complexes of trivalent oxygenated phosphorus compounds with cytochrome P-450 and cytochrome P-420: the origin of double Soret Spectra. Chem Biol Interact 21:137–154

Danni O, Chiarpotto E, Aragno M, Biasi F, Comoglio A, Belliardo F, Dianzani MU, Poli G (1991) Lipid peroxidation and irreversible damages. Synergism between carbon tetrachloride and 1,2-dibromoethane in isolated rat hepatocytes. Toxicol Appl Pharmacol 110:216–222
Danni O, Aragno M, Tamagno E, Ugazio G (1992) In vivo studies on halogen compound interactions. IV. Interaction among different halogen derivatives with and without synergistic action on liver toxicity. Res Comm Chem Pathol Pharmacol 76:355–366
Dianzani MU (1954) Uncoupling of oxidative phosphorylation in mitochondria from fatty livers. Biochim Biophys Acta 14:514–532
Dianzani MU (1972) Liver steatosis induced by white phosphorus. Morgagni 5:1–24
Dianzani MU (1975) Toxic liver injury by protein synthesis inhibitors. In: Popper H, Schaffner E (eds) Progress in liver disease. Grune and Stratton, New York, p 232
Dianzani MU (1978) Biochemical aspects of fatty livers. In: Slater TF (eds) Biochemical mechanisms of liver injury. Academic, New York, p 145
Dianzani MU (1979a) Reactions of the liver to injury: fatty liver. In: Farber E, Fisher M (eds) Toxic injury of the liver. Decker, New York, p 327
Dianzani MU (1979b) Biological activity of methyl glyoxal and related aldehydes. In: Wolstenholme GEW (ed) Submolecular pathology and cancer. Elsevier, Amsterdam, p 245 (Ciba Foundation Symposium 63)
Dianzani MU (1981) Role of sulphydryl compounds in protection against liver injury. In: Recent advances in 2-MPG treatment of liver diseases, p 11
Dianzani MU (1982) Biochemical effects of saturated and unsaturated aldehydes. In: McBrien DCH, Slater TF (eds) Free radicals, lipid peroxidation and cancer. Academic, London, p 129
Dianzani MU (1985) Lipoperoxidation in ethanol-poisoning: a critical reconsideration. Alcohol Alcohol 20:161–173
Dianzani MU (1988) Role of free radical-mediated reactions in ethanol-induced liver damage. In: Nordmann R, Ribière C, Rouache H (eds) Alcohol toxicity and free radical mechanisms. Pergamon, Oxford, p 35
Dianzani MU (1991a) Free radical pathology in alcohol-induced liver injury. In: Palmer TN (ed) Alcoholism: molecular perspectives. Plenum, New York, p 35
Dianzani MU (1991b) Dietary prooxidants. In: Dreosti IE (ed) Trace elements, micronutrients and free radicals. Humana, New York, p 77
Dianzani MU (1992) Biochemical aspects of fatty liver. In: Meeks RG, Harrison SD, Bull RJ (eds) Hepatotoxicology. CRC Press, Boca-Raton, p 327
Dianzani MU, Gravela E (1975) Inhibition of protein synthesis in carbon tetrachloride-induced liver injury. In: Keppler D (ed) Pathogenesis and mechanisms of liver cell necrosis. MTP, Lancaster, pp 225–228
Dianzani MU, Poli G (1985) Lipid peroxidation and haloalkylation in CCl_4-induced liver injury. In: Poli G, Cheeseman KH, Dianzani MU, Slater TF (eds) Free radicals in liver injury. IRL Press, Oxford, p 149
Dianzani MU, Paradisi L, Barrera G, Rossi MA, Parola M (1989) The action of 4-hydroxynonenal on the plasmamembrane enzymes from rat hepatocytes. In: Beaumont PC et al. (eds) Free radicals, metal ions and biopolymers. Richelieu Press, London, pp 329–339
Dianzani MU, Paradisi L, Parola M, Barrera G, Rossi MA (1990) Action of the aldehydes derived from lipid peroxidation on isolated liver plasmamembranes. In: Crastes de Paulet A et al. (eds) Free radicals, lipoproteins and membrane lipids. Plenum, New York, pp 171–181
Dianzani MU, Muzio G, Biocca ME, Canuto RA (1991) Lipid peroxidation in fatty liver induced by caffeine in rats. Int J Tissue React 13:79–85
Diaz Gomez MI, Castro JA (1980) Nuclear activation of carbon tetrachloride and chloroform. Res Commun Chem Pathol Pharmacol 27:191–194
Dillard CJ, Hu ML, Tappel AL (1991) Vitamin E, Diethylmaleate and bromotrichloromethane interactions in oxidative stress in vivo. Free Radic Res Biol Med 10:51–60

Di Luzio NR (1964) Prevention of the acute ethanol-induced fatty liver by the simultaneous administration of antioxidants. Life Sci 3:113–120
Donohue TM, Tuma DJ, Sorrell MF (1983) Binding of metabolically derived acetaldehyde to hepatic proteins in vitro. Lab Invest 49:226–229
Esterbauer H, Cheeseman KH, Dianzani MU, Poli G, Slater TF (1982) Separation and characterization of the aldehydic products of lipid peroxidation stimulated by ADP-Fe^{2+} in rat liver microsomes. Biochem J 208:129–140
Fazio VM, Barrera G, Martinotti S, Farace MG, Giglioni B, Frati L, Manzari V, Dianzani MU (1992) 4-Hydroxynonenal, a product of cellular lipid peroxidation, which modulates c-myc and globin gene expression in K562 cells. Cancer Res 52:4866–4871
Fazio VM, Barrera G, Muraca R, Rinaldi M, Ciafré AA, Lazzari M, Dianzani MU, Farace MG (1993) Differentiating agents and cancer therapy. Role of cellular lipid peroxidation and its product 4-hydroxy-nonenal in the control of cell proliferation and differentiation. In: Goldstein A, Garaci E (eds) Combination therapy 2, Plenum Press, New York, pp 105–114
Forni LG, Packer JE, Slater TF, Willson RL (1983) Reaction of the trichloromethyl and halothane-derived peroxy radicals with unsaturated fatty acids: a pulse radiolysis study. Chem Biol Interact 45:171–177
Forrester LM, Neal GE, Judah DJ, Glancey MJ, Wolf CR (1990) Evidence for involvement of multiple forms of cytochrome P-450 in aflatoxin B_I metabolism in human liver. Proc Natl Acad Sci USA 87:8306–831
French SW, Wong K, Juli L, Albano E, Hagbjork AL, Ingelman-Sundberg M (1993) Effect of ethanol on cytochrome P 450 2EI (CYP2EI) lipid peroxidation and serum protein adduct formation in relation to liver pathology pathogenesis. Exp Mol Pathol 58:61–75
Fridovich I (1989) Oxygen radicals from acetaldehyde. Free Radic Biol Med 7:557–558
Gabriel L, Bonelli G, Dianzani MU (1977) Inhibition of colchicine binding to rat liver tubulin by aldehydes and by linoleic acid hydroperoxide. Chem Biol Interact 19:101–109
Ghoshal AK, Porta EA, Hartroft WS (1971) Isotopic studies on the absorption and distribution of white phosphorus in rats. Exp Mol Pathol 14:212–219
Glenn JL, Opalka E, Tischer K (1963) The incorporation of labeled palmitic acid into the phospholipids of normal and fatty livers. J Biol Chem 238:1249–1253
Hashimoto S, Recknagel RO (1968) No chemical evidence of hepatic lipid peroxidation in acute ethanol toxicity. Exp Mol Pathol 8:225–242
Heimberg M, Watkin ML, Tookes R (1964) Carbon tetrachloride hepatotoxicity: the direct action of CCl_4 on the liver. J Pharmacol Exp Ter 145:92–101
Inatomi N, Kato S, Ito D, Lieber CS (1989) Role of peroxisomal fatty acid beta-oxidation in ethanol metabolism. Biochem Biophys Res Commun 163:418–423
Jukkola A, Niemelä O (1989) Covalent binding of acetaldehyde to type III collagen. Biochem Biophys Res Commun 159:163–169
Kamimura S, Gaal K, Britton RS, Bacon BR, Triadafilopoulos G, Tsukamoto H (1992) Increased 4-hydroxynonenal levels in experimental alcoholic liver disease: association of lipid peroxidation with liver fibrogenesis. Hepatology 16:448–453
Kato S, Kawase T, Alderman J, Inatomi N, Lieber CS (1990) Role of xanthine oxidase in ethanol-induced lipid peroxidation in rats. Gastroenterology 98:203–210
Kawase T, Kato S, Lieber CS (1989) Lipid peroxidation and antioxidant defence systems in rat liver after ethanol feeding. Hepatology 10:815–820
Kera Y, Ohbora Y, Komura S (1988) The metabolism of acetaldehyde and not acetaldehyde itself is responsible for in vivo ethanol-induced lipid peroxidation in rats. Biochem Pharmacol 37:3633–3638
Kiss Z, Criley KS, Rossi MA, Anderson WB (1992) Selective inhibition by 4-hydroxynonenal of sphingosine stimulated phospholipase D in NIH 3T3 cells. Biochim Biophys Acta 1124:300–302
Kodama M, Inoue F, Akao M (1990) Enzymatic and non-enzymatic formation of free radicals from aflatoxin B_I. Free Radic Res Commun 10:137–142

Kroncke KD, Fricker G, Meier PJ, Gerok W, Wieland T, Kurz J (1986) Alpha-amanitin uptake into hepatocytes. Identification of hepatic membrane transport systems used by amatoxins. J Biol Chem 261:12562–12567

Levy GN, Brabec MJ (1984) Binding of carbon tetrachloride metabolites to rat hepatic mitochondrial DNA. Toxicol Lett 22:229–234

Lieber CS, De Carli L (1991) Hepatotoxicity of ethanol. J Hepatol 12:394–401

Lieber CS, Rubin E, De Carli LM, Misra P, Gang H (1970) Effects of pyrazole on hepatic function and structure. Lab Invest 22:615–621

Lombardi B, Recknagel RO (1962) Interference with secretion of triglycerides by the liver as a common factor in toxic liver injury. With some observations on choline deficiency fatty liver. Am J Pathol 40:571–586

Maellaro E, Del Bello B, Casini AF, Comporti M, Ceccarelli D, Muscatello U, Masini A (1990) Early mitochondrial disfunction in bromobenzene treated mice: a possible factor of liver injury. Biochem Pharmacol 40:1491–1497

Montanaro L, Sperti S, Stirpe F (1973) Inhibition by ricin of protein synthesis in vitro. Ribosomes as the target of the toxin. Biochem J 136:677–687

Mourelle M, Meza MA (1989) Colchicine prevents D-galactosamine-induced hepatitis. J Hepatol 8:165–172

Müller A, Sies H (1982) Role of alcohol dehydrogenase activity and of acetaldehyde in ethanol-induced ethane and pentane production by isolated perfused rat liver. Biochem J 206:154–156

Müller B, Dargel R (1984) Structural and functional impairment of mitochondria from rat livers chronically injured by thioacetamide. Acta Pharmacol Toxicol 55:126–132

Munday R (1982) Studies on the mechanism of toxicity of the mycotoxin, sporidesmin. I. Generation of superoxide radical by sporidesmin. Chem Biol Interact 41:361–374

Nagelkerke JF, Dogterom P, De Bont HJGM, Mulder J (1989) Prolonged high intracellular free calcium concentrations induced by ATP are not immediately cytotoxic in isolated hepatocytes. Changes in biochemical parameters implicated in cell toxicity. Biochem J 263:347–353

Niemelä O, Israel Y (1992) Hemoglobin-acetaldehyde adducts in human alcohol abusers. Lab Invest 67:246–252

Nordmann R, Giudicelli Y, Beaugé F, Clément M, Ribière C, Rouach H, Nordmann J (1973) Studies on the mechanisms involved in the iso-propanol-induced fatty liver. Biochim Biophys Acta 326:1–2

Nordmann R, Ribière C, Rouach H (1992) Implication of free radical mechanisms in ethanol-induced cellular immunity. Fe Radic Biol Med 12:219–240

Olsnes S, Pihl H (1973) Isolation and properties of Abrin: a toxin inhibiting protein synthesis. Evidence for different biological functions of its two constituent peptide chains. Eur J Biochem 35:179–185

Olsnes S, Stirpe F, Sandvig K, Phil Q (1982) Isolation and characterization of Viscumin, a toxic lectin from viscum album L (mistletoe). J Biol Chem 257:13263–13270

Paradisi L, Panagini C, Parola M, Barrera G, Dianzani MU (1985) Effects of 4-hydroxy-nonenal on adenylate cyclase and 5'-nucleotidase activities in rat liver plasma membrane. Chem Biol Interact 53:209–217

Parola M, Leonarduzzi G, Biasi F, Albano E, Biocca ME, Poli G, Dianzani MU (1992a) Vitamin E dietary supplementation protects against carbon tetrachloride-induced chronic liver damage and cirrhosis. Hepatology 16:1014–1021

Parola M, Muraca R, Dianzani I, Barrera G, Leonarduzzi G, Bendinelli P, Piccoletti R, Poli G (1992b) Vitamin E dietary supplementation inhibits transforming growth factor $Beta_1$ gene expression in the rat liver. FEBS 308:267–270

Parola M, Pinzani M, Casini A, Albano E, Poli G, Gentilini A, Gentilini P, Dianzani MU (1993) Stimulation of lipid peroxidation in 4-hydroxynonenal treatment increases procollagen I(I) gene expression in human liver fat-storing cells. Biochim Biophys Res Commun 494:1044–1050

Perin A, Scalabrino G, Sessa A, Arnaboldi A (1974) In vitro inhibition of protein synthesis in rat liver as a consequence of ethanol metabolism. Biochim Biophys Acta 366:101–108

Poggi M, Di Luzio NR (1964) The role of the liver and adipose tissue in the pathogenesis of the ethanol induced fatty liver. J Lipid Res 5:437–445

Poli G, Gravela E, Albano E, Dianzani MU (1979) Studies on fatty liver isolated hepatocytes. II. The action of carbon tetrachloride on lipid peroxidation, protein and lipoprotein synthesis and secretion. Exp Mol Pathol 30:116–127

Poli G, Albano E, Biasi F, Chiarpotto E, Dianzani MU (1983) In vitro evidence for CCl_4 metabolites covalently bound to lipoprotein micelles. FEBS 160:187–190

Poli G, Albano E, Biasi F, Cecchini G, Carini R, Bellomo G, Dianzani MU (1985a) Lipid peroxidation stimulated by carbon tetrachloride or iron and hepatocyte death: protective effect of vitamin E. In: Poli G, Cheeseman KH, Dianzani MU, Slater TF (eds) Free radicals in liver injury. IRL Press, Oxford, p 207

Poli G, Dianzani MU, Cheeseman KH, Slater TF, Lang J, Esterbauer H (1985b) Separation and characterization of the aldehydic products of lipid peroxidation stimulated by carbon tetrachloride or ADP-iron in isolated rat hepatocytes and rat liver microsomal suspensions. Biochem J 227:629–638

Poli G, Albano E, Dianzani MU (1987) The role of lipid peroxidation in liver damage. Chem Physiol Lipids 45:117–142

Poli G, Cheeseman KH, Biasi F, Chiarpotto E, Dianzani MU, Esterbauer H, Slater TF (1989) Promethazine inhibits the formation of aldehydic products of lipid peroxidation but not covalent binding resulting from the exposure of rat liver fractions to CCl_4-induced damage to liver microsomal enzymes: comparative studies in vitro using microsomes and isolated liver cells. Chem Biol Interact 37:13–24

Recknagel RO, Ghoshal AK (1966) Lipoperoxidation as a vector in carbon tetrachloride hepatotoxicity. Lab Invest 15:132–156

Recknagel RO, Lombardi B, Scotz MC (1960) A new insight into pathogenesis of carbon tetrachloride fat infiltration. Proc Soc Exp Biol Med 104:608–610

Recknagel RO, Lombardi B (1961) Studies of biochemical changes in subcellular particles of rat liver and their relationship to a new hypothesis regarding the pathogenesis of carbon tetrachloride fat accumulation. J Biol Chem 236:564–569

Ross D, Albano E, Nilsson U, Moldeus P (1984) Thiyl radicals formation during peroxidase-catalyzed metabolism of acetaminophen in the presence of thiols. Biochem Biophys Res Commun 125:109–115

Rossi MA, Garramone A, Dianzani MU (1988a) Stimulation of phospholipase C activity by 4-hydroxy-nonenal: influence of GTP and calcium concentration. Int J Tissue React 10:321–325

Rossi MA, Garramone A, Dianzani MU (1988b) Effect of 4-hydroxy-2,3-trans-nonenal, a lipid peroxidation product, on hepatic phospholipase C. Med Sci Res 17:257–258

Rossi MA, Fidale F, Garramone A, Esterbauer H, Dianzani MU (1990) Effect of 4-hydroxyalkenals on hepatic phosphatidyl inositol-4,5 biphosphate phospholipase C. Biochem Pharmacol 39:1715–1719

Rossi MA, Fidale F, Garramone A, Dianzani MU (1991) Modulation of phosphatidylinositol-4,5-diphosphate (PIP_2) phospholipase C activity by 4-hydroxyalkenals. In: Columbano A et al. (eds) Chemical carcinogenesis, vol. 2. Plenum Press, New York, pp 349–355

Rossi MA, Di Mauro C, Dianzani MU (1993) Action of lipid peroxidation products on phosphoinositide specific phospholipase C. Mol Aspects Med 14:273–279

Salvador RA, Atkins C, Haber S, Conney AH (1970) Changes in the serum concentration of cholesterol, triglycerides and phospholipids in the mouse and rat after administration of either chlorcyclizine or phenobarbital. Biochem Pharmacol 19:1463–1469

Schofield RF, Schumann WC, Kumaran K, Landau BR (1982) Effects of clofibrate and ethanol on the pathways of initial fatty acid oxidation. Biochem Pharmacol 31:2121–2123

Sergent O (1993) Stress oxydatif induit par l'ethanol dans les hepatocytes de rat en culture. Thèse de doctorat, Université de Rennes, France, pp 1–152

Shinozuka H, Martin JT, Farber E (1973) The induction of fibrillar nucleoli in rat liver cells by D-galactosamine and their subsequent reformation into normal nucleoli. J Ultra-structural Res 44:279–292

Shull KH (1962) Hepatic phosphorylase and adenosine triphosphate levels in ethionine-treated rats. J Biol Chem 237:1734–1735

Slater TF (1972) Free radicals mechanisms in tissue injury. Pion, London, p 1

Slater TF, Sawyer BC, Sträuli BC (1964) Changes in liver nucleotide concentrations in experimental liver injury. II. Acute ethanol poisoning. Biochem J 93:267–270

Smuckler EA, Koplitz M (1974) Thioacetamide-induced alterations in nuclear RNA transport. Cancer Res 34:827–838

Sperti S, Montanaro L, Mattioli A, Stirpe F (1973) Inhibition by ricin of protein synthesis in vitro: 60 S ribosomal subunit as the target of the toxin. Biochem J 136:813–815

Srivastava SP, Chen NQ, Holtzman DL (1990) The in vitro NADPH-dependent inhibition by CCl_4 of the ATP-dependent calcium uptake of hepatic microsomes from male rats. Studies on the mechanism of the inactivation of the hepatic microsomal pump by the $CCl_3^{\bullet}$ radical. J Biol Chem 265:8392–8399

Stirpe F, Gasperi-Campani A, Barbieri L, Montanaro L, Lorenzoni F, Sperti S, Bonetti E (1978) Inhibition of protein synthesis by modeccin, the toxin of *Modecca digitata*. FEBS 85:65–67

Thayer WS (1984) Inhibition of mitochondrial fatty acid oxidation in pentenoic acid-induced fatty liver. A possible model for Reye's syndrome. Biochem Pharmacol 33:1187–1194

Tomasi A, Albano E, Lott KAK, Slater TF (1980) Spin trapping of free radical products of CCl_4 activation by using pulse radiolysis and high energy radiation procedures. FEBS Lett 122:303–306

Tomasi A, Albano E, Dianzani MU, Slater TF, Vannini V (1983a) Metabolic activation of 1,2-dibromoethane to a free radical intermediate by rat liver microsomes and isolated hepatocytes. FEBS Lett 160:191–194

Tomasi A, Billing S, Garner A, Slater TF, Albano E (1983b) The metabolism of halothane by hepatocytes: a comparison between free radical spin trapping and lipid peroxidation in relation to cell damage. Chem Biol Interact 46:353–368

Tomasi A, Albano E, Biasi F, Slater TF, Vannini V, Dianzani MU (1985) Activation of chloroform and related trihalomethanes to free radical intermediates in isolated hepatocytes and in the rat in vivo as detected by the ESR-spin trapping technique. Chem Biol Interact 55:303–316

Tomasi A, Albano E, Banni S, Botti B, Corongiu F, Dessì MA, Iannone A, Vannini V, Dianzani MU (1987) Free radical metabolism of carbon tetrachloride in rat liver mitochondria. A study of the mechanism of activation. Biochem J 246:313–317

Torrielli MV, Baccino FM, Zuretti MF, Pernigotti L, Gabriel L (1973) Influenza delle catecolamine sulle lesioni epatiche sperimentali. Metabolismo 9:91–99

Torrielli MV, Gabriel L, Dianzani MU (1978) Ethanol-induced hepatotoxicity: experimental observations on the role of lipid peroxidation. J Pathol 126:11–25

Towner RA, Janzen EG, Zhang YK, Yashamiro S (1993) Study of the inhibitory effect of new spin traps on in vivo CCl_4-induced hepatotoxicity in rats. Free Radic Biol Med 14:677–681

Ugazio G, Koch RR, Recknagel RO (1973) Reversibility of liver damage in rats rendered resistant to carbon tetrachloride by prior carbon tetrachloride administration: bearing on the lipoperoxidation hypothesis. Exp Mol Pathol 18:281–289

Wang CJ, Hsu JD, Lin JK (1991a) Suppression of aflatoxin B_1-induced hepatotoxic lesions by crocetin (a natural carotenoid). Carcinogenesis 12:1807–1810

Wang CJ, Shiow SL, Lin JK (1991b) Effects of crocetin on the hepatotoxicity and hepatic DNA binding of aflatoxin B_1 in rats. Carcinogenesis 12:459–462

Webb JL (1966) Enzymes and metabolic inhibitors, vol. 2. Academic, New York, pp 615–656

Wooles WR, Weymouth RJ (1968) Prevention of the ethanol-induced maintenance of hepatic lipid oxidation. Lab Invest 18:709–714
Worrall S, De Jersey J, Shanley BC, Wilce PA (1991) Detection of stable acetaldehyde-modified proteins in the livers of ethanol-fed rats. Alcohol Alcohol 26:437–444
Wu DF, Cederbaum AI (1992) Presence of functionally active cytochrome P-450 II E I in plasma membranes of rat hepatocytes. Hepatology 15:515–524
Xu DS, Jennett RB, Smith SL, Sorrell MF, Tuma DJ (1989) Covalent interactions of acetaldehyde with the actin/microfilament system. Alcohol and Alcoholism 24:281–289
Zidenberg-Cherr S, Olin KL, Villanueva J, Tang A, Phinney SD, Halsted CH, Keen CL (1991) Ethanol-induced changes in hepatic free radical defense mechanism and fatty acid composition in the miniature pig. Hepatology 13:1185–1192

CHAPTER 9

Choline Deficiency: An Important Model for the Study of Hepatotoxicity

A.K. GHOSHAL

A. Introduction

The membrane components of the cells of both plants and animals contain choline as a base of phospholipid lecithin. *Deprivation* of choline from the diet of animals (rats have been studied very extensively) causes acute and chronic damage, not unlike, in some respects, that seen after the *introduction* of toxic drugs, e.g., carbon tetrachloride. Deprivation of no other nutrients from the diet of rats has such a fast action as choline. When rats are given a diet devoid only of choline, their liver triglycerides accumulate within 8h, nuclear membrane lipid peroxidation is detected within 24h, DNA alterations within 48h, increased phospholipase A_2 (PLA_2) activity within 72h, cell death within 5 days and cell proliferation from 7 days. Eventually rats develop hepatocellular carcinoma after 1 year. Unlike lipotrope deficiency, liver cirrhosis is not a regular feature of "pure" choline deprivation, unless the food is also devoid of vitamin B_{12}. Choline deficiency is rare in humans except in some parts of the world, e.g., Africa, south China. Even in China, choline deficiency is complicated by other factors such as the contamination of the food with aflatoxin B_1, or the presence of a dietary deficiency of Ca^{2+}. However, metabolic imbalance in certain disease conditions or the action of certain drugs might precipitate a condition whereby the membrane might be deprived of choline, thus altering the lecithin content.

This dietary model, in which no toxic agent or carcinogen is used, provides an excellent opportunity to study acute liver cell injury and liver cancer development without the interference of a xenobiotic. The model highlights the possible role of phospholipase A_2 (PLA_2) and of endogenous as well as exogenous free radicals in the development of cell death and cancer.

Choline was discovered more than a century ago (STRECKER 1862). However, its deficiency syndrome was discovered accidentally by BEST and HUNTSMAN (1932) while working on depancreatized dog with insulin. Insulin could control blood sugar in depancreatized dog but the liver became fatty. The fat could be removed by feeding the dog with raw pancreas. The active compound turned out to be the choline in lecithin. Choline is a positively charged quaternary ammonium compound and the base of the phospholipid lecithin. Eventually it was found that methionine, betaine, vitamin B_{12}, folic acid, pantothenic acid, riboflavin, pyridoxine and inositol were also effective, to varying degrees, in the removal of the fat, although to a lesser extent than was choline (BEST et al. 1953/1954). BEST et al. (1935) called this fat removal or prevention "lipotropism," the fat-removing ability "lipotropic" and the compounds that have the capacity to remove the fat "lipotropes."

Since the discovery of the fat-removing ability of choline, much research has been focused on its mechanism. Innumerable papers and review articles have been published since 1932 dealing with the mechanism of fat accumulation in the liver of rats and other animals by choline deficiency.

In order to generate rapid and heavy deposition of fat in the liver, not only choline but also methionine, vitamin B_{12} and folic acid were removed from the diet. Thus, increasing emphasis in this area of research has been on lipotrope deficiency, rather than choline deficiency. BEST et al. (1953/1954) pointed out at an early stage in this research that removal of methionine from the diet leads to loss of appetite with considerable loss of body weight (GHOSHAL and FARBER 1993). In nutritional experiments, growth of the animal should not be compromised. It is well known in "nutritional pathology" that the patterns of changes in body weight can radically change the nature and extent of induced disease.

The modified choline devoid diet, only deficient in choline and not of any other of the known lipotropes, was developed by YOUNG et al. (1956) as a modification of the diet of RIDOUT et al. (1954). This is the diet we (GHOSHAL and FARBER 1984) and LOMBARDI and SHINOZUKA (1979) have used. This diet, called "choline devoid diet" (CD), is quite different from the various lipotrope-deficient diets used before and after 1956 by several other investigators. The latter are not only lipotrope deficient but also differ in their fat and protein content or composition. At the end of the 1970s, the study of choline deficiency took quite a different turn with the availability of a model to study carcinogenesis and cell injury without the interference of any xenobiotic.

B. Hepatotoxicity by Dietary Manipulation – Not by Addition but by Depletion

The almost exclusive emphasis in this area of research between 1932 and late 1970s, with two exceptions, was on "choline deficiency" and fatty liver. COPELAND and SALMON (1946) first reported the occurrence of carcinoma in the rat liver by "choline deficiency." This finding was very exciting, because the occurrence of cancer by eliminating something from the diet and not by the addition of an outside agent was unexpected. Similar findings were reported later in mice by BUCKLEY and HARTROFT (1955). With the discovery of aflatoxin B in 1958 and of its carcinogenic effects shortly thereafter, the significance of a CD diet was thrown into total disarray because the peanut meal used in the lipotrope deficiency studies was very likely contaminated with aflatoxin B_1 (SALMON and NEWBERNE 1963; NEWBERNE 1965). These observations concerning possible contamination with aflatoxin completely changed the direction of the studies on diet and liver disease including liver cancer, with an ever-

Table 1. Temporal sequence of early alterations in the rat liver exposed to a choline devoid diet

Time exposed to CD diet	Alterations
8 h	Triglyceride (triacylglycerol) accumulation
1 day	Nuclear lipid peroxidation
2 days	DNA damage
3 days	Phospholipase A_2 activation
5 days	Mitochondrial lipid peroxidation
6 days	Cell death and cell proliferation
10 weeks	Initiation

Note: Microsomal lipid peroxidation can be detected only when PLA_2 activation in the microsomes is inhibited.

increasing focus on the diets as modulators (promoters, co-carcinogens, etc.) of carcinogenesis (SHINOZUKA et al. 1979; SHINOZUKA and LOMBARDI 1980; NEWBERNE et al. 1983) rather than as a primary effector.

In our laboratory (GHOSHAL and FARBER 1984), the diet used was only devoid of choline and the diet was monitored for the possible presence of contaminating carcinogens. It was found to be free of aflatoxin B_1 (less than 0.2 ppb), volatile nitrosamines, nitrates and nitrites, 2-acetylaminofluorene and malonaldehyde. Using this diet with male Fischer 344 young adult (120–150 g body wt.) rats, we showed a sequence of liver aberrations which occur in a very reproducible manner. The temporal sequence of events is shown in Table 1. These step by step developments of liver aberrations are discussed in Sect. E. The most exciting and interesting contribution of this "pure" CD diet is that it causes liver cancer by the absence of something in the diet and not by the introduction of any outside agent.

C. Absence of Choline in an Otherwise Complete Diet – An Excellent Model for the Study of Liver Cell Death and Liver Cancer

The diet which was used by our laboratory and by Lombardi and coworkers was first introduced by YOUNG et al. (1956). In this diet, unlike lipotrope-deficient diets, adequate amounts of vitamin B_{12} and folic acid and a minimal amount of methionine (1800 mg/kg diet) were added. This amount of methionine is sufficient for the growth of young adult rats. The diet was virtually devoid only of choline. The control choline-supplemented (CS) diet was the same except for being supplemented by choline bitartrate (Table 2).

With this new purified CD diet, SHINZOUKA et al. (1979) demonstrated that rat liver initiated by a carcinogen can be promoted when rats are exposed to this diet for several weeks. The CD diet also induces liver cell proliferation (GIAMBARRESI et al. 1982). The promoting ability of the CD diet was assigned

Table 2. Choline devoid diet as modified by YOUNG et al. (1956)

Ingredients	Grams per kilogram
Alcohol-extracted peanut meal[a]	90
Soy protein isolate[a]	80
Casein, vitamin-free	10
L-Cysteine	2
Corn starch	100
Dextrin	100
Sucrose	413
Cellulose	10
Corn oil	50
Primex (hydrogenated vegetable oil)	10
Vitamin mix (AIN-76A vitamin mixture)[a]	10
Salt mix (AIN-76 salt mix)[a]	35

[a] Differ slightly from the diet originally used (GHOSHAL and FARBER 1984). All the changes described in Table 1 including liver cancer have been reproduced several times with this diet.

to liver cell proliferation. This was the first step for the re-entry of CD diets into carcinogenesis research. In 1983 it was shown simultaneously from our laboratory (GHOSHAL and FARBER 1983, 1984) and from Poirier's laboratory (MIKOL et al. 1983) and later from Lombardi's laboratory (YOKOYAMA et al. 1985) that a devoid of choline without any added carcinogen induced more than a 50% incidence of hepatocellular carinoma in male rats within 2 years.

As with any carcinogen, either chemical xenobiotic or otherwise, a complete carcinogen will both initiate and promote. What is the mechanism of initiation due to the diet where something has been taken out and not added? The present-day paradigm is that chemical carcinogens initiate by damaging the DNA. A round of cell proliferation is required to fix the damage in the DNA, whatever its nature. Cell proliferation is there but how is DNA damaged by exposure to CD diet?

Based on the early reproducible changes (Table 1) in the liver, a hypothesis has been proposed on the mechanism of carcinogenesis by CD diet (Fig. 1). That free radicals can attack and alter DNA was shown by in vitro experiments from several laboratories (SLAGA et al. 1981; EMERIT and CERUTTI 1982; AMES 1983). In vivo experiments conducted in our laboratory clearly showed the generation of free radicals, as indicated by the appearance of nuclear lipid peroxidation within 24h after a CD diet was begun and DNA alterations within 48h. Cell proliferation was evident within 6 days. The early temporal sequence of events after CD diet feeding are most probably sufficient to initiate the liver cells in the carcinogenic process. Initiated cells are further altered by feeding the CD diet.

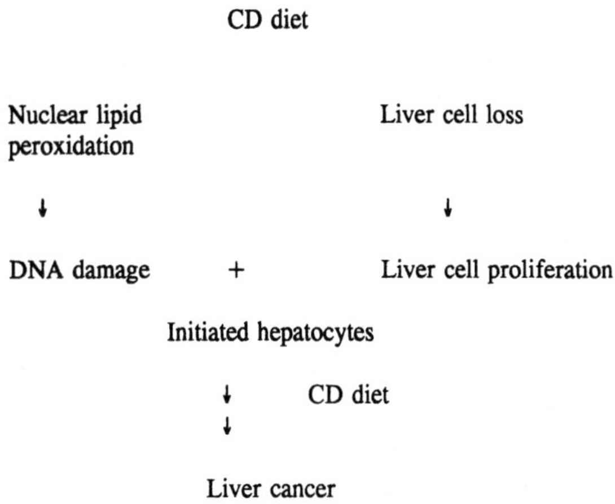

Fig. 1. Liver carcinogenesis with CD: a possible mechanism

I. Choline Deficiency Model and Cell Death

The choline deficiency (CD) model offers for the first time an opportunity to study liver cell death in vivo without the interference of an xenobiotic and with a reaction sequence that is moderately slow and thus analyzable. In the CD model, early temporal changes before liver cell death start with fat accumulation, nuclear lipid peroxidation. DNA alterations and PLA_2 activation. Preteratment with several agents can inhibit all these early aberrations excepting fat accumulation. This suggests that at least in CD induced liver cell death fat accumulation may not be involved. However, involvement of fat accumulation may not be totally ignored, since it may be argued that accumulation of fat might set the stage in some way for the later events, e.g., lipid peroxidation, DNA damage, to become effective in the final killing of the cell. The critical experiment which may clarify this is to shown that fat accumulation is inhibited without inhibiting the subsequent aberrations and eventual cell death. So far, this has not been accomplished.

Lipid peroxidation, DNA damage, PLA_2 induction and cell death can all be inhibited if CD diet feb rats are pretreated with Ca^{2+}, Sr^{2+}, *tert*-nitrosobutane (a spin trap agent), α-phenyl-*tert*-butylnitrone (a spin trap agent), or AD_5 (free radical scavenger). It might be possible that free radical generation, lipid peroxidation and subsequent DNA damage are sufficient to cause cell death. However, induction of phospholipase A_2 activity occurs in this model before cell death occurs. Is it a chain reaction leading to cell death or is free radical generation the prime cause and the others just innocent bystanders in respect to cell death?

It has been shown by Ghazarian et al. (1994) that cell death can be prevented by the administration of an effective inhibitor of phospholipase A_2, PBx (an oligomer of prostaglandin B_1 ($n = 6$)) even after the occurrence of lipid peroxidation and DNA damage. Whether PLA_2 alone is responsible for cell death or whether it is in the downstream of a chain reaction initiated by free radicals has yet to be shown. A definitive experiment whereby free radical generation and DNA damage can be inhibited without inhibiting PLA_2 induction has to be devised. The results may give a chear-cut answer.

II. Choline Deficiency and Liver Cancer

The observation that rats exposed to a CD diet without any added carcinogen develop a 100% incidence of hepatic nodules and a 50% incidence of hepatocellular carcinoma (GHOSHAL and FARBER 1983, 1984) suggests that the CD diet is a complete carcinogenic regimen. SHINOZUKA et al. (1979) have already established that, when rat liver cells are initiated by a chemical carcinogen, 5 or 6 weeks of CD diet can increase the incidence of liver cancer. CD diet is a complete carcinogenic regimen; therefore, it is both initiator and promoter. Complete carcinogenic regimens are frequently additive.

The ability of CD diet to initiate rat liver has been shown in our laboratory (GHOSHAL et al. 1987). After exposure to CD diet alone for 9–10 weeks, initiated hepatocytes were monitored by the appearance of γ-glutamyltransferase (γ-GT) positive foci after the imposition of a strong selection procedure for resistant hepatocytes, a phenomenon induced by many chemical carcinogens (SOLT and FARBER 1976; TSUDA et al. 1980). These resistant hepatocytes are precursors of hepatocyte nodules and these in turn are known sites of origin for hepatocellular carcinoma (SOLT et al. 1977, 1983). However, as indicated, unlike many hepatocarcinogens, it takes about 10 weeks of exposure for a CD diet to induce initiated hepatocytes (GHOSHAL et al. 1987).

Why does it take 10 weeks instead of a few days to generate initiated cells in choline deficiency? With a CD diet, DNA damage occurs within 48 h. Cell proliferation is detected after the cells begin to die at 4.5–5 days. It is possible that the cells with DNA damage are undergoing cell death either before or after initiation. This destruction of DNA-damaged cells goes on until the magnitude of cell death diminishes at about 10 weeks of CD feeding (RUSHMORE et al. 1987).

There is another explanation which may be worth discussing. To generate a resistant hepatocyte, DNA damage and a round of cell proliferation to fix that damage may not be sufficient. Along with DNA damage, other changes may be necessary to generate hepatocytes which are resistant to death by a genotoxic agent and other causes such as a CD diet. When a carcinogen is given to the animals, not only DNA damage but also other changes necessary to induce the resistant property occur simultaneously. In choline deficiency the changes occur step by step, which might be a possible basis for the slow generation of "ultimate" resistant hepatocytes.

Apart from DNA alterations, the alterations in the cell membranes might contribute to the resistant property. In our laboratory it has been shown that polyunsaturated fatty acids of the cellular membrane are replaced by monounsaturated and saturated fatty acids, which are not susceptible to lipid peroxidation (KAPOOR et al. 1992). Our experiments were done for only up to 3 days. At present, we do not know whether the changes can continue, until a critical change occurs, terminating in resistant hepatocytes.

D. Lipotrope Deficiency Versus Choline Deficiency

In a recent article, GHOSHAL and FARBER (1993) have discussed the differences between choline deficiency and lipotrope deficiency and why the symptoms of lipotrope deficiency cannot be accepted as choline deficiency syndromes. The table as modified from GHOSHAL and FARBER (1993) indicating the differences of syndromes between the two diets is given here (Tabel 3). One major difference is that rats on a lipotrope deficiency diet do not gain weight. It was pointed out long ago by BEST et al. (1953/1954) that because of lack of methionine in the lipotrope-deficient diet the rats consuming the diet lose their appetite. As mentioned before, the patterns of changes in body weight can radically change the nature and extent of induced disease.

E. Step by Step Development of Liver Aberration

It has been mentioned before that the initiation process in carcinogenesis by chemical carcinogen occurs so rapidly that there is a possibility that many steps (if there are many steps) may occur simultaneously. If that is the case, it is almost impossible to study the mechanism of he initiation process, unless the

Table 3. Choline deficiency versus lipotrope deficiency

Consequences	Choline devoid	Lipotrope deficient
Body weight	Weight gain as control	Loss of weight
Fatty liver	First detectable fat accumulation in zone 1 (periportal)	First starts to accumulate in zone 3 (centrilobular) of the liver
Necrosis	Early (5–6 days) focal and widespread, at least 50% of hepatocytes within 2 weeks	Late liver cell death secondary to fatty cysts
"Fatty cysts" lipodiastermata	Not seen	Regularly seen after many weeks of LD diet
Fibrosis and cirrhosis	Very infrequent, even after 2 years	A common feature almost in every rat
Status of P450 (MFO) in the liver	Remains unaltered	Depression of P450 (MFO)
Hepatocellular carcinoma	Frequent – at least 50%–70% of male rats by 2 years	Uncertain

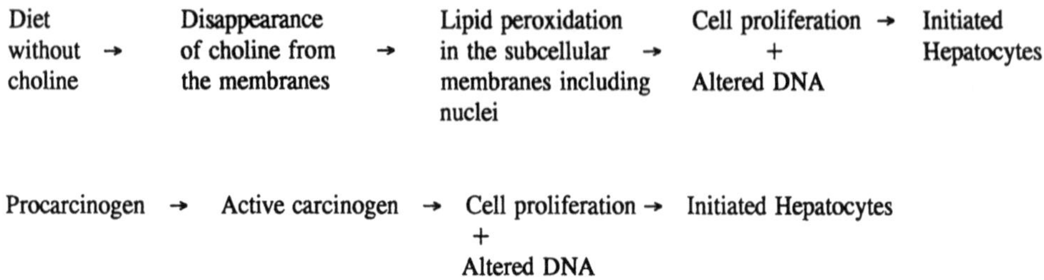

Fig. 2. Similarity between CD-induced and chemical carcinogen induced initiation

steps involved are slowed down and segregated. It seems that the choline deficiency model may offer this possibility.

The separation of PLA_2 activation from lipid peroxidation and DNA damage before cell death and initiation has already been achieved (GHAZARIAN et al. 1994). The role of DNA damage, membrane alterations, fat accumulation, cell death and cell proliferation are there to be segregated and studied for their relevance to initiation in the carcinogenic process.

F. Hypothesis of Choline Deficiency Induced Hepatocarcinoma

It has been studied extensively how cancer might develop in the liver with chemical carcinogens. In the CD model, a hypothesis for initiation has been proposed by Ghoshal and Farber which is remarkably similar to chemical carcinogen induced initiation. Figure 2 depicts the hypothesis of initiation by the CD diet and chemical carcinogens.

G. Conclusions

1. The choline deficiency model shows that cancer can be developed by dietary imbalance without the apparent need for a xenobiotic.
2. This model reveals that there are more steps in the initiation process which can be studied without the interference of an outside agent.
3. This model may turn out to be an excellent tool for the study of cell death in vivo.

References

Ames B (1983) Dietary carcinogens and anticarcinogens. Science 211:1256–1264
Best CH, Huntsman ME (1932) The effects of the components of lecithin upon deposition of fat in the liver. J Physiol (Lond) 75:405–412
Best CH, Huntsman ME, Ridout JH (1935) The lipotropic effect of proteins. Nature 735:821–822
Best CH, Lucas CC, Ridout JH (1953–1954) The lipotropic factors. Ann NY Acad Sci 57:646–653

Buckley GF, Hartroft WS (1955) Pathology of choline deficiency in the mouse. Arch Pathol 59:185–197

Copeland DH, Salmon WD (1946) The occurrence of neoplasms in the liver, lungs and other tissues of rats as a result of prolonged choline deficiency. Am J Pathol 22:1059–1081

Emerit I, Cerutti PA (1982) Tumor promoter phorbol-12-myristate-13-acetate induces a clastogenic factor in human lymphocytes. Proc Natl Acad Sci USA 79:7509–7513

Ghazarian DM, Ghoshal AK, Farber E (1994) In vivo free radical Generation in the rat liver by a choline devoid diet and its role in relation to phospholipase A_2 activation. Proc Am Assoc Cancer Res 35:609

Ghosal AK, Farber E (1983) Induction of liver cancer by a diet deficient in choline and methionine (CMD). Proc Am Assoc Cancer Res 24:98

Ghoshal AK, Farber E (1984) The induction of liver cancer by dietary deficiency of choline and methionine without added carcinogens. Carcinogenesis 5:1367–1370

Ghoshal AK, Farber E (1993) Choline deficiency, lipotrope deficiency and development of liver disease including liver cancer: a new perspective. Lab Invest 68:255–260

Ghoshal AK, Rushmore TH, Farber E (1987) Initiation of carcinogenesis by a dietary deficiency of choline in the absence of added carcinogens. Cancer Lett 36:289–296

Giambarresi LK, Katyal SL, Lombardi B (1982) Promotion of liver carcinogenesis in the rat by a choline-devoid diet: role of liver cell necrosis and regeneration. Br J Cancer 46:825–829

Kapoor R, Ghoshal AK, Farber E (1992) Changes in fatty acid composition of phospholipids from liver microsomes and nuclei in rats fed a choline-free diet. Lipids 27:144–146

Lombardi B, Shinozuka H (1979) Enhancement of 2-acetylfluorene liver carcinogenesis in rats fed a choline-devoid diet. Int J Cancer 23:565–570

Mikol YB, Hoover KL, Creasia D, Poirier LA (1983) Hepatocarcinogenesis in rats fed methyl-deficient amino-acid defined diets. Carcinogenesis 4:1619–1629

Newberne PM (1965) Carcinogenicity of aflatoxin-contaminated peanut meals. In: Wogan GN (ed) Mycotoxins in foodstuffs. MIT Press, Cambridge, MA, pp 187–208

Newberne PM, Nauss KM, de-Camergo JLV (1983) Lipotropes, immunocompetence and cancer. Cancer Res 43:2426s–2434s

Ridout JH, Lucas CC, Patterson JM, Best CH (1954) Changes in chemical composition during the development of cholesterol fatty livers. Biochem J 58:297–301

Rushmore TH, Ghazarian DM, Subramanyan V, Farber E, Ghoshal AK (1987) Probable free radical effects on rat liver nuclei during early hepatocarcinogenesis with a choline-devoid low methionine diet. Cancer Res 47:6731–6740

Salmon WD, Newberne PM (1963) Occurrence of hepatomeas in rats fed diets containimg peanut meal as a major source of protein. Cancer Res 23:571–575

Shinozuka H, Lombardi B (1980) Synergistic effect of a choline-devoid diet and phenobarbital in promoting the emergence of foci of γ-glutamyltranspeptidase-positive hepatocytes in liver of carcinogen treated rats. Cancer Res 40:3846–3849

Shinozuka H, Sells MA, Katyal SL, Sell S, Lombardi B (1979) Effects of choline-devoid diet on the emergence of γ-glutamyltranspeptidase-positive hepatocytes in liver of carcinogen treated rats. Cancer Res 39:2515–2521

Slaga TJ, Klein-Szanto AJP, Triplet LL, Yotti LP, Trosko JE (1981) Skin tumor-promoting activity of benzoyl peroxide, a widely used free radical generating compound. Science 213:1023–1025

Solt DB, Farber E (1976) New principle for the analysis of chemical carcinogenesis. Nature 283:701–703

Solt DB, Medline A, Farber E (1977) Rapid emergence of carcinogen-induced hyperplastic lesions in a new model for the sequential analysis of liver carcinogenesis. Am J Pathol 88:595–618

Solt DB, Cayama E, Tsuda H, Enomoto X, Lee G, Farber E (1983) Promotion of liver cancer development by brief exposure to 2-acetylaminofluorene plus partial hepatectomy or carbon tetrachloride. Cancer Res 43:188–191

Strecker A (1862) Einige neue Bestandtheile der Schweingalle. Ann Chem Pharm 123:353–363

Tsuda H, Lee G, Farber E (1980) Induction of resistant hepatocytes as a new principle for a possible short-term in vitro test for carcinogens. Cancer Res 40:1157–1164

Yokoyama S, Sells MA, Reddy TV, Lombardi B (1985) Hepatocarcinogenic and promoting action of a choline-devoid diet in the rat. Cancer Res 45:2834–2842

Young RJ, Lucas CC, Patterson JM, Best CH (1956) Lipotropic dose-response studies in rats: comparisons of choline, betaine and methionine. Can J Biochem Physiol 34:713–720

CHAPTER 10

Immune Mechanisms and Liver Toxicity

I.R. MACKAY

A. Introduction and Overview of Drug-Mediated Hepatotoxicity

Adverse reactions to drugs are divided into those that are predictable, frequent, dose related and reliably reproducible in experimental animals, and those that are idiosyncratic, non-dose related and non-reproducible in experimental animals. It is important to note that more idiosyncratic drug reactions are attributable predominantly or entirely to pharmacokinetic variations or enzyme polymorphisms or deficiencies than to abnormal immunological reactions, the subject of this chapter. Examples of the former include slow acetylation of hydralazine, slow sulphoxidation of *d*-penicillamine or inefficient oxidation of drugs by cytochrome P450 enzymes. Nonetheless, immune-mediated adverse reactions to drugs is a fascinating albeit poorly understood aspect of immunopathology. The scene is opacified by diversity of initiating mechanisms, limitations of current methods for immunological investigation and imprecise correlations between the observed immune response and the histopathology in affected tissues. In particular, assays in vitro in which lymphocytes are exposed to the culprit drug may be unrevealing, either because the immune response is directed to a drug metabolite present in low abundance in vivo rather than to the drug itself, or the drug acts in some indirect way to modify the immunological system rather than acting as an antigen per se.

General features of immune-mediated hepatotoxicity include the following. (a) The liver may be the only tissue involved, as pertains for drugs that are metabolized by hepatocellular enzymes, or hepatitis may be part of a multisystemic reaction; (b) hepatocellular injury may be accompanied by other features of immunopathy including fever, rash and eosinophilia; (c) the clinical expression may be predominantly hepatocellular, resembling viral hepatitis, or cholestatic, resembling biliary obstruction, or mixed; (d) the liver lesions resolve over a variable period when the drug is withdrawn; (e) re-exposure to the culprit drug elicits the same features, but more rapidly; (f) histopathological features vary in degrees of hepatocellular necrosis, cholestasis, inflammatory infiltration, tissue eosinophilia, steatosis and granulomas.

The liver is one of the more susceptible tissues of the body to immune-mediated drug reactions, others being skin, blood cells, kidney, lung and intestine; the less susceptible are brain, heart, bone and exocrine and endocrine glands. Susceptibility depends on (a) the tissue being a site in which drugs are enzymatically degraded (liver) or excreted (kidney); (b) the presence of antigen-presenting cells, e.g. Kupffer cells in the liver, dendritic cells in the skin or macrophages in the blood and lungs; and (c) the tissue being one wherein cells are readily exposed to the drug, e.g. circulating blood cells and liver. Tissues in which adverse immune-mediated drug reactions are infrequent lack these susceptibility features.

B. Functional Aspects of the Immune System

A functionally efficient immune system effects a brisk eliminative response to foreign (non-self) substances and maintains a tolerance or inertness to autologous (self) constituents. However, an inflexible commitment to this desirable dichotomy of function is impossible, given the resemblances in nature between foreign and autologous molecules. Thus the possibility for error is ever present, resulting either in an underreaction to infectious agents, or an unwanted response to self (autoimmunity), or to ubiquitous allergens, foods or drugs.

I. Immune Repertoire

The immune repertoire is established in embryonic life in the primary lymphoid organs, the thymus and bone marrow (ROSE and MACKAY 1992). The progenitors of immunocytes are lymphoid stem cells that originate in the bone marrow. Precursors of B lymphocytes differentiate within the bone marrow itself to mature B lymphocytes, and precursors of T lymphocytes differentiate within the thymus. During differentiation, precursor cells undergo various rearrangements of germ-line genes that encode for the specific antigen receptor molecule on the lymphocyte surface. For B lymphocytes this is the same molecule as that providing the antigen-binding site on circulating immunoglobulins, and for T lymphocytes the receptor is formed by two covalently linked polypeptide chains, either an α and β chain (mostly), or γ and δ chains for a minor subset of T cells. T lymphocytes are generated by proliferation and diversification in the embryonic thymic cortex under the influence of various stimuli, including molecules encoded by the major histocompatibility complex (MHC) that are presented on cortical epithelial cells. Such positively selected thymocytes will possess antigen receptors tailored to recognize a wide range of small (nona)-peptides. These thymocytes enter the thymic medulla wherein they are negatively selected by being exposed to self-antigens expressed with an MHC molecule on bone marrow-derived dendritic cells; intrathymic exposure to the self-antigen induces apoptosis. Survivors of groups of T lymphocytes purged of cells with reactivities against major self antigens exit as naive T cells to the periphery.

The selection of T cells in the thymus results in a large repertoire of cells that in postnatal life recognize one or another foreign peptide antigen. If such were to include a drug metabolite, susceptibility to an adverse immune response to that drug, if subsequently encountered, would be pre-ordained. Thymic T cells acquire functional specificities that are defined by the presence of particular cell surface molecules. The two major classes are *helper* T cells marked by the CD4 surface molecule, and *cytotoxic* cells marked by the CD8 surface molecule. CD4 helper T cells differentiate in the periphery into subclasses Th1 and Th2, which differ according to their release of different sets of lymphokines. Immunocytes that leave primary lymphoid organs, bone marrow or thymus, are "naive": they have a high threshold for stimulation due inter alia to a low expression of activation molecules on their cell surface. Stimulation by antigen induces phenotypic changes that specify an activated state, and a capacity for immunological memory. These alterations include a conversion of the cell surface CD45RA molecule on naive T cells to the CD45RO molecule, and an increased expression of adhesion molecules that facilitate intercellular interactions and circulatory pathways, including facilitated entry into inflamed tissues (MACKAY 1993).

There are various tolerogenic processes that determine non-responsiveness or "inertia" in the immune system, either to self or foreign antigens. (a) Cells with a receptor for a particular antigenic determinant may not exist in the repertoire due to absence of genetic programming, which may pertain for many drug molecules; (b) the process of negative selection, which occurs in primary lymphoid organs, deletes lymphocytes with anti-self reactivity; (c) in the periphery, exposure of naive T cells to high concentrations of antigen can be tolerogenic; (d) the lack of an essential co-stimulatory signal for T cells, normally delivered by "professional" antigen-presenting cells, may be inhibitory; (e) a subset of T lymphocytes, still not clearly identified, may function to suppress the activation of other immunocytes. Usually, and fortunately, drugs do not evoke a strong immunological response, for any one or other of the above reasons. Perhaps for those drugs that are administered orally, there is developed a process equivalent to the "oral tolerance" that exists for food antigens, and presumably dependent on tolerogenic processes generated in the intestinal lymphoid tissue.

II. Major Histocompatibility Complex

The major histocompatibility complex (MHC) is a complex set of gene loci encoding polymorphic molecules that create a unique marker of "self". MHC molecules – HLA in humans – are heterodimers that bind nonapeptides in such a way as to facilitate their recognition by the T-cell receptor. MHC class I molecules are encoded by HLA A, B and C alleles which (a) exist on most tissue cells; (b) present intracellular (endogenous), e.g. viral antigens; and (c) engage CD8 T cells. MHC class II molecules are encoded by HLA DR, DQ and DP alleles which (a) exist (normally) only on antigen-presenting cells

(APCs); (b) present extracellular (exogenous) antigens after initial uptake by the APCs; and (c) engage CD4 T cells.

III. Afferent Limb of the Immune Response

The immune response resembles a neural arc with an afferent (inductive) and an efferent (effector) limb. Consideration of the afferent limb begins with the antigen. This is either a complex macromolecule that may undergo proteolysis in the blood stream prior to phagocytosis or a simple molecule such as a drug which forms a complex with a host protein. Antigenic molecules are internalized and degraded by antigen-presenting cells, including dendritic cells in lymph nodes and skin, macrophages in the liver (Kupffer cells), spleen and lungs and, notably, the B lymphocyte. B cells can function as APCs in a highly focussed way via capture of antigens by specific immunoglobulin receptors which are the self-same molecules that are secreted as circulating antibodies; antigen presentation by B cells becomes significant whenever there is sustained amplification of a specifically reactive population of B cells, as in chronic inflammation.

The next step is the engagement by the APC of a responsive CD4+ helper T cell. There is an ensuing proliferation of helper T cells with an increased expression of "activation" molecules on their surface, and secretion of various lymphokines, including interleukin-2 (IL-2), that amplify the immune response. Activated CD4+ helper T cells differentiate into functional subsets, Th1 and Th2 (MOSMANN and COFFMAN 1989); Th1 cells secrete IL-2 and interferon-γ which mediates inflammatory delayed-type hypersensitivity (DTH) responses, whilst Th2 cells secrete stimulatory lymphokines for B-cell proliferation and differentiation, IL-4, IL-5, IL-6 and IL-10, thereby influencing levels, isotypes and subclasses of antibodies. The tipping of the CD4 response more towards Th1 or Th2 appears to influence the mode of expression of allergies and autoimmune disease. CD4+ve T-cell clones from patients with drug-induced allergic hepatitis were shown to respond to stimulation with an antigenic liver protein preparation by a high production of IL-5, and this was held to account for the accompanying eosinophilia (TSUTSUI et al. 1992).

Alternatively, an antigenic moiety derived from a drug could associate in the cell cytoplasm with a class I MHC molecule prior to its expression on the cell surface, so that any drug that is metabolized intracellularly could be so presented for recognition by CTLs and thereby elicit direct cytolytic effects. If, as is believed, CD8+ve CTLs require "help" from activated CD4+ve helper cells, then both sets of T cells, CD4 and CD8, would need to be induced by the drug antigen via independent MHC class I and class II pathways.

B cells usually recognize larger and conformational epitopes of a "native" antigen by a recognition structure which is the binding site of immunoglobulin (Ig) molecules, IgM and IgD, on the B-cell membrane. B-cell activation usually requires "helper" signals from CD4 T lymphocytes. B cells exist as different classes according to the functionally different isotype of immunoglobulin (Ig) they produce, IgD, IgM, IgG, IgA and IgE. Expression of these isotypes is dictated by gene-switching events during B-cell development, dependent on particular T-cell signals. IgE secretion by B cells, which is influenced by IL-5, is linked to the eosinophilia often seen in drug responses affecting the liver. Whether the same or different T-cell signals influence IgE secretion and recruitment of eosinophils is uncertain. An eosinophilic response is beneficial in the case of parasite infections, but the role of eosinophils in allergic responses is undetermined.

IV. Efferent Limb of the Immune Response

The efferent limb serves normally to dispose of foreign antigenic material, via processes that include complement-dependent effects of humoral antibody, lymphokines released by helper CD4 T cells and cytolysis by CD8 T cells (Fig. 1). Damaging immune reactions are traditionally classified into types I–IV (MACKAY 1994).

IgE-mediated (type 1) reactions determine immediate hypersensitivity reactions including the classical allergies. Various drugs, penicillin for example,

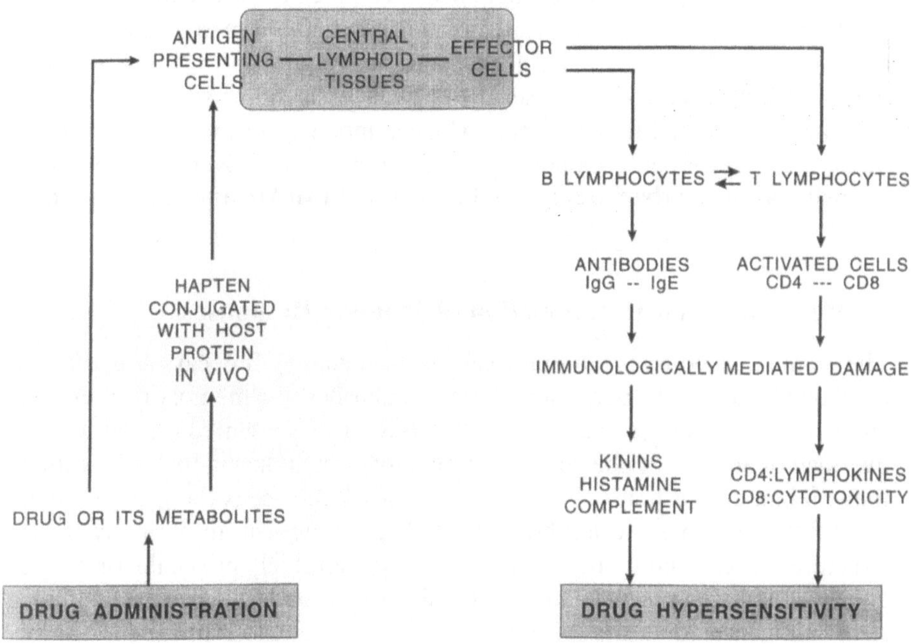

Fig. 1. An outline of inductive (afferent) and effector (efferent) arms of immune responses in drug hypersensitivity reactions. The afferent arm may be activated by the drug or a metabolite conjugated with a host protein. The efferent arm includes B and T lymphocytes which interact in effector pathways. (Modified from MACKAY 1994, with permission of Churchill Livingstone)

can elicit IgE antibodies and cause type 1 reactions, but it is not clear whether any of the drugs that cause hypersensitivity reactions in the liver do so by an IgE response. The occurrence of intrahepatic and blood eosinophilia with hepatic sensitivity reactions to some drugs suggests that an IgE-dependent effect may operate. *IgG-mediated (type 2) reactions* depend on antibodies which effect complement-dependent cytolysis. Such antibodies could be induced either by a drug as such, or by a drug acting as a hapten after combining with a protein carrier. *Immune complex-mediated (type 3) reactions* are expressed as vasculitis, rashes, glomerulonephritis and polyarthritis; the experimental counterpart is the Arthus reaction which occurs when antibody reacts with antigen at a local site and provokes an inflammatory reaction. Drug reactions attributable to this process occur usually several days after initial exposure.

T-cell-mediated (type 4) reactions are exemplified by the accelerated response after initial application of "sensitizing" chemicals to the skin, e.g. dinitrochlorobenzene (DNCB) or nickel. These chemicals may combine with proteins of epithelial cells to form an immunogenic complex that is transferred to regional lymph nodes, or directly presented to T cells in situ by antigen-presenting dendritic cells in the skin. Familiar examples of type 4 reactions include the Mantoux tuberculin reaction, contact sensitivity reactions and the rejection of organ grafts. Drugs that elicit T-cell-mediated reactions in viscera would be those that can accumulate in organs of metabolism or excretion such as the liver and kidney. A particular histological feature indicative of a T-cell-mediated inflammatory response in the liver, or in other sites, is the non-caseating granuloma. It is uncertain which component of the T-cell response induces formation of granulomatous reactions in the liver, as seen with phenylbutazone, carbamazepine and allopurinol (MCMASTER and HENNIGAR 1981).

V. Regulation and Dysregulation of Immune Responses

The immune response is physiologically self-regulating. It decays as antigen is eliminated, but may be perpetuated or re-established as a memory response by antigen which is either retained in the body or re-presented. An excess or overload of antigen can be "counterstimulatory" by inducing tolerance rather than an immune response. Another regulatory influence is the generation of an antibody response to antibody itself. The *idiotype* of an antibody is the structure represented by the binding site of the antibody molecule, or by the equivalent antigen receptor on B or T cells. An antibody can become directed to the antigen-binding site (idiotype) on the antibody molecule and is known as anti-idiotypic antibody. Idiotypic antibody can have a regulatory role in various settings (MACKAY 1988), including antibodies generated to chemical agents (ERLANGER et al. 1986). Suppressor T lymphocytes can have downregulatory effects, either by virtue of being anti-idiotypic to the antigen receptor on B cells or other T cells, or by effects of the "counteractive" lymphokines that they secrete (DEL PRETE et al. 1994). Defects of these regulatory influences are claimed to facilitate autoimmune reactions and hypersensitivity responses to drugs. Immunoregulatory processes may be compromised by a direct effect of the drug itself, since certain types of drug reaction including some that affect the liver appear to involve mechanisms other than a direct stimulation by an antigenic drug of a specific immune response. For example, α-methyldopa induces an autoimmune haemolytic anaemia after some months in a small proportion of recipients (WORRLEDGE 1973), hydralazine and procainamide induce lupus reactions (HESS 1988; RUBIN 1989) and an autoimmune-like hepatitis is induced by certain drugs (vide infra). As one process, lupus-inducing drugs in common are susceptible to oxidation by myeloperoxidase from activated neutrophils (JIANG et al. 1994); this could release labile reactive metabolites with various activities including dysregulatory effects at the lymphocyte surface.

C. Genetic Determinants of Adverse Drug Reactions

Genetic influences on predisposition to immune-mediated drug reactions would be expected, but well-documented familial occurrences are few (HOFT et al. 1981; GENNIS et al. 1991). Genetic predisposition could depend on immunological and/or pharmacokinetic influences, exemplified by reactions to phenytoin in 3 siblings from a family of 12 with fever, rash lymphadenopathy, eosinophilia and anicteric hepatitis; there was an incapacity of affected subjects to detoxify metabolites of phenytoin in vitro (GENNIS et al. 1991). Polymorphisms of drug metabolism may act in combination with the immune response to influence adverse reactions, since those at risk for hydralazine lupus (RUBIN and TAN 1992) are slow acetylators of the drug due to an inherited deficiency of the acetyl transferase enzyme (PERRY et al. 1970), and those at risk for reactions to *d*-penicillamine have an enzyme deficiency that impairs sulphoxidation and disposal of the drug (EMERY and PANAYI 1989). Involvement of MHC class II (HLA) genes is exemplified by polymyositis/myasthenia gravis in recipients of *d*-penicillamine among whom there is an excess of HLA DR4 (HOLLINGSWORTH et al. 1992), whereas in "naturally occurring" polymyositis the MHC association is HLA DR3. In 13 cases of drug-induced CAH reported by LINDBERG et al. (1975), there was an excess of females (10:3), and a raised frequency of HLA-B8 over population controls, 42% versus 23%; however, among 38 cases of hepatitic drug reactions attributed to nitrofurans (25 acute, 13 chronic), there were high frequencies of various autoimmune serological reactions, but no increased frequency of HLA B8 or DR3 was evident (STRICKER et al. 1988). Studies among mouse strains exposed to the hepatotoxin carbon tetrachloride indicated that both MHC and non-MHC determinants of susceptibility were operative, presumably at stages including drug distribution, intracellular degradation and conjugation, and the inflammatory response after cellular injury (BHATHAL et al. 1983; BEISEL et al. 1984). Equivalent differences would be expected in humans.

D. Liver in Relation to Adverse Drug Reactions

I. Intrahepatic Metabolism of Drugs by Microsomal Enzymes

1. Cytochrome P450 Oxidases (CYP450)

The CYP450 enzymes are a genetically diverse superfamily that can interact with numerous structurally different molecules (WATKINS 1990). A given drug may be catalysed by one or more CYP450s, whereas other substances may be catalysed by multiple CYP450 enzymes (KOOP and TIERNEY 1990). The catalytic process involves oxidation by addition of one atom of molecular oxygen (O_2) to the substrate, with reduction of the other atom to water. CYP450 enzymes are readily inducible so that their cellular concentration is increased by exposure to diverse chemicals, as well as hormones intrinsic to the animal. Different CYP450s are encoded by unique genes which are distributed among different chromosomes. The CYP450 superfamily is divided into gene families according to a level of homology in amino acid sequence of 40%. Among the many members of the CYP450 enzyme family, there are a few that are known to participate in hepatic hypersensitivity drug reactions, which are listed in the recent review by LEEDER and OKEY, Chap. 6, this volume.

2. UDP Glucuronosyl Transferases

A family of microsomal enzymes, uridine diphosphoglucuronoside glucuronosyl transferases (UGT), catalyses the conjugation of various endogenous and exogenous substrates, including bilirubin, with glucuronic acid. Various isoenzymes of this family with distinct but overlapping specificities have been isolated (JAKOBY 1994). Numerous drugs are conjugated by these enzymes prior to excretion by the liver, so that a potential exists for a UGT-drug complex to elicit a liver sensitivity reaction. As an example of the participation of UGT in the formation of a neoantigen, it was shown by molecular cloning that the antigen reactive with liver-kidney microsomal antibody type 3, sometimes associated with hepatitis delta virus infection, is a member of the UGT1 family of enzymes (PHILLIPP et al. 1994).

3. Carboxyl Esterases

Esterases are abundant enzymes in the microsomal fraction of liver cells that are active over a wide range of lipophilic xenobiotics and natural substances. A carboxyl esterase has been implicated in immune reactions in halothane hepatitis (vide infra).

II. Intrahepatic Immune Processes

1. Initiation of Immune-Mediated Drug Reactions in the Liver

Drugs that cause hepatic hypersensitivity reactions are those that are biodegraded in the liver to yield a sensitizing metabolite. In some instances the drug itself or a metabolite, by reason of pharmacological idiosyncrasy, initially causes toxic liver injury and so facilitates the formation by the drug or a metabolite of an adduct with a liver protein, and thereby a potential antigenic complex (Pohl 1990). Whether this complex is more likely presented by the MHC class I pathway to CD8 cytotoxic T cells or by the MHC class II pathway by Kupffer cells to CD4 helper T cells is unknown, but, assuming that appropriately responsive CD8 or CD4 T cells exist in the immune repertoire, a potentially damaging immune response will be induced. The relative utilization of the exogenous class II or endogenous class I pathways of antigen presentation (Unanue 1992) has been scarcely explored in drug sensitivity reactions, and more investigation is called for. Whichever pathway is induced will influence the particular effector process(es) that is recruited (see above), but T-cell-dependent hepatocellular damage (type 4) is the most likely outcome, either CD4 T cells with release of various toxic cytokines including interferon-γ, tumor necrosis factor, etc., or CD8 T cells that are directly cytolytic.

2. Regulatory and Dysregulation of Intrahepatic Immune Reactions

Immune responses are intrinsically self-regulating. The waning of an immune response is due to degradation and decay of the provoking antigen. Hence drug reactions tend to be transient, but a "memory" response will be established, perhaps due to prolonged retention of antigen in phagocytic or dendritic cells, with a low level of restimulation of the immune response (Mackay 1993). This may explain accelerated reactions on rechallenge with the same or even a related drug, even after long intervals. Apart from decay of the antigenic stimulus, there are intrinsically downregulatory processes generated within the immune system itself, including anti-idiotypic reactions (Mackay 1988), and immune suppression. Anti-idiotypic reactions are illustrated by the case of chemical ligands that can act as agonists for receptor structures. Antibodies can be raised to such ligands, and when antibodies (anti-idiotypic antibodies) are raised against antibodies to the ligand, these will mimic the natural ligand (agonist) and activate the receptor. Anti-idiotypic antibodies are capable of regulating drug-induced reactions, at least in experimental models, as in mercury-induced autoimmune disease (vide infra). Immune suppression by T cells decreases the intensity and duration of immune responses dependent on activated T or B cells (Gershon 1974). Such activity is best exemplified by the adoptive transfer in experimental models of immune suppressive effects. Although a clear isolation in vitro of a suppressor T cell with unambiguous cell-surface markers is still lacking (CD8 has been long used as a putative marker for suppressor T cells in man), functional suppressor T-cell effects are evident and may operate through anti-idiotypic effects, or by the release of inhibitory rather than stimulatory lymphokines.

III. Infrequency of Hepatic Hypersensitivity Drug Reactions

Hepatitis due to drug hypersensitivity is, fortunately, infrequent, given the very high number of case exposures. In Australia, correlations have been made between drug reactions reported to the Adverse Drug Reactions Advisory Committee (ADRAC) and numbers of prescriptions written for a particular drug. For flucloxacillin, for example, over 720000 prescriptions were written over 4 years (1984–1988), and 50 cases, 1/15000 prescriptions, of sensitivity reactions were reported. For the amoxycillin-clavulanic acid combination (augmentin), the frequency was 1/250000 prescription (WONG et al. 1991); similarly in France, the estimated frequency of reactions due to augmentin was below 1/100000 exposed persons (LARREY et al. 1992). For halothane, the cited rate for severe hepatosensitivity is only about 1/10000 exposed persons, with added risks conferred by female gender, obesity and previous exposure. Actual monitoring of all treated patients could yield higher frequencies, since results for 1081 consecutive patients in Canada treated with flutamide, an anti-androgen used for prostate cancer, disclosed 0.36% with liver functional abnormalities and 0.18% with clinical manifestations (GOMEZ et al. 1992). The infrequency of hepatic drug sensitivity reactions could be explained by (a) a low capacity of MHC molecules to bind potential epitopes derived from drugs; (b) the T-cell repertoire lacking cells with receptors for epitopes derived from drugs; (c) precursors of drug-reactive T cells, even if present, being unable to engage appropriate antigen-presenting cells in the liver; (d) drug-reactive T cells undergoing tolerance rather than immunogenic reponses to the drug; or (e) the response to the drug being expressed only as a non-pathogenic and even unrecognized antibody response, rather than a pathogenic T-cell response.

IV. Immunopathology of Hepatic Hypersensitivity Drug Reactions

Hypersensitivity drug reactions affecting the liver can have both hepatitic and cholestatic components. One or the other usually predominates, with the level of expression on the liver cell surface of a drug-related neoantigen determining either hepatocellular necrosis (high expression) or functional changes including impaired secretion of bile (low expression). Alternatively the type of cytokines released may determine damage either to liver cells or biliary ductular cells. Histological appearances usually reflect the coexistence of toxic injury and an immune-mediated process with acute lesions, steatosis and/or hepatocellular necrosis that may be focal, submassive or massive; there are

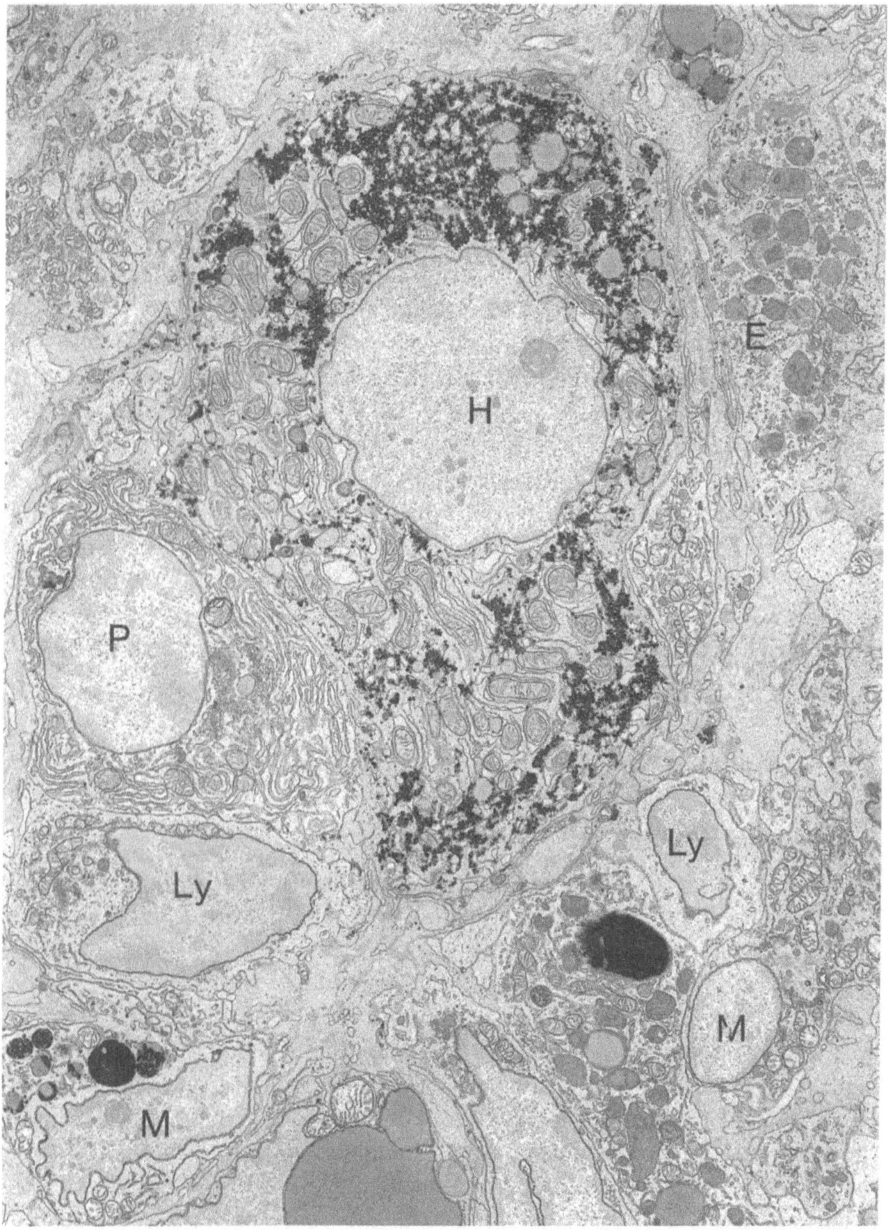

Fig. 2. A photoelectron micrograph from a liver biopsy in a case of drug-induced hepatotoxicity illustrating multiplicity of potential effector processes. The target hepatocyte (*H*) is in contiguity with a plasma cell (*P*), an eosinophil (*E*), macrophages (*M*) and lymphocytes (*Ly*) (×7500). [Illustration kindly provided by Dr. M. James Phillips (PHILLIPS et al. 1987) and reproduced with permission of Raven Press]

inflammatory changes as seen in viral hepatitis, and with the degree of necrosis often exceeding that expected from the clinical signs or biochemical tests. Other changes include portal and sinusoidal mononuclear and eosinophilic infiltration, piecemeal necrosis, bile duct lesions and granulomas. In chronic lesions there is more prominent periportal piecemeal necrosis, and appearances simulate those seen in autoimmune or prolonged viral hepatitis; when exposure to the drug is of long duration or repetitive and hepatic injury indolent and asymptomatic, liver scarring or cirrhosis will occur. When the biliary excretory system is the prime site of injury, appearances range from "pure" cholestasis to acute or chronic cholangiolitis with ductular necrosis, simulating those seen in stage 1 of primary biliary cirrhosis (PBC), e.g. with chlorpromazine and certain other drugs (Klatskin and Kantor 1972; Phillips et al. 1987; King and Blitzer 1990). Rarely there may be progressive ductular loss and biliary cirrhosis (Moradpour et al. 1994). Antimitochondrial antibody (AMA) was reported in three instances of drug-induced cholangiohepatitis attributed to halothane, chlorpromazine or sulphonamide (Klatskin and Kantor 1972), but there are no well-documented examples of PBC being initiated by exposure to a drug. Morphological features do not clarify the nature of effector mechanisms of hepatic hypersensitivity reactions, illustrated by an electron micrograph from a case of propyl thiouracil hepatitis in which a damaged hepatocyte is seen in close juxtaposition to a plasma cell, a lymphocyte, a macrophage and an eosinophil (Fig. 2).

V. Drug-Altered Neoantigen – The Halothane Paradigm

1. Halothane Hepatitis

Halothane (2-bromo-2 chloro-1,1,1-trifluoroethane) was introduced as an anaesthetic agent in 1956. Soon thereafter there were reports of fatalities with jaundice and hepatic necrosis. A threefold greater incidence of fatal hepatic necrosis of 7.1 versus 2.4/100000 cases after multiple halothane anaesthetic exposures, versus non-halothane expsoures, was recorded by the United States National Halothane Study (1966). Although the mortality rate was high, over 40%, there was no residual liver disease in survivors.

The manner whereby a neoantigen might be generated by halothane exposure involves consideration of two metabolic pathways for biotransformation of halothane: both operate through CYP450 and both generate reactive metabolites which could bind covalently to liver cell macromolecules. The oxidative pathway, which is stimulated by high oxygen tension, leads to the generation of trifluoroacetic acid (TFA), whereas the reductive pathway, which is stimulated by hypoxic conditions, leads to the generation of fluoride and the 2-chloro-1,1,1-trifluoroethyl radical (Neuberger and Kenna 1987). Halothane hepatotoxicity illustrates the principle that drugs can cause an idiosyncratic hepatotoxic reaction in either of two ways. There is a milder form that develops in some 20% of patients due to cytotoxic effects of halothane metabolites, and a severe form in 1 in 10000 patients due to an immune response to metabolite-altered liver proteins (RAY and DRUMMOND 1991).

2. Immunological Investigations of Halothane Hepatitis

In early studies, peripheral blood lymphocytes of 10 of 15 subjects with halothane hepatitis proliferated after exposure to halothane in vitro (PARONETTO and POPPER 1970), a finding that was not confirmed (MOULT and SHERLOCK 1975). Antibodies in serum included those with reactivity to a liver kidney microsomal antigen (WALTON et al. 1976) and those with reactivity to the cell membrane of hepatocytes isolated from rabbits dosed with halothane (VERGANI et al. 1980). The latter observation led to the concept of a "halothane-altered liver antigen," which was further developed using a leucocyte migration test wherein peripheral blood leucocytes from patients with halothane hepatosensitivity were tested against homogenates of liver from rabbits dosed with halothane. Of 12 subjects tested, 8 gave abnormal results, but the positive results were variable, in that migration was inhibited in 4, and increased in 4 (VERGANI et al. 1978). The antigenicity of halothane-altered liver was shown for the serum of patients with halothane sensitivity by specific reactivity with the cell surface membrane of hepatocytes of halothane-anaesthetized rabbits, according to immunofluorescence, and the rendering of liver hepatocytes susceptible to antibody-dependent (K-cell) killing (VERGANI et al. 1980; MIELE-VERGANI et al. 1980).

3. Detection of Antibodies to TFA Conjugates

A TFA-conjugated molecule with potential antigenicity may be created by the hepatic metabolism of halothane. Assays to investigate this have included ELISA (KENNA et al. 1984), immunohistochemical staining (SATOH et al. 1985; HUBBARD et al. 1989) and Western immunoblotting (NEUBERGER and KENNA 1987); further data based on these assays is cited by KENNA et al. (1987), POHL et al. (1989) and MARTIN et al. (1990). The findings are that the serum of patients with halothane hepatitis is reactive with polypeptides separated from homogenates of liver obtained from halothane-exposed animals. By immunoblotting, the reactive components had estimated molecular weights of 100, 76, 59, 57 and 54 kDa. These components were considered to represent neoantigens derived from the covalent binding to microsomal polypeptides of the hapten trifluoracetyl chloride derived from the oxidative metabolism of halothane, and to constitute part of the pathogenic response in halothane hepatitis. The validity of this concept would depend on observations that corresponding components were not evident when sera from subjects exposed to halothane, with or without hepatitis, were exposed to an equivalently treated liver preparation from animals not pretreated with halothane. Of the various microsomal polypeptides recognized by immunoblotting, the 100-kDa and the 76-kDa components were the most frequently identified (KENNA et al.

1987, 1988a). The same neoantigens could be induced by halothane in human liver, as well as in rabbit liver, according to results with liver tissue from patients in whom death occurred shortly after halothane anesthesia (Kenna et al. 1988b).

One of the microsomal trifluoroacetylated polypeptide neoantigens, the 59-kDa component, recognized by antibodies in halothane hepatitis, was isolated by chromatography from liver microsomes of halothane-treated rats; antibodies raised to this polypeptide enabled the native protein to be purified from liver microsomes of untreated rats and to be identified as a microsomal carboxylesterase isozyme (Satoh et al. 1989). Enflurane similarly induced adducts similar to the 59-kDa molecule that reacted with sera of patients with halothane hepatitis, in keeping with the cross-sensitization between halothane and enflurane (Christ et al. 1988). In a further report, serum antibodies of patients with halothane hepatitis reacted with native carboxylesterase purified from human liver, thus behaving as true autoantibodies (Smith et al. 1993). Another of the liver microsomal neoantigens, the 57-kDa component, reactive with sera of patients with halothane hepatitis has been identified as protein disulphide isomerase, by ELISA, using either trifluoroacetylated or native 57-kDa proteins (Martin et al. 1993).

The data on neoantigenic adducts between TFA and liver microsomal proteins, if corroborated, would have important general implications for drug-induced hypersensitivity damage to the liver. Thus sensitization to any agent that is processed by liver microsomal enzymes, and which could form neoantigenic adducts, should be demonstrable by techniques such as immunoblotting and/or ELISA, using tissues of animals exposed to that agent. For example, acetaldehyde derived from alcohol metabolism may similarly form neoantigenic adducts with liver proteins, and so generate immune responses that contribute to alcoholic liver disease (Mackay 1995).

VI. Native Liver Antigens – The Liver-Kidney Microsomal (LKM) System

There is another seemingly different (and more widely validated) set of observations on hepatic hypersensitivity reactions in which the culprit drug induces an autoantibody that reacts with drug-disposing microsomal organelles, but the ensuing reactivity is with a *native* rather than a *drug-altered* antigen. Notably, there is no requirement in the antibody "readout" for liver protein to be complexed with the culprit drug. The first such "readout" was anti-liver-kidney microsomal (anti-LKM) antibody by immunofluorescence, described in a subset of autoimmune hepatitis (Rizzetto et al. 1973; Homberg et al. 1987), and subsequently called anti-LKM-1. Other types of anti-LKM, associated with drug reactions, were designated as anti-LKM-2, and a type associated with delta hepatitis virus infection of the liver was designated as anti-LKM-3.

1. Hepatitis with Anti-LKM-2

Hepatitis with anti-LKM-2 was reported by CRIVELLI et al. (1983) and HOMBERG et al. (1985). The latter authors described 157 cases of hepatic drug sensitivity reactions that included cases with various "anti-organelle" antibodies, to nuclei (ANA), smooth muscle (SMA), mitochondria (AMA) and microsomes (LKM), in response to drugs that included clometacin (ANA and SMA), fenofibrate (SMA), papaverine (SMA) and tienilic acid (anti-LKM). Tienilic acid, which is 2,3-dichloro-4-(2-thenoyl) phenoxy acetic acid (ticrynofen), is a diuretic and uricosuric and is highly hepatosensitizing (ZIMMERMAN et al. 1984).

2. Identification of LKM as Cytochrome P450 Species

The LKM antigen was recognized by BEAUNE et al. (1987) as a CYP450 isoform by studying 20 anti-LKM-2 sera from patients with hepatitis due to tienilic acid. These sera were tested by immunoblotting concurrently with isoform-specific antisera to CYP450 raised in rabbits against electrophoresed preparations of human liver microsomes, and preparations of CYP450s including types 5, 8 and 9. The immunoblots showed that both human anti-LKM and the rabbit antiserum to CYP450-8 reacted specifically with a component corresponding to P450-8, now identified as CYP450 2C9. The antisera did not react with CYP450 isoforms other than 2C9, and sera of non-hepatitic individuals treated with tienilic acid were not reactive. Antisera to LKM-2 specifically inhibited enzymatic activity dependent on 5-hydroxylation of tienilic acid, a reaction mediated by P450 2C9, but did not inhibit activity dependent on other isoforms of CYP450. These results suggested that 5-hydroxylation of tienilic acid in human liver microsomes could lead to the formation of reactive metabolites that could bind to microsomal proteins, and that an immunogenic constituent of CYP450 that was altered by the metabolite could migrate to the liver cell surface. Thus there would be an ensuing production of an antibody reactive not only with the CYP450 protein conjugated with the reactive hapten, but also with the native CYP450 itself. Of particular note, and in contrast with the process proposed for halothane hepatitis, the demonstration of antigenic reactivity did not require a liver cell protein altered by the drug metabolite (Fig. 3).

Both the drug-induced anti-LKM-2 and the spontaneously occurring anti-LKM-1 were shown to recognize a 50-kDa microsomal protein (ALVAREZ et al. 1985; KYRIATSOULIS et al. 1987), but antibodies to LKM-1 and LKM-2 reacted with individual CYP450 isoforms (MANNS et al. 1988; WAXMAN et al. 1988). The reactant for anti-LKM-1 was found to be CYP450 2D6, as judged (a) by the capacity of LKM-1 antisera to inhibit specifically bufuralol-1′-hydroxylation (ZANGER et al. 1988) and (b) the derivation from gene expression libraries by antibody screening of a cDNA that encoded CYP450 2D6 (GUEGUEN et al. 1988). An immunodominant epitope for B cells (antibody) on human CYP450

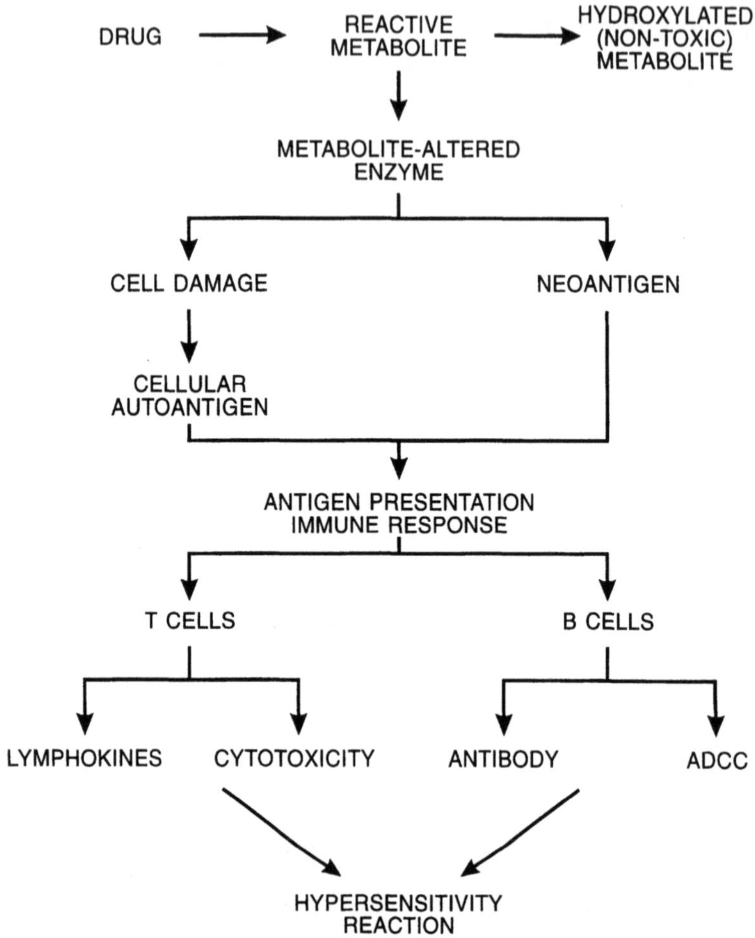

Fig. 3. Hepatic drug reactions may depend on formation of reactive metabolites that can (a) result in direct cellular damage and release of autoantigens or (b) create a neoantigen, e.g. metabolite-altered CYP450. The result may be a response to a native autoantigen, e.g. anti-LKM, or a response to a metabolite-altered enzyme antigen. (Modified from MACKAY 1994, with permission of Churchill Livingstone)

2D6 was found to consist of a highly conserved sequence in the 2D subfamily of CYP450 (MANNS et al. 1991).

3. Antibodies to CYP 1A2 in Drug-Induced Hepatitis

In an infrequently occurring type of drug-induced hepatitis provoked by dihydralazine (MANNS et al. 1990a; BOURDI et al. 1990), there is reactivity of sera with another microsomal antigen, CYP450 1A2, the main enzyme for the metabolism of phenacetin. Such sera react as anti-LKM, but this CYP450 is liver specific, so that the antibodies are better called anti-liver-microsomal (LM) rather than anti-LKM. Antibodies to CYP450 1A2, together with anti-CYP2D6, have been detected in LKM-positive (type 2) autoimmune hepatitis.

Autoantibodies to LM antigen react predominantly with microsomes in perivenous hepatocytes (SACHER et al. 1990; BOURDI et al. 1990) in contrast to anti-CYP450 2D6 (LKM-1), which react homogeneously with the entire liver lobule. The specific reactivity of liver microsomal autoantibodies with CYP450 1A2 is shown by the increased reactivity of anti-CYP450 1A2 sera with microsomes derived from rabbits pretreated with TCDD, an inducer of the CYP450 1A subfamily, and also by the strong reactivity with lysates from COS cells transfected with a vector specifically carrying the full-length human cDNA for CYP450 1A2 (MANNS et al. 1990a).

The identified CYP450 autoantigens 2D6, 2C9 and 1A2 migrate as 50-kDa components by immunoblotting. There are other liver microsomal autoantigens detected by immunoblotting (MANNS et al. 1989; CODONER-FRANCH et al. 1989) that are so far not identified. There is one of 55 kDa that may be a CYP450 enzyme protein, and another of 64 kDa which is of larger size than the hepatic microsomal CYP450s, and may be another enzyme species. As noted earlier, the LKM-3 reactivity seen in cases of hepatitis delta infection is directed against a glucuronosyl transferase enzyme.

4. Inhibition of Enzyme Function by Anti-LKM

Autoimmune sera that react with enzyme autoantigens characteristically inhibit the catalytic activity of the enzyme. In keeping with this, anti-LKM-1 sera (anti-CYP450 2D6) inhibit bufuralol-1′-hydroxylation and the metabolism of sparteine. Since there is a genetic polymorphism with lack of expression of CYP450 2D6 in 5%–10% of Caucasians who are poor metabolizers of drugs dependent on 2D6 (GONZALES et al. 1988), the question arises whether this polymorphism is relevant to formation of anti-LKM-1. However, patients seropositive for anti-CYP450 2D6 express functional enzyme in their livers, and efficiently metabolize drugs that depend on CYP450 2D6 (MANNS et al. 1990b). Also, whilst anti-CYP450 2D6 sera of patients with autoimmune hepatitis inhibit the enzyme in vitro, such patients do metabolize 2D6-dependent-drugs, so that LKM-1 autoantibodies appear not to penetrate the cell membrane to inhibit enzyme function in vivo (MANNS et al. 1990b). The LKM-2 and LM antibodies that react with CYP450 2C9 and 1A2 likewise specifically inhibit the metabolism of drugs dependent on these enzyme in vitro (MANNS et al. 1990a), but apparently not in vivo.

5. Origins of Anti-LKM Reactivity

The occurrence of anti-LKM in "spontaneous" autoimmune hepatitis, drug-induced hepatitis and virus-induced hepatitis (HCV and HDV) raises issues on the origin of this reactivity, such as the creation of a new antigenic determinant by linkage between a P450 enzyme and an extrinsic molecule, whether derived from a drug, virus or other cryptic source. Positive tests for anti-HCV in autoimmune hepatitis, particularly in type 2 cases (anti-LKM-1), is well validated (FUSCONI et al. 1990), but there is a curiously differing geographical distribution of such cases, much higher in southern Europe than elsewhere. The attachment of an extrinsic molecule, derived from a virus or drug, to a CYP450 enzyme is required to initiate an immune response, but thereafter the unaltered CYP450 molecule may be sufficient to sustain the response. We can again note the two possible models for drug-induced hepatitis (vide supra) in which CYP450 enzymes are implicated. One is the "halothane model" in which serum reactivity in vitro requires that the antigen be a halothane-altered molecule, whereas in the "tienilic acid model" the reaction is with a native CYP450 autoantigen. For a CYP450 species to act as an immunogenic stimulus and as a target in an immune response, the enzyme molecule should be expressed on the intact liver cell surface; this was demonstrable for P450 2D6 by LENZI et al. (1984) and LOEPER et al. (1989), but not by GERKEN et al. (1987). Finally the reactant for T cells, essential to the process of immune induction, needs to be identified. The relevant immunogenic nonapeptide derived from the drug-cytochrome complex should associate either with MHC class II molecules to stimulate a CD4 T-cell response, or with MHC class I molecules to stimulate a CD8 (cytotoxic) T-cell response, or both.

VII. Drug-Induced Hepatitis with Reactions to Autoantigens

There is a third type of liver sensitization expressed as an autoimmune response in which the autoantigens are clearly not associated with the metabolic degradation of the drug, as pertains with microsomal enzymes in the liver. First of all, a general comment can be made on drug-induced autoimmune diseases such as lupus induced by hydralazine and haemolytic anaemia by α-methyldopa. In these examples, the autoimmune process usually develops slowly in a variable (usually small) proportion of users of the drug, and is preceded by the characteristic autoantibody, histones in the case of hydralazine- or procainamide-induced lupus (RUBIN 1989), or erythrocytes in the case of α-methyldopa-induced haemolytic anaemia (WORRLEDGE 1973). The autoimmune response is drug specific and disease specific, and the serological reactions and the disease recede when the culprit drug is withdrawn. There is no complementary relationship between the autoantibody and the inducing drug, so that the immune response is directed at a native autoantigen, nuclear or erythrocyte, rather than a host protein altered by the drug. Finally, demonstration of autoantibody in vitro does not require the presence of the drug in the test system. The effector mechanism for these drug-associated diseases appears to be humoral antibody, presumably with formation of immune complexes in lupus reactions associated with hydralazine or procaine amide, or complement-dependent haemolytic reactions with α-methyldopa.

In the case of the liver, the classical example of drug-induced autoimmunity is hepatitis induced by oxyphenisatin (REYNOLDS et al. 1971). This simulated in most respects spontaneous autoimmune lupoid-type hepatitis, with serological reactions to nuclear and smooth muscle antigens. The disease receded after treatment with prednisolone, or spontaneously when the drug was withdrawn, with a few cases of long-term drug usage being followed by scarring and cirrhosis of the liver (LINDNER et al. 1975). A similar autoimmune-like hepatitic disease was later reported with other drugs including α-methyldopa (TOGHILL et al. 1974), nitrofurantoin (IWARSON et al. 1979) and possibly others (MADDREY and BOITNOTT 1991). A recent explanation for drug-induced autoimmunity is the model induction experimentally of MHC class II molecules on thyroid epithelial cells that normally lack MHC class II (TAKORABET et al. 1995); this process may occur in vivo and involve hepatocytes.

E. Experimental Models of Drug-Induced Immune-Mediated Disease

Given that drug-induced immune-mediated disease in humans is relatively rare and idiosyncratic, models in animals will be infrequent. The closest models are the multisystem diseases induced in rats, mice and rabbits by heavy metals, particularly mercury or gold (DRUET et al. 1989; GOLDMAN et al. 1991). In the model in Brown-Norway (BN) rats, repeated low doses of mercuric chloride $HgCl_2$ induce glomerulonephritis of a mixed type due to antibodies to glomerular basement membrane and/or deposited immune complexes, an increase in levels both of CD4 T cells and B cells, high serum levels of IgG and IgE, and multiple autoantibodies against DNA, nucleolar components (fibrillarin and laminin) and collagen types II and IV. The same disease occurs in mice after either $HgCl_2$ or gold salts (GOTER ROBINSON et al. 1986). These diseases are characteristically self-regulatory since, after 2 weeks, there is regression attributed to the operation of immune suppression networks dependent either on anti-idiotypic antibodies or regulatory cytokines released by T cells (GOLDMAN et al. 1991). Susceptibility is strain dependent among rats and mice, with H-2s mice being highly susceptible and H-2d mice resistant. Non-MHC genes are also implicated (GOLDMAN et al. 1991). Heavy metal immune disease does not occur in animals deprived of T cells, suggesting that T-cell influences are critical in drug-related immune disease in humans. One of the earliest detectable abnormalities, within 3 days, is an increased expression of MHC class II molecules on the surface of B cells (DUBEY et al. 1991), and this effect may be critical to pathogenesis.

Three interpretations of pathogenesis have been offered by GOLDMAN et al. (1991). First, T cells are hyperstimulated by chemically modified MHC class II molecules, which provide an allogeneic-type stimulus; second, T-cell receptors modified by the chemical acquire specificity for normally tolerated MHC class II molecules; or third, the chemical expressed on the surface of both T and B cells creates "superadhesins" that enhance T- and B-cell interactions.

As with other autoimmune expressions, imbalance of the CD4 Th1 and Th2 subsets may be important in experimental heavy metal immune diseases, since data from the $HgCl_2$ rodent models indicate that Th2 cells play the predominant role, with potent activation of autoantibody-secreting B cells.

F. Laboratory Investigation of Immune-Mediated Hepatic Drug Reactions

I. General Laboratory Investigations

Any occurrence of a hepatitis-like or cholestatic illness in adults should prompt the possibility of drug-related liver disease with enquiry for recent drug or anaesthetic exposures. Laboratory investigations may reveal neutrophilia and/or eosinophilia. The abnormalities of liver function tests include increases in serum levels of transaminase enzymes, alkaline phosphatase or γ-glutamyl transpeptidase which improve after withdrawal of the suspected drug. Positive serological tests for autoantibodies to nuclei, smooth muscle, microsomes and mitochondria will disclose those hepatic drug reactions that simulate autoimmune hepatitis: an antinuclear reaction generally will have a homogeneous pattern, an anti-smooth muscle reaction will have specificity for actin, and a liver-kidney microsomal reaction by immunofluorescence can be investigated by immunoblotting on cell homogenates to reveal components at a molecular weight of 50 kDa (usually), or 55 or 64 kDa. Liver biopsy comes into consideration when the biochemical indices fail to improve after 4 weeks, and histological features suggestive of a drug reaction include eosinophilia, steatosis, biliary ductular damage or granulomas. If a culprit drug among several others needs to be specifically identified, then oral challenge can be performed (with extreme caution); the challenge dose should be small and be followed by frequent (e.g. daily) monitoring of blood levels of transaminase enzymes and blood eosinophilia.

II. Drug-Specific Immunological Investigations

Specific immunological investigation to identify definitively a culprit liver-sensitizing drug are usually not rewarding. Circulating antibodies are seldom demonstrable, either because the drug must become conjugated in vivo with proteins to form the immunogenic complex for B cells, and/or the drug is degraded to reactive metabolites. Hence selection of an appropriate reactant for an in vitro assay is difficult. Intradermal skin-prick or scratch tests have proven informative for detecting drug sensitivities mediated by anaphylactic (type 1, IgE-mediated) reactions, in particular those due to anaesthetic agents or penicillin derivatives, but such tests have not proven useful for the diagnosis of liver sensitivity reactions (MACKAY 1994).

1. Detection of T-Cell-Mediated Reactions

Tests for T-cell-mediated reactivity of drugs could include in vivo procedures that are used to demonstrate T-cell-mediated responses in other settings, i.e. a "patch test" to the skin as used in contact sensitivity to nickel, or intradermal injection as in a tuberculin test, but again these test formats have not been revealing in confirming drug reactions affecting the liver. In vitro procedures to detect activated T cells depend on the suspect drug provoking cultured T lymphocytes either to undergo a mitogenic response, or to release indicator lymphokines into the culture fluid.

In practice, mitogenesis is the procedure that is generally used to investigate T-cell reactivity to sensitizing drugs. However, this type of assay cannot be done as a "casual" laboratory procedure. The expertise and resources of a specialized immunology laboratory are required. Peripheral blood lymphocytes are gradient separated, after which 10^5 viable lymphocytes are exposed in culture to various concentrations of the suspect drug or a metabolite. After 3 days in culture, there is added tritium-labelled thymidine, which becomes incorporated into nuclei of mitogenically stimulated T lymphocytes, and after 2 days the lymphocytes are harvested and counted for incorporated radioactivity. Precautions include the following. The test drug should be fully solubilized; repetitive mitogenesis readouts are required to control for the inherent variability in such assays; the establishment of a dose-response relationship is essential; there should be inclusion of a positive control with a plant mitogen, e.g. phytohaemagglutinin (PHA), and a negative control; and there should be repetition of an early negative test, since this may become positive later. Lymphocyte stimulation assays for drug hypersensitivity often give "false-negative" results, but a well-validated positive result should establish the existence of a drug sensitivity (Houwerzijl et al. 1977). In the event, very few of the recorded examples of drug sensitivity in the medical literature include an immunological laboratory confirmation of specific drug sensitivity reaction, some exceptions being a reaction to carbamazepine (Houwerzijl et al. 1977), erythromycin estolate (Cooksley and Powell 1977), nifedipine (Rotmensch et al. 1980), erythromycin ethylsuccinate (Victorino and Maria 1985) and allopurinol (Braden et al. 1994).

There are procedures recommended to improve the sensitivity of T-cell mitogenesis assays to identify drug sensitivity. One is the selection of a drug metabolite; for example, in a case of allopurinol-induced hepatic hypersensitivity, the metabolite oxypurinol induced greater proliferation than the parent drug, allopurinol (Braden et al. 1994). Another is the addition to the assay system of a prostaglandin inhibitor, indomethacin (Victorino and Maria 1985; Victorino et al. 1992), to reduce the effect of prostaglandin-producing suppressor cells, and another is to use drug metabolites rather than intact drugs as stimulators. This may be achieved by stimulating T cells with metabolite-containing serum (Berg et al. 1979), or urine, as exemplified by a case of diclofenac-induced immune-mediated haemolysis (Salama et al. 1991). In this case, reactivity of serum antibodies with erythrocytes required the presence of urine that presumably contained a trace metabolite of diclofenac, since the presence of the drug itself, or its known metabolites in the test system, was ineffective. In many cases, however, the reactive drug metabolites that generate antigenicity are not identifiable (LEEDER and OKEY, Chap. 6, this volume).

III. Pharmacological Idiosyncrasy

Apart from immunological considerations, there may also be a requirement for assessing pharmacological idiosyncrasy. Thus in cases of idiosyncratic reactions, investigations have included incubation of lymphocytes of the susceptible individual, and their relatives, with the suspected drug and a rodent microsomal system to generate the reactive metabolite which can be tested against blood leucocytes. Patients with reactions to halothane, diphenylhydantoin, barbiturates or nitrofuratoin have been investigated in this way (SHEAR and SPIELBERG 1988). This approach is illustrated by the family referred to above in which three siblings developed a transient hypersensitivity reaction to phenytoin with fever, rash, lymphadenopathy and anicteric hepatitis (GENNIS et al. 1991). Oxidative metabolites from phenytoin were prepared using murine hepatic microsomes and these were used to challenge peripheral blood mononuclear leucocytes over 16h, with a cell viability readout. There was demonstrable toxicity of phenytoin metabolites for leucocytes for the three affected siblings, and also for leucocytes of four unaffected siblings. Thus an inherited abnormality in a detoxification pathway, phenytoin in the above instance, may be combined with an immunological response initiated by toxic products of degradation of the drug. LEEDER and OKEY (Chap. 6, this volume), discuss the combined influences of pharmacological idiosyncrasy and immunological dysfunction in several exemplary situations.

References

Alvarez F, Bernard O, Homberg JC, Kreibich G (1985) Anti-liver-kidney microsome antibody recognizes a 50000 molecular weight protein of the endoplasmic reticulum. J Exp Med 161:1231–1236

Beaune P, Dansette PM, Mansuy D et al. (1987) Human anti-endoplasmic reticulum autoantibodies appearing in a drug-induced hepatitis are directed against a human liver cytochrome P-450 that hydroxylates the drug. Proc Natl Acad Sci USA 84:551–555

Beisel KW, Ehrinpreis MN, Bhathal PS, Mackay IR, Rose NR (1984) Genetics of carbon tetrachloride-induced liver injury in mice. II. Multigenic regulation. Br J Exp Pathol 65:125–131

Berg PA, Schuff-Werner P, Henning H (1979) Immune reactions to drugs and metabolites in man. In: Eddleston ALWF, Weber JCP, Williams R (eds) Immune reactions in liver disease. Pitman Medical, Tunbridge Wells, pp 247–258

Bhathal PS, Rose NR, Mackay IR, Whittingham S (1983) Genetics of carbon tetrachloride liver injury in mice. I. Morphological and functional studies. Br J Exp Pathol 64:524–533

Bourdi M, Larrey D, Nataf J et al. (1990) Anti-liver endoplasmic reticulum autoantibodies are directed against human cytochrome P-4501A2. J Clin Invest 85:1967–1973

Braden GL, Warzynski MJ, Golightly M, Ballow M (1994) Cell-mediated immunity in allopurinal-indiced hypersensitivity. Clin Immunol Immunopathol 70:145–151
Codoner-Franch P, Paradis K, Gueguen M, Bernard O, Costesek AA, Alvarez F (1989) A new antigen recognized by anti-liver-kidney microsome antibody (LKMA). Clin Exp Immunol 75:354–358
Christ DD, Kenna JG, Kammerer W et al. (1988) Enflurane metabolism produces covalently-bound liver adducts recognized by antibodies from patients with halothane hepatitis. Anesthesiology 69:833–838
Cooksley WGE, Powell LW (1977) Erythromycin jaundice: diagnosis by an in vitro challenge test. Aust NZ J Med 7:291–293
Crivelli D, Lavarini C, Chiaberge E et al. (1983) Microsomal autoantibodies in chronic infection with HBsAg associated delta agent. Clin Exp Immunol 54:232–238
Del Prete G, Maggi E, Romagnani S (1994) Biology of disease. Human Th1 and Th2 cells: functional properties, mechanisms of regulation, and role in disease. Lab Invest 70:299–306
Druet P, Pelletier L, Rossert L, Druet E, Hirsch F, Sapin C (1989) Autoimmune reactions induced by metals. In: Kammuller ME, Bloksma N, Seinen W (eds) Autoimmunity and toxicology: immune dysregulation induced by drugs and chemicals. Elsevier, Amsterdam, pp 347–362
Dubey C, Bellon B, Hirsch F, Kuhn J, Vial MC, Goldman M, Druet P (1991) Increased expression of class II major histocompatibility complex molecules on B cells in rats susceptible or resistant to $HgCl_2$-induced autoimmunity. Clin Exp Immunol 86:118–123
Emery P, Panayi GS (1989) Autoimmune reactions to d-penicillamine. In: Kammuller ME, Bloksma N, Seinen W (eds) Autoimmunity and toxicology: immune dysregulation induced by drugs and chemicals. Elsevier, Amsterdam, pp 167–182
Erlanger BF, Cleveland WL, Wassermann N et al. (1986) The auto-anti-idiotypic route to antireceptor antibodies. Ann NY Acad Sci 475:219–226
Fusconi M, Lenzi M, Ballardini G et al. (1990) Anti-HCV testing in autoimmune hepatitis and primary biliary cirrhosis. Lancet 336:823 (letter)
Gennis MA, Vemuri R, Burns EA, Hill JV, Miller MA, Spielberg SP (1991) Familial occurrences of hypersensitivity to phenytoin. Am J Med 91:631–634
Gerken G, Manns M, Ramadori G, Poralla T, Dienes HP, Meyer zum Büschenfelde K-H (1987) Liver membrane autoantibodies in chronic active hepatitis: studies on mechanically and enzymatically isolated rabbit hepatocytes. J Hepatol 5:65–74
Gershon RK (1974) T cell control of antibody production. Contemp Top Immunol 3:1–40
Goldman M, Druet P, Glechmann E (1991) Th2 cells in systemic autoimmunity: insights from allogeneic diseases and chemically-induced autoimmunity. Immunol Today 12:223–227
Gomez J-L, Duport A, Conan L, Tremblay M, Suburu R, Lemay M, Labrie F (1992) Incidence of liver toxicity with the use of flutamide in prostate cancer patients. Am J Med 92:465–470
Gonzales FJ, Skoda RC, Kimura S et al. (1988) Characterization of the common genetic defect in humans deficient in debrisoquine metabolism. Nature 331:442–446
Goter Robinson CJ, Balazs T, Egorov IK (1986) Mercuric chloride-, gold sodium thiomalate- and D-penicillamine-induced antinuclear antibodies in mice. Toxicol Appl Pharmacol 86:159–169
Gueguen M, Meunier-Rotival M, Bernard O, Alvarez F (1988) Anti-liver kidney microsome antibody type I recognizes cytochrome P450 from the IID subfamily. J Exp Med 168:801–806
Hess E (1988) Drug-related lupus. N Engl J Med 318:1460–1462
Hoft RH, Bunker JP, Goodman HI (1981) Halothane hepatitis in three pairs of closely related women. N Engl J Med 304:1023–1024
Hollingsworth PN, Thomas R, Dawkins RL (1992) Autoimmune diseases of muscle. In: Rose NR, Mackay IR (eds) The autoimmune diseases II. Academic, Orlando, pp 317–343

Homberg JC, Abuaf N, Helmy-Khalil S et al. (1985) Drug induced hepatitis associated with anti-cytoplasmic auto-antibodies. Hepatology 5:722–727

Homberg JC, Abuaf N, Bernard O et al. (1987) Chronic active hepatitis associated with anti-liver/kidney microsome antibody type I: a second type of "autoimmune" hepatitis. Hepatology 7:1333–1339

Houwerzijl J, DeGast GC, Nater JP, Esselink MT, Nieweg HO (1977) Lymphocyte stimulation tests and patch tests in carbamazepine hypersensitivity. Clin Exp Immunol 29:272–277

Hubbard AK, Roth TP, Schuman S, Gandolfi AJ (1989) Localization of halothane-induced antigen *in situ* by specific anti-halothane metabolite antibodies. Clin Exp Immunol 76:422–427

Iwarson S, Lindberg J, Lunden P (1979) Nitrofurantoin-induced chronic liver disease. Clinical course and outcome of five cases. Scand J Gastroenterol 14:497–502

Jakoby WB (1994) Detoxification: conjugation and hydrolysis. In: Arias IM, Boyer JL, Fausto N, Jakoby WB, Schachter D, Shafritz DA (eds) The liver: biology and pathobiology, 3rd edn. Raven, New York, pp 429–442

Jiang X, Khursigara G, Rubin RL (1994) Transformation of lupus-inducing drugs to cytotoxic products by activated neutrophils. Science 266:810–813

Kenna JG, Neuberger J, Williams R (1984) An enzyme linked immunosorbent assay for detection of antibodies against halothane altered hepatocyte antigens. J Immunol Methods 75:3–14

Kenna JG, Neuberger JM, Williams R (1987) Identification by immunoblotting of three halothane induced liver microsomal antigens recognized by antibodies in sera from patients with halothane hepatitis. J Pharmacol Exp Ther 242:733–740

Kenna JG, Neuberger J, Williams R (1988a) Evidence for expression in human liver of halothane induced neoantigens recognized by antibodies in sera from patients with halothane hepatitis. Hepatology 8:1635–1641

Kenna JG, Satoh H, Christ DD, Pohl LR (1988b) Metabolic basis for a drug hypersensitivity: antibodies in sera from patients with halothane hepatitis recognize liver neoantigens that contain the trifluoroacetyl group derived from halothane. J Pharmacol Exp Ther 245:1103–1109

King PD, Blitzer BL (1990) Drug-induced cholestasis: pathogenesis and clinical features. Semin Liver Dis 10:316–321

Klatskin G, Kantor FS (1972) Mitochondrial antibody in primary biliary cirrhosis and other diseases. Ann Intern Med 77:533–541

Koop DR, Tierney DJ (1990) Multiple mechanisms in the regulation of ethanol-inducible cytochrome P450IIE1. Bioassays 12:429–435

Kyriatsoulis A, Manns M, Gerken G et al. (1987) Distinction between natural and pathological autoantibodies by immunoblotting and densitometric subtraction: liver-kidney microsomal antibody (LKM) positive sera identify multiple antigens in human liver tissue. Clin Exp Immunol 70:53–60

Larrey D, Vial T, Micaleff A, Babany G, Morichan Beauchant M, Michel H, Benhamou JP (1992) Hepatitis associated with amoxycillin-clavulanic acid combination. Report of 15 cases. Gut 33:368–371

Lenzi M, Bianchi FB, Cassani F, Pisi E (1984) Liver cell surface expression of the antigen reacting with liver-kidney microsomal antibody (LKM). Clin Exp Immunol 55:36–40

Lindberg J, Lindholm A, Lundin P, Iwarson S (1975) Trigger factors and HL-A antigens in chronic active hepatitis. Br Med J 4:77–79

Lindner H, du Bosque G, Dammermann R, Klöppel G, Krause D (1975) Phenolisatin-induzierte Lebererkrankungen. Sicherung der Pathogenese durch Reexposition und Langzeitbeobachtung bei 14 Patientinnen. Dtsch Med Wochenschr 100:2530–2535

Loeper J, Descatoire V, Amouyal G, Letteron P, Larrey D, Pessayre D (1989) Presence of covalently bound metabolites on rat hepatocyte plasma membrane proteins after administration of isaxonine, a drug leading to immunoallergic hepatitis in man. Hepatology 9:675–678

Mackay IR (1988) The idiotype network: implications for autoimmunity, infections, cancer, aging and vaccines. In: Arias IM, Jakoby WB, Popper H, Schachter D, Shafritz DA (eds) The liver: biology and pathobiology, 2nd edn. Raven, New York, pp 1259–1268
Mackay CR (1993) Immunological memory. Adv Immunol 53:217–265
Mackay IR (1994) The immunological mediation of drug reactions affecting the liver. In: Farrell GC (ed) Drug-induced liver disease. Churchill Livingstone, Edinburgh, pp 61–81
Mackay IR (1994) Contemporary concepts of immunological function. Alcohol Alcohol, Suppl 2, pp 413–423
Maddrey WC, Boitnott JK (1991) Drug-induced chronic active hepatitis. In: Krawitt EL, Wiesner RH (eds) Autoimmune liver diseases. Raven, New York, pp 219–232
Manns M, Kyriatsoulis A, Amelized Z et al. (1988) Relationship between the target antigen of liver-kidney microsomal (LKM) autoantibodies and rat isoenzymes of cytochrome P450. J Clin Lab Anal 2:245–248
Manns M, Johnson EF , Griffin ICJ, Tan EM, Sullivan KKF (1989) The major antigen of liver kidney microsomal autoantibodies in idiopathic autoimmune hepatitis is cytochrome P450 dbl. J Clin Invest 83:1066–1072
Manns M, Griffin KJ, Quattrochi LC, Sacher M, Thaler H, Tukey RH, Johnson EF (1990a) Identification of cytochrome P450 1A2 as a human autoantigen. Arch Biochem Biophys 280:229–232
Manns M, Zanger U, Gerken G, Sullivan KF, Meyer zum Büschenfelde K-H, Meyer UA, Eichelbaum M (1990b) Patients with autoimmune hepatitis type II express functionally intact cytochrome P450 db1 which is inhibited by LKM-1 autoantibodies in vitro but not in vivo. Hepatology 12:127–132
Manns MP, Griffin KD, Sullivan KF, Johnson EF (1991) LKM-1 autoantibodies recognize a short linear sequence in P450IID6, a cytochrome P-450 monooxygenase. J Clin Invest 88:1370–1378
Martin JL, Kenna G, Pohl LR (1990) Antibody assays for the detection of patients sensitized to halothane. Anaesth Analg 70:145–149
Martin JL, Kenna JG, Martin BM, Thomassen D, Reen GF, Pohl LR (1993) Halothane hepatitis patients have serum antibodies that react with protein disulfide isomerase. Hepatology 18:858–863
McMaster KR, Hennigar GR (1981) Drug-induced granutomatous hepatitis. Lab Invest 44:61–73
Mieli-Vergani G, Vergani D, Tredger J et al. (1980) Lymphocyte cytotoxicity to halothane altered hepatocytes in patients with severe hepatic necrosis following halothane anaesthesia. J Lab Clin Med 4:49–51
Mosmann TR, Coffman RL (1989) TH1 and TH2 cells: different patterns of lymphokine secretion lead to different functional properties. Annu Rev Immunol 7:145–173
Moult PJA, Sherlock S (1975) Halothane-related hepatitis. A clinical study of twenty-six cases. Q J Med 44:99–114
Mouradpour D, Altorfer J, Flury R, Greminger P, Meyenberger C, Jost R (1994) Chlorpromazinc-induced vanishing bile duct syndrome leading to biliary cirrhosis. Hepatology 20:1437–1441
National Halothane Study (1966) Summary of the national halothane study: possible association between halothane anaesthesia and post-operative hepatic necrosis. J Am Med Assoc 197:123–134
Neuberger J, Kenna JG (1987) Halothane hepatitis: a model of immune mediated drug hepatotoxicity. Clin Sci 72:263–270
Paronetto F, Popper H (1970) Lymphocyte stimulation induced by halothane in patients with hepatitis following exposure to antigen. N Engl J Med 283:2–280
Perry HM Jr, Tan EM, Carmody S, Sakamoto A (1970) Relationship of acetyl transferase activity to antinuclear antibodies and toxic symptoms in hypersensitive patients treated with hydralazine. J Lab Clin Med 76:114–125

Phillipp T, Durrazzo M, Trautwein C, Alex B, Straub P, Lamb JG, Johnson EF, Tukey RH, Manns MP (1994) Regulation of uridine diphosphate glucuronosyl transferases by LKM-3 antibodies in chronic hepatitis D. Lancet 344:578–581

Phillips MJ, Powell A, Patterson J, Valencia P (1987) Drug and toxic effects. In: The liver: an atlas and text of ultrastructural pathology. Raven, New York, pp 159–238

Pohl LR (1990) Drug-induced allergic hepatitis. Semin Liver Dis 10:305–315

Pohl LR, Kenna JG, Satoh H, Christ DD, Martin JL (1989) Neoantigens associated with halothane hepatitis. Drug Metabol Rev 20:206–207

Ray DC, Drummond GB (1991) Halothane hepatitis. Br J Anaesth 67:84–89

Reynolds TB, Peters RL, Yamada S (1971) Chronic active and lupoid hepatitis caused by a laxative, oxyphenisatin. N Engl J Med 280:813–820

Riley RJ, Leeder JS (1995) In vitro analysis of metabolic predisposition to drug hypersensitivity reactions. Clin Exper Immunol 99:1–6

Rizzetto M, Swana G, Doniach D (1973) Microsomal antibodies in active chronic hepatitis and other disorders. Clin Exp Immunol 15:3331–3344

Rose NR, Mackay IR (1992) The immune response in autoimmunity and autoimmune disease. In: Rose NR, Mackay IR (eds) The autoimmune diseases II. Academic, Orlando, pp 1–26

Rotmensch HH, Roth A, Liron M, Rubenstein A, Gefel A (1980) Lymphocyte sensitization in nifedipin-induced hepatitis. Br Med J 281:976–977

Rubin RL (1989) Autoimmune reactions induced by procainamide and hydralazine. In: Kammuller ME, Bloksma N, Seinen W (eds) Autoimmunity and toxicology: immune dysreglation induced by drugs and chemicals. Elsevier, Amsterdam, pp 119–150

Rubin RL, Tan E (1992) B-cell epitopes in natural and induced autoimmunity. In: Rose NR, Mackay IR (eds) The autoimmune diseases II. Academic, Orlando, pp 173–212

Sacher M, Blumel P, Thaler H, Manns M (1990) Chronic active hepatitis associated with vitiligo, nail dystrophy, alopecia and a new variant of LKM antibodies. J Hepatol 10:364–369

Salama A, Göttsche B, Mueller-Eckhardt C (1991) Autoantibodies and drug- or metabolite-dependent antibodies in patients with diclofenac-induced immune haemolysis. Br J Haematol 77:546–549

Satoh H, Gillette JR, Davies HW, Schulick RD, Pohl LR (1985) Immunochemical evidence of trifluoroacetylated cytochrome P450 in the liver of halothane-treated rats. Mol Pharmacol 28:468–474

Satoh H, Martin BM, Schulick AH, Christ DD, Kenna SG, Pohl LR (1989) Human anti-endoplasmic reticulum antibodies in sera of halothane hepatitis patients are directed against a trifluoroacetylated carboxylesterase. Proc Natl Acad Sci USA 86:322–326

Shear NH, Spielberg SP (1988) Anticonvulsant hypersensitivity syndrome. In vitro assessment of risk. J Clin Invest 82:1826–1832

Smith GCM, Kenna JG, Harrison DJ, Tew D, Wolf CR (1993) Autoantibodies to hepatic microsomal carboxylesterase in halothane hepatitis. Lancet 342:963–964

Stricker BHCh, Blok APR, Claas FHJ et al. (1988) Hepatic injury associated with the use of nitrofurans: a clinicopathological study. Hepatology 8:599–606

Takorabet L, Ropers A, Raby C, Charreire J (1995) Phenothiazine induces de novo MHC class II antigen expression on thyroid epithelial cells. A new mechanism for drug-induced autoimmunity. J Immunol 154:3593–3602

Tsutsui H, Terano Y, Sakagami C, Hasegawa I, Mizoguchi Y, Morisawa S (1992) Drug-specific T cells derived from patients with drug-induced allergic hepatitis. J Immunol 149:706–716

Toghill PJ, Benton P, Brown RC, Matthews HL (1974) Methyldopa liver damage. Br Med J 3:545–548

Unanue E (1992) Cellular studies on antigen presentation by class II MHC molecules. Curr Biol 4:63–69

Vergani D, Eddleston A, Tsantoulas D et al. (1978) Sensitisation to halothane altered liver components in severe hepatic necrosis after halothane anaesthesia. Lancet I:801–803

Vergani D, Mieli-Vergani G, Alberti A, Neuberger J, Eddleston A, Davis M (1980) Antibodies to the surface of halothane altered rabbit hepatocytes in patients with severe halothane associated hepatitis. N Engl J Med 303:66–71

Victorino RMM, Maria VA (1985) Modifications of the lymphocyte transformation test in a case of drug-induced cholestatic hepatitis. Diagn Immunol 3:177–181

Victorino RM, Maria VA, Pinto LA (1992) Evidence for prostaglandin-producing suppressor cells in drug-induced liver injury and implications in the diagnosis of drug sensitization. Clin Exp Immunol 87:132–137

Walton B, Simpson BR, Strunin L, Doniach D, Perrin J, Appleyard AJ (1976) Unexplained hepatitis following halothane. Br Med J 1:1171–1176

Watkins BP (1990) Role of cytochromes P-450 in drug metabolism and hepatoxicity. Semin Liver Dis 10:235–250

Waxman DJ, Lapenson DP, Krishnan M, Bernard O, Kreibich G, Alvarez F (1988) Antibodies to liver/kidney microsome 1 in chronic active hepatitis recognize specific forms of hepatic cytochrome P450. Gastroenterology 95:1326–1331

Wong FS, Ryan J, Dabkowski P, Dudley FJ, Sewell RB, Smallwood RA (1991) Augmentin-induced jaundice. Med J Aust 154:698–701

Worrledge SM (1973) Immune drug-induced hemolytic anemia. Semin Hematol 10:327–333

Zanger UM, Hauri HP, Loeper J, Homberg J-C, Meyer UA (1988) Antibodies against human cytochrome P450 db1 in autoimmune hepatitis type II. Proc Natl Acad Sci USA 85:8256–8260

Zimmerman HJ, Lewis JH, Ishak KG, Maddrey WC (1984) Ticrynafen-associated hepatic injury. Analysis of 340 cases. Hepatology 4:315–323

CHAPTER 11

Hepatic Encephalopathy

A.S. Basile

A. Introduction

Hepatic encephalopathy (HE) is a complex neuropsychiatric syndrome characterized by global CNS dysfunction resulting in impaired consciousness and coma. The association of the syndrome with acute or chronic liver failure implicates a plethora of metabolic abnormalities and gut-derived toxins in its pathogenesis. Thus, it is difficult to ascribe the neurological and psychiatric manifestations of HE to the presence of a single agent or changes in a particular metabolic pathway. The manifestations of HE are determined by two principle components of the underlying liver disease: hepatocellular failure and systemic shunting of portal venous contents (Basile et al. 1991b). Significant portal venous shunting is often found in chronic liver disease. HE occurs most frequently in this setting, where it is a milder, more persistent and episodic variant of the syndrome. In contrast, fulminant hepatic failure (FHF) has no vascular component. HE associated with FHF shows an acute onset with delirium progressing to deep coma. While delirium and seizures are generally uncommon in HE, they may occur during the rapid evolution of HE due to FHF (Pappas 1986). Although some of the characteristics of HE associated with acute or chronic liver failure result from fundamental differences in the mechanism of pathogenesis, many findings regarding the pathogenesis and treatment of the syndrome are held in common. Finally, it is important to recognize that while many of the animal models of liver failure used in research emphasize one or the other component of liver failure, most clinical cases tend to have a mixture of both. Although a single, perfect animal model of this syndrome does not exist, the animal models in use have nonetheless provided valuable insights into the pathogenesis of HE and allowed for the testing of new therapeutic modalities.

I. Clinical Manifestations of Hepatic Encephalopathy

The clinical features of HE include a broad spectrum of fluctuating psychiatric and neurological abnormalities which are nonspecific and occur in other metabolic encephalopathies or sedative overdose. In general, the changes in neurological status reflect alterations in personality, cognition, consciousness and neuromuscular function which can be conveniently graded into four

Table 1. Clinical stages of hepatic encephalopathy

Stage	Mental state	Neuromuscular state
I	Mild confusion, euphoria, depression, decreased attention, slowed analytical ability, irritability, sleep inversion	Mild incoordination, impaired handwriting
II	Drowsiness, lethargy, gross deficits in analytical ability, obvious personality changes, inappropriate behavior, intermittent disorientation, low-frequency EEG abnormalities	Asterixis, ataxia, dysarthria, paratonia, apraxia
III	Somnolent but rousable, unable to perform analytical tasks, disorientation to time/place, amnesia, rage, slurred speech	Hyperreflexia, muscle rigidity, fasciculations, abnormal Babinski's sign, seizures (rare)
IV_a	Coma	Oculovestibular responses lost, response to painful stimuli lost
IV_b	Deep coma	Decerebrate postures, no response to painful stimuli

main stages for routine clinical assessment (Basile et al. 1991b; Conn 1993) (Table 1).

The earliest abnormalities in psychiatric and cognitive function associated with HE include personality changes, euphoria, irritability and apathy, which may not be readily detectable during a conventional clinical assessment (Gazzard et al. 1986). As the encephalopathy worsens, dysphasia and perseveration along with intellectual deterioration and disorientation are manifested, reflecting altered forebrain function and central information processing. Simple psychometric tests such as the subtraction of serial 7's, Mini Mental Status Examination, handwriting and the Reitan Trails test part A (Conn 1993) are useful in detecting and quantifying subtle defects in mental function in early stages (O-II) of HE.

A variety of neuromuscular abnormalities are also associated with HE. Decreased spontaneous movement and fixed stare often accompany the most characteristic neurological abnormality in HE: asterixis (liver flap or flapping tremor, Conn 1993). Asterixis differs from tremor in that it is: intermittent; of lower frequency; and bilaterally asynchronous. Other neurological disorders include exaggeration of deep tendon reflexes, muscle rigidity, sustained ankle clonus, fasciculations, ataxic gait, decerebrate postures and bizarre facial expressions. Deficits in consciousness are evidenced in HE, with hypersomnia an early manifestation of the syndrome. Hypersomnia can progress to inversion of sleep rhythm, then to a coma which resembles normal sleep (stage IV_a), but may advance to complete unresponsiveness to painful stimuli (stage IV_b). Progression from the early stages of HE to coma may occur over a period of hours, regardless of therapy or may cease and/or reverse at any stage.

Common precipitants of HE in patients with chronic liver disease include: protein loading (10%), azotemia (29%), GI hemorrhage (18%), electrolyte imbalances (11%), sedatives/analgesics (24%), constipation (3%) or infection (3%) (CONN 1993). When HE appears spontaneously (i.e., without obvious precipitants) in patients with decompensated cirrhosis, it is attributed to deteriorating hepatocellular function and the prognosis is grave. While proper management of precipitants is crucial for the clinician, an understanding of the mechanisms by which these factors precipitate HE would provide further insights into its pathogenesis and, ultimately, the development of new treatments for the syndrome.

II. Neuropathological Changes in Hepatic Encephalopathy

1. Anatomy

HE is considered a reversible metabolic encephalopathy, thereby excluding changes in neuronal morphology from the development of the syndrome. No significant changes in neuron structure in HE have been observed at the light or electron microscope levels (CONN 1993). In contrast, the development of Alzheimer type II astrocytes, characterized by large pale nuclei and nuclear inclusions, are a hallmark of patients succumbing from chronic liver disease with prolonged or recurrent episodes of coma (BASILE et al. 1991b). The mechanisms underlying the development of type II astrocytosis and its role in the pathogenesis of HE are discussed in Sect. B.I.1.

The gross anatomy of postmortem brains from patients with acute HE is normal, except for generalized edema in 50% of these patients (O'BRIEN et al. 1987). Patients with chronic, nonalcoholic liver disease may have cerebral edema and cortical atrophy despite not being overtly encephalopathic (BERNTHAL et al. 1987). These morphological abnormalities are associated with decreased performance on psychometric tests and correlate with the degree of liver dysfunction. Although it appears that liver failure itself mediates the CNS atrophy, the mechanisms responsible for these changes are unknown. Further, it is not clear that morphological as opposed to metabolic changes are directly involved in the pathogenesis of HE (BERNTHAL et al. 1987), as psychomotor deficits in subclinical HE can be reversed with standard therapies (MORGAN et al. 1989) despite brain atrophy.

The lack of significant alterations in neuron morphology, the presence of minor astrocytic changes in the early stages of HE and the clinical impression that this syndrome is potentially reversible are compatible with the concept of a metabolic encephalopathy.

2. Electrophysiology

The electroencephalographic (EEG) changes associated with this syndrome are not specific for HE. The EEG assessment indicates a generalized slowing, with initial suppression of the α rhythm (Conn 1993). An unstable, high-voltage α rhythm appears as the syndrome progresses, with paroxysmal, triphasic waves of 5–7 cps beginning bilaterally in the frontal and temporal regions and spreading posteriorly. Finally, the overall amplitude of the EEG decreases, and bilaterally synchronous 2- to 3-cps waves are found primarily over the frontal lobes. Global electrophysiological recording techniques such as the EEG are useful for monitoring HE, particularly when combined with frequency analysis (De Groot et al. 1985).

The recording of evoked responses has not been widely applied to humans with HE. While abnormal visual and somatosensory evoked responses (VER and SER) may occur in preclinical (latent) HE and are certainly observed in overt HE (Casellas et al. 1985), they do not correlate well with the clinical stage of HE in patients (Johansson et al. 1989) and suffer from considerable inter- and intraindividual variability in the amplitudes and latencies of the components of the evoked responses. Presently, evoked responses are most useful as research tools in animal models of HE, where individual variables can be minimized by rigid control over electrode placement. It is hoped that their future clinical application may become more widespread (Davies et al. 1990).

B. Involvement of Neurotoxins in the Pathogenesis of Hepatic Encephalopathy

Although HE is associated with hepatic failure, it is fundamentally a neuropsychiatric syndrome. This reflects the role of the CNS in translating metabolic imbalances and the presence of toxins into behavioral manifestations through altered neurotransmission. These alterations reflect changes in neuronal polarization, neurotransmitter metabolism, receptor sensitivity and basic oxidative metabolism in neurons and glia. Many of the substances or metabolic changes present in liver failure are innocuous by themselves and would not engender any pathologies in a normal individual. However, normal CNS function succumbs to the cumulative effects of these toxins in liver failure. Neurotoxic agents and metabolic alterations putatively involved in the pathogenesis of HE (Sherlock and Dooley 1993) are as follows:

1. Of colonic origin
2. Nitrogenous
3. Produced wholly or in part by intestinal bacteria
4. Present in portal venous blood
5. Metabolized by a normal liver
6. Able to enter the CNS
7. Able to alter CNS function
8. Occur in concentrations correlated with the severity of HE

Finally, toxic agents involved in the pathogenesis of HE should possess the general characteristics outlined in Table 2.

Table 2. Neuroactive agents implicated in the pathogenesis of hepatic encephalopathy

Direct	Indirect (via)
Ammonia	Ammonia (synergist, increases glutamine levels, inhibits oxidative metabolism)
GABA[a]	
Endogenous Benzodiazepines[a]	Tryptophan (alters serotonin turnover)
Fatty acids[b]	
Tryptophan[b]	Phenylalanine, tyrosine (enhances false neurotransmitter synthesis[b])
Mercaptans[b]	
Phenol[b]	

[a] While GABA and endogenous benzodiazepines can directly influence neuronal activity, their sources remain unclear.
[b] The role of these agents in the pathogenesis of HE is questionable due to a lack of evidence for their presence in the CNS or unphysiological toxic concentrations.

I. Ammonia

The principal nitrogenous toxin involved in the pathogenesis of HE is ammonia. Ammonia has direct and indirect neurotoxic properties, and while hyperammonemia is not equivalent to HE it is a major contributor to its development. The GI tract, particularly the colon, is a major source of blood ammonia, generated principally by the action of bacteria containing urea- or amino acid oxidases (CONN 1993). Ammonia is normally converted in the liver to urea by via the Krebs-Henseleit cycle. However, in liver failure ammonia metabolism shifts to skeletal muscle and brain where ammonia is coupled to glutamate, forming glutamine.

Clinical evidence of a role for ammonia in HE is based on the accumulation of ammonia in liver failure and its ability to enter the brain (CONN 1993). Studies of cirrhotics ingesting ammoniagenic compounds such as amino acids, urea or ammonia-releasing resins (GABUZDA et al. 1952) suggested an association between ammonia accumulation and encephalopathy. In addition, CSF levels of the ammonia metabolites glutamine and α-ketoglutaramate correlate well with the clinical severity of HE (VERGARA et al. 1974; OEI et al. 1979). Moreover, present therapies for HE (e.g., lactulose, lactitol and non-absorbable antibiotic administration, reduction of alimentary protein loads) decrease plasma ammonia levels by eliminating the colonic sources of ammonia production (CONN 1993). This is followed (after several hours or days) by the amelioration of HE.

Ammonia has manifold effects on the CNS, including changes in glial function, electrophysiology and oxidative metabolism.

1. Glial Interactions

Ammonia significantly alters glial morphology and function. Acute exposure to ammonia results in compensatory biochemical and morphological changes supporting ammonia detoxification. Norenberg (1977) indicated that pathological changes in astrocyte subcellular structure (hypertrophy of mitochondria and endoplasmic reticulum) occurred before the development of overt encephalopathy in animal models. Patients with chronic hyperammonemia due to congenital defects in urea cycle enzymes and rodents in hyperammonemic states develop Alzheimer type II astrocytosis (Cooper and Plum 1987), the nature of which is consistent with degenerative glial changes. Similar changes are observed in primary cultures of astrocytes exposed to 5–10 m*M* ammonia (Gregorios et al. 1985a,b). Exposing astrocytes to ammonia in vitro decreases levels of glutaminase, glutamic acid dehydrogenase, succinic dehydrogenase and glutamate, and increases glutamine synthetase, aspartate aminotransferase and glutamine (Subbalakshmi and Murthy 1983). However, the effects of ammonia on oxidative metabolism in astrocytes are unclear. Although no changes in the malate-aspartate shunt or in CO_2 production from either pyruvate or glucose are noted in astrocytes treated chronically with 3 m*M* ammonia in vitro (Fitzpatrick et al. 1988), other studies report decreased cellular ATP levels and glycogenolysis (Dombro et al. 1993).

These ammonia-induced changes in astrocyte morphology and metabolism may be relevant to the pathogenesis of HE. Ammonia causes significant decreases in the ability of cultured astrocytes to take up glutamate and GABA (Norenberg et al. 1985). These changes are also manifested in intact brain and brain slice preparations (Tossman et al. 1987; Butterworth et al. 1991; Wysmyk et al. 1992) (Table 3) from animal models of acute and chronic liver failure, and could contribute to the neurotransmitter alterations observed in HE. Hyperammonemia also causes astrocytic swelling, which may contribute to the cerebral edema observed in FHF and alterations in blood-brain barrier permeability (Norenberg et al. 1991).

2. Electrophysiological Changes

Electrophysiological and biochemical studies of single neurons and isolated synaptic networks have shown that ammonia inactivates Cl^- extrusion pumps. The resulting elevation of intracellular Cl^- impairs inhibitory postsynaptic potential (IPSP) formation (Raabe 1987), transiently increasing excitatory phenomena. This phenomenon could be involved in the production of seizures in hyperammonemic states (at blood concentrations of 1–1.7 m*M*, Iles and Jack 1980). At even higher concentrations (>2 m*M*), acute ammonia exposure suppresses excitatory synaptic transmission, causing presynaptic conduction blocks, interfering with excitatory neurotransmitter release and generally depressing neuronal electrical activity (Raabe 1987).

While the CSF concentrations of ammonia required to alter inhibitory neurotransmission (200–800 μM) are within the range commonly observed in congenital hyperammonemia (200–400 μM), they are generally higher than

Table 3. Brain levels of neurotransmitter amino acids and glutamine in hepatic encephalopathy

Sampling	Basal Glu	Stim Glu	Gln	Basal GABA	Stim GABA
Human, CLF					
1. Frontal cortex	↔		250%↑	↔	
Human, FHF					
2. Frontal cortex	61%↑			↔	
Rat, CCl_4					
3. Hippocampus (synaptosomes)					140%↑
Rat, PCS					
4. Whole brain	↔		160%↑	↔	
5. ECF	54%↑	23%↑	470%↑	↔	73%↑
Rat, PCS/HAL					
4. Whole brain	↔		230%↑	65%↑	
Rat, TAA					
6. Brain	35%↓			↔	
CSF	65%↑			95%↑	
7. Astrocytes					83%↑

CLF, chronic liver failure (cirrhosis); FHF, fulminant hepatic failure; CCl_4, carbon tetrachloride; PCS, portacaval shunt; HAL, hepatic artery ligation; TAA, thioacetamide; ECF, extracellular fluid; CSF, cerebrospinal fluid; stim, stimulated; 1, Lavoie et al. (1987); 2, Record et al. (1976); 3, Diaz-Munoz and Tapia (1988); 4, Mans et al. (1979); 5, Tossman et al. (1987); 6, Swain et al. (1992); 7, Albrecht and Rafalowska (1987).

the concentrations of ammonia observed in patients with subcomatose HE ($100\,\mu M$, Iles and Jack 1980). The correlation between plasma levels is even poorer. Furthermore, it is not clear if neurons throughout the brain are equally sensitive to ammonia inhibition of IPSP formation. Alger and Nicoll (1983) reported that ammonia did not selectively block IPSP formation in hippocampal pyramidal cells at concentrations below $2\,mM$. Indeed, ammonia may have minimal effect on IPSP formation in the cerebral cortex, where IPSPs terminate spontaneous neuronal activity rather than occurring independently at resting membrane potentials. IPSPs which terminate excitatory activity are not sensitive to the presence of ammonia (Raabe 1987). Finally, many of the changes in the EEG and VER induced by hyperammonemia are not characteristic of those observed in HE (Pappas et al. 1984; Jones et al. 1987). The electrophysiological effects of ammonia in normal animals or on preparations of normal neurons are quite different from the electrophysiological changes that occur in animal models of HE. Some animal models have normal IPSPs, despite chronically elevated plasma ammonia concentrations (Raabe and Onstad 1985). This may result from the development of Cl^- pump tolerance to the persistently increased levels of ammonia (Raabe 1987), although the change in activity of these pumps has never been confirmed by direct measurement. The recent observation that ammonia at concentrations of less than $1\,mM$ enhances GABA-gated Cl^- currents in cortical neurons

(TAKAHASHI et al. 1993) suggests that there is a continuum of electrophysiological effects of ammonia, with an enhancement of inhibitory neurotransmission at low concentrations (consistent with the lethargy observed in the early stages of HE), followed by disinhibition at higher (0.75–1.5 m*M*) concentrations. This phenomenon may underlie the development of seizures in patients with FHF, who display a rapid increase in ammonia levels in the absence of ammonia "tolerance." Although complete suppression of electrical activity could occur at the highest ammonia concentrations (>2 m*M*), these levels are not found in patients suffering strictly from liver failure.

3. Changes in Oxidative Metabolism

Hyperammonemia is also involved in alterations of cerebral energy metabolism, although the precise nature of the metabolic changes is unclear. Oxygen consumption is decreased in animals with portacaval shunts (HINDFELT et al. 1977; NIETO et al. 1980), and cerebral glucose consumption is reduced at plasma ammonia levels of 1 m*M* (JESSY et al. 1991). The latter change is correlated with CNS glutamine concentrations (JESSY et al. 1991), suggesting that the metabolic consequences of hyperammonemia may be related to elevated levels of glutamine, a hypothesis supported by the observation that suppression of glutamine synthesis ameliorates some of the cerebral metabolic abnormalities observed in hyperammonemia (HAWKINS and JESSY 1991; HAWKINS et al. 1993).

Since many of these metabolic changes are also observed in patients with liver failure but without encephalopathy, their contribution to HE is unclear (PLUM and HINDFELT 1976). While significant decreases in cerebral blood flow and oxygen metabolism are observed in hyperammonemic animals (GJEDDE et al. 1978), at least one study reports increased brain glucose metabolism (LOCKWOOD et al. 1986). Moreover, the issue has been raised whether changes in cerebral energy status are the result rather than the cause of ammonia-induced encephalopathy (CROSSLEY et al. 1983).

4. Summary

While a significant body of information indicates that elevations in brain and plasma levels of ammonia occur in liver failure, and that ammonia modulates neuronal function, evidence that hyperammonemia is *solely* responsible for the development of HE is lacking. This conclusion is based on the following observations:

1. There is a poor correlation between plasma ammonia levels and the severity of HE. Normal or near normal concentrations of arterial ammonia are found in patients with coma (SHERLOCK 1958) while arterial ammonia levels are increased in many patients with chronic liver disease without signs of overt encephalopathy.

2. Progressive, acute ammonia intoxication is characterized by a preconvulsive, lethargic state, seizures and postictal coma (ILES and JACK 1980). While seizures are common in congenital hyperammonemia syndromes (FLANNERY et al. 1982), they are relatively rare in acute liver failure (PAPPAS 1986) and higly unusual in patients with chronic liver failure.
3. EEG alterations in patients with chronic liver failure administered ammonium acetate were not typical of HE (COHN and CASTELL 1966).
4. Hemodialysis of patients in hepatic coma due to acute or chronic liver failure yields inconsistent results. Although significant reductions in plasma ammonia levels are achieved using a variety of dialysis techniques (OPOLON 1980), enhancement of neurological function occurs in less than 50% of the patients so treated.
5. Many of the neurotoxic effects of ammonia occur at concentrations substantially higher than observed in humans with HE (ILES and JACK 1980).
6. Finally, the nature of ammonia intoxication does not reproduce the subtle changes in personality and mentation, and the sleep inversion that are significant components of HE due to chronic liver failure.

II. Synergistic Neurotoxins

Plasma concentrations of free fatty acids (ZIEVE 1985), mercaptans (methanethiol and dimethylsulfide) and phenol (ZIEVE and BRUNNER 1985) are increased by an average of 150%–400% in patients with acute and chronic liver disease. These compounds are directly neuro- and gliatoxic (NORENBERG and NORENBERG 1986), and their comagenic potency is synergistically enhanced by ammonia (ZIEVE and BRUNNER 1985).

Despite their direct neurotoxicity, the toxic concentrations of these substances are 4–15 times higher than levels observed in patients with liver failure (ZIEVE et al. 1984). Furthermore, mercaptans cause abnormalities in VER and behavior (with the evocation of seizures) that bear no resemblence to those recorded in animals with HE (PAPPAS et al. 1984; JONES et al. 1987). In many cases, brain or plasma levels of these substances do not correlate with the severity of HE (BLOM et al. 1991). Finally, there is some concern that the techniques used initially to measure plasma mercaptan levels may artifactually generate mercaptans via methionine degradation (TANGERMAN et al. 1985).

While the neuropsychiatric manifestations of HE may result from the synergistic interactions of multiple metabolic abnormalities (including agents other than mercaptans, fatty acids, phenols and ammonia), the relevance of the comagenic potential (the penultimate result of organ system failure) of these "synergistic neurotoxins" to the spectrum of neurological changes characteristic of HE is nil.

C. Neurotransmitter Involvement in the Pathogenesis of Hepatic Encephalophathy

I. γ-Aminobutyric Acid

One of the fundamental characteristics of HE is global CNS depression. Thus, it is logical that enhanced function of inhibitory neurotransmitter systems may play a role in HE. SCHAFER and JONES (1982) postulated that plasma levels of gut-derived GABA would increase in liver failure. GABA would then enter the CNS through a permeabilized blood-brain barrier, enhancing GABAergic neurotransmission and inhibiting neuronal function. Since this initial postulate much effort, employing electrophysiological, neurochemical and behavioral techniques, has been expended in testing this hypothesis and determining the precise role of GABAergic neurotransmission in the pathogenesis of HE.

1. Electrophysiology

Electrophysiological evidence for the involvement of GABAergic neurotransmission in the pathogenesis of HE was initially provided by measurements of VERs in animal models. The development of HE in animal models of FHF was associated with alterations in the VER pattern similar to those observed following the administration of encephalopathic doses of barbiturates, diazepam or muscimol (SCHAFER et al. 1984; BASILE et al. 1991b). These changes were normalized by the administration of bicuculline, isopropylbicyclo phosphorothionate and flumazenil, concurrent with ameliorations of the neurological manifestations of HE (GAMMAL et al. 1990; BASILE et al. 1991b). Comparable results were obtaîned by recording the activity of single neurons from rabbits with HE. These Purkinje neurons were three to five times more sensitive to inhibition by $GABA_A$ receptor-selective depressants than neurons from control animals (BASILE et al. 1988). The hypersensitivity to depressants observed in this animal model of HE appeared to result from the presence of endogenous benzodiazepine receptor agonists.

2. Neurochemistry and Pharmacology

Complementary neurochemical investigations have provided mixed support for the role of GABAergic systems in HE. While initial radioligand-binding studies of the $GABA_A$-benzodiazepine receptor complex in HE indicated an increase in receptor density in several animal models of HE (SCHAFER et al. 1983) and in humans with cirrhosis (FERENCI et al. 1988), more recent investigations have failed to confirm that the density of either GABA or benzodiazepine receptors is altered in HE (BASILE et al. 1989, 1991b). It is now believed that this apparent increase in $GABA_A$ receptor density resulted from the tissue preparation technique (ROSSLE et al. 1989), suggesting that an agent is present in liver failure (e.g., a benzodiazepine receptor agonist) which alters the physicochemical properties of the receptor such that a greater density of $GABA_A$ receptor remains in the membrane. While an increased density of $GABA_A$ receptors would be unusual in the face of increased CNS GABA levels, one would not necessarily expect a compensatory decrease to occur either. Unlike catecholamine or opiate receptor subtypes, the density of $GABA_A$-benzodiazepine receptors is decreased only in the presence of high levels of agonists for periods of time (several weeks, MILLER et al. 1988) that are usually longer than the lifetime of many animal models of HE. Thus, the cumulative evidence indicates that the density of the $GABA_A$ receptor complex is unchanged in HE.

An alternative mechanism by which GABAergic neurotransmission could be enhanced in HE involves increased CNS GABA concentrations. Enteric bacteria, the gut wall or the liver itself release GABA into the plasma, where its concentrations increase as a result of impaired hepatic extraction (SCHAFER et al. 1980; SCHAFER and JONES 1982). GABA then enters the CNS along its concentration gradient by crossing a permeabilized blood-brain barrier. While early reports indicated that plasma levels of GABA or taurine were elevated in animals with liver failure several hours before the onset of overt HE (SCHAFER et al. 1980; BASILE et al. 1991b) and in patients with HE due to acute or chronic liver failure (MINUK et al. 1985), plasma GABA levels are not uniformly elevated (MADDISON et al. 1986), and when increased do not always correlate with the severity of encephalopathy (LOSCHER et al. 1991). Furthermore, the increases in blood-brain barrier permeability observed in acute liver failure (HOROWITZ et al. 1983) which lead to increased permeability of GABA-like substances (BASSETT et al. 1990) may be model-and compound-specific (ZENEROLI et al. 1982), and often do not occur until the end stages of liver disease.

Nonetheless, synaptic GABA concentrations may be elevated in HE through other mechanisms within the CNS. These include decreased GABA catabolism due to inhibition of GABA-transaminase activity (FERENCI et al. 1984a), or activation of arginine conversion to GABA (ALBRECHT et al. 1990), although basal CNS GABA levels are either unchanged or increased in humans who died of liver failure (RECORD et al. 1976) or animal models of liver failure (ZIMMERMANN et al. 1989; BUTTERWORTH and GIGUERE 1986) (Table 3). In contrast, increased release of GABA has been observed from glia, brain slices and intact brain of two animal models of HE (ALBRECHT and RAFALOWSKA 1987; TOSSMAN et al. 1987; WYSMYK et al. 1992). This may result from decreased rates of glial reuptake (NORENBERG et al. 1985), or the loss of negative feedback regulation of GABA release resulting from the loss of presynaptic $GABA_B$ receptors (OJA et al. 1993).

Other humoral factors can act to enhance GABAergic neurotransmission. As previously noted, ammonia (<1 mM) increases GABA-gated Cl^- currents (TAKAHASHI et al. 1993). Recently, the presence of benzodiazepine receptor ligands with agonist properties in peripheral tissues, body fluids and brains of animal models of FHF and humans with HE (MULLEN et al. 1986, 1990; BASILE et al. 1989, 1991a,b) has been reported. The brain and plasma levels of these agonists correlate with the severity of HE (MULLEN et al. 1990; YURDAYDIN et al. 1993; BASILE et al. 1994), and occur in concentrations sufficient to occupy ≈30% of the benzodiazepine receptors, further enhancing GABAergic neurotransmission (BASILE et al. 1990). The presence of benzodiazepine receptor agonists in HE was suggested by the ability of benzodiazepine receptor antagonists (such as flumazenil and Ro 14-7437) to improve the behavioral and electrophysiological manifestations of HE in animal models of FHF and patients with HE (BASILE et al. 1988, 1991b; GAMMAL et al. 1990; SCOLLO-LAVIZZARI and STEINMANN 1985). While the chemical structure and absolute concentrations of these agents have yet to be fully determined, they may play a unique role not only in the pathogenesis of HE but in other neuropsychiatric disorders, such as idiopathic recurrent stupor (ROTHSTEIN et al. 1992), anxiety and seizure disorders.

3. Behavior

Finally, a substantial body of behavioral information suggests that GABAergic neurotransmission is enhanced in HE. The seizure threshold to bicuculline or 3-mercaptopropionic acid is increased in two animal models of HE due to FHF (BASILE et al. 1991b). Since both bicuculline and 3-mercaptopropionic acid induce seizures by reducing GABAergic tone, these findings are consistent with the presence of increased GABAergic neurotransmission in HE. Benzodiazepine receptor antagonists such as flumazenil, Ro 15-4513, Ro 15-3505 and CGS-8216 improve some of the behavioral manifestations of HE in animal models (GAMMAL et al. 1990; YURDAYDIN et al. 1993) at doses that display little or no intrinsic activity. It should be noted that benzodiazepine receptor antagonists are not universally effective in reversing the behavioral effects of HE in animal models or man (STEINDL and FERENCI 1990; BASILE et al. 1991b; POMIER-LAYRARGUES et al. 1994) and, when they do, the effects of single doses are transient (GAMMAL et al. 1990; YURDAYDIN et al. 1993). Nonetheless, their selectivity for the benzodiazepine receptor and the rapidity of their effectiveness (within 5 min after administration) are consistent with their ability to displace endogenous agonists from the benzodiazepine receptor.

4. Summary

Interdisciplinary studies provide strong evidence for a functional increase in GABAergic neurotransmission in patients with HE and in animal models. Presently, the mechanistic details of this involvement remain unclear.

1. VER and single neuron electrophysiology indicates that GABAergic neurotransmission is enhanced in HE.
2. No consistent changes in $GABA_A$ receptors are found in HE using well-washed tissue preparations.

3. The enhancement of GABAergic neurotransmission may result from increased levels of GABA and/or benzodiazepine receptor agonists in the synapse. The source of these agonists remains unclear, but in the case of GABA, may result from decreased rates of glial reuptake.
4. Behavioral evidence and controlled clinical trials of benzodiazepine receptor antagonists suggest that endogenous benzodiazepine receptor ligands may be involved in the pathogenesis of HE.

II. Excitatory Amino Acids

An alternative explanation for the CNS depression present in HE entails a decrease in the activity of excitatory neurotransmitter pathways. As glutamate is the primary excitatory neurotransmitter in the mammalian CNS, this system is the logical focus of studies of the role of impaired excitatory neurotransmission in HE. Detoxification of ammonia in the CNS by coupling to glutamate increases glutamine while depleting glutamate levels (Cooper and Plum 1987). Thus, alterations in glutamate neurotransmission would occur secondarily to ammonia intoxication. This hypothesis was supported by reports of decreased glutamine synthetase and glutaminase activity in animal models and in necropsy samples from cirrhotic humans (Hertz et al. 1987; Lavoie et al. 1987). Consistent with the reduction of enzyme activity, glutamate and aspartate levels are decreased in whole brain, brain regions or CSF in animals (Butterworth and Giguere 1986; Swain et al. 1992) and in patients that died in hepatic coma (Record et al. 1976; Lavoie et al. 1987) (Table 3). While these studies of total CNS glutamate concentrations were unable to distinguish between neurotransmitter and metabolic glutamate pools, subsequent investigations reported increased levels of free glutamate in human CSF (Therrien and Butterworth 1991) and in animal models of HE (Tossman et al. 1987). This probably results from ammonia-induced decreases in astrocytic reuptake of glutamate (Norenberg et al. 1985; Butterworth et al. 1989), as opposed to increased neurotransmitter release.

If free glutamate levels are chronically elevated in liver failure, compensatory decreases in the density or affinity of glutamate receptors might result. Initial observations supported this proposal, with small to moderate decreases in the density of [^{3}H]glutamate binding to selected brain regions from rabbits with HE due to FHF (Ferenci et al. 1984a) (Table 4). This study did not discriminate between glutamate receptor subtypes, and could reflect interactions of [^{3}H]glutamate with transporters and enzymes. Unfortunately, the results of more recent investigations have not unequivocally determined which glutamate receptor subtypes are altered in animal models of liver failure. The density of [^{3}H]glutamate binding to the NMDA receptor subtype was moderately decreased in one study with no changes in AMPA or kainate receptor subtypes (Peterson et al. 1990), while studies of other animal models indicated no change in the density of NMDA receptors, but significant decreases

Table 4. Changes in the density of glutamate receptors in hepatic encephalopathy

Subject	Radioligand	Brain region	Density change
1. Rabbit	[^{3}H]Glutamate	Cortex	↔
GalN		Hippocampus	39%↓
		Cerebellum	22%↓
	[^{3}H]Kainate	Cortex	33%↓
2. Rat	[^{3}H]Glutamate	Brain	10%–39%↓
PCS	[^{3}H]Kainate		↔
	[^{3}H]AMPA		↔
3. Rabbit	[^{3}H]MK-801	Cortex	↔
HDV		Hippocampus	↔
		Striatum	↔
4. Dog	[^{3}H]Glutamate	Cortex	↔
PCE	[^{3}H]MK-801		↔
	[^{3}H]Kainate		37%↓
	[^{3}H]AMPA		100%↓

No changes in radioligand affinity for glutamate receptor subtypes were observed in any study. GalN, galactosamine; PCS, portacaval shunt; HDV, hepatic devascularization; PCE, encephalopathy associated with congenital protacaval shunt; AMPA, amino-3-hydroxy-5-methyl-4-isoxazolepropionic acid. MK801, (+)-5-methyl-10,11-di-hydro-5H-dibenzo[*a*,*d*]cyclohepten-5,10-imine maleate; 1, Ferenci et al. (1984a,b); 2, Peterson et al. (1990); 3, deKnegt et al. (1993); 4, Maddison et al. (1991).

in the density of kainate and AMPA receptors (Maddison et al. 1991; deKnegt et al. 1993). While the absence of change in the densities of glutamate receptor subtypes does not preclude the involvement of glutamatergic neurotransmitter systems in the pathogenesis of HE, it is clear that more work must be done to clarify the nature of the changes in glutamate receptor dynamics in liver failure.

Finally, glutamate is not the only excitatory glutamatergic agent that could be involved in the pathogenesis of HE. Quinolinic acid is derived from tryptophan and can be synthesized by the liver or macrophages. In view of the elevated levels of tryptophan observed in liver failure (Table 5), it was hypothesized the quinolinic acid synthesis could be enhanced, increasing excitatory neurotransmission or causing excitotoxicity. Early reports indicated that quinolinic acid is elevated in the brains of patients with HE and animal models of hyperammonemia (Moroni et al. 1986a,b). Subsequent studies indicate that CNS quinolinic acid levels are only elevated in animal models and patients in stage IV of HE due to FHF (Basile et al. 1995a,b). The increase in CNS quinolinic acid levels may result from increased blood-brain permeability to peripherally produced quinolinic acid in the end stages of acute liver failure, as it is not observed in patients who died from chronic liver failure. Moreover, the absolute levels of quinolinic acid observed in liver failure are far below those necessary to cause neurotoxicity, although they may enhance excitatory neurotransmission in the end stages of liver failure and promote seizure development.

Table 5. Representative brain levels of aromatic amino acids in hepatic encephalopathy

Subject	Tyrosine	Tryptophan	Phenylalanine
1. Human, FHF	670%↑	275%↑	700%↑
2. Human, CLF	71%↑	–	130%↑
3. Rat, PCS	320%↑	75%↑	980%↑

FHF, fulminant hepatic failure; CLF, chronic liver failure (cirrhosis); PCS, portacaval shunt; –, not determined. Amino acid levels measured in frontal cortex of human subjects with FHF or CLF, and in whole brain of rats with PCS. 1, RECORD et al. (1976); 2, BERGERON et al. (1989a); 3, MANS et al. (1979).

A pathogenic mechanism for HE invoking a reduction in excitatory neurotransmitter function would be consistent with some of the early manifestations of HE. While basal glutamate levels in the brain are decreased in liver failure, these may reflect changes in metabolic, as opposed to neurotransmitter, pools of glutamate. Indeed, the efficacy of glutamatergic neurotransmission may be maintained or increased as a result of decreased glial uptake and normal receptor density. Additional investigations are needed to solve this apparent paradox and to determine what role, if any, excitatory neurotransmitters play in the development of HE.

III. Aromatic Amino Acids and Monoamine Neurotransmitters

A hallmark of liver failure is the increased ratio of the aromatic amino acids (AAA) tyrosine, phenylalanine and free tryptophan relative to the levels of the branched chain amino acids (BCAA) valine, leucine and isoleucine. These aromatic amino acids are known to be the precursors of catecholamine and indoleamine neurotransmitters. AAA transport into the CNS is facilitated in liver failure (JAMES et al. 1978), leading to elevated brain concentrations in animal models (MANS et al. 1979) and humans with HE (RECORD et al. 1976) (Tabel 5). The precise mechanism by which AAAs alter CNS function is unclear. Tryptophan is directly neurotoxic, albeit at extremely high doses (2–10 g/kg, HUET et al. 1981). AAAs have been hypothesized to indirectly alter CNS function by serving as a substrate for the synthesis of "false" neurotransmitters such as tyramine, phenethylamine, phenylethanolamine and octopamine, which would deplete catecholamine and indoleamine neurotransmitter levels. However, depletion of norepinephrine (NE) levels by 90% following the direct administration of octopamine caused no significant alterations in behavior (ZIEVE and OLSEN 1977). Further reduction of NE produces sedation and decreased motor activity, but not a neurological syndrome resembling HE. Indeed, false neurotransmitters are low-potency catecholamine receptor agonists (SAAVEDRA 1989). Thus, residual catecholamine neurotransmitter function could remain despite a decrease in primary neurotransmitter levels. Moreover, plasma and brain levels of false neurotransmitters are either decreased in patients and animal models of liver disease, or are not correlated with the stage of HE (YONEKURA et al. 1991). Thus, while false neurotransmitters may lower CNS catecholamine levels, the extent of this depletion, in concert with their intrinsic agonist properties, is insufficient to induce significant behavioral alterations, let alone the manifestations of HE.

Since serotonergic neurons in the midbrain reticular system are involved in the maintenance of consciousness and trophotropism (JOUVET 1973), serotonin may be involved in the sleep inversion and altered consciousness observed in HE. Concentrations of the serotonin precursor tryptophan increase in liver failure and may enhance serotonin synthesis (Table 6). While most reports indicate that serotonin levels are only moderately elevated in liver failure (RECORD et al. 1976; YURDAYDIN et al. 1990; BERGERON et al. 1989b), significant increases in the concentrations of the serotonin metabolite 5-HIAA are consistently observed in HE, suggesting enhanced rates of serotonin turnover (Tabel 6). While the increase in 5-HT turnover may correlate with the severity of HE (YURDAYDIN et al. 1990), there are no corresponding changes in the density or affinity of 5-HT_1 or 5-HT_2 receptors (BENGTSSON et al. 1989). Elucidation of serotonin's involvement (if any) in the pathogenesis of HE awaits further investigation.

Levels of NE in the CNS are slightly increased in liver failure (Table 6) (BERGERON et al. 1989b; YURDAYDIN et al. 1990). These observations do not support a depletion of NE by false neurotransmitters or a role in HE. Simi-

Table 6. Representative brain.catecholamine and indoleamine levels in hepatic encephalopathy

Subject	NE	DA	5-HT	5-HIAA
1. Human, FHF	–	–	↔	87%↑
2. Human, CLF	211%↑	↔	↔	↔
3. Rat, PCS	24%↑	↔	29%↑	130%↑
4. Rat, TAA	54%↓	↔	↔	160%↑

FHF, fulminant hepatic failure; CLF, chronic liver failure; PCS, protacaval shunt; TAA, thioacetamide treatment; NE, norepinephrine; DA, dopamine; 5-HT, serotonin; 5-HIAA, 5-hydroxyindole acetic acid; –, not determined; 5-HT and 5-HIAA levels in human, FHF subjects were determined in frontal cortex. NE and DA concentratios in human, CLF patients determined in caudate, while 5-HT and 5-HIAA levels were measured in frontal cortex. Neurotransmitter levels in PCS rat were measured in whole brain. NE levels in TAA rat were measured in hippocampus, while DA, 5HT and 5-HIAA concentrations were determined in striatum. 1, RECORD et al. (1976); 2, BERGERON et al. (1989b); 3, MANS et al. (1979); 4, YURDAYDIN et al. (1990).

larly, dopamine (DA) levels in animal models and patients with HE are mostly unchanged (Mans and Hawkins 1986; Bergeron et al. 1989b). Although DA receptor density is decreased in some models of liver failure (Baraldi et al. 1983), this may have no functional relevance, as the activity of postsynaptic DA-sensitive adenylate cyclase is normal in rabbits with FHF (Ferenci et al. 1986). The lack of involvement of DA in the pathogenesis of HE is further supported by the absence of consistent effects of the dopaminergic agents L-DOPA (Michel et al. 1980) or bromocriptine (Uribe et al. 1983) in ameliorating HE in patients with chronic liver disease. In summary, these findings strongly suggest that catecholamine neurotransmitters, their amino acid precursors and trace amines make no significant contribution to the pathogenesis of HE.

D. Conclusions

The impact of acute or chronic liver failure on CNS function is significant and is manifested in the syndrome of hepatic encephalopathy. Of the myriad metabolic abnormalities and potential neurotoxins that result from liver failure, concerted investigations over the past 4 decades have narrowed the field. Hyperammonemia directly and indirectly gives rise to a broad spectrum of CNS abnormalities, and should be considered a major factor in the pathogenesis of HE. However, investigations of patients with congenital hyperammonemia in the absence of significant liver failure and animals rendered hyperammonemic have made it clear that ammonia alone cannot account for many of the manifestations of HE. These additional manifestations result from changes in neurotransmitter systems. The primary neurotransmitter altered in HE is the GABAergic system, although our understanding of its role in HE is still evolving. Although most of the neurotoxins observed in liver failure (e.g., mercaptans, false neurotransmitters) may not have a significant role in the pathogenesis of HE, their effect on peripheral organ systems may feed back to influence CNS function. Indeed, new neuromodulators are being invoked in the pathogenesis of HE (benzodiazepine receptor agonists). It is hoped that continued investigation of the changes in CNS function accompanying liver failure may yield new therapeutic modalities aimed at directly correcting these neurochemical abnormalities.

References

Albrecht J, Rafalowska U (1987) Enhanced potassium stimulated γ-aminobutyric acid release by astrocytes derived from rats with hepatogenic encephalopathy. J Neurochem 49:9–11

Albrecht J, Hilgier W, Rafalowska U (1990) Activation of arginine metabolism to glutamate in rat brain synaptosomes in thioacetamide-induced hepatic encephalopathy: an adaptive response? J Neurosci Res 25:125–130

Alger BE, Nicoll RA (1983) Ammonia does not selectively block IPSPs in rat hippocampal pyramidal cells. J Neurophys 49:1381–1391

Baraldi M, Zeneroli ML, Ricci P, Caselgrandi E, Ventura E (1983) Down regulation of striatal dopamine receptors in experimental hepatic encephalopathy. Life Sci 32:1417–1425

Basile AS, Gammal S, Mullen K, Jones EA, Skolnick P (1988) Differential responsiveness of cerebellar Purkinje neurons to GABA and benzodiazepine receptor ligands in an animal model of hepatic encephalopathy. J Neurosci 8:2414–2421

Basile AS, Gammal SH, Jones EA, Skolnick P (1989) The $GABA_A$ receptor complex in an experimental model of hepatic encephalopathy: evidence for elevated levels of an endogenous benzodiazepine receptor ligand. J Neurochem 53:1057–1063

Basile AS, Ostrowski NL, Gammal SH, Jones EA, Skolnick P (1990) The $GABA_A$ receptor complex in hepatic encephalopathy: autoradiographic evidence for the presence of an endogenous benzodiazepine receptor ligand. Neuropsychopharmacology 3:61–71

Basile AS, Hughes RD, Harrison PM, Murata Y, Pannell L, Jones EA, Williams R, Skolnick P (1991a) Elevated brain concentrations of 1,4-benzodiazepines in fulminant hepatic failure. N Engl J Med 325:473–478

Basile AS, Jones EA, Skolnick P (1991b) The pathogenesis and treatment of hepatic encephalopathy: evidence for the involvement of benzodiazepine receptor ligands. Pharmacol Rev 43:27–71

Basile AS, Harrison PM, Hughes RD, Gu ZQ, Pannell L, McKinney A, Jones EA, Williams R (1994a) Relationship between plasma benzodiazepine receptor ligand concentrations and severity of hepatic encephalopathy. Hepatology 19:112–121

Basile AS, Saito K, Al-Mardini H, Record CO, Hughes RD, Williams R, Li Y, Heyes MP (1995a) The relationship between plasma and brain quinolinic acid levels and the severity of hepatic encephalopathy. Gastroenterology 108:818–823

Basile AS, Saito K, Li Y, Heyes MP (1995b) The relationship between plasma and brain quinolinic acid levels and the severity of hepatic encephalopathy in animal models of fulminant hepatic failure. J Neurochem 64:2607–2614

Bassett ML, Mullen KD, Scholz B, Fenstermacher JD, Jones EA (1990) Increased brain uptake of γ-aminobutyric acid in a rabbit model of hepatic encephalopathy. Gastroenterology 98:747–757

Bengtsson F, Bugge M, Hall H, Nobin A (1989) Brain $5\text{-}HT_1$ and $5\text{-}HT_2$ binding sites following portacaval shunt in the rat. Res Exp Med 189:249–256

Bergeron M, Pomier-Layrargues G, Butterworth RF (1989a) Aromatic and branched chain amino acids in autopsied brain tissue from cirrhotic patients with hepatic encephalopathy. Metab Brain Dis 4:169–176

Bergeron M, Reader TA, Layrargues GP, Butterworth RF (1989b) Monoamines and metabolites in autopsied brain tissue from cirrhotic patients with hepatic encephalopathy. Neurochem Res 14:853–859

Bernthal RE, Hays A, Tarter RE, Van Thiel D, Lecky J, Hegedus A (1987) Cerebral CT scan abnormalities in cholestatic and hepatocellular disease and their relationship to neuropsychologic test performance. Hepatology 7:107–114

Blom HJ, Ferenci P, Grimm G, Yap SH, Tangerman A (1991) The role of methanethiol in the pathogenesis of hepatic encephalopathy. Hepatology 13:445–454

Butterworth RF, Giguere JF (1986) Cerebral amino acids in portal systemic encephalopathy: lack of evidence for altered γ-aminobutyric (GABA) function. Metab Brain Dis 1:221–228

Butterworth RF, Lavoie J, Peterson C, Cotman CW, Szerb JC (1989) Excitatory amino acids and hepatic encephalopathy. In: Butterworth RF, Pomier-Layrargues G (eds) Hepatic encephalopathy. Pathophysiology and treatment. Humana, Clifton, p 417

Butterworth RF, Le O, Lavoie J, Szerb JC (1991) Effect of portacaval anastomosis on electrically stimulated release of glutamate from rat hippocampal slices. J Neurochem 56:1481–1484

Casellas P, Sagales T, Calzada MD, Accarino A, Vargas V, Guarneri L (1985) Visual evoked potetials in hepatic encephalopathy. Lancet I:394–395

Cohn R, Castell DO (1966) The effect of acute hyperammonemia on the electroencephalogram. J Lab Clin Med 68:195–205

Conn HO (1993) Hepatic encephalopathy. In: Schiff L, Schiff ER (eds) Diseases of the liver, vol 2. Lippincott, Philadelphia, p 1036

Cooper AJ, Plum F (1987) Biochemistry and physiology of brain ammonia. Physiol Rev 67:440

Crossley IR, Wardle EMM, Williams R (1983) Biochemical mechanisms of hepatic encephalopathy. Clin Sci 64:247–252

Davies MG, Rowan MJ, MacMathuna P, Keeling PWN, Weir DG, Feely J (1990) The auditory P300 event-related potential: an objective marker of the encephalopathy of chronic liver disease. Hepatology 12:688–694

De Groot GH, Schalm SW, De Vlieger M, van der Rijt CCD (1985) Objective measurement of hepatic encephalopathy by means of spectral analysis of the electroencephalogram (EEG). Brain Res 360:298–303

deKnegt RJ, Kornhuber J, Schalm SW, Rusche K, Riederer P, Tan J (1993) Binding of the ligand [^{3}H]MK-801 to the MK-801 binding site of the N-methyl-D-aspartate receptor during experimental encephalopathy from acute liver failure and from acute hyperammonemia in the rabbit. Metab Brain Dis 8:81–94

Diaz-Munoz M, Tapia R (1988) Regional brain GABA metabolism and release during hepatic coma produced in rats chronically treated with carbon tetrachloride. Neurochem Res 13:37–44

Dombro RS, Hutson DG, Norenberg MD (1993) The action of ammonia on astrocyte glycogen and glycogenolysis. Mol Chem Neuropathol 19:259–268

Ferenci P, Pappas SC, Munson PJ, Jones EA (1984a) Changes in glutamate receptors on synaptic membranes associated with hepatic encephalopathy or hyperammonemia in the rabbit. Hepatology 4:25–29

Ferenci P, Pappas SC, Munson PJ, Henson K, Jones EA (1984b) Changes in the status of neurotransmitter receptors in a rabbit model of hepatic encephalopathy. Hepatology 4:186–191

Ferenci P, Jones EA, Hanbauer I (1986) Lack of evidence for impaired dopamine receptor function in experimental hepatic encephalopathy. Neurosci Lett 65:60–64

Ferenci P, Riederer P, Jellinger K, Schafer DF, Jones EA (1988) Changes in cerebral receptors for γ-aminobutyric acid in patients with hepatic encephalopathy. Liver 8:225–230

Fitzpatrick SM, Cooper AJL, Hertz L (1988) Effects of ammonia and β-methylene-DL-aspartate on the oxidation of glucose and pyruvate by neurons and astrocytes in primary culture. J Neurochem 51:1197–1203

Flannery DB, Hsia YE, Wolf B (1982) Current status of hyperammonemia syndromes. Hepatology 2:495–506

Gabuzda G, Phillips GB, Davidson CS (1952) Reversible toxic manifestations in patients with cirrhosis of the liver given cation-exchange resins. N Engl J Med 246:124–130

Gammal S, Basile AS, Geller D, Skolnick P, Jones EA (1990) Reversal of the behavioral and electrophysiological abnormalities of an animal model of hepatic encephalopathy by benzodiazepine receptor ligands. Hepatology 11:371–378

Gazzard BG, Price H, Dawson AM (1986) Detection of hepatic encephalopathy. Postgrad Med J 62:163–166

Gjedde A, Lockwood AH, Duffy TE, Plum F (1978) Cerebral blood flow and metabolism in chronically hyperammonemic rats: effect of an acute ammonia challenge. Ann Neurol 3:325–330

Gregorios JB, Mozes LW, Norenberg LOB, Norenberg MD (1985a) Morphologic effects of ammonia on primary astrocyte cultures. I. Light microscopic studies. J Neuropathol Exp Neurol 44:391–403

Gregorios JB, Mozes LW, Norenberg MD (1985b) Morphologic effects of ammonia on primary astrocyte cultures. II. Electron microscopic studies. J Neuropathol Exp Neurol 44:404–414

Hawkins RA, Jessy J (1991) Hyperammonemia does not impair brain function in the absence of net glutamine synthesis. Biochem J 277:697–703

Hawkins RA, Jessy J, Mans AM, DeJoseph MR (1993) Effect of reducing brain glutamine synthesis on metabolic symptoms of hepatic encephalopathy. J Neurochem 60:1000–1006

Hertz L, Murthy CR, Lai JC, Fitzpatrick SM, Cooper AJ (1987) Some metabolic effects of ammonia on astrocytes and neurons in primary cultures. Neurochem Pathol 6:97–129

Hindfelt B, Plum F, Duffy TE (1977) Effect of acute ammonia intoxication on cerebral metabolism in rats with porto-caval shunts. J Clin Invest 59:386–394

Horowitz ME, Schafer DR, Molnar P, Jones EA, Blasberg EG, Patlak CS, Waggoner JS, Fenstermacher JD (1983) Increased blood-brain barrier transfer in a rabbit model of acute liver failure. Gastroenterology 84:1003–1011

Huet PM, Pomier-Layrargues G, Duguay L, Du Souich P (1981) Blood-brain transport of tryptophan and phenylalanine: effect of portacaval shunt in dogs. Am J Physiol 241:G163–G169

Iles JF, Jack JJB (1980) Ammonia: assessment of its action on postsynaptic inhibition as a cause of convulsions. Brain 103:555–578

James JH, Escourrou J, Fischer JE (1978) Blood-brain neutral amino acid transport activity is increased after portacaval anastomosis. Science 200:1395–1397

Jessy J, DeJoseph MR, Hawkins RA (1991) Hyperammonaemia depresses glucose consumption throughout the brain. Biochem J 277:693–696

Johansson U, Andersson T, Persson A, Eriksson LS (1989) Visual evoked potential – a tool in the diagnosis of hepatic encephalopathy? J Hepatol 9:227–233

Jones DB, Mullen KD, Roessle M, Maynard T, Jones EA (1987) Hepatic encephalopathy: application of visual evoked responses to test hypotheses of its pathogenesis in rats. J Hepatol 4:118–126

Jouvet M (1973) Serotonin and sleep in the cat. In: Barchas J, Usdin E (eds) Serotonin and behavior. Academic Press, New York, p 385

Lavoie J, Giguere J-F, Layrargues GP, Butterworth RF (1987) Amino acid changes in autopsied brain tissue from cirrhotic patients with hepatic encephalopathy. J Neurochem 49:692–697

Lockwood AH, Ginsberg MD, Rhoades HM, Gutierre MT (1986) Cerebral glucose metabolism after portocaval shunting in the rat. Pattern of metabolism and implications for the pathogenesis of hepatic encephalopathy. J Clin Invest 78:123–131

Loscher W, Kretz FJ, Karavias T, Dillinger U (1991) Marked increases of plasma gamma-aminobutyric acid concentrations in cirrhotic patients with portacaval shunts are not associated with alterations of cerebral functions. Digestion 49:212–220

Maddison JE, Yau D, Stewart P, Farrell GC (1986) Cerebrospinal fluid γ-aminobutyric acid levels in dogs with chronic portosystemic encephalopathy. Clin Sci 71:749–753

Maddison JE, Watson WEJ, Dodd PR, Johnston GAR (1991) Alterations in cortical [^{3}H]kainate and α-[^{3}H]amino-3-hydroxy-5-methyl-4-isoxazolepropionic acid binding in a spontaneous canine model of chronic hepatic encephalopathy. J Neurochem 56:1881–1888

Mans AM, Hawkins RA (1986) Brain monoamines after portacaval anastomosis. Metab Brain Dis 1:45–52

Mans AM, Saunders SJ, Kirsch RE, Biebuyck JF (1979) Correlation of plasma and brain amino acid and putative neurotransmitter alterations during acute hepatic coma in the rat. J Neurochem 32:285–292

Michel H, Solere M, Granier P, Cauvet G, Bali JP, Pons F, Bellet-Hermann H (1980) Treatment of cirrhotic hepatic encephalopathy with L-dopa. A controlled trial. Gastroenterology 79:207–211

Miller LG, Greenblatt DJ, Barnhill JG, Shader RI (1988) Chronic benzodiazepine administration. I. Tolerance is associated with benzodiazepine receptor downregulation and decreased γ-aminobutyric $acid_A$ receptor function. J Pharmacol Exp Ther 246:170–176

Minuk GY, Winder A, Burgess ED, Sargeant EJ (1985) Serum γ-aminobutyric acid levels in patients with hepatic encephalopathy. Hepatogastroenterology 32:171–174

Morgan MY, Alonso M, Stanger LC (1989) Lactitol and lactulose for the treatment of subclinical hepatic encephalopathy in cirrhosis patients. J Hepatol 8:208–217

Moroni F, Lombardi G, Carla V, Lal S, Etienne P, Nair NPV (1986a) Increase in the content of quinolinic acid in cerebrospinal fluid and frontal cortex of patients with hepatic failure. J Neurochem 47:1667–1671

Moroni F, Lombardi G, Carla V, Pellegrini D, Carassale GL, Cortesini C (1986b) Content of quinolinic acid and of other tryptophan metabolites increases in brain regions of rats used as experimental models of hepatic encephalopathy. J Neurochem 46:869–874

Mullen KD, Martin JV, Bassett ML, Mendelson WB, Jones EA (1986) Hepatic encephalopathy: a syndrome modulated by an endogenous benzodiazepine ligand? Hepatology 6:1221

Mullen KD, Szauter KM, Kaminsky-Russ K (1990) "Endogenous" benzodiazepine activity in physiological fluids of patients with hepatic encephalopathy. Lancet II:81–83

Nieto C, Arias J, Alsasua A, Garcia d Jalon PD (1980) Changes in brain oxidative metabolism in rats with portocaval shunt. Experientia 36:1403–1404

Norenberg (1977) A light and electron microscopic study of experimental portal-systemic (ammonia) encephalopathy. Lab Invest 36:618–627

Norenberg LOB, Norenberg MD (1986) Synergism of hepatic coma toxins in primary astrocyte cultures. Proc Int Cong Neuropathol 10:48

Norenberg MD, Mozes LW, Papendick RE, Norenberg LOB (1985) Effect of ammonia on glutamate, GABA and rubidium uptake by astrocytes. Ann Neurol 18:149

Norenberg MD, Baker L, Norenberg LO, Blicharska J, Bruce-Gregorios JH, Neary JT (1991) Ammonia-induced astrocyte swelling in primary culture. Neurochem Res 16:833–836

O'Brien CJ, Wise RJS, O'Grady JG, Williams R (1987) Neurological sequelae in patients recovered from fulminant hepatic failure. Gut 28:93–95

Oei LT, Kuys J, Lombarts AJP, Goor C, Endtz LJ (1979) Cerebrospinal fluid glutamine levels and EEG findings in patients with hepatic encephalopathy. Clin Neurol Neurosurg 81:59–63

Oja SS, Saransaari P, Wysmyk U, Albrecht J (1993) Loss of $GABA_B$ binding sites in the cerebral cortex of rats with acute hepatic encephalopathy. Brain Res 629:355–357

Opolon P (1980) Large-pore hemodialysis in fulminant hepatic failure. In: Brunner G, Schmidt FW (eds) Artificial liver support. Springer, Berlin Heidelberg New York, pp 141–146

Pappas SC (1986) Fulminant hepatic failure. In: Bayless TM (ed) Current therapy in gastroenterology and liver disease, vol 2. Mosby, St Louis, p 383

Pappas SC, Ferenci P, Schafer DF, Jones EA (1984) Visual evoked potentials in a rabbit model of hepatic encephalopathy. II. Comparison of hyperammonemic encephalopathy, postictal coma, and coma induced by synergistic neurotoxins. Gastroenterology 86:546–551

Peterson C, Giguere J-F, Cotman CW, Butterworth RF (1990) Selective loss of N-methyl-D-aspartate-sensitive L-[^{3}H]glutamate binding sites in rat brain following portacaval anastomosis. J Neurochem 55:386–390

Plum F, Hindfelt B (1976) The neurological complications of liver disease. In: Vinken PH, Bruyn GW (eds) Handbook of clinical neurology, vol 27. Elsevier, New York, p 349

Pomier-Layrargues G, Giguere JF, Lavoie J, Perney P, Gagnon S, D'Amour M, Wells J, Butterworth RF (1994) Flumazenil in cirrhotic patients in hepatic coma: a randomized double-blind placebo-controlled crossover trial. Hepatology 19:322–337

Raabe W (1987) Neurophysiology of ammonia intoxication. In: Butterworth R, Pomier-Layrargues G (eds) Hepatic encephalopathy. Pathophysiology and treatment. Humana, Clifton, p 49
Raabe W, Onstad G (1985) Porta-caval shunting changes neuronal sensitivity to ammonia. J Neurol Sci 71:307–314
Record CA, Buxton B, Chase RA, Curzon G, Murray-Lyon IM, Williams R (1976) Plasma and brain amino acids in fulminant hepatic failure and their relationship to hepatic encephalopathy. Eur J Clin Invest 6:387–394
Rossle M, Mullen KD, Jones EA (1989) Cortical benzodiazepine receptor binding in a rabbit model of hepatic encephalopathy: the effect of Triton X-100 on receptor solubilization. Metab Brain Dis 4:203–212
Rothstein JD, Guidotti A, Tinuper P, Cortelli P, Avoni P, Plazzi G, Lugaresi E, Schoch P, Montagna P (1992) Endogenous benzodiazepine receptor ligands in idiopathic recurring stupor. Lancet 340:1002–1004
Saavedra J (1989) False neurotransmitters. In: Trendelenburg U, Weiner N (eds) Catecholamines, vol II. Springer, Berlin Herdelberg New York, p 427
Schafer DF, Jones EA (1982) Hepatic encephalopathy and the γ-aminobutyric acid neurotransmitter system. Lancet I:18–20
Schafer DF, Thakur AK, Jones EA (1980) Acute hepatic coma and inhibitory neurotransmission: increase in γ-aminobutyric acid levels in plasma and receptors in brain. Gastroenterology 79:1123
Schafer DF, Pappas SC, Brody LE, Jacobs R, Jones EA (1984) Visual evoked potentials in a rabbit model of hepatic encephalopathy. I Sequential changes and comparisons with drug-induced comas. Gastroenterology 86:540–545
Schafer DRT, Fowler JM, Munson PJ, Thakur AK, Waggoner JG, Jones EA (1983) Gamma-aminobutyric acid and benzodiazepine receptors in an animal model of fulminant hepatic failure. J Lab Clin Med 102:870–880
Scollo-Lavizzari G, Steinmann E (1985) Reversal of hepatic coma by benzodiazepine antagonist (Ro 15-1788). Lancet I:1324
Sherlock S (1958) Pathogenesis and management of hepatic coma. Am J Med 24:805–813
Sherlock S, Dooley J (1993) Diseases of the liver and biliary system. Blackwell Scientific, London
Steindl P, Ferenci P (1990) Effect of drugs modulating central benzodiazepine receptors on hepatic encephalopathy in rats with thioacetamide-induced liver failure. Gastroenterology 98:A636
Subbalakshmi GYCV, Murthy CRK (1983) Acute metabolic effects of ammonia on the enzymes of glutamate metabolism in isolated astroglial cells. Neurochem Int 5:593–597
Swain MS, Bergeron M, Audet R, Blei AT, Butterworth RF (1992) Monitoring of neurotransmitter amino acids by means of an indwelling cisterna magna catheter: a comparison of two rodent models of fulminant liver failure. Hepatology 16:1028–1035
Takahashi K, Kameda H, Kataoka M, Sangou K, Harata N, Akaike N (1993) Ammonia potentiates $GABA_A$ response in dissociated rat cortical neurons. Neurosci Lett 151:51–54
Tangerman A, Meuwese-Arends MT, Van Tongeren JHM (1985) New methods for the release of volatile sulfur compounds from human serum: its determination by Tenax trapping and gas chromatography and its application in liver diseases. J Lab Clin Med 106:175–182
Therrien G, Butterworth RF (1991) Cerebrospinal fluid amino acids in relation to neurological status in experimental portal-systemic encephalopathy. Metab Brain Dis 6:65–74
Tossman U, Delin A, Eriksson S, Ungerstedt U (1987) Brain cortical amino acids measured by intracerebral dialysis in portacaval shunted rats. Neurochem Res 12:265–269

Uribe M, Garcia-Ramos G, Ramos M, Valverdi C, Marquez MA, Farca A, Guevara L (1983) Standard and higher doses of bromocriptine for severe chronic portal-systemic encephalopathy. Am J Gastroenterol 78:517–522

Vergara J, Plum F, Duffy TE (1974) α-Ketoglutaramate: increased concentrations in the cerebrospinal fluid of patients with hepatic coma. Science 183:81–83

Wysmyk U, Oja SS, Saransaari P, Albrecht J (1992) Enhanced GABA release in cerebral cortical slices derived from rats with thioacetamide-induced hepatic encephalopathy. Neurochem Res 17:1187–1190

Yonekura T, Kamata S, Wasa M, Okada A, Kawata S, Tarui S (1991) Simultaneous analysis of plasma phenethylamine, phenylethanolamine, tyramine and octopamine in patients with hepatic encephalopathy. Clin Chim Acta 199:91–98

Yurdaydin C, Hortnagl H, Steindl P, Zimmermann C, Ferenci P (1990) Increased serotoninergic and noradrenergic activity in hepatic encephalopathy in rats with thioacetamide-induced acute liver failure. Hepatology 21:695–700

Yurdaydin C, Gu ZQ, Nowak G, Fromm C, Holt AG, Basile AS (1993) Benzodiazepine receptor ligands are elevated in an animal model of hepatic encephalopathy: relationship between brain concentration and severity of encephalopathy. J Pharmacol Exp Ther 265:565–571

Zeneroli ML, Iuliano E, Racagni G, Baraldi M (1982) Metabolism and brain uptake of γ-aminobutyric acid in galactosamine-induced hepatic encephalopathy in rats. J Neurochem 38:1219–1222

Zieve L (1985) Encephalopathy due to short- and medium-chain fatty acids. In: McCandless DW (ed) Cerebral energy metabolism and metabolic encephalopathy. Plenum, New York, p 163

Zieve L, Brunner G (1985) Encephalopathy due to mercaptans and phenols. In: McCandless DW (ed) Cerebral energy metabolism and metabolic encephalopathy. Plenum, New York, p 179

Zieve L, Olsen RL (1977) Can hepatic coma be caused by a reduction of brain noradrenaline and dopamine? Gut 18:688–691

Zieve L, Doizaki WM, Lyftogt C (1984) Brain and blood methanethiol and ammonia concentrations in experimental hepatic coma and coma due to injections of various combinations of these substances. J Lab Clin Med 104:655–664

Zimmermann C, Ferenci P, Pifl C, Yurdaydin C, Ebner J, Lassmann H, Roth E, Hortnagl H (1989) Hepatic encephalopathy in thioacetamide-induced acute liver failure in rats: characterization of an improved model and study of amino-acidergic neurotransmission. Hepatology 9:594–601

CHAPTER 12

Liver Drug Reactions and Pregnancy

F. TREVISANI and D.H. VAN THIEL

In the general population, iatrogenic liver injury accounts for less than 2% of all identified cases of hepatic dysfunction (BJORNBOE et al. 1967; KOFF et al. 1970). The epidemiologic impact of iatrogenic liver injury is considerably more important, however, when the mortality due to liver disease is considered. Specifically, the case-fatality rate for drug-induced hepatic injury ranges from a minimum figure of 10% to a high of 50% of cases, depending upon the specific drug involved (ZIMMERMAN 1978).

The mechanisms whereby drugs induce hepatic injury and the clinical as well as histologic characteristics of drug-associated hepatotoxicity are described in several other chapters of this volume. The focus of this chapter is on the potential influence of pregnancy on the susceptibility for diagnosis, outcome and treatment of drug-induced liver disease. With this perspective, an awareness of the effect of a normal pregnancy on hepatic function is a fundamental requisite for any approach to the problem of gestation-associated hepatic dysfunction.

A. The Liver in Normal Pregnancy

Pregnancy is characterized by a panoply of physiological changes which occur sequentially and adapt the body to the specific needs of this unique condition. The key factors promoting these changes are the increased production of estrogens and progesterone initially by the corpus luteum and later by the placenta. Normal liver has both estrogen and progesterone receptors (VAN THIEL and GAVALER 1987). Thus, it is not particularly surprising that several physiological changes in both hepatic histology and function take place during the course of pregnancy, when the levels of these hormones change dramatically. Besides the obvious increases in sex hormone production, both hemodynamic and metabolic modifications occur during pregnancy and contribute to the changes in hepatic structure and function seen during pregnancy.

I. Liver Histology

The liver does not change its shape or consistency during pregnancy. Nonetheless, nonspecific cellular and subcellular modifications in hepatocyte structure are observed. These include an increased variability in hepatocyte size, an augmented cytoplasmic content of fat vacuoles, proliferation of both the smooth and rough endoplasmic reticulum as well as peroxisomes and an enlargement of the mitochondria. Moreover, the Kupffer cells become larger (RUSTGI et al. 1993). The critical role played by sex steroids in the etiology of these changes in hepatic structure is confirmed by their presence in nonpregnant women using oral contraceptives.

II. Liver Perfusion and Function

Although both blood volume and cardiac output increase 30%–50% during pregnancy, hepatic perfusion remains unaltered (MUNNELL and TAYLOR 1947). Therefore, a 20%–35% fall in the fraction of the cardiac output delivered to the liver occurs as pregnancy progresses (RUSTGI et al. 1987). Hepatic protein synthesis increases during pregnancy such that, despite an expanded plasma volume, the concentration of most circulating proteins (α_1-, α_2- and β-globulins) increases during pregnancy. Consequently, the serum concentrations of α_1-antitrypsin (serum proteases), ceruloplasmin, transferrin and fibrinogen increase. α_1-Fetoprotein levels increase markedly as a result of its synthesis by fetal tissue. A noticeable exception to this rule is the serum albumin level, which progressively declines to a level 60% of normal at the end of pregnancy. This hypoalbuminemia associated with normal pregnancy is attributable almost in its entirety to the increase in plasma volume that occurs during pregnancy. A reduced albumin synthesis rate, reported to occur in women taking oral contraceptives, may contribute minimally to these findings (HONGER and ROSSING 1969; RAMCHARAN et al. 1976). Antithrombin III levels, like albumin, decline during pregnancy and with the use of oral contraceptives. In contrast, the prothrombin time and the levels of proteins associated with a normal prothrombin time do not change during the course of a normal pregnancy.

The flux of lipids from peripheral fat stores to the liver increases over the course of pregnancy. Consequently, the hepatic synthesis of triglycerides, cholesterol, phospholipids, very low-density (VLDL), low-density (LDL) and high-density (HDL) lipoproteins increase. This results in a progressive increase in the levels of each of these lipid components of serum.

The biliary excretion of cholesterol during pregnancy increases to a greater extent than does that of phospholipids (VAN THIEL and GAVALER 1987). This and an impaired hepatic bile acid and water excretion lead to a supersaturation of hepatic bile which accounts substantially for the propensity of gravid women to develop gallstones.

The maximal excretory capacity of the liver for organic anions, such as bilirubin, bile acids and Bromosulphalein, is impaired by sex steroids. Specifically, estrogens inhibit the canalicular excretion of organic anions without affecting conjugation of such substances by hepatic cellular phase II enzymes. Conversely, progesterone depresses phase II reactions, leading to an accumulation in plasma of unconjugated organic ions (such as bilirubin) while conjugated organic acids such as bile acids are excreted normally (VAN THIEL and GAVALER 1987). The results of a simultaneous exposure to increased concentrations of both steroids is that many pregnant women have plasma levels of unconjugated bilirubin at the upper limit of the normal range and a mild increase in the level of circulating bile acids.

Beginning around the 7th month of pregnancy, the serum alkaline phosphatase activity progressively increases two- to fourfold. This increase in alkaline phosphatase activity is due to an enhanced production of placental and skeletal isoenzymes (KREEK 1987; VAN THIEL and GAVALER 1987). γ-Glutamyl transpeptidase (GGT), transaminases and 5-nucleotidase plasma levels do not change during the course of a normal pregnancy. Rarely, these levels may decline slightly as a result of hemodilution.

Table 1. Changes in liver function and histology associated with normal pregnancy

Histology	
Hepatocytes	Increased variability in morphology Increased fat content (vacuoles) Proliferation of smooth and rough endoplasmic reticulum Enlargement of mitochondria
Kupffer cells	Hypertrophy
Synthetic function parameters	
Albumin	20%–25% reduction (hemodilution)
α_1-Globulins	50% increase
α_2-Globulins	50% increase
β-Globulins	50% increase
Prothrombin time	No change
Excretory function parameters	
Total bilirubin	No change
Unconjugated bilirubin	Slight increase
Bile acids	Slight increase
Bile salt flow	Increase in storage capacity and 27% reduction in transport maximum
Cholestasis parameters	
Alkaline phosphatase	100%–400% increase (hepatobiliary fraction unchanged)
Gamma-glutamyl transpeptidase	No change or slight reduction
5-Nucleotidase	No change or slight reduction
Hepatocytonecrosis parameters	
Transaminases	No changes or slight reduction (hemodilution)
Tumoral markers	
α-Fetoprotein	Marked increase (fetal production)
Xenobiotic metabolism	
High-clearance xenobiotics	Reduced extraction
Low-clearance xenobiotics	Variable changes

The altered laboratory profile of hepatic function may persist for several months after delivery. A summary of many of the pregnancy-induced changes in various parameters used to assess the liver is reported in Table 1.

B. Effects of Pregnancy on the Risk of Experiencing a Drug-Induced Hepatic Injury

In theory, pregnancy should enhance the risk of an individual experiencing an iatrogenic hepatitis by different ways (Table 2).

I. Specific Pre-Marketing Risk/Benefit Evaluation of Drugs

Worldwide, more than 1000 new drugs are introduced yearly onto the market (NEWTON and NEWTON 1988). The pre-marketing evaluation of these drugs is directed at collecting data on both their effectiveness and safety before the drug becomes clinically available. As pregnant women are usually excluded from drug studies, due to the putative risk of teratogenic effects, the safety of most drugs used by pregnant women can be predicted only from the experience with the drug in experimental animal models. If one assumes that both the metabolism of some drugs (BERTHOU et al. 1988; LE BOT et al. 1988) and hepatocyte susceptibility to drug-associated injury (MARTELLI et al. 1990) in nonpregnant and pregnant humans and animals differ, this strategy does not allow one to assess the potential of any drug to either be safe or produce injury in a pregnant woman.

II. Risk of Exposure to Hepatotoxic Drugs

The use of all drugs during pregnancy should be reduced primarily to avoid any possible teratogenic effects that the use of a drug may have. However, both the many antecedent and pregnancy-related conditions make the use of certain drugs very common during pregnancy. A list of drugs commonly used during pregnancy is shown in Table 3. In two series of 1000 pregnant women

Table 2. Factors which may affect the risk of experiencing a drug-induced hepatic injury during pregnancy

No specific pre-marketing evaluation of drugs
Change in the probability of exposure to hepatotoxic drugs
Changes in pharmacokinetics
Change in the intrinsic liver vulnerability due to:
– Increased production of hepatotoxic intermediates
– Cholestatic effect of sexual hormones
– Propensity to hepatic vascular lesions
– Possible deficiency of protective factors (hepatic glutathione, vitamin E)
– Increased lipid metabolism and relative deficiency of carnitine

Table 3. Drugs and medications used during pregnancy

Control of uterine contractions: β-sympathomimetic agents (hexaprenaline, ritrotidine hydrochloride, terbutaline), methyl-ergonovine maleate, nifedipine, oxytocin, prostaglandins

Infectious diseases: acyclovir, amphotericin, aztreonam, cephalosporins, chloroquine, erytromycin, ethambutol, isoniazid, lindane, mebendazole, metronidazole, miconazole, nitrofurantoin, nystatin, penicillins, pyrantel, quinidine, rifampicin, sulfonamides, tetracyclines, trimetoprim, vancomycin, zidovuline

Gastrointestinal and hepatic disorders: antacids, chlorpormazine, cyclizin, doxylamine, H_2-receptor antagonists, hydroxyzine, lactulose, meclizine, penicillamine, perphenazine, prochlorperazine, promethazine, *S*-adenosyl-*l*-methionine, sulfasalazine, trimethobenzamide, ursodeoxycholic acid

Fever, pain and inflammation: acetaminophen, aspirin, codeine, gold salt, ibuprofen, indomethacin, meperidine, morphine

General anesthesia and local anesthetics: bupivacaine, cyclopropane, halothane, enflurane, isoflurane, lidocaine, mepivacaine, methoxyflurane, procaine, tetracaine, thiopental

Neurologic and psychiatric diseases: amitriptyline, carbamazepine, chlordiazepoxide, diazepam, imipramine, lithium, nitrazepam, nortriptyline, penicillamine, phenobarbital, phenothiazines, phenytoin, trimethadione, valproic acid

Metabolic and hormonal disorders: clomiphene, corticosteroids, estrogens, insulin, methimazole, progestins, propylthiouracil, thyroid hormones

Cardiovascular diseases: β-blockers, captopril, coumarins, digoxin, dopamine, enalapril, furosemide, heparin, methyldopa, nifedipine, procainamide, quinidine, thiazides, verapamil

Pulmonary diseases: albuterol, corticosteroids, cromolyn, ephedrine, epinephrine, guaifenesin, metaproterenol, terbutaline, theophylline

Cancer: azathioprine, chlorambucil, cisplatin, cyclophosphamide fluorouracil, melphalan, methotrexate, procarbazine, vincristine

Immunosuppressant agents: azathioprine, corticosteroids, cyclosporine

Other agents: amphetamines, antihistamines, barbiturates, caffeine, cocaine, chlormezanone, heroin, naloxone, thioureas, vitamins

recruited in the 1970s, the prevalence of women taking medications other than iron was 83% and 72%, respectively (Eskes et al. 1988). Similar figures have been reported by others (Brocklebank et al. 1978; Doering and Steward 1982; Lewis and Zimmerman 1986). These medications are taken for several different reasons which, in order of frequency, are a need to inhibit or stimulate uterine contractility; treat an infectious disease or digestive tract dysfunction; manage pain and fever; provide general anesthesia; treat a neurologic or psychiatric disease and control a metabolic or hormone-associated disorder (Eskes et al. 1988). Obstetricians head the list of physicians prescribing drugs to pregnant women followed by general practitioners and anesthesiologists. Importantly, the percentage of women who self-administer drugs is rather high (12% and 7%, respectively). In addition, it has been estimated that, in the Western world, 8%–15% of women of childbearing age occasionally or repeatedly use illicit drugs (ADAMS et al. 1989; KHALSA and GFROERER 1991).

Thus pregnancy does not reduce but rather increases the likelihood of a normal young adult woman taking medication. Indeed, it clearly enhances the likelihood of exposure to certain drugs such as tokolytics, analgesics, anesthetics, antiemetics and laxatives. In contrast, drugs with proven or suspected teratogenicity are taken less often than is the case for the nonpregnant state. In general, because many drugs share potential hepatotoxicity with teratogenicity, it can be assumed that the management of pregnancy reduces the likelihood of experiencing an iatrogenic liver injury.

III. Pharmacokinetics

Drug absorption and handling may be influenced greatly by pregnancy. This section will summarize the known and theoretical effects of pregnancy on the pharmacokinetics of drugs.

1. Absorption

Gastric emptying and intestinal transit times are delayed during pregnancy (LIND and HYTTEN 1969; PARRY et al. 1970; VAN THIEL and SHADE 1986). Although there is no evidence that this influences the kinetics of drug absorption, in theory, pregnancy could enhance the absorption of most substances as a result of providing more time for this process to occur. Conversely, for drugs partially cleared by the stomach and gut (i.e., chlorpromazine), a reduced systemic bioavailability would be expected, Delayed gastric emptying could result in an accumulation of drugs given in repeated fragmented doses, leading to the administration of a "toxic" amount of drug as the stomach empties (ESKES et al. 1988).

Due to the increased respiratory activity and pulmonary perfusion that occurs during pregnancy (ESKES et al. 1988), an accelerated absorption of drugs administered by aerosol can occur in pregnant women. Similarly, since blood flow to the skin, nasal (FABRICANT 1960) and vaginal (ESKES et al. 1988) mucosa is increased, drug administration through these routes can also have an enhanced bioavailability unless local metabolism of the agent in question is also an important process.

2. Distribution

The increased plasma volume (up to 50% by the third trimester) and a major expansion of the extravascular fluid space leads to a 7–81 increment of total body water during pregnancy (ESKES et al. 1988). This represents a greatly enlarged volume of distribution for water-soluble drugs. Fat stores increase by 3–4 kg during pregnancy, thereby also enhancing the volume of distribution of fat-soluble agents.

As the plasma albumin concentration falls, the total plasma concentration of drugs highly bound to albumin also declines. A proportional increase in the unbound fraction should result if the dose of the drug is not altered. However, because the total clearance of high-clearance drugs is proportional to the circulating free fraction, the level of free drug does not actually increase in most cases. The increased metabolism of the drug may ultimately result in a new steady state characterized by a lower total and normal free plasma level (LEVY and YACOBI 1974; WOSILAIT 1974). In the last trimester of pregnancy, the accelerated mobilization of fat deposits produces a marked increase in circulating non-esterified fatty acids, which can compete with many xenobiotics for plasma protein binding. Finally, the progressive increase in the fetal to maternal plasma albumin concentration ratio observed throughout pregnancy (KRAUER et al. 1980) may affect the proportion of highly albumin-bound drug distributed in the two compartments of the fetal maternal unit.

3. Hemodynamics and Drug Clearance

As stated above, the fraction of the cardiac output reaching the liver declines by 20%–35% during the course of a normal pregnancy. This, together with the expansion of both the blood and extravascular volumes, reduces the concentration of solutes in plasma. Thus an impaired metabolism of high-clearance drugs, whose metabolism is blood flow dependent, is observed (HAWKER 1993). In contrast, the effect of pregnancy on the hepatic metabolism of "enzyme-limited" (low extraction) substances is not readily predictable.

Estrogen administration and pregnancy are associated with a reduced activity of enzymes such as hepatic glucuronyltransferase in rats (BROCK and VORE 1982). Progestational agents induce hepatic mixed oxidase function (VORE and MONTGOMERY 1980). These opposite influences on the various enzymatic systems involved in drug biotransformation favor the production of metabolites, some of which are toxic.

As reported above (Sect. A.II), the maximum rate of hepatic transport of organic anions is impaired during pregnancy and the plasma levels of sulfated and glucoronidated lipophilic endo- and xenobiotics increase (VAN THIEL and GAVALER 1987). It can be assumed that these changes in plasma levels occur also for drugs that share the same excretory pathways.

In contrast to hepatic blood flow, renal blood flow almost doubles and the glomerular filtration rate increases from about 100ml/min to 170ml/min during the course of a normal pregnancy (DAVISON and NOBLE 1981; DUNLOP 1981). It is likely that these changes speed the elimination of water-soluble drugs removed primarily by the kidneys (KRAUER et al. 1980).

4. Maternal-Placental-Fetal Unit

It should be noted that during pregnancy the "total" metabolism of a xenobiotic is influenced by the presence of the placenta and other fetal organs, which transform the body into a complex unit, the so-called maternal-placental-fetal unit. While the impact on the biotransformation processes of the fetal liver is rather low, due to the large difference in the hepatic mass of the mother and fetus, the impact upon metabolism by the placenta is not negligible. The placenta has a large battery of enzymatic systems for the oxidation, reduction, hydrolysis and conjugation of xenobiotics. Moreover, it acts as an impedence barrier to the translocation of water-soluble molecules from mother to fetus and vice versa. Small (<300 daltons) lipophilic agents readily cross the placenta along their concentration gradients, while larger (>100 daltons) molecules are transferred less readily (PIERCE and COHEN 1988).

The many pregnancy-induced changes in drug metabolism act in combination such that the kinetics of any given drug can be influenced to a very different degree or direction. As a matter of fact, for most drugs, plasma levels are lower and disposal rates are accelerated during pregnancy. Acetaminophen metabolism is increased in the third trimester of pregnancy, resulting in a 58% raise in apparent clearance and a 28% reduction in the elimination half-life of the drug with respect to nonpregnant women (MINERS et al. 1986). Decreased plasma concentrations of carbamazepine and elevated levels of its metabolites suggest an accelerated metabolism of this drug during pregnancy (CHRISTIANSEN et al. 1977). Similar conclusions can be reached for a number of antibiotics and digoxin (HIRSCH et al. 1974; PHILIPSON 1979; ROGERS et al. 1972). The clearance of valproic acid (NAU et al. 1981), phenobarbital and phenytoin (DAM et al. 1979) may be increased during pregnancy. However, not all authors report similar results (PEIKER and TRAEGER 1974; ROWLAND et al. 1990).

Not all drugs obey the general rule of an accelerated biotransformation rate during pregnancy. Pharmacokinetic studies have demonstrated an impaired metabolism of promazine, pethidine (meperidine) and cortisol (CRAWFORD and RUDOFSKI 1966; VORE et al. 1978). In addition, it has been shown that oral contraceptives depress antipyrine metabolism (CARTER et al. 1973; HOMEIDA et al. 1978; O'MALLEY et al. 1972) and increase morphine and temazepam clearance (WATSON et al. 1986; STOEHR et al. 1984).

In conclusion, pregnancy-induced altered xenobiotic handling on the one hand can reduce the clinical effectiveness of certain drugs and, on the other hand, can expose the maternal organism to an abnormally elevated amount of drug or metabolite and favor metabolic pathways producing potentially toxic products (see also Sect. B.IV).

IV. Liver Vulnerability

Theoretically, sex steroids predispose the liver to the adverse effects of drugs in many different ways. Estrogens induce microsomal enzyme systems, which, in turn, increase the production of hepatotoxic intermediates from parenteral drugs such as acetaminophen, α-methyldopa, nitrofurantoin and isoniazid (PESSAYRE and LARREY 1991; WATKINS 1990). The accelerated acetaminophen metabolism occurring in the third trimester of pregnancy leads to an 88% increase in glutathione-derived conjugates (MINERS et al. 1986), leading to an increased risk of glutathione depletion, if very high or repeated doses of acetaminophen are used. Indeed, it has been found that pregnant mice, with initially normal hepatic concentrations of glutathione, are uniquely susceptible to acetaminophen hepatotoxicity (LARREY et al. 1986). Microsomal enzyme induction is also a risk factor for halothane-associated hepatitis during pregnancy (RAY and DRUMMOND 1991). Moreover, the sex-steroid-induced interference with bile secretion can cooperate with certain drugs to produce cholestasis. Thus the risk for the development of an acute drug-induced cholestasis during pregnancy is increased (HAWKER 1993). Finally, since several different hepatic vascular lesions may complicate either a normal pregnancy or oral contraceptive use (VALLA and BENHAMOU 1988), pregnancy is thought to predispose women to the adverse effects of certain drugs such as methotrexate, azathioprine, vitamin A and some antineoplastic drugs, either proven or suspected of causing vascular lesions of the liver (HAWKER 1993). However, it needs to be noted that all these substances also manifest teratogenicity that precludes their use during pregnancy in most cases.

Deficiencies of protective factors such as hepatic glutathione and vitamin E may ensue during pregnancy due either to inappropriate nutrition or repeated administration of drugs with pregnancy-enhanced glutathione-dependent inactivation. Moreover, experimental data suggest a reduced ability of pregnant mice to replace the glutathione consumed as a result of acetaminophen metabolism (LARREY et al. 1986). Because of the impaired auto protection mechanisms, not only toxic but also immunoallergic reactions become more probable under these circumstances. The latter, in fact, are initiated by the covalent binding of the reactive metabolics to plasma membrane proteins.

An accelerated metabolic turnover of lipids (Sect. A.II) and a deficiency of carnitine, an essential cofactor in the transport of fatty acids into mitochondria for oxidation (EVERSON et al. 1982), are known to occur in pregnancy. They represent the background for the development of "spontaneous" acute fatty liver of pregnancy and magnify the effects of drugs that inhibit oxidation of fatty acids by mitochondria, such as tetracycline and valproic acid, or interfere with the action of lysosomal phospholipases, such as amiodarone and perhexiline maleate. A drug-induced fatty infiltration of the liver (steatosis or phospholipidosis) results when these drugs are used and can progress to hepatic failure more easily in pregnant women than in nonpregnant women. Indeed, pregnancy has been found to be a predisposing factor for tetracycline-associated toxicity (LEWIS and ZIMMERMAN 1986; PASSAYRE and LARREY 1991).

C. Liver Drug Reactions Occurring During Pregnancy

It is generally held that pregnant women run the same risk of having an adverse drug reaction as do nonpregnant women (FALLON 1988; LEWIS and ZIMMERMAN 1986; RIELY 1993). However, based on the preceding, it is probable that drug-induced hepatic injury occurring during pregnancy is an underrecognized problem. Many factors make a correct assessment of this issue difficult to obtain. First, there is a scarcity of epidemiologic studies addressing maternal as opposed to fetal adverse effects. Second, the usual methods used to obtain a history of drug exposure may fail during pregnancy (BODENDORFER et al. 1979). Specifically, some women refuse to take even prescribed drugs during pregnancy fearing that their fetus might be harmed. In contrast, others use drugs unknown to their physicians to alleviate common complaints related to pregnancy and deny using such agents when specifically questioned about drug use for fear that the agent being used will be denied them. Both categories of patients are reluctant to admit their behavior. Third, mild drug-induced abnormalities of liver tests (i.e., increase in bilirubin and alkaline phosphatase occurring during pregnancy) may be attributed to the physiological changes associated with pregnancy. This results in a "camouflage effect." Fourth, liver diseases which are unique to pregnancy can mimic toxic drug reactions. Finally, a "long latency" between the initiation of drug use and the onset of an adverse drug reaction (FLETCHER and GRIFFIN 1991) may result in the association being missed or the reaction occurring after delivery and not being recognized as a pregnancy-associated drug reaction.

As a matter of fact, it should be understood that any drug that can cause liver injury in the nonpregnant state can also do so during pregnancy.

I. Antibiotics

Up to 50% of pregnant women use antibiotics at some time during their pregnancy. Since the early 1960s, high doses of intravenous tetracycline have been associated with acute fatty liver of pregnancy (SCHULTZ et al. 1963). More recently, HAGUE et al. (1983) reported that, among 128 cases of acute fatty liver, 31% had received tetracycline and almost all cases occurring before the 28th gestational week were associated with the use of high intravenous doses of the drug. Like acute fatty liver of pregnancy, which characteristically occurs late in the third trimester, tetracycline-associated fatty infiltration of the liver is more common in women with preeclampsia. It also occurs more frequently in women having more than one fetus (BORHANMANESH et al. 1973; DAVIS and KAUFMAN 1966). The fetal liver may experience the same hepatic damage as the mother as a result of tetracycline exposure (DEINHARDT and GUST 1982). Of interest, the regular oral use of tetracycline for acne before pregnancy has been found to be associated with an increased risk of hepatic injury during pregnancy (WENK et al. 1981). The authors of this report hypothesized that the antibiotic is stored in bonex as complexes with calcium apatite, which is released into the plasma if gestational acidosis, osteomalacia or hyperparathyroidism occur. The maternal and fetal mortality rate associated with acute fatty liver due to tetracycline use is considerable, reaching 85% of cases (LEWIS and ZIMMERMAN 1986).

Hypersensitivity and probably intrinsic drug toxicity determine the presence or absence of erythromycin-induced liver injury. It has been estimated that as many as 5% of pregnant women use this antibiotic during their pregnancy (BROCKLEBANK et al. 1978). In one study, 10% of pregnant women given erythromycin estolate for at least 3 weeks manifested a subclinical and reversible liver injury (McCORMACK et al. 1977). The putative susceptibility of pregnant women to erythromycin estolate-induced hepatotoxicity needs to be confirmed by assessing the incidence of these same adverse effects in nonregnant women taking equal amounts and for equal periods of treatment. Cholestatic jaundice has been reported in one pregnant woman using triacetyloleandomycin (LEWIS and ZIMMERMAN 1986). It is of interest to note that oral contraceptives predispose women to hepatic injury with this drug (ZIMMERMAN 1978).

Although theoretically anticipated, an increased toxicity of isoniazid (INH) during pregnancy has not been demonstrated in a cohort of 1300 pregnant women (SNIDER et al. 1980). Instead, despite the knowledge that up to 20% of recipients of INH can develop at least one laboratory abnormality consistent with liver injury while using INH, none of these women did so. This surprising result can be explained, at least in part, by the relationship linking increasing age to isoniazid toxicity (LEWIS and ZIMMERMAN 1986). Nonetheless, some authors have reported severe hepatocellular injury occurring in pregnant women taking isoniazid (LEWIS and ZIMMERMAN 1986). In the general population, the factors predicting a lethal evolution of isoniazid-induced hepatic injury are 2 months or more of treatment, a serum bilirubin level above 20mg/dl, the presence of clotting abnormalities and a female gender.

II. Antiemetics

Cholestatic jaundice has been reported to occur in pregnant women using phenothiazines for the control of nausea and vomiting (HALL 1956; STEVEN 1981). Pregnancy is well known to be associated with an increased incidence of nausea and vomiting (HALL 1956). Both hydroxyzine and perphenazine can cause cholestasis in pregnancy (LEWIS and ZIMMERMAN 1986). Fortunately, the prognosis for such cases is generally good, with a complete recovery occurring within 2 months.

III. Anesthetics and Analgesics

Reports of chloroform-induced hepatitis were among the initial reports of adverse drug reactions occurring in pregnant women (LITTLE and WESTONE

1964; SHEEHAN 1950). Thereafter, liver reactions to halothane and methoxyflurane were reported (HOLDEN and SHERLINE 1972; RUBINGER et al. 1975). In each such case, an elevation of the plasma bilirubin level above 20 mg/dl has been a predictor of death (ZIMMERMAN 1978).

The use of prescribed, as well as nonprescribed, analgesic and anti-inflammatory drugs is exceedingly common among pregnant women (LEWIS and ZIMMERMAN 1986). Salicylates and acetaminophen are the most frequently used such agents with acetaminophen alone or in combination accounting for over 60% of the analgesic drugs taken during pregnancy. Both of these drugs can cause liver injury through different mechanisms (LEWIS and ZIMMERMAN 1986). Despite the theoretical increased susceptibility to drug-induced liver injury during pregnancy (Sect. B.IV), only a few cases of hepatic injury due to an overdose of acetaminophen have been reported (HAIBACH et al. 1984; KURZEN 1990; MCELHATTON et al. 1990; STOKES 1984). Aspirin hepatotoxicity is a dose-dependent phenomenon, which results in a mild or moderate and rapidly reversible increase in transaminases in about 97% of the patients experiencing this adverse effect (LEWIS and ZIMMERMAN 1986). The difficulty in interpreting a transient moderate hypertransaminasemia ensuing during pregnancy explains why no cases of aspirin-related liver injury have been reported in pregnant women.

IV. Anticonvulsants

In rats, the dose-dependent maternal toxicity and mortality of orally and intravenously administered phenytoin increases as pregnancy proceeds (ROWLAND et al. 1990). In pregnant women, the adverse effects of phenytoin include hepatitis and cholestasis (ZIMMERMAN 1978). In evaluating the laboratory abnormalities of individuals taking phenytoin, it should be remembered that one-third of subjects using phenytoin experience an increase in alkaline phosphatase as a result of an increased release of the bone isoenzyme occurring as a result of a relative vitamin D deficiency associated with phenytoin use (WILLIAMS et al. 1984). The suspected teratogenicity of valproic acid precludes its clinical use in pregnancy (ZIMMERMAN and ISHAK 1982).

V. Other Agents

Fulminant hepatic failure occurring during pregnancy has been reported with the use of propylthiouracil (MORRIS et al. 1989), quinidine phenylethylbarbituate (BOURLIERE et al. 1988) and chlormezanone (BOURLIERE et al. 1992).

Corticosteroids can produce fatty infiltration of the liver, but there is no convincing evidence that this effect is harmful to pregnant women, even when administered at high dosage and associated with the use of other immunosuppressant agents (MORENO et al. 1991).

Chenodeoxycholic acid treatment of gallstones is frequently followed by a moderate elevation of serum transaminase levels in about one-third of cases (SHOENFIELD and LACKIN 1981). Liver injury occurs with chenodeoxycholic acid in pregnant baboons (MCSHERRY et al. 1976). Although specific information is lacking in humans, these findings and a potential teratogenicity contraindicate its use in pregnancy.

D. Clinical Presentation and Diagnostic Approach to Hepatic Injury in Pregnancy

It has been estimated that 1 in 1500 pregnancies is complicated by jaundice. Of these, only 1%–2% can be related to the use of medications (LEWIS and ZIMMERMAN 1986). The diagnostic evaluation of liver dysfunction seen in pregnancy does not differ from that utilized by physicians caring for nonpregnant patients. However, in evaluating pregnancy-associated hepatic dysfunction, the physician must be aware of the physiological changes in liver function, perfusion, laboratory tests, as well as the unique hepatic diseases associated with pregnancy such as pruritus gravidarum, intrahepatic cholestasis of pregnancy, acute fatty liver of pregnancy or the liver dysfunction that accompanies hyperemesis gravidarum, preeclampsia/eclampsia and HELLP (hemolysis, elevated liver enzymes and low platelet count) syndrome. Some of these unique problems associated with pregnancy can occur at any time during pregnancy while others are much more likely to occur only late in pregnancy (RUSTGI et al. 1993). Besides these, many other liver diseases not unique to pregnancy need to be differentiated from putative drug-induced hepatic injury seen during pregnancy. These include acute viral hepatitis, an exacerbation of antecedent chronic liver disease or porphyria, cholangitis, ischemic liver injury occurring as a result of shock or anoxia, Budd-Chiari syndrome, veno-occlusive disease, granulomatous liver diseases, gallstone disease and others.

Jaundice, pruritus, loss of appetite, dyspepsia and fatigue are often the first indicators of liver dysfunction whether the individual is pregnant or not. Other symptoms include abdominal pain/discomfort (mainly in the upper right quadrant), fever, nausea, vomiting and weight loss. Hepatic dysfunction can also occur in the absence of any presenting symptoms as occurs typically with hepatitis C.

The physical examination of an individual suspected of having liver disease must include a search for icterus, spider angioma, palmar erythema, abdominal venous dilatation, changes in size and consistency of the liver and spleen, and the presence of peripheral edema, ascites and asterixis. It should be remembered that spider nevi and palmar erythema occur in 70% of women who have a normal pregnancy; thus their finding alone does not suggest liver disease. Because the physical examination of the liver does not change during pregnancy, either palpable hepatomegaly or an abnormal liver consistency should suggest the presence of hepatic disease in a pregnant woman.

The usual initial laboratory studies utilized to assess the presence or absence of liver dysfunction include a determination of the serum levels of bilirubin, transaminase, albumin, globulins, alkaline phosphatase, GGT and the prothrombin time. When clinical findings or laboratory investigations suggest the presence of liver disease, additional studies must be performed to distinguish between the various possible hepatic disorders. Invasive diagnostic procedures not essential for a diagnosis and the many radiographic and radionuclide scans normally used to assess hepatic disease should be avoided during pregnancy.

A diagnosis of drug-induced hepatic injury requires that several particular criteria be met. These include: (1) exposure to the putative offending drug, (2) the time span between drug exposure and hepatic injury is compatible with a cause-effect relationship, (3) the clinical characteristics of the disease and liver histology are compatible with a drug-induced hepatic injury and (4) all other causes of liver damage have been ruled out. Additional important evidence is that improvement or resolution of the disease process occurs after the suspected drug is discontinued. It should be kept in mind, however, that recovery may take months and that the hepatic injury can progress for several months despite drug withdrawal (HAWKER 1993). The only criterion which can establish a specific diagnosis of a drug reaction for certain is relapse of the disease when the patient is "rechallenged" with the putative etiologic agent. In many cases and, certainly all those with severe hepatic injury or if another drug can be substituted for the offending agent, a rechallenge is not possible and the causal relationship between the use of a drug and the observed hepatic injury remains only presumptive. If a diagnosis of a drug-induced hepatic injury remains equivocal after completion of a noninvasive diagnostic workup, a liver biopsy is indicated. An ultrasound-guided approach easily overcomes any technical difficulty that might occur related to the upward and displacement of the liver by the gravid uterus. With few exceptions (i.e., phospholipidosis in amiodarone- or perhexiline-induced hepatitis), the microscopic features of drug-related injuries are rather nonspecific. Nevertheless, hepatic histology in such cases is helpful by demonstrating a histologic picture compatible with the suspected toxic agent in question or will direct the physician to an alternative diagnosis.

E. Treatment

Chemical injury of the liver occurring during pregnancy should be managed in a conservative way. In general, it should be managed as is the routine for nonpregnant patients. Specifically, immediate cessation of the suspected drug is mandatory and, if needed, supportive treatment should be started with attention to the possibility of hypoglycemia, bleeding and renal failure.

Except for acetaminophen poisoning (JANES and ROUTLEDGE 1992), there is no established specific treatment for liver drug reactions. Nonetheless, the use of acetylcysteine is recommended in all cases to replete glutathione stores.

When cholestasis dominates the clinical picture, cholestyramine, which traps hydrophopic material present in bile within the gut lumen, may be beneficial. On the other hand, it can disrupt the absorption of fat-soluble vitamins and the sex hormone homeostasis of pregnancy (KREEK 1970). Moreover, it may aggravate frequent gastrointestinal consequences of pregnancy (LAATIKAINEN 1978). Phenobarbital has been shown to partially reverse the estrogen-induced reduction in bile flow (KREEK 1987) that occurs during pregnancy and may improve cholestatic drug reactions in both pregnant and nonpregnant women (TREVISANI et al. 1988). However, the use of phenobarbital provides only limited benefit in the cholestasis associated with pregnancy (LAATIKAINEN 1978), and specific information on its use in pregnant women with drug-induced cholestasis is not available. Considering the depressant effect of phenobarbital on the central nervous system of the fetus, barbiturates are not widely used in pregnancy. *S*-Adenosyl-L-methionine (SAMe) is known to antagonize the cholestatic effect of ethynylestradiol without interfering with hormonal kinetics (DI PADOVA et al. 1982). Doses of 800mg/day of SAMe can improve the pruritus and biochemical measures of liver injury in cholestatic pregnant women without having any apparent adverse effect on the fetus (FREZZA et al. 1984). Therefore, this treatment represents a potentially useful approach to the clinical management of cholestasis influenced by medication and seen during pregnancy. The beneficial effect of ursodeoxycholic acid administration in the treatment of the cholestasis of pregnancy (PALMA et al. 1992) has encouraged the initiation of clinical trials on the use of this agent in individuals with iatrogenic cholestasis. The parenteral administration of vitamin K is recommended whenever prolonged cholestasis is present in a pregnant woman to prevent hypoprothrombin liver occurring in the fetus.

Liver transplantation is an option in the management of acute hepatic failure, which occurs in a pregnant woman (BOURLIERE et al. 1992; FAIR et al. 1990; MERRITT et al. 1991; MORENO et al. 1991; OCKNER et al. 1990). If a potentially life-threatening acute liver disease shows no signs of clinical improvement, this option should be considered even in a pregnant woman. Both mother and child have survived cases of drug-induced fulminant hepatic failure occurring in pregnant women who have required liver transplantation (BOURLIERE et al. 1988, 1992). A favorable outcome has been reported in a case of HBsAg-positive fulminant hepatic failure associated with the use of erythromycin in a pregnant woman (MERRITT et al. 1991).

F. Prevention

In clinical practice, the prevention of iatrogenic disease occurring during pregnancy is based on two different strategies. First, the selection of any treatment must consider not only the potential teratogenic effect but also the potential for an harmful effect for the mother. Several reviews of the pertinent literature can help the physician in making a choice (Beeley 1981; Berkowitz et al. 1981; Lewis and Zimmerman 1986; Witter and King 1984). Second, the use of "new" drugs for any condition during pregnancy should be avoided unless they are indispensable for managing an otherwise untreatable serious disease process. In conclusion, it is unrealistic to expect that pharmacologic agents can be avoided during pregnancy. Therefore, the potential for drug-induced liver diseases needs to be remembered. Because of methodologic problems, the data available concerning liver-associated drug reactions occurring in pregnant women remain a burning and somewhat neglected medical problem.

References

Adams E, Gfroerer JC, Rouse BA (1989) Epidemiology of substance abuse including alcohol and cigarette smoking. Ann NY Acad Sci 562:14–20

Beeley L (1981) Adverse effects of drugs in the later pregnancy. Clin Obstet Gynecol 8:275–290

Berkowitz RL, Coustan DR, Mochizuki TK (1981) Handbook for prescribing medications during pregnancy. Little Brown, Boston

Berthou F, Ratanasavanh D, Alix D, Carlhant D, Riche C, Guillouzo A (1988) Caffeine and theophylline metabolism in newborn and adult human hepatocytes: comparison with adult rat hepatocytes. Biochem Pharmacol 37:3691–3700

Bjornboe M, Iverson O, Olsen S (1967) Infected hepatitis jaundice in a municipal hospital during a five-year period. Acta Med Scand 182:491–501

Bodendorfer TW, Briggs GG, Gunning GE (1979) Obtaining drug exposure histories during pregnancy. Am J Obstet Gynecol 135:490–495

Borhanmanesh F, Haghighi P, Hekmat K, Rezaizadeh K, Ghavami AG (1973) Viral hepatitis during pregnancy: severity and effect on gestation. Gastroenterology 64:304–312

Bourliere M, Bernuau J, Rueff B, Benhamou JP (1988) Quinidine phenylethylbarbiturate-induced fulminant hepatitis in pregnant women. J Hepatol 6: 214–216

Bourliere M, Le Treut YP, Manelli JC, Botta-Fridlund D, Bertolino JG, Boubli L, Sanson D, Pol B, Briscot R, Gautheir AP (1992) Chlormezanone-induced fulminant hepatitis in pregnant women: successful delivery and liver transplantation. J Gastroenterol Hepatol 7:339–341

Brock WJ, Vore M (1982) Hepatic morphine and estrone glucuronyltransferase activity and morphine biliary excretion in the isolated perfused rat liver. Drug Metab Dispos 10:336–343

Brocklebank J, Raj WA, Federspiel CF, Shaffner W (1978) Drug prescribing during pregnancy. Obstet Gynecol 132:235

Carter DE, Goldman JM, Bressler R, Huxtable RJ, Christian CD, Heine MW (1973) Effect of oral contraceptives on drug metabolism. Clin Pharmacol Ther 13:22–31

Christiansen J, Mygind K, Munck O, Dam M (1977) Plasma levels of antiepileptic drugs in pregnancy. Epilepsia 18:295–301

Crawford JS, Rudofsky S (1966) Some alterations in the pattern of drug metabolism associated with pregnancy, oral contraceptives and the newly born. Br J Anesth 38:446–454

Dam M, Christiansen J, Munck O, Mygind KI (1979) Anti-epileptic drugs: metabolism in pregnancy. Clin Pharmacokinet 4:53–62

Davis JS, Kaufman RH (1966) Tetracycline toxicity: a clinicopathologic study with special reference to liver damage and its relationship to pregnancy. Am J Obstet Gynecol 95:523–529

Davison JM, Noble MCB (1981) Serial changes in 24-hour creatinine clearance during normal menstrual cycles and the first trimester of pregnancy. Br J Obstet Gynaecol 88:10–17

Deinhardt F, Gust ID (1982) Viral hepatitis. Bull WHO 60:661–691

Di Padova C, Tritapepe R, Cammareri G, Humpel M, Stramentinoli G (1982) S-Adenosyl-methionine antagonizes ethynylestradiol-induced bile cholesterol supersaturation in humans without modifying the estrogen plasma kinetics. Gastroenterology 82:223–227

Doering PL, Steward RB (1978) The extent and character of drug consumption during pregnancy. J Am Med Assoc 239:843–846

Dunlop W (1981) Serial changes in renal hemodynamics during normal human pregnancy. Br J Obstet Gynaecol 88:1–9

Eskes TKAB, Niijdam WS, Buys MJRM, van Rossum JM (1988) Prospective study of the use of medication during pregnancy in the Netherlands. In: Eskes TKAB, Finster M (eds) Drug therapy during pregnancy. Butterworths, London, p 1

Everson GT, McKinley C, Lawson M, Johnson M, Kern F Jr (1982) Gallbladder function in the human female: effect of the ovulatory cycle, pregnancy and contraceptive steroids. Gastroenterology 82:711–719

Fabricant ND (1960) Sexual functions and the nose. Am J Med Sci 239:498–502

Fair J, Klein AS, Feng T, Merritt WT, Burdick JF (1990) Intrapartum orthotopic liver transplantation with successful outcome of pregnancy. Transplantation 3:534–535

Fallon HJ (1988) Liver diseases. In: Burrow GN, Ferris TF (eds) Medical complications during pregnancy. Saunders, Philadelphia, p 318

Fletcher AP, Griffin GP (1991) International monitoring for adverse drug reactions of long latency. Adverse Drug React Toxicol Rev 10:209–230

Frezza M, Pozzato G, Chiesa L, Stramentinoli G, Di Padova C (1984) Reversal of intrahepatic cholestasis of pregnancy in women after high dose S-adenosyl-L-methionine administration. Hepatology 4:274–278

Hague WM, Fenton DW, Duncan SLB, Slater DN (1983) Acute fatty liver of pregnancy. J R Soc Med 76:652–661

Haibach H, Akter JE, Muscato MS, Cary PL, Hoffman MF (1984) Acetaminophen overdose with fetal demise. Am J Clin Pathol 82:240–242

Hall RE (1956) The treatment of hyperemesis gravidarum with chlorpromazine. Am J Obstet Gynecol 71:215–219

Hawker F (1993) Drugs and the liver. In: Hawker F (ed) The liver. Saunders, London, p 250

Hirsch HA, Herbst S, Lang R, Dettli L, Gablinger A (1974) Transfer of a new cephalosporin antibiotic to the fetus and the amniotic fluid during a continuous infusion (steady state) and single repeated intravenous injections to the mother. Arch Gynakol 216:1–14

Holden TE, Sherline DM (1972) Hepatitis and hepatic failure in pregnancy. Obstet Gynecol 40:586–593

Homeida M, Halliwell M, Branch RA (1978) Effects of an oral contraceptive on hepatic size and antipyrine metabolism in premenopausal women. Clin Pharmacol Ther 24:228–232

Honger PE, Rossing N (1969) Albumin metabolism and oral contraception. Clin Sci 36:41–45

Janes J, Routledge P (1992) Recent developments in the management of paracetamol (acetaminophen) poisoning. Drug Safety 7:170–177

Khalsa JF, Gfroerer J (1991) Epidemiology and health consequences of drug abuse among pregnant women. Semin Perinatol 15:265–270

Koff RS, Gardner R, Harinasuta U (1970) Profile of hyperbilirubinemia in free hospital populations. Clin Res 18:680–687

Krauer B, Karuer F, Hytten FE (1980) Drug disposition and pharmacokinetics in the maternal-placental-fetal units. Pharmacol Ther 10:301–328
Kreek MJ (1970) Binding of estradiol and other steroids to cholestyramine. Fed Proc 29:781–786
Kreek MJ (1987) Female sex steroids and cholestasis. Semin Liver Dis 7:8–23
Kurzen RB (1990) Can acetaminophen excess result in maternal and fetal toxicity? South Med J 83:953–955
Laatikainen T (1978) Effects of cholestyramine and phenobarbital on pruritus and serum bile acid levels in cholestasis of pregnancy. Am J Obstet Gynaecol 132: 501–506
Larrey D, Letteron P, Foliot A, Descatoire V, Degott C, Geneve J, Tinel M, Pessayre D (1986) Effects of pregnancy on the toxicity and metabolism of acetaminophen in mice. J Pharmacol Exp Ther 237:283–291
Le Bot MA, Begue JM, Kernaleguen D, Robert J, Ratanasavanh D, Airiau J, Riche C, Guillouzo A (1988) Different cytotoxicity and metabolism of doxorubicin, daunorubicin, epirubicin, esorubicin and idarubicin in cultured human and rat hepatocytes. Biochem Pharmacol 37:3877–3887
Levy G, Yacobi A (1974) Effect of plasma protein binding on elimination of warfarin. J Pharm Sci 63:805–806
Lewis JH, Zimmermann HJ (1986) Drug-induced jaundice during pregnancy. In: Rustgi WK, Cooper JN (eds) Gastrointestinal and hepatic complications in pregnancy. Wiley, New York, p 226
Lind T, Hytten FE (1969) Blood glucose following oral loads of glucose, maltose and starch during pregnancy. Proc Nutr Soc 28:64A
Little DM Jr, Wetstone HJ (1964) Anesthesia and the liver. Anesthesiology 25: 815–824
Martelli A, Allavena A, Robbiano L, Mattioli F, Brambilla G (1990) Comparison of the sensitivity of human and rat hepatocytes to the genotoxic effects of metronidazole. Pharmacol Toxicol 66:329–334
McCormack WM, George H, Donner A, Kodgis LF, Alpert S, Lowe EW, Kass EH (1977) Hepatotoxicity of erythromycin estolate during pregnancy. Antimicrob Agents Chemotherapy 12:630–635
McSherry CK, Morrissey KP, Suarm RL, May PS, Niemann WH, Gleen F (1976) Chenodeoxycholic acid induced liver injury in pregnant and neonatal baboons. Ann Surg 184:490–499
Merritt WT, Dickstein R, Beattie C, Burdick J, Klein A (1991) Liver transplantation during pregnancy: anesthesia for two procedures in the same patient with successful outcome of pregnancy. Transplant Proc 23:1996–1997
Miners JO, Robson RA, Birkett DJ (1986) Paracetamol metabolism in pregnancy. Br J Clin Pharmac 22:359–362
Moreno EG, Garcia GI, Gomez SR, Gonzales-Pinto I, Loinaz SC, Ibanez AJ, Perez Cerda F, Riano D, Colina E, Cisneros C (1991) Fulminant hepatic failure during pregnancy successfully treated by orthotopic liver transplantation. Transplantation 52:923–926
Morris CV, Goldstein RM, Cofer JB, Salomon H, Klintmalm GB (1989) An unusual presentation of fulminant hepatic failure secondary to propylthiouracil therapy. Clin Transplant 311–314
Munnell EW, Taylor CH (1947) Liver blood flow in pregnancy – hepatic vein catheterization. J Clin Invest 26:952–956
Nau H, Wittfoht W, Kuhnz W, Klinkmuller K, Rating D, Helge H (1981) Stable isotope-labelled analogues as probes into the pharmacokinetics and teratogenicity of valproic acid and primidone. 9th conference of the European Teratology Society, Sandoz, Basel, p 60
Newton M, Newton E (1988) Complications of drug therapy in gynecology and obstetrics. In: Newton M, Newton E (eds) Complication of gynecologic and obstetric management. Saunders Philadelphia, p 405

Ockner SA, Brunt EM, Cohn SM, Krul ES, Hanto DW, Peters MG (1990) Fulminant hepatic failure caused by acute fatty liver of pregnancy treated by orthotopic liver transplantation. Hepatology 11:59–64

O'Malley K, Stevenson IH, Crooks J (1972) Impairment of human drug metabolism by oral contraceptive steroids. Clin Pharmacol Ther 13:552–557

Palma J, Reyes H, Ribalta J, Iglesias J, Gonzales MC, Hernandez I, Alvarez C, Molina C, Danitz AM (1992) Effects of ursodeoxycholic acid in patients with intrahepatic cholestasis of pregnancy. Hepatology 15:1943–2047

Parry E, Shields R, Turnbull AC (1970) Transit time in the small intestine in pregnancy. J Obstet Gynecol Br Commonwealth 77:900–901

Peiker G, Traeger A (1974) Pharmacokinetics of phenobarbital in pregnancy. Zentralbl Gynakol 96:577–582

Pessayre D, Larrey D (1991) Drug-induced liver injury. In: McIntyre N, Benhamou JP, Bircher J, Rizzetto M, Rodes J (eds) Oxford textbook of clinical hepatology. Oxford University Press, Oxford, p 875

Philipson A (1979) Pharmacokinetics of antibiotics in pregnancy and labor. Clin Pharmacokinet 4:297–309

Pierce RJ, Cohen H (1988) Anesthesia considerations and complications in obstetric and gynecologic surgery. In: Newton M, Newton E (eds) Complications of gynecologic and obstetric management. Saunders, Philadelphia, p 480

Ramcharan S, Sponzilli EE, Wingerd JC (1976) Serum protein fraction. Effects of oral contraceptives and pregnancy. Obstet Gynecol 48:211–215

Ray DC, Drummond G (1991) Halothane hepatitis. Br J Anesth 67:84–99

Riely CA (1993) The liver in pregnancy. In: Schiff L, Shiff ER (eds) Diseases of the liver, 7th edn. Lippincott, Philadelphia, p 1411

Rogers MC, Willerson JT, Goldblatt A, Smith TW (1972) Serum digoxin concentrations in the human fetus, neonate and infant. N Engl J Med 287:1010–1013

Rowland JR, Binkerd PE, Hendricks AG (1990) Developmental toxicity and pharmacokinetics of oral and intravenous phenytoin in the rat. Reprod Toxicol 4:191–202

Rubinger D, Davidson JT, Melmed RN (1975) Hepatitis following the use of methoxyflurane in obstetric analgesia. Anesthesiology 43:593–595

Rustgi VK, Fagiuoli S, Van Thiel DH (1993) The liver in pregnancy. In: Rustgi VK, Van Thiel DH (eds) The liver in systemic disease. Raven, New York, p 267

Schultz JC, Adamson JS, Workman WW, Norman TD (1963) Fatal liver disease after intravenous administration of tetracycline in high dosage. N Engl J Med 269:999–1004

Sheehan HL (1950) Delayed chloroform poisoning. Br J Anesth 22:204–207

Shoenfield LJ, Lackin JM (1981) The Steering Committee, the National Cooperative Gallstone Study Group. Chenodiol (chenodeoxycholic acid) for dissolution of gallstones: the national cooperative gallstone study: a controlled trial of efficacy and safety. Ann Intern Med 95:257–282

Snider DE Jr, Layde PM, Johnson MW, Lyle MA (1980) Treatment of tuberculosis during pregnancy. Am Rev Respir Dis 122:65–79

Steven MM (1981) Pregnancy and liver disease. Gut 22:592–614

Stoehr GP, Kroboth PD, Juhl RP, Wender DB, Phillips JP, Smith RB (1984) Effect of oral contraceptives on triazolam, temazepam, alprazolam and lorazepam kinetics. Clin Pharmacol Ther 36:683–690

Stokes IM (1984) Paracetamol overdose in the second trimester of pregnancy: case report. Br J Obstet Gynaecol 91:286–288

Trevisani F, Pancione L, Bernardi M, Mazzetti M, Gasbarrini G (1988) Beta-lactam antibiotic-induced cholestasis: synergistic effect of phenobarbitone plus corticosteroid treatment. Ital J Gastroenterol 20:134–136

Valla D, Benhamou JP (1988) Drug-induced vascular and sinusoidal lesions of the liver. Baillieres Clin Gastroenterol 2:481–500

Van Thiel DH, Gavaler JS (1987) Pregnancy associated sex steroid and effects on the liver. Semin Liver Dis 7:1–7

Van Thiel DH, Schade RR (1986) Pregnancy: its physiologic course, nutrient course and effects on gastrointestinal function. In: Rustgi VK, Cooper JN (eds) Gastrointestinal and hepatic complications in pregnancy. Wiley, New York, p 1

Vore M, Montgomery C (1980) The effect of estradiol-17β treatment on the metabolism and abiliary excretion of phenytoin in the isolated perfused rat liver and in vivo. J Pharmacol Exper Ther 215:71–76

Vore M, Bauer J, Pascucci V (1978) The effect of pregnancy on the metabolism of [^{14}C]phenytoin in the isolated perfused rat liver. J Pharmacol Exp Ther 206:438–662

Watson KJR, Ghabrial H, Mashford ML (1986) The oral contraceptive pill increases morphine clearance but does not increase hepatic blood flow. Gastroenterology 90:1779 (abstract)

Watkins PB (1990) Role of cytochrome P450 in drug metabolism and hepatotoxicity. Semin Liver Dis 4:235–250

Wenk RE, Gebhardt FC, Bhagavan BS, Bhagavan BS, Lustgarten JA, McCarthy EF (1981) Tetracycline-associated fatty liver of pregnancy, including possible pregnancy risk after chronic dermatologic use of tetracycline. J Reprod Med 6:135–141

Williams C, Netzloff M, Folkers L, Vargas A, Garnica A, Frias J (1984) Vitamin D metabolism and anti-convulsivant therapy: effect of sunshine on incidence of osteomalacia. South Med J 77:834–836

Witter FR, King TM (1984) Drugs and the management of chronic diseases in the pregnant patients. In: Stern L (ed) Drug use in pregnancy. ADIS Health Science, Sydney, p 190

Wosilait WD (1974) An analysis of the effect of hypoalbuminemia on the amount of free drug in plasma for drugs bound at two sets of sites. Res Commun Chem Pathol Pharmacol 9:681–688

Zimmerman HJ (1978) Hepatotoxicity. The adverse effects of drugs and other chemicals on the liver. Appleton Century Crofts, New York

Zimmerman HJ, Ishak KJ (1982) Valproate-induced hepatic injury: analysis of 23 fatal cases. Hepatology 2:592–597

CHAPTER 13

Pediatric Hepatic Drug Reactions

E.A. Roberts

A. Classification of Drug Hepatotoxicity

Children are considered less susceptible to drug hepatotoxicity than adults. This is thought to be due to differences in their hepatic drug metabolism which protect against drug hepatotoxicity. However, most children take fewer medications than adults. Children are less likely to be obese; they generally do not smoke or drink. Drug hepatotoxicity does occur in children, and adolescents may be at equivalent risk for drug hepatotoxicity as adults. Difficulties in diagnosing drug hepatotoxicity in children, and consequent underreporting of these adverse drug reactions, may also contribute to the perceived rarity of pediatric hepatic drug reactions.

The biochemical basis of drug hepatotoxicity has been examined for many of the drugs causing liver damage in children. The mechanism of such drug hepatotoxicity often involves abnormalities in drug biotransformation which lead to increased production of toxic metabolite(s) or inadequate cytoprotective defenses. In children abnormal drug biotransformation is frequently due to an abnormal drug-metabolizing enzyme, inherited as a genetic trait. This pharmacogenetic defect becomes apparent only if the appropriate drug is administered. The target of the toxic metabolite determines the clinical features of the drug hepatotoxicity. Damage to hepatocellular organelles may cause cytotoxicity directly. Damage to hepatocellular membranes may initiate an immune response leading to an immunoallergic reaction similar to a hypersensitivity reaction. Damage to other cells composing the liver may lead to other patterns of hepatotoxicity.

In order to characterize drug hepatotoxicity on the basis of predictability, hepatotoxic agents should be categorized as follows: intrinsic hepatotoxin, contingent hepatotoxin and hepatotoxin eliciting an immunoallergic response. The intrinsic hepatotoxin is a predictable poison. Environmental xenobiotics are examples of intrinsic hepatotoxins. The contingent hepatotoxin causes hepatotoxicity only when hepatic drug metabolism has become abnormal to favor generation of toxic metabolites or to undermine detoxification pathways or other cytoprotective mechanisms. Hepatic drug biotransformation may be abnormal on an acquired or genetic basis. This category encompasses the category denoted as "metabolic idiosyncrasy" by others. A hepatotoxin eliciting an immunoallergic response causes hepatotoxicity accompanied by fever, eosinophilia and atypical lymphocytosis or hepatic granulomatosis: these findings imply some degree of dependency on the host immune response. These mechanisms are poorly understood and have been designated rather imprecisely as "hypersensitivity." Elaboration of autoantibodies, such as anti-liver/kidney microsomal antibodies, is another type of immunoallergic reaction. Some chemicals can act as different types of hepatotoxin under different circumstances. If the details of hepatic biotransformation are established for a given chemical, then it is possible to predict circumstances in which that chemical would function as a contingent hepatotoxin. Unfortunately, especially in the case of genetic defects, it is not always possible to identify abnormal hepatic biotransformation until after drug-induced hepatotoxicity has occurred. To the affected individual, the hepatotoxicity appears totally unpredictable.

B. Specific Drugs Causing Hepatotoxicity in Children

I. **Acetaminophen** (Intrinsic Hepatotoxin, Contingent Hepatotoxin)

A single large dose of acetaminophen is profoundly hepatotoxic in children as well as in adults. Acetaminophen is usually metabolized via sulfation and glucuronidation. The mechanism for acetaminophen hepatotoxicity involves production of a toxic metabolite (JOLLOW et al. 1973; MITCHELL et al. 1973a,b; POTTER et al. 1973). If a very large amount is taken, the glucuronidation and sulfation pathways are saturated, and an otherwise minor pathway through cytochromes P450 becomes quantitatively important. The product of this pathway is a highly reactive species *N*-acetyl-*p*-benzoquinoneimine (NAPQI) (MINER and KISSINGER 1979), a potent electrophile. It is conjugated by glutathione to form mercapturic acid, excreted in the urine. When cellular reserves of glutathione are used up, NAPQI reacts with cellular proteins. The clinical course of acute acetaminophen toxicity is distinctive. Immediately after the drug is taken, nausea and vomiting occur. These symptoms subside and then there is an asymptomatic interval of 1–2 days before hepatic damage becomes clinically apparent. At that point, jaundice with elevated serum aminotransferases and coagulopathy develops. Finally coma and renal failure may develop. Serum aminotransferases may be extremely high but still do not necessarily predict outcome.

The acute type of hepatotoxicity typically occurs in toddlers who ingest large numbers of pills from the medicine cabinet or in suicidal teenagers. There is an important second pattern of acetaminophen hepatotoxicity in children which is more subtle, a type of therapeutic misadventure. In these cases relatively large doses of acetaminophen (approximately 30–70 mg/kg) are administered at regular intervals (usually every 2–4 h) for 2–3 days, or longer, before hepatotoxicity becomes evident. Acute liver failure develops, but without the usual systemic signs of toxicity. The classic asymptomatic interval does not occur. Serum concentrations of acetaminophen are frequently *not* in a toxic range. Diagnosis is elusive unless a very meticulous drug history is taken. The acute liver failure may be attributed to other possible etiologies. The nomogram for treatment with *N*-acetylcysteine, commonly used in treatment of an acute overdose, does not easily apply in such situations. The estimate of the lethal per-kilogram dose (140mg/kg) is based on observations in adults and is probably not accurate for children. Estimating the elimination half-life of acetaminophen may be helpful. In general, it seems reasonable to treat with *N*-acetylcysteine as soon possible.

Young children appear to be quite resistant to acetaminophen hepatotoxicity and tend to recover when it does occur (MEREDITH et al. 1978; PETERSON and RUMACK 1981; RUMACK 1984). This may be due to differences in acetominophen metabolism in children. The elimination half-life is essentially the same in children and adults, although interindividual variation ranges as much as 1–3.5h (PETERSON and RUMACK 1978). The elimination half-life is somewhat longer (2.2–5.0h) in neonates. In early childhood, by contrast to adolescence and adulthood, sulfation predominates over glucuronidation (MILLER et al. 1976). The switch to the adult pattern occurs around 12 years of age. Nevertheless, in newborns urinary metabolites reflecting intermediates generated by cytochromes P450 can be found (LEDERMAN et al. 1983; ROBERTS et al. 1984). In vitro studies with fetal human hepatocytes have shown that these cytochrome P450-generated intermediates can be formed and conjugated to glutathione as early as at 18 weeks of gestation with a rate of formation approximately 10% of that in adult human hepatocytes. Among phase II detoxification processes only sulfation of acetaminophen can be detected in the human fetal liver cells (ROLLINS et al. 1979). Studies have shown less susceptibility to acetaminophen hepatotoxicity in the 11-day-old rat than in the adult rat (GREEN et al. 1984). In other studies, hepatocytes from young rats were found to have a higher basal capacity for synthesizing glutathione than those from older rats and also to be able to increase synthesis when glutathione was depleted (LAUTERBURG et al. 1980). It is possible that human infants have a greater capacity for synthesis of glutathione than adults.

Despite this relative resistance to this type of hepatotoxicity, young children can develop severe hepatotoxicity from acetaminophen. Some of these reports represent acute poisoning (ARENA et al. 1978; LIEH-LAI et al. 1984; HICKSON et al. 1983, 1989). Therapeutic misadventure due to inappropriate dosing is more common; it is sometimes described as "chronic" overdosage but the time frame for this chronicity is comparatively short, usually a few days (NOGEN and BREENER 1978; AGRAN et al. 1983; CLARK et al. 1983; GREENE et al. 1983; SWETNAM and FLORMAN 1984; SMITH et al. 1986; BLAKE et al. 1988; DE-NARDO et al. 1988; HENRETIG et al. 1989). The type of ingestion has not always been apparent despite histologically proven hepatotoxicity (WEBER and CUTZ 1980). Acetaminophen hepatotoxicity has also occurred in infants less than 2 months old (GREENE et al. 1983).

Hepatotoxicity and extreme prolongation of the elimination half-life of acetaminophen have also been found in infants born after maternal self-poisoning with acetaminophen (Lederman et al. 1983; Roberts et al. 1984).

Chronic alcoholics are more sensitive to acetaminophen than nonalcoholics and can develop subacute acetaminophen hepatotoxicity after taking ordinary therapeutic doses chronically (Seeff et al. 1986). Cytochrome P450 2E1, which is induced by ethanol, as well as P450 1A2, is capable of metablizing acetaminophen (Raucy et al. 1989) and thus enhances its toxicity. Adolescents drinking alcohol regularly may be at risk for this type of enhanced acetaminophen hepatotoxicity.

The antiviral drug zidovudine has been reported to increase acetaminophen hepatotoxicity, possibly by competing for glucuronidation pathways and forcing a switchover to the pathways mediated by cytochromes P450 (Shriner and Goetz 1992). Gunn rats, which are deficient in bilirubin UDP-glucuronosyl transferase, are more susceptible to acetaminophen hepatotoxicity than normal rats (De Morais and Wells 1988). Children with Crigler-Najjar syndrome or Gilbert's syndrome, usually not diagnosed until adolescence, may be more susceptible to acetaminophen hepatotoxicity, but this has not been proven conclusively.

II. **Phenytoin** (Contingent Hepatotoxin/Hepatotoxin-Eliciting Immunoallergic Response)

Phenytoin-induced hepatitis is not uncommon in children. It is the only drug-induced hepatitis mentioned specifically among adverse drug reactions in a large prospective study of adverse drug reactions in children (Mitchell et al. 1988). There are 17 cases of phenytoin hepatotoxicity reported in the literature (Powers and Carson 1987) and an additional 9 cases in children in whom hepatic dysfunction was incidental to other organ system involvement (Shear and Spielberg 1988).

Phenytoin hepatotoxicity presents as a hepatitic process associated with a drug hypersensitivity syndrome. Serum aminotransferases are elevated, and the patient may be moderately jaundiced. In severe cases clinical features of hepatic failure (coagulopathy, ascites, altered level of consciousness) are also present. The drug hypersensitivity syndrome typically includes fever, rash (such as morbiliform rash, Stevens-Johnson syndrome or toxic epidermal necrolysis), lymphadenopathy, leukocytosis, eosinophilia and atypical lymphocytosis. Histopathological examination of the liver shows spotty necrosis of hepatocytes, along with features reminiscent of mononucleosis in some case or of viral hepatitis in others. Parenchymal cholestasis may complicate more severe hepatocellular injury, and granulomas are sometimes found (Mullick and Ishak 1980). Reports of a diphenylhydantoin-induced cholestatic hepatitis are unconvincing. In severe cases treatment with high-dose corticosteroids has appeared effective in some patients, although this has not been tested in a controlled trial and anecdotal reports do not consistently show a clear benefit.

A toxic metabolite may be the cause of phenytoin hepatotoxicity. Phenytoin is metabolized via an arene oxide intermediate which is ordinarily metabolized and detoxified by epoxide hydrolase. This hypothesis has been investigated in vitro with lymphocytes, which are easy to isolate and retain most phase II detoxification pathways. When lymphocytes from persons who have developed the drug hypersensitivity syndrome to phenytoin are incubated in vitro in medium containing the intermediate metabolites of phenytoin generated by a murine microsomal system, these lymphocytes are killed to a greater extent than lymphocytes from normal control subjects (SPIELBERG et al. 1981a). If lymphocytes from normal individuals are pretreated with chemicals which inhibit cellular epoxide hydrolase, these lymphocytes become similar to those from affected individuals (SPIELBERG et al. 1981b). Studies of parents indicate an intermediate sensitivity to the toxic metabolite(s), consistent with an inherited defect in drug detoxification. Instead of only causing cell death, the toxic metabolite may bind to certain cellular proteins and create haptens for initiating an immune response. This may account for the features of a drug hypersensitivity syndrome clinically and for positive immune challenges noted by others (KLECKNER et al. 1875; KAHN et al. 1984). The finding of hepatic granulomas in some patients with phenytoin hepatotoxicity corroborates the importance of immune mechanisms in this adverse reaction. Phenytoin thus appears to be a contingent hepatotoxin which is capable of eliciting an immunoallergic response.

Three of four children reported with fatal diphenylhydantoin hepatotoxicity were taking phenobarbital at the same time. As in vitro studies indicate that some patients who cannot detoxify toxic intermediates of phenytoin are similarly sensitive to phenobarbital, this dual treatment may have made the hepatotoxicity worse. One further patient was switched from phenytoin to phenobarbital and then relapsed; he improved when high-dose corticosteroids were given along with the phenobarbital (POWERS and CARSON 1987).

III. **Valproic Acid** (Contingent Hepatotoxin?)

Valproic acid is an eight-carbon, branched fatty acid used as an anticonvulsant. It causes hepatotoxicity mostly in children (ZAFRANI and BERTHELOT 1982). A certain proportion of patients, estimated at 11% overall (POWELL-JACKSON et al. 1984), develop abnormal serum aminotransferases usually within a short time of starting treatment. This dose-responsive biochemical abnormality resolves when the dose of valproic acid is decreased. Rarely, some patients develop progressive liver failure which may resemble Reye's syndrome clinically (GERBER et al. 1979; SUCHY et al. 1979). This severe hepatotoxicity usually does not improve when the drug is withdrawn and is frequently fatal in children (ZAFRANI and BERTHELOT 1982; ZIMMERMAN and ISHAK 1982; POWELL-

JACKSON et al. 1984; DREIFUSS et al. 1987; SCHEFFNER et al. 1988). It cannot be predicted by regular monitoring of serum aminotransferases and other liver function tests (GREEN 1984). The time from initiating treatment with valproic acid to onset of liver disease is usually less than 4 months, but longer duration of treatment does not preclude hepatotoxicity. Specific risk factors in children include age under 2 years, multiple anticonvulsant treatment along with valproic acid, and coexistent medical problems such as severe developmental delay or congenital abnormalities (DREIFUSS et al. 1987). Hyperammonemia, usually not associated with liver failure, is another metabolic adverse effect of valproic acid (COULTER and ALLEN 1981; KONDO et al. 1992a). In one child with Down's syndrome, however, hyperammonemia was associated with hepatotoxicity and other systemic toxicities of valproic acid (KANE et al. 1992).

The clinical presentation of the severe hepatotoxicity resembles hepatitis: malaise, anorexia, nausea and vomiting. Seizure control may deteriorate during this time. Coagulopathy often develops early. Clinical jaundice tends to develop later, along with other signs of progressive hepatic insufficiency such as ascites and hypoglycemia. Death due to liver failure, complicated by renal failure or infection, is frequent. Liver transplantation has been performed. Liver histology reviewed in one large series (ZIMMERMAN and ISHAK 1982) shows evidence of extensive hepatocellular necrosis, sometimes zonal. Remaining hepatocytes appear extremely damaged. Acidophilic bodies, ballooned hepatocytes and cholangiolar proliferation may be present. Microvesicular steatosis is common in addition to the features of cell necrosis. The mitochondria in hepatocytes may be so prominent on light microscopy that the hepatocytes have a granular, eosinophilic appearance. In cases presenting clinically like Reye's syndrome, fever, coagulopathy, progressive loss of consciousness, severe acidosis and variably abnormal aminotransferases are present, but the patient is not jaundiced (GERBER et al. 1979). Hepatocellular necrosis, as well as microvesicular fat, is found on histological examination of the liver, unlike the histological findings of Reye's syndrome. The succinate dehydrogenase stain, reflecting mitochondrial function, is negative in Reye's syndrome but positive in drug-induced Reye's-like hepatotoxicity. By electron microscopy, mitochondrial changes associated with valproic acid toxicity differ from those found in Reye's syndrome.

The mechanism of this severe hepatotoxicity appears to involve generation of toxic metabolite(s) plus some type of metabolic idiosyncrasy rendering the individual susceptible. Metabolic idiosyncrasy is probable not only because severe hepatotoxicity is rare but because toxic ingestions do not necessarily lead to liver necrosis (SCHNABEL et al. 1984). Valproic acid is extensively metabolized in the liver (EADIE et al. 1988). Glucuronidation is a major pathway of biotransformation. Since it is fatty acid, valproic acid also can undergo mitochondrial or peroxisomal β-oxidation. Mitochondrial metabolism is the more important. Valproic acid passes through the mitochondrial membrane spontaneously and is converted to its coenzyme A (CoA) thioester in the mitochondrial matrix. The major product of mitochondrial metabolism, 2-propylpentanoyl-CoA, can be hydrolyzed to form valproic acid again or conjugated to carnitine and excreted (LI et al. 1991). Two other pathways, ω- and ω_1-hydroxylation, are associated with microsomes, that is, with cytochromes P450.

Valproic acid and more specifically its partially unsaturated metabolite 4-en-valproic acid (4-en-VPA) are related structurally to two known hepatotoxins: hypoglycin, which is associated with Jamaican vomiting sickness, a Reyes-like hepatopathy with microvesicular steatosis, and 4-pentenoic acid, which causes microvesicular steatosis in rat liver and inhibits β-oxidation. 4-en-VPA is produced by δ-dehydrogenation, which is a minor pathway of valproic acid metabolism. In rat liver a cytochrome P450-associated pathway has been described in which 4-en-valproate is formed directly from valproic acid (RETTIE et al. 1987). Formation of 4-en-VPA has also been demonstrated in a primate model (RETTENMEIER et al. 1986) and in patients with liver failure associated with valproic acid treatment. Several metabolites of valproic acid including 4-en-VPA have been shown to be toxic to isolated rat hepatocytes (KINGSLEY et al. 1983). Administration of 4-en-VPA to rats caused accumulation of microvesicular fat in hepatocytes along with changes in hepatocyte organelles, including mitochondrial abnormalities and elaboration of myeloid bodies (KESTERSON et al. 1984). In the same model 4-en-VPA caused inhibition of β-oxidation, although not to the same extent as hypoglycin (GRANNEMAN et al. 1984). Valproic acid and 4-en-VPA have been shown to be toxic to human liver cells in in vitro testing. Increased susceptibility to 4-en-VPA and VPA toxicity was demonstrated in weanling compared to adult rats and in liver tissue from younger patients (FISHER et al. 1994). 4-en-VPA, but not 2-en-VPA, has also been shown to deplete glutathione in the rat (KASSAHUN et al. 1994). Thus valproic acid and its metabolite(s) are capable of causing adverse changes in liver cell metabolism which may lead to observed features of this hepatotoxicity. Similarities and differences in these metabolic toxicities compared to the toxic effects of hypoglycin and 4-pentenoic acid reflect the complexity of this metabolic system.

Investigations of valproic acid metabolism in patients with severe hepatotoxicity indicate that β-oxidation is inhibited (BÖHLES et al. 1982; KOCHEN et al. 1983; EADIE et al. 1990), but the step in β-oxidation at which the apparent block has occurred varies from person to person (EADIE et al. 1990). Increased amounts of 4-en-VPA have been measured in some cases (KOCHEN et al. 1983; DICKINSON et al. 1985; KEULEN and KOCHEN 1985). In one case increased propylglutaric acid, the product of a cytochrome P450-associated pathway, was also found (EADIE et al. 1990). These observations suggest β-oxidation is inhibited and alternative pathways including those associated with cytochromes P450 and δ-dehydrogenation are utilized producing 4-en-VPA and other metabolites. Valproic acid itself can inhibit mitochondrial β-oxidation. People having anomalous mitochondrial β-oxidation may be more susceptible to this adverse metabolic effect of valproic acid (APPLETON et al. 1990). Inherited variation in branched-chain amino acid metabolism may also be important (ANDERSON et al. 1994). Studies of valproic acid toxicity in vitro in human liver slices indicate important interindividual variation in susceptibility to toxicity (FISHER et al. 1991). An intercurrent environmental problem, such as a viral illness, might additionally inhibit β-oxidation. Experimental data in the ornithine transcarbamylase-deficient mouse support the hypothesis of an intrinsic metabolic defect in the mitochondrion. The ornithine transcarbamylase-deficient mouse develops hepatocellular necrosis and microvesicular steatosis at doses of valproic acid which do not affect the normal control adversely (QURESHI et al. 1985). These data may provide a clue to possible metabolic abnormalities in humans. Ornithine transcarbamylase deficiency may be one such definable abnormality and has been suspected in some patients (HJELM et al. 1986; KAY et al. 1986). Another child with deficient cytochrome *c* oxidase and valproic acid hepatotoxicity has been reported (CHABROL et al. 1994). Administration of drugs which strongly induce cytochromes P450 (such as phenytoin, phenobarbital or carbamazepine) could magnify the effect of inhibiting mitochondrial β-oxidation and shunting into cytochrome P450-associated pathways (LEVY et al. 1990).

In summary, valproic acid is an example of a drug in which juvenile patterns of drug metabolism may enhance the risk of drug hepatotoxicity, conventional concomitant drug treatment induces potentially noxious pathways of valproic acid metabolism, and undiagnosed genetic variation in hepatocellular metabolism may also increase the risk of production of toxic metabolites. Valproic acid appears to be a contingent hepatotoxin. Valproic acid hepatotoxicity has a hepatitic pattern and may be very severe in some persons. In the severe form of hepatotoxicity mitochondrial β-oxidation is inhibited, and pathways capable of producing toxic products may assume more importance quantitatively. Interindividual variation in mitochondrial function may determine susceptibility to inhibition of β-oxidation. Although inhibition of β-oxidation has important adverse consequences in itself, it does not appear sufficient to explain all the features of valproic acid hepatotoxicity. The toxic metabolite 4-en-VPA appears to inhibit β-oxidation further and cause direct cellular damage. However, the exact mechanism of valproic acid hepatotoxicity remains uncertain. Detoxification processes, namely conjugation to glutathione, may also be important in humans (KASSAHUN et al. 1991). Enhanced production of 4-en-VPA due to induction of cytochromes P450 by drugs such as diphenylhydantion or carbamazepine may also contribute. Elevated valproic acid concentrations may also affect its own metabolism (ANDERSON et al. 1992; KONDO et al. 1992b).

Decreased serum carnitine has been found in valproic acid hepatotoxicity (BÖHLES et al. 1982; MURPHY et al. 1985). Serum carnitine is also low in patients treated chronically, without any clinical evidence of hepatotoxicity (MURPHY et al. 1985; MATSUDA et al. 1986; BEGHI et al. 1990). In one study, administration of carnitine to children receiving valproic acid normalized acyl-

/free carnitine ratios but did not affect certain biochemical features associated with abnormal mitochondrial β-oxidation (KOSSAK et al. 1993). Conjugation to carnitine is a minor metabolic pathway for valproic acid (MILLINGTON et al. 1985). It seems unlikely that this pathway is important for the development of hepatotoxicity. It is not known whether carnitine repletion is effective as treatment for severe hepatotoxicity, but limited reported experience suggests it is not (LAUB et al. 1986; MURPHY et al. 1993). Recent studies suggest that administration of carnitine plus pantothenic acid can reverse the inhibition of β-oxidation caused by valproic acid in mouse pup liver (THURSTON and HAUHART 1992). Pantothenic acid acid and carnitine are both important in the production of acetyl CoA, depleted by valproic acid in this model. Whether these supplements would benefit young patients receiving valproic acid remains to be determined.

IV. **Isoniazid** (Contingent Hepatotoxin?)

Isoniazid (INH) has been associated with a wide spectrum of hepatotoxicity in adults (MADDREY and BOITNOTT 1973; MITCHELL et al. 1976). The most common abnormality is asymptomatic elevation of serum aminotransferases. Overt symptoms of hepatitis (fatigue, anorexia, nausea and vomiting) indicate severe disease; mortality is >10% in patients with jaundice (ZIMMERMAN 1990). INH hepatotoxicity is generally considered to be more common in adults than in children; however, there are numerous reports of INH hepatotoxicity, including fatal hepatic necrosis, in children either being treated for tuberculosis or receiving prophylaxis (RUDOY et al. 1973; CASTEELS-VAN DAELE et al. 1975; LITT et al. 1976; VANDERHOOF and AMENT 1976; PESSAYRE et al. 1977; WALKER and PARK-HAH 1977). In large studies of children receiving INH alone as prophylaxis against tuberculosis, the incidence of INH hepatotoxicity (indicated by abnormal serum aminotransferases) was 7% in a series of 369 children (BEAUDRY et al. 1974) and 17.1% in 239 patients aged 9–14 years (SPYRIDIS et al. 1979). This is nearly equivalent to the incidence in adults. Hepatic dysfunction is common in children being treated with INH plus rifampicin for tuberculosis. Thirty-six of 44 patients receiving INH plus rifampicin had some elevation of serum aminotransferases and 15 patients (42%) of these were jaundiced (TSAGAROPOULOU-STINGA et al. 1985). In another study, 37% had hepatotoxicity including four of seven children <17 months old (MARTINEZ-ROIG et al. 1986). These children received conventional doses of INH and rifampicin, as well as brief sequential courses of streptomycin and ethambutal. As in adults, hepatotoxicity typically developed in the first 2–3 months of treatment. Children with more severe tuberculosis seem to be at greater risk for hepatotoxicity, especially when tuberculous menigitis occurs (O'BRIEN et al. 1983).

Isoniazid hepatotoxicity appears to be due to a toxic metabolite, but the mechanism has not yet been determined. Metabolism by cytochromes P450 may also be implicated since rifampicin, a potent inducer of the P450 3A subfamily, may also enhance INH toxicity (Pessayre et al. 1977). Acetylation via the polymorphic *N*-acetyltransferase (NAT-2) is important in INH metabolism but whether rapid or slow acetylators are at greater risk for INH hepatotoxicity remains uncertain. If acetylisoniazid or its derivatives are toxic, rapid acetylators should be at greater risk for INH hepatotoxicity (Mitchell et al. 1976). This has not been confirmed in adults (Gurumurthy et al. 1984) or in children (Martinez-Roig et al. 1986). Hydrazine, derived from INH via a cytochrome P450-associated pathway, has been proposed as the toxic agent (Lauterburg et al. 1985; Sarma et al. 1986). Free plasma concentrations of hydrazine are higher in slow acetylators than in rapid acetylators (Beever et al. 1982). If hydrazine is the toxic intermediate, then hepatotoxicity from INH should be worse in slow acetylators. Multiple reports in children again show no clear pattern of hepatotoxicity in relation to acetylator status (Seth and Beotra 1989). Variable effects of coadministered drugs and individual patterns of drug metabolism may account for the lack of a clear pattern of susceptibility to INH hepatotoxicity.

V. **Halothane** (Hepatotoxin-Eliciting Immunoallergic Response)

Halothane hepatotoxicity is classically hepatitic and shows two major clinical patterns. One is asymptomatic hepatitis indicated only by abnormal serum aminotransferases in the 1st or 2nd week after the anesthetic exposure. The other pattern is severe hepatitis with extensive hepatocyte necrosis and liver failure (Moult and Sherlock 1975). Halothane is commonly used in pediatric anesthetic practice. Large retrospective studies in children estimate the incidence is at approximately 1:80000–1:200000 (Wark 1983; Warner et al. 1984), in contrast to 1:4000–1:30000 in adults (Farrell et al. 1985). Eight cases have been documented in detail in children aged 11 months to 15 years, all of whom had multiple exposures to halothane. One child died of fulminant liver failure but all others recovered (Kenna et al. 1987; Hassall et al. 1990; Wark 1991). In addition, there are three cases of halothane hepatitis found retrospectively (Wark 1983; Warner et al. 1984) and three further children who succumbed to fulminant hepatic failure after halothane (Campbell et al. 1977; Inman and Mushin 1978; Psacharopoulos et al. 1980). A further nine possible cases are difficult to evaluate because of inadequate data or concomitant complicated systemic disease.

Halothane is metabolized by various cytochromes P450 and toxic metabolites are generated (DeGroot and Noll 1983; Farrell 1988; Pohl et al. 1988). Reductive metabolism generates a toxic intermediate identified as a chlorotrifluoroethyl radical which leads to lipid peroxidation, and oxidative metabolism generates a trifluoroacetyl (TFA) intermediate which can acetylate cellular membranes, thus generating TFA adducts. This oxidative pathway appears to be associated with hepatocellular membrane damage and immune phenomena typical of the clinical hepatotoxicity syndrome. TFA adducts can be identified with fluorescent-tagged antibodies in rats, mainly in hepatocytes in Rappaport zone 3 after phenobarbital pretreatment and also on the hepatocyte plasma membrane (SATOH et al. 1985; SATOH et al. 1989; MARTIN et al. 1993; GUT et al. 1993). Antibodies to these neoantigens have been identified in sera from adults with halothane hepatitis (KENNA et al. 1988a). Further studies have shown that neoantigens analogous to these neoantigens derived from halothane-treated animals are expressed in human liver in individuals exposed to halothane (KENNA et al. 1988b). Elaboration of TFA-associated neoantigens in rat and human hepatocytes in vitro has recently been reported (VANPELT and KENNA 1994; ILYIN et al. 1994). Studies in rats also suggest that factors such as gender and previous exposure to specific inducers of cytochromes P450 may influence the expression of halothane-associated neoantigens (KENNA et al. 1990). Kupffer cells may play a role in the process by which the TFA adducts initiate an immune response (CHRISTEN et al. 1991). HLA phenotype may be important (BERSON et al. 1994). Children may be less likely to form these neoantigens because they tend to be more immunotolerant than adults.

VI. **Carbamazepine** (Contingent Hepatotoxin/Hepatotoxin-Eliciting Immunoallergic Response)

Carbamazepine is a dibenzazepine derivative, similar structurally to imipramine in that it has fundamentally a tricyclic chemical structure. Although granulomatous hepatitis is reported in adults, in children the usual clinical picture has been hepatitis, sometimes associated with a drug hypersensitivity syndrome similar to that of phenytoin. Two children had a mononucleosis-like illness consisting of rash, lymphadenopathy, hepatosplenomegaly and neutropenia (LEWIS and ROSENBLOOM 1982; BRAIN et al. 1984). A girl treated at the Hospital for Sick Children (Toronto) presented with fever, rash, incipient liver failure, lymphopenia and eosinophilia. Rechallenge of her lymphocytes in vitro with metabolites of carbamazepine provided evidence of defective detoxification mechanisms. An infant boy also was seen at this hospital with only a hepatitic type of toxicity from carbamazepine. Three other children with drug hypersensitivity to carbamazepine (where hepatitis was not the dominant clinical feature) were described (SHEAR and SPIELBERG 1988). Severe hepatotoxicity has also been reported in children. One child died with progressive liver failure when carbamazepine was not stopped soon enough (ZUCKER et al. 1977). Four children with fatal acute liver failure were taking carbamazepeine, phenytoin and primidone (SMITH et al. 1988). More recently severe hepatitis was reported in three children taking only carbamazepine: one recovered with corticosteroid treatment but the others died or required liver transplant (HADZIC et al. 1990).

Like phenytoin and phenobarbital, carbamazepine may be metabolized via arene oxides. These intermediates are ordinarily detoxified by epoxide hydrolase. Persons with an inherited metabolic idiosyncrasy, possibly involving an abnormal epoxide hydrolase, may be unable to detoxify active metabolite(s) of carbamazepine and thus develop hepatotoxicity. The same metabolic idiosyncrasy which renders them susceptible to carbamazepine hepatotoxicity places them at risk for phenytoin and phenobarbital hepatotoxicity. This may explain the fatal hepatotoxicity reported in children on multiple antiepileptics, since primidone contains phenobarbital (Smith et al. 1988).

VII. **Phenobarbital** (Contingent Hepatotoxin)

Phenobarbital hepatitis is comparatively rare. When it occurs, it is usually associated with a multisystemic drug hypersensitivity syndrome, but it may dominate the clinical picture (McGeachy and Bloomer 1953; Evans et al. 1976; Shapiro et al. 1980). Six of 12 patients reported in the world literature were children. Three additional children, a girl aged 3 years and boys aged 10 and 18 months, have been treated at the Hospital for Sick Children (Toronto); all had severe hepatic dysfunction with coagulopathy or ascites but ultimately survived (Roberts et al. 1990). In most cases with clinically significant hepatotoxicity, jaundice began within 8 weeks of starting phenobarbital, along with generalized rash and fever. Eosinophilia and other systemic involvement may occur. Usually the liver disease was moderately severe but self-limited; however, one child died of fulminant hepatic failure. One child developed chronic liver disease.

The mechanism of phenobarbital-induced hepatotoxicity remains unclear. Results from in vitro rechallenge of lymphocytes indicate an inherited defect in detoxification of an active metabolite. Phenobarbital may also be metabolized via arene oxide intermediates, which are typically detoxified via epoxide hydrolase. In in vitro rechallenge, if lymphocyte epoxide hydrolase is inhibited, the extent of cytotoxicity of metabolites generated from phenobarbital, as from phenytoin, increases (Spielberg et al. 1981b).

Persons who develop hepatotoxicity from phenobarbital typically develop adverse reactions from other barbiturates. Sedation for a diagnostic procedure in a child is an important opportunity for such a drug exposure. Additionally, persons who develop hepatitis from phenobarbital may also be likely to develop hepatitis from carbamazepine or phenytoin.

VIII. Antineoplastic Drugs

Many drugs used to treat neoplasia in childhood can cause hepatotoxicity (Menard et al. 1980; Perry 1982; Sznol et al. 1987). Drug hepatotoxicity is difficult to evaluate because these drugs are rarely used separately and patients receiving them are often susceptible to many types of liver damage. A hepatitic pattern, often asymptomatic with elevation in serum aminotransferases and no other evidence of severe liver toxicity, is common. Antineoplastic drugs which frequently produce asymptomatic elevation of aminotransferases include nitrosoureas, 6-mercaptopurine, cytosine arabinoside, *cis*-platinum and dacarbazine (DTIC). Cyclophosphamide may cause a hepatitic reaction: it appears to be dose related (HONJO et al. 1988). Adriamycin, dactinomycin and vinca alkaloids are infrequently associated with hepatotoxicity. However, several patients treated at the Hospital for Sick Children (Toronto) with dactinomycin have developed severe hepatic dysfunction, with extremely elevated serum aminotransferases and coagulopathy, all of which resolved spontaneously off drug. Irradiation may enhance hepatotoxicity of dactinomycin (McVEAGH and EKERT 1975). Adriamycin given together with 6-mercaptopurine may increase the hepatotoxic potential of 6-mercaptopurine (MINOW et al. 1976).

L-Asparaginase has been associated with more severe damage characterized by severe steatosis, hepatocellular necrosis and fibrosis. This is usually reversible after the L-asparaginase is stopped (PRATT and JOHNSON 1971). L-Asparaginase is an intrinsic hepatotoxin: the most likely mechanism of hepatotoxicity is profound interference with hepatocellular protein metabolism. Mithramycin has been associated with acute hepatic necrosis (KENNEDY 1970). Thrombocytopenia and acute liver failure have been reported in an 18-year-old patient receiving carboplatin (HRUBAN et al. 1991).

Veno-occlusive disease is associated with antineoplastic drugs. Veno-occlusive disease presents acutely with an enlarged tender liver, ascites or unexplained weight gain, and jaundice; serum aminotransferases may be elevated. Thioguanine is a classic cause of veno-occlusive disease and its toxicity may be enhanced by drug interactions with other antineoplastic drugs (PENTA et al. 1977). Other antineoplastic agents including cytosine arabinoside, busulfan, DTIC and carmustine (BCNU) have been associated with veno-occlusive disease at conventional or high doses (ROLLINS 1986). Currently, veno-occlusive disease most frequently develops after allogeneic bone marrow transplantation. Irradiation by itself can lead to veno-occlusive disease (EVANS et al. 1976) possibly because endothelial cells lining hepatic sinusoids are more sensitive to radiation than hepatocytes. The combination of irradiation and chemotherapy in conditioning regimens may lead to earlier development of veno-occlusive disease than after single-agent (irradiation or chemical) injury (McDONALD et al. 1985). Methotrexate plus cyclosporine (as prophylaxis for graft-versus-host disease) in patients prepared for bone marrow transplant by a regimen using busulfan and cyclophosphamide led to a higher incidence of jaundice and veno-occlusive disease than methylprednisolone and cyclosporine prophylaxis in a busulfan-methotrexate regimen (ESSELL et al. 1992). Clinical predictors of likelihood for development of veno-occlusive disease in children have not yet been identified, although ongoing hepatitis prior to transplant may increase susceptibility to hepatic damage. Veno-occlusive disease due to dacarbazine appears to involve damage to endothelial cells through production of toxic metabolite(s) in the endothelial cells; glutathione appears to protect against toxicity (DELEVE and KAPLOWITZ 1991).

IX. Pemoline

Although pemoline has been associated with asymptomatic elevation of aminotransferases (Sampson 1975) and in one study liver biopsy revealed steatosis and focal hepatocellular necrosis (Tolman et al. 1973), more recent reports describe acute hepatitic reactions of variable severity (Elitsur 1990; Pratt and Dubois 1990). The largest series documenting hepatitis included one patient who died with fulminant hepatic failure (Nehra et al. 1990); males predominated. Two other deaths associated with hepatic dysfunction while on pemoline have been reported. Both patients were boys: one may have had previous chronic liver disease and the other may have taken an overdose of pemoline (Jaffe 1989). Three cases have recently been seen at the Hospital for Sick Children (Toronto) in the past few years: a young boy with anicteric hepatitis with serum aminotransferases elevated 20 times the upper limits of normal, another boy with clinical jaundice and hepatitis, and a further case of fulminant hepatic failure in an adolescent boy. Both children with hepatitis recovered after the drug was stopped, but the patient with fulminant hepatic failure required liver transplant. The mechanism of this hepatotoxicity is not known. Aminotransferases should be monitored during treatment with pemoline. If aminotransferases become elevated, pemoline should be discontinued.

X. Sulfonamides (Contingent Hepatotoxin, Hepatotoxin-Eliciting Immunoallergic Response)

Any sulfonamide can cause hepatotoxicity. Children are most commonly treated with these drugs for otitis media and upper respiratory infections or for inflammatory bowel disease. Sulfanilamide, trimethoprim-sulfamethoxazole and pyrimethamine-sulfadoxine have all been reported as causing significant hepatotoxicity (Dujovne et al. 1967; Shear et al. 1986; Zitelli et al. 1987). Sulfasalazine has been associated with severe liver disease in adolescents and young adults (Sotolongo et al. 1978; Losek and Werlin 1981; Ribe et al. 1986). In some cases acute liver failure occurred, sometimes fatal. The spectrum of sulfa-associated liver toxicity also includes asymptomatic elevation of serum aminotransferases and granulomatous hepatitis. A bland cholestatic pattern has sometimes been reported (Ghishan 1983; Kowdley et al. 1992). In general, sulfa-hepatotoxicity is associated with a systemic hypersensitivity reaction. Fever, significant rash, periorbital edema, atypical lymphocytosis, lymphadenopathy and renal dysfunction with proteinuria all may occur. However, the incidence of hepatotoxicity associated with erythromycin/sulfisoxazole is not clear.

Sulfonamide hepatotoxicity is due to elaboration of an electrophilic toxic metabolite in the liver. The toxic metabolite appears to be a reactive species, possibly the nitroso, derived from the hydroxylamine metabolite of the particular sulfonamide (RIEDER et al. 1989; CRIBB et al. 1990). The hydroxylamine metabolite of sulfamethoxazole has been identified in humans, and microsomes prepared from human liver specimens generate this metabolite in the presence of NADPH (CRIBB and SPIELBERG 1992). Some patients who developed sulfa-hepatotoxicity have been shown to be slow acetylators (in the rapid/slow polymorphism for NAT-2) as well as being unable to detoxify this reactive metabolite. Upon in vitro rechallenge of their lymphocytes with sulfonamide metabolites generated by murine microsomes, the patient's lymphocytes show significantly more cytotoxicity than control lymphocytes (SHEAR et al. 1986). Glutathione appears to be important for detoxifying the toxic intermediate (SHEAR and SPIELBERG 1985; RIEDER et al. 1988).

XI. **Aspirin** (Intrinsic Hepatotoxin?)

Hepatotoxicity had been associated with high-dose aspirin treatment. Hepatotoxicity is dose dependent, and not limited to patients with rheumatoid disease. Approximately 60% of the 300 reported cases have been in patients with juvenile rheumatoid arthritis (not all children) and a further 10% have occurred in children with acute rheumatic fever (BENSON 1983). Rheumatological diseases may predispose to aspirin hepatotoxicity. Chronic inflammation may generate oxygen radicals (PARKE 1987).

In most cases salicylate hepatotoxicity has hepatitic features with anorexia, nausea, vomiting, abdominal pain and elevated serum aminotransferases (SEAMAN et al. 1974; ZUCKER et al. 1975; DOUGHTY et al. 1980; BARRON et al. 1982; HAMDAN et al. 1985). Hepatomegaly, sometimes tender, is present. Progressive signs of liver damage such as jaundice and coagulopathy are rare. Even in uncomplicated cases serum aminotransferase levels may be greater than 1000 IU (DOUGHTY et al. 1980). In some cases encephalopathy (not related to Reye's syndrome) has been present (PETTY et al. 1978; ULSHEN et al. 1978). Liver histology typically shows a nonspecific picture with acute, focal hepatocellular necrosis (SEAMAN et al. 1974). Clinical and laboratory abnormalities resolve when aspirin is stopped.

XII. **Propylthiouracil** (Contingent Hepatotoxin?, Hepatotoxin-Eliciting Immunoallergic Response)

Five cases of prophylthiouracil (PTU) hepatotoxicity have been reported in children and three additional children with PTU hepatotoxicity have been treated at the Hospital for Sick Children (Toronto): all were girls (PARKER 1975; REDDY 1979; GARTY et al. 1985; JONAS and EDISON 1988). The clinical presentation includes nonspecific symptoms of hepatitis such as anorexia, nausea, vomiting and jaundice. Aminotransferases are moderately elevated.

Symptoms typically begin within 2–3 months of starting treatment, but in one child treated at the Hospital for Sick Children (Toronto) liver disease began at least 9 months after starting treatment and in one reported case liver disease was not apparent until 15 months after beginning PTU (Maggiore et al. 1989). Asymptomatic elevation of aminotransferases may be the earliest sign of hepatotoxicity, and these should be checked regularly throughout the first 3–6 months of treatment.

Several cases of PTU-associated liver disease in adults have been called "chronic active hepatitis," but data presented do not satisfy rigorous diagnostic criteria. A more convincing case of PTU hepatotoxicity associated with "chronic active hepatitis" has been reported in a child who developed urticaria during treatment with methimazole and non-icteric hepatomegaly with elevated aminotransferases after more than 1 year of treatment with PTU (Maggiore et al. 1989). Liver biopsy revealed portal inflammation and moderate piecemeal necrosis; stopping the PTU and treating with corticosteroids led to prompt clinical improvement in the liver disease. Anti-smooth muscle antibodies and anti-liver/kidney microsomal (anti-LKM1) antibodies were not detected. (Anti-LKM antibodies should be checked whenever PTU-induced chronic active hepatitis is suspected because autoimmune thyroid disease is more likely to occur with autoimmune hepatitis type 2.)

XIII. Erythromycin

All forms of erythromycin are potentially hepatotoxic (Zafrani et al. 1979; Keeffe et al. 1982; Funck-Brentano et al. 1983; Diehl et al. 1984; Derby et al. 1993). The clinical presentation is similar regardless of which erythromycin ester is involved: anorexia, nausea, jaundice and abdominal pain, predominantly in the right upper quadrant. The overall clinical appearance is that of a mixed hepatitic-cholestatic process, which may be severe enough to suggest biliary tract obstruction. Hepatomegaly, sometimes accompanied by splenomegaly, appears to be common in children (Funck- Brentano et al. 1983). A single report of erythromycin ethylsuccinate hepatotoxicity in a child described relatively mild, self-limited disease (Phillips 1983).

XIV. Methotrexate (Intrinsic Hepatotoxin, Contingent Hepatotoxin?)

Chronic low-dose treatment with methotrexate, as used in psoriasis or certain connective tissue diseases, frequently causes hepatic fibrosis with steatosis (Whiting-O'keefe et al. 1991). The histological appearance may be similar to that of alcoholic hepatitis with fibrosis. Cirrhosis can develop, and liver transplantation has been performed in some adult patients treated for psoriasis (Gilbert et al. 1990). Although this toxicity has been studied more in adults than in children, it is still a risk for children (Keim et al. 1990). It is difficult to screen for liver damage by biochemical testing. Serum aminotransferases may not reflect ongoing liver damage and may be normal even after the development of cirrhosis or fibrosis (NEWMAN et al. 1989). Risk factors for the likely development of liver disease proposed for adults (advanced age, chronic ethanol use, obesity, diabetes mellitus and renal insufficiency) (ZACHARIAE et al. 1980) cannot be applied to children, with the possible exception of obesity. Although daily administration of methotrexate appears more prone to cause hepatotoxicity, weekly pulse doses are also associated with the development of hepatic fibrosis (SHERGY et al. 1988). Higher cumulative doses are more likely to be associated with hepatotoxicity, but liver damage has sometimes been found at low cumulative doses. The cumulative dose at which hepatotoxicity becomes likely in children has not been determined.

Regular histological examination of the liver during prolonged treatment with methotrexate has been customary. Liver biopsy prior to treatment and at regular, perhaps yearly, intervals during prolonged treatment has been advocated, but this may involve a considerable number of invasive procedures for a child. For adults with rheumatoid arthritis, regular monitoring of liver function tests may be a reasonable alternative (KREMER et al. 1994). For children, the surveillance strategy should be individualized for each patient. A pretreatment baseline biopsy. especially if there is reason to suspect ongoing liver disease, and liver biopsies at regular intervals thereafter may be indicated.

Methotrexate is also associated with acute hepatitis. High-dose methotrexate treatment used in some antineoplastic treatment regimens may produce acute hepatitis as shown by a sudden rise in aminotransferases (PEREZ et al. 1979; JOLIVET et al. 1983; BANNERJEE et al. 1988). After chronic treatment for malignancy, usually at comparatively low doses, hepatic damage may be relatively mild, with some steatosis and fibrosis (HARB et al. 1983). However, an early report documents severe liver disease with ascites, hepatosplenomegaly and transient jaundice; histological features included evidence of hepatocellular damage, some inflammatory infiltrates and extensive fibrosis (TAFT 1965). Steatosis or portal fibrosis has been found on liver biopsies from children with acute lymphoblastic leukemia, treated with various drugs including methotrexate (TOPLEY et al. 1979). In a small study of liver histology after maintenance high-dose methotrexate for 1–2 years, portal fibrosis was found in more than half of the patients, but this was neither severe nor accompanied by clinical liver disease (McINTOSH et al. 1977).

The mechanism of methotrexate toxicity is unknown although a toxic metabolite has been postulated. The poorly soluble metabolite 7-hydroxymethotrexate has been detected after treatment with high-dose regimens and may be associated with renal toxicity from methotrexate. A single study in rats suggests that 7-hydroxymethotrexate may be associated with cholestasis due to precipitation of bile constitutents (BREMNES et al. 1991).

How this relates to clinical acute hepatotoxicity is not clear since cholestasis is not predominant. The mechanism of chronic hepatotoxicity may differ from that of acute toxicity.

XV. Estrogens: Oral Contraceptive Pill

Hepatic vein thrombosis (Budd-Chiari syndrome) has been associated with use of oral contraceptives (Lewis et al. 1983; Maddrey 1987). It has been reported in adolescents (Lockhat et al. 1981; Valla et al. 1986; Barnet and Joffe 1991). Other disorders associated with hepatic vein thrombosis, such as paroxysmal nocturnal hemoglobinuria, circulating lupus anticoagulant and congenital disorders of coagulation proteins, should be excluded. Early diagnosis is preferable, but clinical presentation may be subtle with only gradual increase in abdominal girth due to ascites and nonspecific changes in liver function tests.

XVI. Ketoconazole (Contingent Hepatotoxin?)

Unlike amphotericin, the oral antifungal drug ketoconazole causes significant hepatotoxicity. The initial major report of ketoconazole hepatotoxicity in the United States included two children (a 17-year-old boy and a 5-year-old boy, both with chronic mucocutaneous candidiasis) among 54 reported occurrences of which 33 (including both these children) were considered probable or possible cases of ketoconazole-induced hepatotoxicity (Lewis et al. 1984). Presenting symptoms included jaundice and hepatitis (anorexia, nausea, vomiting, malaise) and occurred on average after 6–8 weeks of treatment (range: 5 days to 6 months).

XVII. Haloperidol

Haloperidol may cause hepatotoxicity. Cholestasis dominates the clinical picture, although some degree of hepatocellular damage and eosinophilia may be present (Fuller et al. 1977; McCreadie and MacDonald 1977). A prolonged severe bland cholestatic reaction, mimicking extrahepatic bile duct obstruction, may develop in children (Dincsoy and Saelinger 1982). One such case has been seen in a 10-year-old boy at the Hospital for Sick Children (Toronto).

XVIII. Amiodarone

Amiodarone is an iodinated benzofuran derivative used for the treatment of cardiac arrhythmias, used occasionally in children. Lamellar inclusion bodies, similar to those found in genetic phospholipid storage diseases, are found in the lungs, lymph nodes, peripheral blood leukocytes and liver of patients taking amiodarone chronically (POUCELL et al. 1984; DAKE et al. 1985). These may also be found in children taking amiodarone.

Amiodarone-induced hepatotoxicity, with hepatomegaly and abnormal serum aminotransferases, may develop within 1 month of treatment or after 1 year of treatment. Hepatotoxic changes mimicking acute alcoholic hepatitis have been described in adults, but not in children (SIMON et al. 1984; GENEVE et al. 1989; LEWIS et al. 1989). Severe amiodarone hepatotoxicity had been reported in a child (YAGUPSKY et al. 1985). It presented as rapidlly progressive hepatic failure beginning after 2 months of treatment at a relatively high dose of amiodarone (9mg/kg per day).

XIX. **Nitrofurantoin** (Hepatotoxin-Eliciting Immunoallergic Response)

In adults nitrofurantoin has been associated with features of chronic active hepatitis (SHARP et al. 1980). Fatal cholestatic hepatitis with severe pulmonary toxicity has been reported in a teenaged girl (MULBERG and BELL 1993).

XX. **Retinoids**

The retinoid used for treatment of cystic acne (13-*cis*-retinoic acid, isotretinoin) has been associated with severe teratogenicity (FERNHOFF and LAMMER 1984). Hepatotoxicity associated with isotretinoin and etretinate is variable, generally with a hepatitic pattern, as evidenced by asymptomatic elevations in serum aminotransferases (ROENIGK 1988).

XXI. **Azathioprine** (Contingent Hepatotoxin?)

Azathioprine is a potent immunosuppressive drug which consists of 6-mercaptopurine linked to an imidazole side-chain. It is effectively a prodrug for 6-mercaptopurine. Since its introduction in the 1960s, azathioprine has been associated with hepatotoxicity, including in children (MALEKZADEH et al. 1972), but these early studies cannot be analyzed easily due to underdiagnosed concomitant viral liver disease in these patients. In adults azathioprine hepatotoxicity had been characterized mainly by cholestasis or a hepatitic-cholestatic picture (DAVIS et al. 1980; JEURISSEN et al. 1990). Liver biopsy in one case showed centrilobular ballooning of hepatocytes and canalicular cholestasis (DEPINHO et al. 1984). More recently azathioprine hepatotoxicity has been described in orthotopic liver transplant recipients: endothelial cell damage, as well as hepatocyte damage and cholestasis, was noted (STERNECK et al. 1991). Nodular regenerative hyperplasia associated with chronic use of azathioprine has been reported (DUVOUX et al. 1991).

XXII. Cocaine

Cocaine hepatotoxicity has not yet been reported in children, but adolescents are conceivably at risk. A clinically severe hepatitic reaction has been reported in five young adults: the predominant histological finding was extensive zonal necrosis of hepatocytes in Rappaport zone 3 with zone 1 steatosis (Perino et al. 1987; Wanless et al. 1990). The histological pattern of hepatic injury in humans is consistent with generation of a toxic metabolite, probably by cytochromes P450. Glutathione appears to protect against cocaine-induced hepatic injury (Boelsterli and Goldlin 1991). Ethanol and phenobarbital-type inducers increase cocaine hepatotoxicity. However, recent observations suggest that metabolism via cytochrome P450 3A-associated enzymes is critical (Pellinen et al. 1994). Studies in primary cultures of human hepatocytes also demonstrate that ethanol potentiates the toxicity of cocaine to hepatocytes, leading to depletion of cellular glycogen stores and glutathione (Ponsoda et al. 1992).

References

Agran PF, Zenk KE, Romansky SG (1983) Acute liver failure and encephalopathy in a 15-month-old infant. Am J Dis Child 137:1107–1114

Anderson GD, Acheampong AA, Wilensky AJ, Levy RH (1992) Effect of valproate dose on formation of hepatotoxic metabolites. Epilepsia 33:736–742

Anderson GD, Acheampong AA, Levy RH (1994) Interaction between valproate and branched-chain amino acid metabolism. Neurology 44:742–744

Appleton RE, Farrell K, Applegarth DA, Dimmick JE, Wong LT, Davidson AG (1990) The high incidence of valproate hepatotoxicity in infants may relate to familial metabolic defects. Can J Neurol Sci 17:145–148

Arena JM, Rourk MH Jr, Sibrack CD (1978) Acetaminophen: report of an unusual poisoning. Pediatrics 61:68–72

Bannerjee AK, Lakhani S, Vincent M, Selby P (1988) Dose-dependent acute hepatitis associated with administration of high dose methotrexate. Hum Toxicoll 7:561–562

Barnet B, Joffe A (1991) Hepatic vein thrombosis in a teenager: a case report. J Adolesc Health 12:60–62

Barron KS, Person DA, Brewer EJ (1982) The toxicity of non-steroidal anti-inflammatory drugs in juvenile rheumatoid arthritis. J Rheumatol 9:149–155

Beaudry P, Brickman H, Wise M, MacDougall D (1974) Liver enzyme disturbances during isoniazid chemoprophylaxis in children. Am Rev Respir Dis 110:581–584

Beever IW, Blair IA, Brodie MJ (1982) Circulating hydrazine during treatment with isoniazid and rifampicin in man. Br J Clin Pharmacol 13:599P

Beghi E, Bizzi A, Codegoni AM, Trevisan D, Torri W (1990) Valproate, carnitine metabolism, and biochemical indicators of liver function. Collaborative Group for the Study of Epilepsy. Epilepsia 31:346–352

Benson GD (1983) Hepatotoxicity following the therapeutic use of antipyretic analgesics. Am J Med 75:85–93

Berson A, Freneaux E, Larrey D, Lepage V, Douay C, Mallet C, Fromentry B, Benhamou JP, Pessayre D (1994) Possible role of HLA in hepatotoxicity – an exploratory study in 71 patients with drug-induced idiosyncratic hepatitis. J Hepatol 20:336–342

Blake KV, Bailey D, Zientek GM, Hendeles L (1988) Death of a child associated with multiple overdoses of acetaminophen. Clin Pharm 7:391–397

Boelsterli UA, Goldlin C (1991) Biomechanisms of cocaine-induced hepatocyte injury mediated by the formation of reactive metabolites. Arch Toxicol 65:351–360
Böhles H, Richter K, Wagner-Thiessen E, Shaefer H (1982) Decreased serum carnitine in valproate induced Reye syndrome. Eur J Pediatr 139:185–186
Brain C, MacArdle B, Levin S (1984) Idiosyncratic reactions to carbamazepine mimicking viral infection in children. Br Med J 289:354
Bremnes RM, Smeland E, Huseby N-E, Eide TJ, Aarbakke J (1991) Acute hepatotoxicity after high-dose methotrexate administration to rats. Pharmacol Toxicol 69:132–139
Campbell RL, Small EW, Lesesne HR, Levin KJ, Moore WH (1977) Fatal hepatic necrosis after halothane anesthesia in a boy with juvenile rheumatoid arthritis: a case report Anesth Analg 56:589–593
Casteels-Van Daele M, Igodt-Ameye L, Corbell L, Eeckels R (1975) Hepatotoxicity of rifampicin and isoniazid in children. J Pediatr 86:739–741
Chabrol B, Mancini J, Chretien D, Rustin P, Munnich A, Pinsard N (1994) Valproate-induced hepatic failure in a case of cytochrome c oxidase deficiency. Eur J Pediatr 153:133–135
Christen U, Buergin M, Gut J (1991) Halothane metabolism: Kupffer cells carry and partially process triflouroacetylated protein adducts. Biochem Biophys Res Commun 175:256–262
Clark JH, Russell GJ, Fitzgerald SF (1983) Fatal acetaminophen toxicity in a two year old. J Ind St Med Assoc 76:832–835
Coulter DR, Allen RJ (1981) Hyperammonemia with valproic acid therapy. J Pediatr 99:317–319
Cribb AE, Spielberg SP (1992) Sulfamethoxazole is metabolized to the hydroxylamine in humans. Clin Pharmacol Ther 51:522–526
Cribb AE, Miller M, Tesoro A, Spielberg SP (1990) Peroxidase-dependent oxidation of sulfonamides by monocytes and neutrophils from humans and dogs. Mol Pharmacol 38:744–751
Dake MD, Madison JM, Montgomery CK, Shellito JE, Hinchcliffe WA, Winkler ML, Bainton DF (1985) Electron microscopic demonstration lysosomal inclusion bodies in lung, liver, lymph nodes, and blood leukocytes of patients with amiodarone pulmonary toxicity. Am J Med 78:506–512
Davis M, Eddleston ALWF, Williams R (1980) Hypersensitivity and jaundice due to azathioprine. Postgrad Med J 56:274–275
De Morais SMF, Wells PG (1988) Deficiency in bilirubin UDP-glucuronyl transferase as a genetic determinant of acetaminophen toxicity. J Pharmacol Exp Ther 247:323–331
De-Nardo V, Lapadula G, Soligno O (1988) Hepatic injury and death of a three year old girl due to paracetamol poisoning. Minerva Pediatr 40:571
DeGroot H, Noll T (1983) Halothane hepatotoxicity: relation between metabolic activation, pyrexia, covalent binding, lipid peroxidation and liver cell damage. Hepatology 3:601–606
DeLeve LD, Kaplowitz N (1991) Selective susceptibility of hepatic endothelial cells to dacarbazine toxicity, a model for hepatic veno-occlusive disease. Hepatology 14:161A
DePinho RA, Goldberg CS, Lefkowitch JH (1984) Azathioprine and the liver. Evidence favoring idiosyncratic, mixed cholestatic-hepatocellular injury in humans. Gastroenterology 86:162–165
Derby LE, Jick H, Henry DA, Dean AD (1993) Erythromycin-associated cholestatic hepatitis. Med J Aust 158:600–602
Dickinson RG, Bassett ML, Searle J, Tyrer JH, Eadie MJ (1985) Valproate hepatotoxicity: a review and report of two instances in adults. Clin Exp Neurol 21:79–91
Diehl AM, Latham P, Boitnott JK, Mann J, Maddrey WC (1984) Cholestatic hepatitis from erythromycin ethylsuccinate. Am J Med 765:931–934

Dincsoy HP, Saelinger DA (1982) Haloperidol-induced chronic cholestatic liver disease. Gastroenterology 83:694–700
Doughty R, Giesecke L, Athreya B (1980) Salicylate therapy in juvenile rheumatoid arthritis. Am J Dis Child 134:461–463
Dreifuss FE, Santilli N, Langer DH, Sweeney KP, Moline KA, Menander KB (1987) Valproic acid hepatic fatalities. Neurology 37:379–385
Dujovne CA, Chan CH, Zimmerman HJ (1967) Sulfonamide hepatic injury. Review of the literature and report of a case due to sulfamethoxazole. N Engl J Med 277:785–788
Duvoux C, Kracht M, Lang P, Vernant J-P, Zafrani E-S, Dhumeaux D (1991) Hyperplasie nodulaire régénérative du foie associée à la prise d'azathioprine. Gastroenterol Clin Biol 15:968–973
Eadie MJ, Hooper WD, Dickinson RG (1988) Valproate-associated hepatotoxicity and its biochemical mechanisms. Med Toxicol Adverse Drug Exp 3:85–106
Eadie MJ, McKinnon GE, Dunstan PR, MacLaughlin D, Dickinson RG (1990) Valproate metabolism during hepatotoxicity associated with the drug. QJ Med 77:1229–1240
Elitsur Y (1990) Pemoline (Cylert)-induced hepatotoxicity. J Pediatr Gastroenterol Nutr 11:143–144
Essell JH, Thompson JM, Harman GS, Halvorson RD, Snyder MJ, Johnson RA, Rubinsak JR (1992) Marked increase in veno-occlusive disease of the liver associated with methotrexate use for graft-versus-host disease prophylaxis in patients receiving busulfan/cyclophosphamide. Blood 79:2784–2788
Evans WE, Self TH, Weisbusrt MR (1976) Phenobarbital-induced hepatic dysfunction. Drug Intell Clin Pharm 10:439–443
Farrell G, Prendergast D, Murray M (1985) Halothane hepatitis: detection of a constitutional susceptibility factor. N Engl J Med 313:1310–1314
Farrell GC (1988) Mechanism of halothane-induced liver injury: is it immune or metabolic idiosyncrasy? J Gastroenterol Hepatol 3:465–482
Fernhoff PM, Lammer EJ (1984) Craniofacial features of isotretinoin embryopathy. J Pediatr 105:595–597
Fisher R, Nau H, Gandolfi AJ, Putnam CW, Brendel K (1991) Valproic acid hepatotoxicity in human liver slices. Drug Chem Toxicol 14:375–394
Fisher RL, Saniuk JT, Nau H, Gandolfi AJ, Brendel K (1994) Comparative toxicity of valproic acid and its metabolites in liver slices from adult rats, weanling rats and humans. Toxicol In Vitro 8:371–379
Fuller CM, Yassinger S, Imperato TJ, Ruebner B (1977) Haloperidol-induced liver disease. West J Med 127:515–518
Funck-Brentano C, Pessayre D, Benhamou JP (1983) Hépatites dues à divers dérivés de l'érythromycine. Clin Biol (Paris) 7:362–369
Garty BZ, Kauli R, Ben-Ari J, Lubin E, Nitzam M, Laron Z (1985) Hepatitis associated with propylthiouracil treatment. Drug Intell Clin Pharm 19:740–742
Geneve J, Zafrani ES, Dhumeaux D (1989) Amiodarone induced liver disease. J Hepatol 9:130–133
Gerber N, Dickinson RG, Harland RC, Lynn RK, Houghton D, Antonias JI (1979) Reye-like syndrome associated with valproic acid therapy. J Pediatr 95:142–144
Ghishan FK (1983) Trimethoprim-sulfamethoxazole-induced intrahepatic cholestasis. Clin Pediatr 22:212–214
Gilbert SC, Klintmalm G, Mentor A, Silverman A (1990) Methotrexate-induced cirrhosis requiring liver transplantation in three patients with psoriasis: a word of caution in light of the expanding use of this "steroid sparing" agent. Arch Intern Med 150:889–891
Granneman GR, Wang SI, Kesterson JW, Machinist JM (1984) The hepatotoxicity of valproic acid and its metabolites in rats. II. intermediary and valproic acid metabolism. Hepatology 4:1153–1158

Green MD, Shires TK, Fischer LJ (1984) Hepatotoxicity of acetaminophen in neonatal and young rats. I. Age-related changes in susceptibility. Toxicol Appl Pharmacol 74:116–124

Green SH (1984) Sodium valproate and routine liver function tests. Arch Dis Child 59:813–814

Greene JW, Graft L, Gishan FK (1983) Acetaminophen poisoning in infancy. Am J Dis Child 137:386–387

Gurumurthy PG, Krishnamurthy MS, Nazareth O, Parthasarthy R, Raghupati Sarma G, Somasundaram PR, Tripathy SP, Ellard GA (1984) Lack of relationship between hepatic toxicity and acetylator phenotype in three thousand South Indian patients during treatment with isoniazid for tuberculosis. Am Rev Respir Dis 129:58–61

Gut J, Christen U, Huwyler J (1993) Mechanisms of halothane toxicity: novel insights. Pharmacol Ther 58:133–155

Hadzic N, Portmann B, Davies ET, Mowat AP, Mieli-Vergani G (1990) Acute liver failure induced by carbamazepine. Arch Dis Child 65:315–317

Hamdan JA, Manasra K, Ahmed M (1985) Salicylate-induced hepatitis in rheumatic fever. Am J Dis Child 139:453–455

Harb JM, Werlin SL, Camitta BM, Oechler H, Kamen BA, Blank EL (1983) Hepatic ultrastructure in leukemic children treated with methotrexate and 6-mercaptopurine. Am J Pediatr Hematol Oncol 5:323–331

Hassall E, Israel DM, Gunasekaran T, Steward D (1990) Halothane hepatitis in children. J Pediatr Gastroenterol Nutr 11:553–557

Henretig FM, Selbst SM, Forrest C, Kearney TK, Orel H, Werner S, Williams TA (1989) Repeated acetaminophen overdosing. Clin Pediatr 28:525–528

Hickson GB, Greene JW, Craft LT (1983) Apparent intentional poisoning of an infant with acetaminophen. Am J Dis Child 137:917

Hickson GB, Altemeier WA, Martin ED, Campbell PW (1989) Parental administration of chemical agents: a cause of apparent life threatening events: J Pediatr 83:772–776

Hjelm M, Ds Silva LVK, Seakins IWT, Oberholzer VG, Rolles CJ (1986) Evidence of inherited urea cycle defect in a case of fatal valproate toxicity. Br Med J 292:23–24

Honjo I, Suou T, Hirayama C (1988) Hepatotoxicity of cyclophosphamide in man: pharmacokinetic analysis. Res Commun Chem Pathol Pharmacol 61: 149–165

Hruban RH, Sternberg SS, Meyers P, Fleisher M, Menendez-Botet C, Boitnott JK (1991) Fatal thrombocytopenia and liver failure associated with carboplatin therapy. Cancer Invert 9:263–268

Ilyin GP, Rissel M, Malledant Y, Tanguy M, Guillouzo A (1994) Human hepatocytes express trifluoroacetylated neoantigens after in vitro exposure to halothane. Biochem Pharmacol 48:561–567

Inman WHV, Mushin WW (1978) Jaundice after repeated exposure to halothane: a further analysis of reports to the Committee of Safety of Medicines. Br Med J 2:1455–1456

Jaffe SL (1989) Pemoline and liver function. J Am Acad Child Adolesc Psychiatr 28:457–458

Jeurissen ME, Boerbooms AM, van de Putte LB, Kruijsen MW (1990) Azathioprine induced fever, chills, rash, and hepatotoxicity in rheumatoid arthritis. Ann Rheum Dis 49:25–27

Jolivet J, Cowan KH, Curt GA, Clendeninn NJ, Crabner BA (1983) The pharmacology and clinical use of methotrexate. N Engl J Med 309:1094–1104

Jollow DJ, Mitchell JR, Potter WZ, Davis DC, Gillette JR, Brodie BB (1973) Acetaminophen-induced hepatic necrosis. II. Role of covalent binding in vivo. J Pharmacol Exp Ther 187:195–202

Jonas MM, Edison MS (1988) Propylthiouracil hepatotoxicity: two pediatric cases and review of the literature. J Pediatr Gastroenterol Nutr 7:776–779

Kahn HD, Faguet GB, Agee JF, Middleton HM (1984) Drug-induced liver injury. In vitro demonstration of hypersensitivity to both phenytoin and phenobarbital. Arch Intern Med 144:1677–1679

Kane RE, Kotagel S, Bacon BR, Vogler CA (1992) Valproate use associated with persistent hyperammonemia and mitochondrial injury in a child with Down's syndrome. J Pediatr Gastroenterol Nutr 14:223–227

Kassahun K, Farrell K, Abbott F (1991) Identification and characterization of the glutathione and N-acetylcysteine conjugates of (e)-2-proply-2,4-pentadienoic acid, a toxic metabolite of valproic acid, in rats and humans. Drug Metab Dispos 19:525–535

Kassahun K, Hu P, Grillo MP, Davis MR, Jin LX, Baillie TA (1994) Metabolic activation of unsaturated derivatives of valproic acid — identification of novel gluathione adducts formed through coenzyme A-dependent and -independent processes. Chem Biol Interact 90:253–275

Kay JDS, Hilton-Jones D, Hyman N (1986) Valproate toxicity and ornithine carbamoyltransferase deficiency. Lancet II:1283–1284

Keeffe EB, Reis TC, Berland JE (1982) Hepatotoxicity to both erythromycin estolate and erythromycin ethylsuccinate. Dig Dis Sci 27:701–704

Keim D, Ragsdale C, Heidelberger K, Sullivan D (1990) Hepatic fibrosis and the use of methotrexate for juvenile rheumatoid arthritis. J Rheumatol 17:846–848

Kenna JG, Newberger J, Mieli-Vergani G, Mowat AP, Williams R (1987) Halothane hepatitis in children. Br Med J 294:1209–1211

Kenna JG, Satoh H, Christ DD, Pohl LR (1988a) Metabolic basis for a drug hypersensitivity: antibodies in sera from patients with halothane hepatitis recognize liver neoantigens that contain the trifluoroacetyl group derived from halothane. J Pharmacol Exp Ther 245:1103–1109

Kenna JG, Neuberger J, Williams R (1988b) Evidence for expression in human liver of halothane-induced neoantigens recognized by antibodies in sera from patients with halothane hepatitis. Hepatology 8:1635–1641

Kenna JG, Martin JL, Satoh H, Pohl LR (1990) Factors affecting the expression of trifluoracteylated liver microsomal protein neoantigens in rats treated with halothane. Drug Metab Dispos 18:788–793

Kennedy BJ (1970) Metabolic and toxic effects of mithramycin during tumor therapy. Am J Med 49:494–503

Kesterson JW, Granneman GR, Machinist JM (1984) The hepatotoxicity of valproate in rats. I. Toxicologic, biochemical and histopathologic studies. Hepatology 4:1143–1152

Keulen FP, Kochen W (1985) Hepatotoxität unter Valproinsaure Behandlung. Klin Pädiatr 197:431–436

Kingsley E, Gray P, Tolman KG, Tweedale R (1983) The toxicity of metabolites of sodium valproate in cultured hepatocytes. J Clin Pharmacol 23:178–185

Kleckner HB, Yakulis V, Heller P (1875) Severe hypersensitivity to diphenylhydantoin with circulating antibodies to the drug. Ann Intern Med 83:522–523

Kochen W, Schneider A, Ritz A (1983) Abnormal metabolism of valproic acid in fatal hepatic failure. Eur J Pediatr 14:30–35

Kondo T, Ishida M, Kaneko S, Hirano T, Otani K, Fukushima Y, Muranaka H, Koide N, Yokoyama M, Nakata S et al. (1992a) Is 2-propyl-4-pentenoic acid, a hepatotoxic metabolite of valproate, responsible for valproate-induced hyperammonemia? Epilepsia 33:550–554

Kondo T, Kaneka S, Otani K, Ishida M, Hirano T, Fukushima Y, Muranaka H, Koide N, Yokoyama M (1992b) Associations between risk factors for valproate hepatotoxicity and altered valproate metabolism. Epilepsia 33:172–177

Kossak BD, Schmidt-Sommerfeld E, Schoeller DA, Rinaldo P, Penn D, Tonsgard JH (1993) Impaired fatty acid oxidation in children on valproic acid and the effect of L-carnitine. Neurology 43:2362–2368

Kowdley KV, Keeffe EB, Fawaz KA (1992) Prolonged cholestasis due to trimethoprim sulfamethoxazole. Gastroenterology 102:2148–2150

Kremer JM, Alarcón GS, Lightfoot RWJ, Willkens RF, Furst DF, Williams HJ, Dent PB, Weinblatt ME (1994) Methotrexate for rheumatoid arthritis. Suggested guidelines for monitoring liver toxicity. Arthintis Rheum 37:316–328
Laub MC, Paetzke-Brunner I, Jaeger G (1986) Serum carnitine during valproic acid therapy. Epilepsia 27:559–562
Lauterburg BH, Vaishnav Y, Stillwell WG, Mitchell JR (1980) The effect of age and glutathione depletion on hepatic glutathione turnover in vivo determined by acetaminophen probe analysis. J Pharmacol Exp Ther 213:54–58
Lauterburg BH, Smith CV, Todd EL, Mitchell JR (1985) Pharmacokinetics of the toxic hydrazino metabolites formed from isoniazid in humans. J Pharmacol Exp Ther 235:566–570
Lederman S, Fysh WJ, Tredger M, Gamsu HR (1983) Neonatal paracetamol poisoning: treatment by exchange transfusion. Arch Dis Child 58:631–633
Levy RH, Rettenmeier AW, Anderson GD, Wilensky AJ, Friel PN, Baillie TA, Acheampong A, Tor J, Guyot M, Loiseau P (1990) Effects of polytherapy with phenytoin, carbamazepine, and stiripentol on formation of 4-ene-valproate, a hepatotoxic metabolite of valproic acid. Clin Pharmacol Ther 48:225–235
Lewis IJ, Rosenbloom L (1982) Glandular fever-like syndrome, pulmonary eosinophilia and asthma associated with carbamazepine. Postgrad Med J 58:100–101
Lewis JH, Tice HL, Zimmerman HJ (1983) Budd-Chiari syndrome assoicated with oral contraceptive steroids. Review of treatment of 47 cases. Dig Dis Sci 28:673–683
Lewis JH, Zimmerman HJ, Benson GD, Ishak KG (1984) Hepatic injury associated with ketoconazole therapy. Analysis of 33 cases. Gastroenterology 86:503–513
Lewis JH, Ranard RC, Caruso A, Jackson LK, Mullick F, Ishak KG, Seeff LB, Zimmerman HJ (1989) Amiodarone hepatotoxicity: prevalence and clinicopathologic correlations among 104 patients. Hepatology 9:679–685
Li X, Norwood DL, Mao L-F, Schulz H (1991) Mitochondrial metabolism of valproic acid. Biochemistry 30:388–394
Lieh-Lai MW, Sarnaik AP, Newton JF, Miceli JN, Fleischman LE, Hook JB, Kauffman RE (1984) Metabolism and pharmacokinetics of acetaminophen in a severely poisoned young child. J Pediatr 105:125–128
Litt IF, Cohen MI, McNamara H (1976) Isoniazid hepatitis in adolescents. J Pediatr 89:133–135
Lockhat D, Katz SS, Lisbona R, Mishkin S (1981) Oral contraceptives and liver disease. Can Med Assoc J 124:993–999
Losek JH, Werlin SL (1981) Sulfasalazine hepatotoxicity. Am J Dis Child 135:1070–1072
Maddrey WC (187) Hepatic vein thrombosis (Budd Chiari syndrome): possible association with the use of oral contracptives. Semin Liver Dis 7:32–39
Maddrey WC, Boitnott JK (1973) Lsoniazid hepatitis. Ann Intern Med 79:1–12
Maggiore G, Larizza D, Lorini R, De Giacomo C, Scotta MS, Severi F (1989) PTU hepatotoxicity mimicking autoimmune chronic active hepatitis in a girl. J Pediatr Gastroenterol Nutr 8:547–548
Malekzadeh MH, Grushkin CM, Wright HT, Fine RN (1972) Hepatic dysfunction after renal transplantation in children. J Pediatr 81:279–285
Martin JL, Kenna JG, Martin BM, Thomassen D, Reed GF, Pohl LR (1993) Halothane hepatitis patients have serum antibodies that react with protein disulfide isomerase. Hepatology 18:858–863
Martinez-Roig A, Cami J, Llorens-Teroi J, De La Torre R, Perich F (1986) Acetylation phenotype and hepatotoxicity in the treatment of tuberculosis of children. Pediatrics 77:912–915
Matsuda I, Ohtani Y, Ninoniya N (1986) Renal handling of carnitine in children with carnitine deficiency and hyperammonemia associated with valproate therapy. J Pediatr 109:131–134
McCreadie RG, MacDonald IM (1977) High dosage haloperidol in chronic schizophrenia. Br J Psychiatr 131:310–316

McDonald GB, Sharma P, Matthews DE, Shulman HM, Thomas ED (1985) The clinical course of 53 patients with veno-occlusive disease of the liver after marrow transplantation. Transplantation 39:603–608
McGeachy TE, Bloomer WE (1953) The phenobarbital sensitivity syndrome. Am J Med 14:600–604
McIntosh S, Davidson DL, O'Brien RT, Pearson HA (1977) Methotrexate hepatotoxicity in children with leukemia. J Pediatr 90:1019–1021
McVeagh P, Ekert H (1975) Hepatotoxicity of chemotherapy following nephrectomy and radiation therapy for righ-sided Wilm's tumor. J Pediatr 87:627–628
Menard DB, Gisselbrecht C, Marty H, Reyes F, Dhumeaux D (1980) Antineoplastic agents and the liver. Gastroenterology 78:142–164
Meredith TJ, Newman B, Goulding R (1978) Paracetamol poisoning in children. Br Med J 2:478–479
Miller RP, Roberts RJ, Fischer LF (1976) Acetaminophen elimination kinetics in neonates, children and adults. Clin Pharmacol Ther 19:284–294
Millington DS, Bohan TP, Roe CR, Yergey AL, Liberato DJ (1985) Valproylcarnitine: a novel drug metabolite identified by fast atom bombardment and thermospray liquid chromatography-mass spectroscopy. Clin Chim Acta 145:69–76
Miner DJ, Kissinger PT (1979) Evidence for the involvement of N-acetyl-p-quinoneimine in acetaminophen metabolism. Biochem Pharmacol 28:3285–3290
Minow RA, Stern MH, Casey JH, Rodriguez V, Luna MA (1976) Clinico-pathologic correlation of liver damage in patients treated with 6-mercaptopruine and adriamycin. Cancer 38:1524–1528
Mitchell AA, Lacouture PG, Sheehan JE, Kauffman RE, Shapiro S (1988) Adverse drug reactions in children leading to hospital admission. Pediatrics 82: 24–29
Mitchell J, Zimmerman H, Ishak K, Thorgeirsson UP, Timbrell JA, Snodgrass WR, Nelson SD (1976) Isoniazid liver injury: clinical spectrum, pathology and probable pathogenesis. Ann Intern Med 84:181–196
Mitchell JR, Jollow DJ, Potter WZ, Davis DC, Gillette JR, Brodie BB (1973a) Acetaminophen-induced hepatic necrosis. I. Role of drug metabolism. J Pharmacol Exp Ther 187:185–194
Mitchell JR, Jollow DJ, Potter WZ, Gillette JR, Brodie BB (1973b) Acetaminophen-induced hepatic necrosis. IV. Protective role of glutathione. J Pharmacol Exp Ther 187:211–217
Moult PJ, Sherlock S (1975) Halothane-related hepatitis. A clinical study of twenty-six cases. QJ Med 44:99–114
Mulberg AE, Bell LM (1993) Fatal cholestatic hepatits and multisystem failure associated with nitrofurantoin. J Pediatr Gastroenterol Nutr 17:307–309
Mullick FG, Ishak KG (1980) Hepatic injury associated with diphenylhydantoin therapy. Am J Clin Pathol 74:442–452
Murphy JV, Maquardt KM, Shug AL (1985) Valproic acid associated abnormalities of carnitine metabolism. Lancet I:820–821
Murphy JV, Groover RV, Hodge C (1993) Hepatotoxic effects in a child receiving valproate and carnitine. J Pediatr 123:318–320
Nehra A, Mullick F, Ishak KG, Zimmerman HJ (1990) Pemoline-associated hepatic injury. Gastroenterology 99:1517–1519
Newman M, Auerbach R, Feiner H, Holzman RS, Shupack J, Migdal P, Culubret M, Camuto P, Tobias H (1989) The role of liver biopsies in psoriatic patients receiving long-term methotrexate treatment. Arch Dermatol 125:1218–1224
Nogen AG, Breener JE (1978) Fatal acetaminophen overdosage in a growing child. J Pediatr 92:832–833
O'Brien RJ, Long MW, Cross FS, Lyle MA, Snider DE (1983) Hepatotoxicity from isoniazid and rifampin among children treated for tuberculosis. Pediatrics 72:491–499
Parke DV (1987) Activation mechanisms to chemical toxicity. Arch Toxicol 60:5–15
Parker LN (1975) Hepatitis and propilthiouracil. Ann Intern Med 82:228–229

Pellinen P, Honkakoshi P, Stenback F, Niemitz M, Alhava E, Pelkonen O, Lang MA, Pasanen M (1994) Cocaine N-demethylation and the metabolism-related hepatotoxicity can be prevented by cytochrome P450 3A inhibitors. Eur J Pharmacol 270:35–43
Penta JS, van Hoff DD, Muggia FM (1977) Hepatotoxicity of combination chemotherapy for acute myelocytic leukemia. Ann Intern Med 87:247–248
Perez C, Sutow WW, Wang YM, Pearson HA (1979) Evaluation of overall toxicity of high-dosage methotrexate regimens. Med Pediatr Oncol 6:219–228
Perino LE, Warren GH, Levine JS (1987) Cocaine-induced hepatotoxicity in humans. Gastroenterology 93:176–180
Perry MC (1982) Hepatotoxicity of chemotherapeutic agents. Semim Oncol 9:65–74
Pessayre D, Bentata M, Degott C, Nouel O, Miguet JP, Rueff B, Benhamou JP (1977) Isoniazid-rifampin fulminant hepatitis. A possible consequence of the enhancement of isoniazid hepatotoxicity by enzyme induction. Gastroenterology 72:284–289
Peterson RG, Rumack BH (1978) Pharmacokinetics of acetaminophen in children. Pediatrics 62:877–879
Peterson RG, Rumack BH (1981) Age as a variable in acetaminophen overdose. Arch Intern Med 141:390–393
Petty BG, Zahka KG, Bernstein MT (1978) Aspirin hepatitis associated with encephalopathy. J Pediatr 93:881–882
Phillips KG (1983) Hepatotoxicity of erythromycin ethylsuccinate in a child. Can Med Assoc J 129:411–412
Pohl LR, Satoh H, Christ DD, Kenna J (1988) The immunologic and metabolic basis of drug hypersensitivities. Annu Rev Pharmacol Toxicol 28:367–387
Ponsoda X, Jover R, Castell JV, Gomez-Lechon MJ (1992) Potentiation of cocaine hepatotoxicity in human hepatocytes by ethanol. Toxicol In Vitro 6:155–158
Potter WZ, Davis DC, Mitchell JR, Jollow DJ, Gillette JR, Brodie BB (1973) Acetaminophen-induced hepatic necrosis. III. Cytochrome P-450-mediated covalent binding in vitro. J Pharmacol Exp Ther 187:203–210
Poucell S, Ireton J, Valencia-Mayoral P, Downbar E, Larratt L, Patterson J, Blendis L, Phillips MJ (1984) Amiodarone-associated phospholipidosis of the liver. Light, immunohistochemical and electron microscopic studies. Gastroenterology 86:926–936
Powell-Jackson PR, Tredger JM, Williams R (1984) Hepatotoxicity to sodium valproate: a review. Gut 25:673–681
Powers NG, Carson SH (1987) Idiosyncratic reactions to phenytoin. Clin Pediatr 26:120–124
Pratt CB, Johnson WW (1971) Duration and severity of fatty metamorphosis of the liver following L-asparaginase therapy. Cancer 28:361–364
Pratt DS, Dubois RS (1990) Hepatotoxicity due to pemoline (Cylert). A report of two cases. J Pediatr Gastroenteror Nutr 10:239–241
Psacharopoulos HJ, Mowat AP, Davies M, Portmann B, Silk DBA, Williams R (1980) Fulminant hepatic failure in childhood: an analysis of 31 cases. Arch Dis Child 55:252–258
Qureshi IA, Letarte J, Tuchweber B, Yousef I, Qureshi SR (1985) Heptotoxicology of sodium valproate in ornithine transcarbamylase-deficient mice. Toxicol Lett 25:297–306
Raucy JL, Lasker JM, Lieber CS, Black M (1989) Acetaminophen activation by human liver cytochromes P450IIE1 and P450IA2. Arch Biochem Biophys 271:270–283
Reddy CM (1979) Propylthiouracil and hepatitis: a case report. J Natl Med Assoc 72:1185–1186
Rettenemeier AW, Gordon WP, Prickett KS, Levy RH, Lockard JS, Thummel KE, Baillie TA (1986) Metabolic fate of valproic acid in the rhesus monkey. Formation of a toxic metabolite, 2-n-propyl-4-pentenoic acid. Drug Metab Dispos 14:443–453

Rettie AE, Rettenmeier AW, Howald WN, Baillie TA (1987) Cytochrome P-450-catalyzed formation of delta4-VPA, a toxic metabolite of valproic acid. Science 235:890–893
Ribe J, Benkov KJ, Thung SN, Shen SC, Leleiko NS (1986) Fatal massive hepatic necrosis: a probable hypersensitivity reaction to sulfasalazine. Am J Gastroenterol 81:205–208
Rieder MJ, Uetrecht J, Shear NH, Spielberg SP (1988) Synthesis and in vitro toxicity of hydroxylamine metabolites of sulfonamides. J Pharmacol Exp Ther 244:724–728
Rieder MJ, Uetrecht J, Shear NH, Cannon M, Miller M, Spielberg SP (1989) Diagnosis of sulfonamide hypersensitivity reactions by in-vitro "rechallenge" with hydroxylamine metabolites. Ann Intern Med 110:286–289
Roberts EA, Spielberg SP, Goldbach M, Phillips MJ (1990) Phenobarbital hepatotoxicity in an 8-month-old infant. J Hepatol 10:235–239
Roberts I, Robinson MJ, Mughal MZ, Rutcliffe JG, Prescott LF (1984) Paracetamol metabolites in the neonate following maternal overdose. Br J Clin Pharmacol 18:201–206
Roenigk HH Jr (1988) Liver toxicity of retinoid therapy. J Am Acad Dermatol 19:199–208
Rollins BJ (1986) Hepatic veno-occlusive disease. Am J Med 81:297–306
Rollins DE, von Bahr C, Glaumann H, Moldeus P, Rane A (1979) Acetaminophen: potentially toxic metabolites formed by human fetal and adult liver microsomes and isolated fetal liver cells. Science 205:1414–1416
Rudoy R, Stuemky J, Poley R (1973) Isoniazid administration and liver injury. Am J Dis Child 125:733–736
Rumack BH (1984) Acetaminophen overdose in young children. Treatment and effects of alcohol and other additional ingestants in 417 cases. Am J Dis Child 138:428–433
Sampson P (1975) Scientists meet and compare notes on hyperactive children. J Am Med Assoc 232:1204–1216
Sarma GR, Immanuel C, Kailasam S, Narayama ASL, Venkatesen P (1986) Rifamipicin-induced release of hydrazine from isoniazid – a possible cause of hepatitis during treatment of tuberculosis with regimens containing isoniazid and rifampicin. Am Rev Respir Dis 133:1072–1075
Satoh H, Fukada Y, Anderson DK, Ferrans VJ, Gillette JR, Pohl LR (1985) Immunological studies on the mechanism of halothane-induced hepatotoxicity: immunohistochemical evidence of trifluoroacetylated hepatocytes. J Pharmacol Exp Ther 233:857–862
Satoh H, Martin BM, Schulick AH, Christ DD, Kenna JG, Pohl LR (1989) Human anti-endoplasmic reticulum antibodies in sera of patients with halothane-induced hepatitis are directed against a trifluoroacetylated carboxylesterase. Proc Natl Acad Sci USA 86:322–326
Scheffner D, Konig ST, Rauterberg-Ruland I, Kochen W, Hoffman WJ, Unkelbach ST (1988) Fatal liver failure in 16 children with valproate therapy. Epilepsia 29:530–542
Schnabel R, Rambeck B, Janssen F (1984) Fatal intoxication with sodium valproate. Lancet I:221–222
Seaman WE, Ishak KG, Plotz PH (1974) Aspirin-induced hepatotoxicity in patients with systemic lupus erythematosus. Ann Intern Med 80:1–8
Seeff LB, Cuccherini BA, Zimmerman HJ, Alder E, Benjamin SB (1986) Acetaminophen hepatotoxicity in alcoholics. A therapeutic misadventure. Ann Intern Med 104:399–404
Seth V, Beotra A (1989) Hepatic function in relation to acetylator phenotype in children treated with antitubercular drugs. Ind J Med Res 89:306–309
Shapiro PA, Antonioli DA, Peppercorn MA (1980) Barbiturate-induced submassive hepatic necrosis. Am J Gastroenterol 74:270–273
Sharp JR, Ishak KG, Zimmerman HJ (1980) Chronic active hepatitis and severe hepatic necrosis associated with nitrofurantoin. Ann Intern Med 92:14–19

Shear NH, Spielberg SP (1985) In vitro evaluation of toxic metabolite of sulfadiazine. Can J Physiol Pharmacol 63:1370–1372

Shear NH, Spielberg SP (1988) Anticonvulsant hypersensitivity syndrome. In vitro assessment of risk. J Clin Invest 82:1826–1832

Shear NH, Spielberg SP, Grant DM, Tang BK, Kalow W (1986) Differences in metabolism of sulfonamides predisposing to idiosyncratic toxicity. Ann Intern Med 105:179–184

Shergy WJ, Polisson RP, Caldwell DS, Rice JR, Pisetsky DS, Allen NB (1988) Methotrexate-associated hepatotoxicity: retrospective analysis of 210 patients with rheumatoid arthritis. Am J Med 85:771–774

Shriner K, Goetz MB (1992) Severe hepatotoxicity in a patient receiving both acetaminophen and zidovudine. Am J Med 93:94–96

Simon JB, Manley PN, Brien JF, Armstrong PW (1984) Amiodarone hepatotoxicity simulating alcoholic liver disease. N Engl J Med 311:167–172

Smith DW, Isakson G, Frankel LR, Kerner JA Jr (1986) Hepatic failure following ingestion of multiple doses of acetaminophen in a young child. J Pediatr Gastroenterol Nutr 5:822–825

Smith DW, Cullity GJ, Silberstein EP (1988) Fatal hepatic necrosis associated with multiple anticonvulsant therapy. Aust N Z J Med 18:575–581

Sotolongo RP, Neefe LI, Rudzki C, Ishak KG (1978) Hypersensitivity reaction to sulfasalazine with severe hepatotoxicity. Gastroenterology 75:95–99

Spielberg SP, Gordon GB, Blake DA, Goldstein DA, Herlong HF (1981a) Predisposition to phenytoin hepatotoxicity assessed in vitro. N Engl J Med 305:722–727

Spielberg SP, Gordon GB, Blake DA, Mellits ED, Bross DS (1981b) Anticonvulsant toxicity in vitro: possible role of arene oxides. J Pharmacol Exp Ther 217: 386–389

Spyridis P, Sinantios C, Papadea I, Oreopoulos L, Hadziyannis S, Papadotos C (1979) Isoniazid liver injury during chemoprophylaxis in children. Arch Dis Child 54:65–67

Sterneck M, Wiesner R, Ascher N, Roberts J, Ferrell L, Ludwig J, Lake J (1991) Azathioprine hepatotoxicity after liver transplantation. Hepatology 14:806–810

Suchy FJ, Balistreri WF, Buchino J, Sondheimer JM, Bates SR, Kearns GL, Still JD, Bove KE (1979) Acute hepatic failure associated with the use of sodium valproate. Report of two fatal cases. N Engl J Med 300:962–966

Swetnam SM, Florman AL (1984) Probable acetaminophen toxicity in an 18-month-old infant due to repeated overdosing. Clin Pediatr 23:104–105

Sznol M, Ohnuma T, Holland JF (1987) Hepatic toxicity drugs used for hematologic neoplasia. Semin Liver Dis 7:237–256

Taft LI (1965) Methotrexate induced hepatitis in childhood leukemia. Isr J Med Sci 1:823–827

Thurston JH, Hauhart RE (1992) Amelioration of adverse effects of valproic acid on ketogenesis and liver coenzyme A metabolism by cotreatment with pantothenate and carnitine in developing mice: possible clinical significance. Pediatr Res 31:419–423

Tolman KG, Freston JW, Berenson MM, Samella JJ (1973) Hepatotoxicity due to pemoline. Report of two cases. Digestion 9:532–539

Topley J, Benson J, Squier MV, Chessells JM (1979) Hepatotoxicity in the treatment of acute lymphoblastic leukemia. Med Pediatr Oncol 7:393–399

Tsagaropoulou-Stinga H, Mataki-Emmanouilidou T, Karadi-Kavalioti S, Manios S (1985) Hepatotoxic reactions in children with severe tuberculosis treated with isoniazid-rifampin. Pediatr Infect Dis 4:270–273

Ulshen MH, Grand RJ, Crain JD, Gelfand EW (1978) Hepatotoxicity with encephalopathy associated with aspirin therapy in rheumatoid arthritis. J Pediatr 93;1034–1037

Valla D, Le MG, Poynard T, Zucman N, Rueff B, Benhamou JP (1986) Risk of hepatic vein thrombosis in relation to recent use of oral contraceptives. A case control study. Gastroenterology 90:807–811

Vanderhoof JA, Ament ME (1976) Fatal hepatic necrosis due to isoniazid chemoprophylaxis in a 15-year-old girl. J Pediatr: 88:867–868
Vanpelt FNAM, Kenna JG (1994) Formation of trifluoroacetylated protein antigens in cultured rat hepatocytes exposed to halothane in vitro. Biochem Pharmacol 48:461–471
Walker A, Park-Hah J (1977) Possible isoniazid-induced hepatotoxicity in a two-year-old child. J Pediatr 91:344–345
Wanless IR, Dore S, Gopinath G, Tan J, Cameron R, Heathcote EJ, Blendis LM, Levy G (1990) Histopathology of cocaine hepatotoxicity. Report of four cases. Gastroenterology 98:497–501
Wark H (1991) Halothane hepatitis in children. J Pediatr Gastroenterol Nutr 13:222–223
Wark HJ (1983) Postoperative jaundice in children. Anaesthesia 38:237–242
Warner LO, Beach TP, Gariss JP, Warner EJ (1984) Halothane and children: the first quarter century. Anesth Analg 63:838–840
Weber JL, Cutz E (1980) Liver failure in an infant. Can Med Assoc J 123:112–117
Whiting-O'Keefe QE, Fye KH, Sack KD (1991) Methotrexate and histologic hepatic abnormalities: a meta-analysis. Am J Med 90:711–716
Yagupsky P, Gazala E, Sofer S (1985) Fatal hepatic failure and encephalopathy associated with amiodarone therapy. J Pediatr 107:967–970
Zachariae H, Kragbulle K, Sugaard H (1980) Methotrexate induced liver cirrhosis. Br J Dermatol 102:407–412
Zafrani ES, Berthelot P (1982) Sodium valproate in the induction of unusual hepatotoxicity. Hepatology 2:648–649
Zafrani ES, Ishak KG, Rudzki C (1979) Cholestatic and hepatocellular injury associated with erythromycin esters. Report of nine cases. Dig Dis Sci 24:385–396
Zimmerman HJ (1990) Update of hepatotoxicity due to classes of drugs in common clinical use: non-steroidal drugs, anti-inflammatory drugs, antibiotics, antihypertensives, and cardiac and psychotropic drugs. Semin Liver Dis 10:322–338
Zimmerman HJ, Ishak KG (1982) Valproate-induced hepatic injury. analysis of 23 fatal cases. Hepatology 2:591–597
Zitelli BJ, Alexander J, Taylor S, Miller KD, Howrie DL, Kuritsky JN, Perez TH, Van Thiel DH (1987) Fatal hepatic necrosis due to pyrimethamine-sulfadoxine (Fansidar). Ann Intern Med 106:393–395
Zucker P, Daum F, Cohen MI (1975) Aspirin hepatitis. Am J Dis Child 129:1433–1434
Zucker P, Daum F, Cohen MI (1977) Fatal carbamazepine hepatitis. J Pediatr 91:667–668

CHAPTER 14

Reye's Syndrome

R.R. VARMA

A. Introduction

REYE, MORGAN and BARAL in 1963 in their classic paper described a distinct disease entity in children with characteristic clinicopathologic features (encephalopathy and fatty degeneration of the viscera). Manifestations of the disease included viral prodrome usually characterized by upper respiratory infection followed by severe vomiting after which mental changes and coma eventually occurred. Clinically, biochemically and histologically there was evidence of fatty liver, hypoglycemia and cerebral edema which eventually resulted in the death of 17 of 21 children reported in the series. In 1958, KAPILLA et al. had reported neurologic and hepatic disorders associated with influenza in children who had died following complications of the infection in India. In 1963, JOHNSON et al. who was then working at the Center for Disease Control, United States Public Health Service, and North Carolina State Health Department also described similar cases. However, whereas the Australian patients had been seen over a decade, the cases from North Carolina were clustered within 4 months and had occurred in association with an epidemic of influenza B. The association of chemical toxins with fatty degeneration has been speculated upon since the initial descriptions of the entity. REYE commented on the resemblance of Jamaican vomiting sickness and speculated about the possible role of toxins (REYE et al. 1963; LINNEMAN et al. 1975).

The association of Reye's syndrome with various viruses, especially varicella and influenza, especially influenza B, is well established (RUBIN 1975; TANG et al. 1975; COREY et al. 1976). The peak number of cases are reported in the winter months but sporadic cases may occur at any time of year (CROCKER and OZERE 1979). Varicella-related Reye's syndrome tends to occur in younger children, whereas influenza A, B-associated illness may occur more commonly in older children and young adults (MORSE 1975; VARMA et al. 1979). Less commonly associated viral infections include mumps, adenovirus, echovirus, coxsackievirus A and B and many others (SULLIVAN-BOLYAI and COREY 1981). In Thailand a similar syndrome has been reported in association with aflatoxin toxicity (DHIENSIRI et al. 1979). Some of these patients have no apparent viral infection and salicylate levels are relatively low. In Canada insecticides have been associated with Reye's syndrome and the possibility of insecticide-viral-toxin interaction has been suggested (CROCKER et al. 1974; CROCKER and OZERE 1979). In Malaysia, margosa oil (a long-chain fatty acid compound) toxicity and in Japan *ekiri* syndrome and *Toxischegrippe* (YAMASHITA et al. 1979) have been known to simulate Reye's syndrome, but there appears to be dissimilarities. Hymenoptera toxicity from multiple hornet stings produces an illness which produces some of the features which include hepatic steatosis and enlargement of the mitochondria. The link to salicylates has been suggested and may act as an inhibitor of mitochondrial function and produce additional metabolic changes. Salicylates may act synergistically with viral infections, especially influenza B, varicella and less commonly others.

B. Clinical Features

Reye's syndrome mostly occurs in children, but it has also been reported in adults. Average age at presentation is about 6 years with most children reporting in the 4- to 12-year-old range. The disease affects both sexes equally. Rural and suburban areas seem to exhibit a greater propensity than urban populations (COREY et al. 1976; HEUBI et al. 1987; BARRETT 1986; BALISTRERI and SCHUBERT 1993).

The illness follows a biphasic course. The initial phase is that of a viral prodrome characterized by a febrile illness, usually upper respiratory in nature. There may be a period of apparent recovery, which is then followed by the second phase, during which vomiting occurs. The illness then becomes protracted and pernicious and is followed by mental changes. Neurologic manifestations may occur rapidly. The disease represents a true emergency state which is capable of progressing to irreversible coma within a short period of time. Therefore, early diagnosis and prompt therapy are key to success and to a favorable outcome. Delirium and stupor may occur. Progressive coma follows in severe cases. Seizures, coma and death may occur within a day or two and progression may only take hours. Despite dramatic neurologic manifestations, there are no localizing signs. Liver is slightly or moderately enlarged. Despite coma and liver enlargement, jaundice typically does not occur except in more severe cases. The patients appear well nourished and are usually somewhat obese. Liver chemistries show a hepatocellular injury pattern. Hypoglycemia may be present in children usually under 4 years of age. Cerebrospinal fluid is normal with the exception of an increased opening pressure (SCHUBERT 1972).

A number of diseases may mimic Reye's syndrome (Table 1). For the accurate diagnosis of Reye's syndrome liver biopsy, including special fat stains and electron microscopy, is essential. Without electron microscopy the diagnosis remains questionable. However, in most of the cases liver biopsy can be performed even in the presence of coagulopathy by the use of fresh frozen plasma. In extreme cases it may not be safe. The timing of biopsy is also critical in that more diagnostic features are present within the first 24–48h of mental changes. The neurologic staging of Reye's syndrome is helpful in assessing the severity of illness and determining prognosis. In the 1970s there was considerable confusion about the staging. It was standardized during the Reye's Syn-

Table 1. Reye's-like syndromes

CNS infections	
Meningitis	
Encephalitis	
CNS intoxicants	
Toxic encephalopathy	
Drug ingestion	
Salicylate	Valproate
Tetracycline	Calcium hopantenate (HOPA)
Toxins	
Hypoglycin A	Aflatoxin (*Aspergillus flavus*)
Mushrooms (*Amanita phalloides*)	Pesticides and their emulsifiers
Margosa oil	Chlordane
Pyrrolizidine	Camphor
Methylbromides	Paint
Multiple stings by the oriental hornet	
Metabolic diseases	
Organic acidemias/defects in hepatic fatty acid oxidation (primary or secondary)	
Urea cycle defects	
Mitochondrial	CPS deficiency
	OTC deficiency
Extramitochondrial (Cytosolic)	Arginosuccinic acidemia
	Citrullinemia
	Arginemia
Hereditary fructose intolerance	
Defects in fatty acid metabolism	
Acyl-CoA dehydrogenase deficiencies	
Long-chain	(LCAD)
Medium-chain	(MCAD)
Short-chain	(SCAD)
Systemic carnitine deficiency	
Hepatic carnitine palmitoyltransferase deficiency	
3-OH, 3-methylglutanyl-CoA lyase deficiency	
Offspring of women with acute fatty liver of pregnancy	
Miscellaneous	
Neurogenic bladder or urethral stricture complicated by infection with urease-producing organisms	
Prune belly syndrome	

References: Brusilow and Horowich (1989), Drayna et al. (1981), Hinkle (1994), LaBreque (1979), Martens and Lee (1984), Osterloh et al. (1989), Roe and Coates (1989), Rognstad (1991), Rowe et al. (1988), Schoeman et al. (1991), Seifter and England (1994), Sweetman (1989), Touma and Charpentier (1992).

Table 2. Staging of Reye's syndrome[a]

	I	II	III	IV	V
Level of consciousness	Lethargy, follows verbal commands	Combative/ stupor, verbalizes inappropriately	Coma	Coma	Coma
Posture	Normal	Normal	Decorticate	Decerebrate	Flaccid
Response to pain	Purposeful	Purposeful	Decorticate	Decerebrate	None
Pupillary reaction	Brisk	Sluggish	Sluggish	Sluggish	None
Oculocephalic reflex (doll's eyes)	Normal	Conjugate deviation	Conjugate deviation	Inconsistent or absent	None

[a]Staging in criteria adopted at the NIH Reye's Syndrome Consensus Development Conference held in March 1981. Modified from the criteria proposed by LOVEJOY et al. (1974).

drome Consensus Development conference held at the National Institute of Health in March 1981. The criteria of LOVEJOY et al. (1974) were modified and five stages were given, which are summarized in Table 2. Stages I through III suggest mild to moderate and stages IV and V indicate presence of severe Reye's syndrome.

The Reye's syndrome mimickers of Reye's-like syndromes (BALISTRERI and SCHUBERT 1993) may be more likely under the following circumstances. These are cases presenting at infancy, with recurrent episodes or family history of Reye's syndrome, failure to thrive, developmental delay, history of death of a sibling in early childhood, and Reye's syndrome occurring in nonepidemic or sporadic forms. Under these circumstances, heredofamilial metabolic causes become much more likely and must be excluded. Normal or nearly normal serum aspartate transaminase (AST), alanine transaminase (ALT) levels and clinical jaundice, especially in the setting of relatively mild changes in sensorium, should suggest causes other than Reye's syndrome. In these settings tissue diagnosis is very helpful. In more recent years there has been a decline in the number of cases worldwide and the need for morphologic confirmation has increased.

C. Laboratory Features

Liver chemistries show features of hepatocellular injury. Both serum AST and ALT are elevated but levels tend to be lower than those seen in acute viral hepatitis. Serum levels exceed over 1000 units in a small minority of patients. Prothrombin time is prolonged despite vitamin K injections. Prothrombin time is within 2 s of control in mild cases but is more prolonged with increasing severity. Despite obvious changes in mentation or in the presence of coma, serum bilirubin levels are normal to mildly elevated. Clinical jaundice is uncommon and is usually limited to those with more severe stages of Reye's syndrome. Hypoglycemia is more common in children under the age of 4 years. Hypoglycemia in older children or in adults suggests other possibilities or severe Reye's syndrome.

Blood ammonia levels are elevated, especially if measured within 24h of the onset of encephalopathy (PARTIN 1972; TANG et al. 1975). Almost all patients with eventual progression to stage IV or V coma exhibit initial ammonia levels which reach 300μg/dl or higher, whereas those with levels within 1.5 times of normal on admission are distinctly more likely to have stage I disease (LICHTENSTEIN et al. 1983). Blood ammonia levels rapidly reach peak levels and then decline gradually regardless of the outcome. Other liver chemistries also improve.

Abnormalities of serum lipids and amino acids are noted and include elevated free fatty acids. A more consistent finding is a mild to moderate increase in propionic acid; mild and variable changes in butyrate, isobutyrate, valeric and isovaleric acids may also occur (VARMA et al. 1974). Octanoate and caprylic acids may be elevated. Serum amino acid elevations include those of alanine, glutamine and lysine. Citrulline levels are decreased.

Dicarboxylic acids appear in the serum and urine, and ketopenia and lactic acidemia may be noted. Increased excretion of sebacic (C_{10}), suberic (C_8) and adipic (C_6) acids may occur as peroxisomal β-oxidation cannot proceed beyond the 6 carbon chain. Serum creatinine phosphokinases are elevated. Other metabolic changes include lactic acidemia and hypercatecholaminemia. Salicylates were commonly detected in blood until the association with aspirin was suspected and the recommendation to avoid it in children with viral illness was made. Lumbar puncture may show elevated opening pressure but the spinal fluid itself is unremarkable and helps exclude meningitis and encephalitis. Electroencephalography shows features of metabolic encephalopathy. In severe cases, diffuse slowing and triphasic wave activity is seen. Computed tomography of head shows features of cerebral edema without loss of symmetry. Focal lesions are not present.

D. Diagnostic Criteria for Population Surveys

In the United States, The Center for Disease Control has used the following criteria for case definition. Acute onset of noninflammatory encephalopathy with: microvesicular fatty metamorphosis of the liver diagnosed by biopsy or autopsy; a threefold or greater rise in serum AST, ALT or ammonia; if cerebral spinal fluid is obtained, it must have ≤8 leukocytes/mm^3. These criteria were adopted for epidemiologic and other studies involving large populations. In individual cases, a more detailed evaluation, especially electron microscopic, may be needed.

E. Liver Morphology

In mild cases slight rarefaction of the mitochondria is present along with pleomorphism, swelling and reduction in their number and partial loss of cristae. These changes become more pronounced in severe cases. Ameboid forms appear, cristae may be completely lost, and pleomorphism and loss of mitochondrial dense bodies are more pronounced. These changes reflect the uncoupling of cellular respiration. During recovery large mitochondria divide. Budding and branching forms appear. By the 3rd or 4th day these changes improve and the mitochondrial matrix appears normal or near normal. The varying timing at which liver biopsies were undertaken in various series may in significant part account for the conflicting morphology reported in the literature (PARTIN et al. 1971; HEUBI 1987; TANG et al. 1975; LICHTENSTEIN 1983; BOVE et al. 1975).

Other ultrastructural changes observed in the liver are less specific and consistent. In mild forms, glycogen is abundant but decreases with severity. Proliferation of the smooth endoplasmic reticulum is common. Golgi bodies which contain very low density lipoproteins are generally empty but become filled during recovery. Peroxisomes may be increased in number. Virus particles may be seen. The liver history is nearly normal in children who were biopsied 2 months after illness. The abnormal mitochondrial morphology observed correlates with changes in mitochondrial enzyme levels which are generally decreased but not absent. The reduction in these enzymes results in a variety of changes in carbohydrate, amino acid, fatty acid, ammonia and coagulation metabolism.

F. Brain Morphology

Grossly the brain shows features on cerebral edema. The brain size is increased and flattening of gyri and sulci is present. Tonsillar herniation may be seen. On the cut surface, the cortical and subcortical white matter and gray and white matter are sharply demarcated. The deep white matter is swollen and ventricles are compressed. Morphologic and biochemical studies of the brain tissue in Reye's syndrome patients is limited. Changes in brain tissue occur rapidly and autopsy specimens may not provide reliable results. Brain biopsies performed during cranial surgery to reduce intracranial pressure provided a reliable but limited amount of tissue (PARTIN et al. 1975, 1978, 1979).

Inflammation and necrosis are absent or minimal. The myelin sheath is edematous and contains blebs. Astrocyte swelling and alterations of neuronal mitochondria essentially similar to those observed in the liver are seen. The changes observed in brain morphology obtained during craniectomy may not be identical to those seen at autopsy when additional factors such as hypoxia and tissue autolysis complicate the interpretation and appearance of the brain tissue and enzyme determinations may also not be reliable. Enzyme levels measured in brain specimens obtained antemortem are normal (ROBINSON et al. 1978). In this respect brain tissue differs significantly from liver, where the levels are clearly reduced. The normal enzyme levels in brain tissue may, at least in part, be due to a limited amount of specimens being available to conduct enzyme determinations. Neuronal tissue comprises only a small fraction of the brain cells. Repeating these studies in larger brain tissue specimens obtained antemortem may minimize this probable sampling error but is not practical. Moreover, astrocyte swelling may be the consequence of hyperammonemia rather than a primary event. Disorders of the urea cycle are frequently associated with astrocyte swelling.

Other organs. Fatty infiltration has also been reported in the muscles, lungs, pancreas, renal tubules and myocardial fibrils in Reye's syndrome (BALISTRERI and SCHUBERT 1993).

G. Liver Histology and Electron Microscopy in Reye's Syndrome

In patients with medium-chain acyl CoA dehydrogenase deficiency (MCAD) and long-chain acyl CoA dehydrogenase deficiency (LCAD), liver biopsies are distinct from those seen in Reye's patients. These findings very from normal morphology when the patient is doing well to more severe alterations. Histologically the macro- or microvesicular steatosis, or both, may be present. Inflammatory changes, if present, are minimal. Fibrosis may be scant but in some cases marked fibrosis or even cirrhosis may be detected (TREEM et al. 1986). Ultrastructurally, the liver may be normal or show minimal, nonspecific changes. Mitochondria may be normal or may show crystalloids in the matrix often associated with an increased number of cristae. Enlarged and abnormally shaped mitochondria with condensed appearance due to increased density of the matrix with widening of the intracrystal space may be observed. Liver morphology in short-chain acyl CoA deficiency is less well defined. Short-chain fatty acid levels are mildly abnormal in Reye's syndrome but blood propionic acid levels may be more consistently elevated. However, these levels are not in the range seen in patients with propionic acidemia.

In patients with valproic acid hepatotoxicity, microvesicular steatosis and necrosis are common and cirrhosis may be present (ZIMMERMAN and ISHAK 1982). In urea cycle enzyme deficiencies (Table 3), the liver biopsy is also quite variable. LABRECQUE (1979) reported on a series of 16 patients, 3 with carbamyl phosphate synthetase (CPS) deficiency and the remaining 13 with ornithine transcarbamylase (OTC) deficiency. Liver histology was normal in two children and showed mild microvesicular fatty change in the other. Liver histology was normal in three OTC-deficient patients. In the other ten, morphology showed a wide spectrum, varying from relatively mild nonspecific changes mild to moderate microvesicular steatosis, and inflammation. Fibrosis was less common but in one case bridging fibrosis was seen. Electron microscopy was not undertaken in this study and biopsies were performed at

Table 3. Features of urea cycle disorders

Disorder	Histologic changes	Enzyme deficiency	Amino acids
A. Mitochondrial			
1. *N*-Acetylglutamate[a]	Micro- and macrovesicular steatosis	*N*-Acetylglutamate synthetase	↓ Urine orotic acid
a) CPS deficiency[c]	Microsteatosis	Carbamyl phosphate synthetase	↓ Citrulline ↓ Arginine ↑ Glutamine, alanine
2. OTC deficiency[b]	No steatosis or microsteatosis, focal inflammation, fibrosis	Ornithine transcarbomylase	↑↑ Orotic acid ↑↑ Orotic acid
B. Extramitochondrial (cytasolic)			
3. Citrullinemia[b]	Microvesicular steatosis, focal necrosis	Arginosuccinate synthetase	↑↑ Citrulline ↓ Arginine
4. Arginosuccinic[b] acidurea	Microvesicular steatosis	Arginosuccinase (lyase)	↑↑ Arginosuccinic acid ↓ Citrulline
5. Arginemia[b]	Microvesicular steatosis, ballooning degeneration	Arginase	↑↑ Arginine

[a] Data Limited: mode of inheritance not clear.
[b] X-linked disorder.
[c] Autosomal recessive inheritance.
For references see foot of Table 1.

various stages of illness or while the patients were asymptomatic. The same group undertook another study during which patients with CPS deficiency and their close relatives and two siblings with OTC deficiency underwent liver biopsies, during which EM was also performed. The liver mitochondria showed minimal alterations with essentially normal mitochondria during periods when patients were relatively asymptomatic. Liver mitochondria were normal in CPS-deficient heterozygotes (LATHAM et al. 1984). *N*-Acetylglutamate a (mitochondrial matrix enzyme which is a physiologic activator of carbamyl phosphate synthetase I) deficiency states are rare. Liver biopsy shows micro- and macrovesicular steatosis. Electron microscopy shows irregular-shaped mitochondria which contain intracristae crystallizations (VOCKLEY et al. 1992).

Liver biopsy in patients with salicylate intoxication shows nearly normal histology, and lipid accumulations may be minimal. Mitochondria and peroxisomes appear normal on electron microscopy (PARTIN et al. 1984). Salicylism must also be distinguished from salicylate hepatotoxicity, especially in those patients with associated "collagen vascular diseases."

H. Pathophysiology

Despite an extensive knowledge base, the precise mechanism of Reye's syndrome is not clearly understood. Any theory proposed must adequately explain the following factors: mitochondrial changes especially those observed in the liver, brain and perhaps a more generalized mitochondrial dysfunction; association with viral prodrome, during the initial phase of the biphasic illness; preponderance in children and younger adults even while most viral illnesses associated with the disease affect all ages; role of salicylate use and role of other environmental toxins probably in conjunction with viral illness; reason for dramatic decline in the number of cases; general absence of Reye's syndrome in more than one family member even though most family members have the same viral illness; starvation or near starvation status due to poor oral intake and increased gastrointestinal loss (diarrhea, vomiting) is common and increased lipolysis can be expected.

The precise pathophysiology of Reye's syndrome is not known. Several theories have been proposed. One of the most common is that of a phenomenon that may be related to viral-toxin interaction. Viral illnesses, especially influenza B and varicella, are most likely to be associated. However, any virus infection can potentially result in the development of Reye's syndrome. The implicated antecedent viral illness usually, and uniformly, affects most family members, only one of whom develops Reye's syndrome. In others, the viral prodrome is uncomplicated. What produces the illness in only one, but not in other, family members, and what causes one to develop Reye's syndrome out of several thousand people afflicted by the same virus, remains one of the key unanswered questions.

Several toxins have been suspected and their roles investigated (CROCKER 1974; SAFE 1979). Reye himself noticed the similarity to Jamaican vomiting sickness, which results from the ingestion of unripe fruit of the ackee tree, which contains hypoglycin. Hypoglycin toxicity primarily affects children in a poor state of nutrition and carries a high mortality, causing inhibition of fatty acid oxidation, which then lowers tissue levels of CoA and carnitine, both cofactors necessary for fatty acid oxidation. Hypoglycin toxicity thus results in the development of isovaleric and alfa-methylbutyric acidemias, neither of which have been observed consistently in Reye's syndrome. Other toxins suspected in the inhibition of fatty acid metabolism and the development of Reye's-like syndromes are magosa oil (SINNIAH et al. 1989), valproic acid (KATAFUCHI et al. 1989) and calcium hopantenate (NODA et al. 1988). Sera obtained from Reye's syndrome patients have been the subject of several studies and are summarized in another section.

Hepatic mitochondrial enzymes are consistently decreased but are not absent in patients with Reye's syndrome (Table 4) and result in disturbances to the urea and citric acid cycles, gluconeogenesis and others. Cytosolic enzyme levels are normal. Increased lipolysis further adds to the mitochondrial dysfunction. β-Oxidation is thus compromised or overwhelmed and dicarboxylic acids appear in the serum and urine (TRACEY 1988). Compounds such as dicarboxylic acids are referred to as uncouplers which inhibit mitochondrial phosphorylation, impair ATP formation and have other adverse effects (KANG 1989). What brings about such a cascade of changes is not clear and reduction

Table 4. Mitochondrial enzyme changes in Reye's syndrome[a]

A.	Involving urea cycle
	Carbamyl phosphate synthetase
	Ornithine transcarbamylase
B.	Involving gluconeogenesis
	Pyruvate carboxylase
	Pyruvate dehydrogenase
C.	Involving citric acid cycle
	Citrate synthetase
	Glutamate dehydrogenase
	Succinic dehydrogenase
	Malic dehydrogenase
	Isocitric dehydrogenase
D.	Cytochrome oxidase

[a] Levels generally reduced but not absent.

of hepatic ATP has not been established. That sera obtained from Reye's syndrome patients do have uncoupling potential has been suggested by TONSGARD and GETZ (1985). Accumulation of the products of impaired β-oxidation has been demonstrated by CORKEY (1988), who later (CORKEY 1991) demonstrated elevated plasma cytokines in Reye's syndrome during acute illness and suggested a genetic defect in cytokinoreceptor-modulated signal transduction. Cytokine production is stimulated by viral infection and by aspirin. Similarities of these changes to those observed in patients with long- and medium-chain acyl CoA dehydrogenase deficiencies were implied. The authors used Center for Disease Control criteria (see previous section), and it is not clear if electron microscopy was required for the diagnosis of Reye's syndrome. It is interesting that several of the Reye's-like syndromes, such as valproate, margosa oil and calcium hopantenate, seem to inhibit fatty acid metabolism and may have some common features.

I. Aspirin and Reye's Syndrome

Children dying from salicylate toxicity have cerebral edema and have microvesicular fatty liver without inflammation or necrosis. Electron microscopy does not show any of the characteristics of Reye's syndrome. Despite disturbances in the acid-base balance, coagulopathy and liver dysfunction, there are clinical and other differences. Even histology of the liver may show minimal fat and liver mitochondria are normal. Until 1980 or so, salicylates were detected in most children with Reye's syndrome but levels did not correlate with severity of mental changes.

That various drugs used in the symptomatic treatment of antecedent viral illness may have a role has been a matter of speculation and debate for decades (Reye et al. 1963; Nartens 1984; Taylor et al. 1985). A report of salicylate-treated varicella infection complicated by encephalopathy which antedated Reye's paper may represent the first indication of a potential link between salicylates and Reye's syndrome (Mortimer and Lepow 1962). Reye's syndrome cases were seen in New Zealand in the 1950s and 1960s, but mysteriously almost disappeared in later years. The clinical similarity between Reye's syndrome and salicylate intoxication has further heightened the interest about the role of salicylates. The toxic potential of salicylates is summarized later in this section. In the late 1970s and the early 1980s three case-controlled studies were conducted in the United States, in the states of Ohio (Linneman et al. 1975; Sullivan-Bolyai 1980; Halpin et al. 1982), Arizona (Starko et al. 1980) and Michigan (Waldman et al. 1982). In all three studies the use of aspirin was reported by a significantly higher proportion of children with Reye's syndrome than controls. A great deal of controversy arose as a result of limitations and biases in the design of these and other studies (Young et al. 1984; Remington et al. 1984, 1985; Daniels et al. 1985). The Surgeon General advised against the use of salicylates in children in antecedent viral illnesses. Based on the available data, the United States Public Health Service (Hurwitz et al. 1985, 1987) conducted additional studies which more clearly established the association of salicylate use and subsequent diagnosis of Reye's syndrome. As a result there was a mandate for warning labels on all salicylate-containing products. There was a dramatic decline in the use of baby aspirin and a persistent decline in Reye's syndrome followed. There has been a worldwide decline in the use of aspirin in children and in the number of Reye's syndrome cases seen. This decline may not necessarily be all due to avoidance of salicylates. Parents seem to be more cautious in the use of drugs in general in the symptomatic relief of viral illnesses and in the control of febrile episodes. However, in a small proportion of cases, Reye's syndrome may occur even in those who have not taken salicylates, which therefore cannot account for all cases. Newly diagnosed cases not associated with salicylates may be milder in nature. Salicylates may also adversely affect the course of various organic acidemias such as those associated long-, medium- and perhaps short-chain acyl-CoA dehydrogenase deficiencies and other metabolic disorders and it may be due to their adverse effects on mitochondrial/peroxisomal functions (Deschamps 1991).

In man, salicylates may uncouple mitochondrial respiration, produce mitochondrial swelling and impair ATP formation. Gluconeogenesis may also be impaired. In isolated rat mitochondria, salicylates potentiate Ca^{2+}-induced damage to inner mitochondrial membrane (You 1983; Yoshida et al. 1988; Gutknecht 1992), may directly inhibit oxidative phosphorylation, displace albumin-bound fatty and dicarboxylic acids in the serum, and increase mitochondrial load for CoA-dependent β-oxidation (Tonsgard 1988). Additional studies suggest that salicylates inhibit gluconeogenesis and induce ω-oxidation (Mock 1986; Murphy 1992;

SAKAIDA 1990). Salicylate metabolism may be altered in patients with Reye's syndrome. Salicylate turnover may be prolonged. Aspirin esterase activity may be reduced. Reye's syndrome must be differentiated from salicylate intoxication (ROSENFELD and LIEBHABER 1976; REMINGTON et al. 1985).

J. Animal Models

No available animal model reliably reproduces the biochemical and morphologic features of Reye's syndrome in the human. That is especially frustrating given the fact that in 2 decades numerous investigators have attempted to develop a suitable animal model based on the facts available at the time. Reye suggested that environmental toxin(s) may play a role in the development of the disease and numerous studies published since then have supported that opinion. Despite evidence suggesting a possible role of pesticides, herbicides and surfactants, such agents have not been identified in sufficient quantities in the biologic specimens obtained from patients with Reye's syndrome. BROWNSTEIN (1984) developed an animal model in Balb/cByj mice exposed to indigenous murine viruses. These mice developed a disease with striking similarity to Reye's syndrome. Unfortunately, even the same authors could not reproduce the results during subsequent experiments. The readers are referred to a review of the subject by HEUBI et al. (1987). Please also refer to other sections of this book. Since HEUBI's review, other animal models have been proposed. KUNDU et al. (1991) assessed ω-oxidation of a spectrum of fatty acids in rats and then investigated the effect of aspirin pretreatment. Aspirin increased liver free fatty acids as well as the capacity for ω-oxidation three- to sevenfold, especially of the long chain. Based on a number of experiments, the authors concluded that aspirin was a potent stimulator of ω-oxidation and suggested that there may be multiple enzymes with overlapping substrate specificity. HIDAKA et al. (1991) developed a 4-pentanoic acid induced rat model and found that 16, 16-dimethyl prostaglandin E_2 pretreatment prevented the experimental liver injury resembling that of Reye's syndrome. The relevance of these interesting experiments to human disease and extent to which the changes produced resembled Reye's syndrome is not clear. Study of the effects of agents implicated in the encephalopathy of Reye's syndrome using mouse astrocytes in primary culture provides useful insights for future experiments, but will need additional studies in different animals. The effects of intraperitoneal infections of margosa oil, 4-pentanoic acid, valproic acid, calcium hopantenate and other compounds and the development of seizures and brain edema by KATAFUCHI et al. (1989) had many dissimilarities to Reye's syndrome and aspirin injection did not result in seizures.

K. Reye's Syndrome in Adults

Viral illnesses associated in children with Reye's syndrome also afflict adults. Therefore, Reye's syndrome can be expected to occur at any age. It has been reported in several adults in the literature. Our experience with such children including adolescents led us to look for the disease in adults. Reye's syndrome was diagnosed between 1976 and 1983 in seven adults. All of them were seen at five metropolitan Milwaukee hospitals. Their features were similar to those seen in children. At least five of the seven patients had taken salicylates for antecedent viral illnesses. The diagnosis of Reye's syndrome was more difficult in adults as it was confirmed in only 7 out of 22 patients in whom it was suspected (VARMA et al. 1979; MEYTHALER and VARMA 1987; EDDY et al. 1988; MORSE 1975). Drug abuse and drug-induced hepatotoxicity were two of the most common problems mimicking Reye's syndrome in adults. Therefore, liver biopsy is even more critical in the diagnosis and must be done as much as practically possible. Unlike in children, salicylates are still widely used in adults. Caution is needed in their use in adults during acute viral illnesses, especially on a regular basis. As in children, the occurrence of Reye's syndrome in adults also appears to have decreased in the Milwaukee area. However, in recent years we have encountered resistance in the referral of adults with features suggestive of Reye's syndrome due to managed care restrictions in southeastern Wisconsin. Such practices limit referrals to tertiary care facilities with special areas of expertise.

L. Treatment

The following are the key factors in the successful management:

1. *Early diagnosis and prompt treatment* are likely to improve the chances of survival. Reye's syndrome should be considered in any child with unexplained neurologic symptoms regardless of vomiting. In adults with relatively typical presentation, the possibility of Reye's syndrome should, at least, be considered. A team approach in an ICU setting at a tertiary care facility is essential. Rapid change in sensorium is common and therefore should be expected and therapy planned accordingly.
2. *Cerebral edema* is the most common cause of high mortality and should be treated aggressively. Therefore, control of increased intracranial pressure should be the primary goal of therapy. Correction of metabolic abnormality should be secondary. Close monitoring of intracranial pressure is needed as the mental status deteriorates. Clinical signs may not be reliable. As the intracranial pressure rises, it may approach systemic pressure, resulting in a significant reduction in cerebral perfusion pressure. The aim of therapy is to maintain adequate perfusion pressure, maintain aerobic metabolism and reduce elevated intracranial pressure. Dextrose solution 10%–15% along with appropriate electrolytes is generally used at most centers. It acts as a

mild osmotic agent, reduces the chances of hypoglycemia and may improve lipolysis. We prefer less than maintenance fluid replacement with frequent monitoring of serum osmolarity to just over 300 mOsm because it may reduce the risk of cerebral edema. Others have used normal fluid replacement to minimize renal complications. Whether or not giving normal or less than normal fluid replacement changes the risk of cerebral edema is not established. Frequent monitoring of arterial blood gases, electrolytes, glucose, ammonia and prothrombin time is recommended. Hourly mental status check is indicated. The head of the bed should be elevated; the patient should be kept quiet and unstimulated as much as possible. Several modalities to lower intracranial pressure include intravenous mannitol (drip or bolus), use of respirator to protect airway, hyperventilation, hypothermia, pentobarbital coma, placement of subdural, intraventricular or other devices. In most severe cases craniectomy may be considered if all other measures are unsuccessful. Use of a mannitol drip may be preferable to boluses to reduce the risk of "rebound" rise in intracranial pressure. Protection of airway and hyperventilation appears to be a more accepted initial step.

3. *Management of liver failure* consists of nasogastric suction, cleansing enemas, lactulose with or without neomycin, antacids and H_2-receptor antagonists. Hypokalemia and serious coagulopathy should be corrected. Fresh frozen plasma contains substantial amounts of sodium and should be given with caution.
4. *Correction of metabolic abnormalities:* Exchange transfusion has been used by many centers (PARTIN 1972). Use of fresh blood obtained within 24h is not necessary for this purpose. Saline-washed packed red cells used in conjunction with stored fresh frozen plasma offer an adequate substitute and pose less strain on blood banks (CASPER et al. 1976). In one such patient under our care, peritoneal dialysis was administered continuously for the treatment of preexisting chronic renal failure but was interrupted during periodic exchange transfusions. During the course of treatment computerized EEG was performed for several days and was analyzed separately without knowledge of the patient's clinical status. The EEG changes improved during exchange transfusion on three separate occasions until he recovered (HARRINGTON 1975). Several other therapies have been proposed but their roles remain unclear.

M. Sequelae

Neuropsychiatric deficits have been described in some of the patients who recovered from the bout of Reye's syndrome and appear to be more severe in those with grade IV encephalopathy. Those with Grade V rarely survive. One of our adult patients presenting in grade V survived but remained in a vegetative state several years later when last seen. However, residual deficits are not necessarily limited to patients with severe Reye's syndrome. It is my impression that those treated with exchange transfusion seem to have a more complete recovery and sequelae may be less common.

References

Balistreri WF, Schubert WK (1993) Liver disease in infancy and childhood. In: Schiff L, Schiff ER (eds) Diseases of the liver. Lippincott, Philadelphia, pp 1099–1203

Barrett MJ, Hurwitz ES, Schonberger LB (1986) Changing epidemiology of Reye syndrome in the United States. Pediatrics 77:598–602

Bove KE, McAdams AJ, Partin JC et al. (1975) Hepatic lesions in Reye's syndrome. Gastroenterology 69:685

Brownstein DG, Johnson EA, Smith AL (1984) Spontaneous Reye's like syndrome in BALB/cByJ mice. Lab Invest 51:386–395

Brusilow SW, Horowich AL (1989) Urea cycle enzymes. In: Scriver CR, Beaudet AL, Sly WS et al. (eds) The metabolic basis of inherited disease, 6th edn. McGraw-Hill, New York, pp 629–663

Casper JT, Varma RR, Lewis JD et al. (1976) Exchange transfusion in Reye's syndrome with saline washed red blood cells. Transfusion 16:130–134

Consensus Development Conference (1981) Diagnosis and treatment of Reye's syndrome. JAMA 246:1441–1444

Corey L, Rubin RJ, Hattwick MAW et al. (1976) A national outbreak of Reye's syndrome: its epidemiologic relationship to influenza B. Am J Med 61: 615–625

Corkey BE, Hale DE, Glennon MC et al. (1988) Relationship between unusual hepatic acyl CoA profiles and the pathogenesis of Reye's syndrome. J Clin Invest 82:782–788

Corkey BE, Geschwind JF, Deeney FJ et al. (1991) Ca^{2+} response to interleukin 1 and tumor necrosis factor in cultured human skin fibroblasts: possible implications for Reye syndrome. J Clin Invest 87:778–786

Crocker JFS, Ozere RL (1979) The incidence and etiology of Reye's syndrome in Eastern Canada. In: Crocker JFS (ed) Reye's syndrome II. Grune and Stratton, New York, pp 3–12

Crocker JFS, Rozee KR, Ozere RL et al. (1974) Viral interaction as a cause of fatty visceral changes and encephalopathy in the mouse. Lancet II:22–24

Crocker JFS, Renten KW, Lee SH et al. (1986) Biochemical and morphological characteristics of a mouse model of Reye's syndrome induced by the interaction of influenza B virus and chemical emulsifier. Lab Invest 54:32–40

Daniels SR, Greenberg RS, Ibrahim MA (1985) Scientific uncertainties in the studies of salicylate use and Reye's syndrome. JAMA 249:1311–1316

Deschamps D, Fisch C, Fromenty B et al. (1991) Inhibition by salicylic acid of the activation and thus oxidation of long chain fatty acids: possible role in the development of Reye's syndrome. J Phamacol Exp Ther 259:894–904

Dhiensiri K, Sinavatana P, Lertsookprasert S et al. (1979) Reye's syndrome in Northeastern Thailand. In: Crocker JFS (ed) Reye's syndrome II. Grune and Stratton, New York, pp 77–100

Drayna CJ, Titcomb CP, Varma RR et al. (1981) Hyperammonemic encephalopathy in neurogenic bladder complicated by infection. N Engl J Med 304:766–768

Eddy AD, Heiselman DE, Bradford JC (1988) Acute encephalography in a 62-year-old woman with a viral syndrome. Ann Emerg Med 17:1234–1242

Gutknecht J (1992) Aspirin, acetaminophen and proton transport through phospholipid bilayers and mitochondrial membranes. Mol Cell Biochem 114:3–8

Halpin TJ, Holtzhauer FJ, Campbell RJ et al. (1982) Reye's syndrome and medication use. JAMA 248:687–691

Harrington GJ (1975) Electroencephalopgraphic monitoring of exchange transfusion in Reye's syndrome. In: Pollack JD (ed) Reye's syndrome. Grune and Stratton, New York, pp 61–64

Heubi JE, Partin JC, Partin JS et al. (1987) Reye's syndrome: current concepts. Hepatology 7:155–164

Hidaka T, Inokuchi T, Nakamura Y et al. (1991) Prevention of 4-pentanoic acid induced liver injury in rats by 16,16-dimethyl PgE_2. Exp Mol Pathol 55:135–142

Hinkle PC (1994) Mitochondria. In: Arias IM, Boyer JL, Fausto N et al (eds) The liver: biology and pathobiology, 3rd edn. Raven, New york, pp 309–317

Hurwitz ES, Barrett MJ, Bergman D et al. (1985) Public health service study on Reye's syndrome and medication. N Engl J Med 313:849–857

Hurwitz ES, Barrett MJ, Bergman D et al. (1987) Public health service of Reye's syndrome and medication: report of the main study. JAMA 257:1905–1911

Johnson GM, Scurletis TR, Carrol NB (1963) A study of sixteen fatal cases of encephalitis-like disease in North Carolina children. N C Med J 24:464–473

Kang ES, Matsuo N, Ngai T et al. (1989) Serum lipolytic activity in Reye's syndrome. Clin Chim Acta 184:107–114

Kang ES, Johnson SB, Holman RT (1991) Fatty acid composition of hepatic triglycerides in Reye's syndrome: implications for hepatic desaturase abnormalities. Clin Chim Acta 204:167–177

Kapila CC, Kaul S, Kapur SC et al. (1958) Neurologic and hepatic disorders associated with influenza. Br Med J 2:1311–1314

Katafuchi Y, Yoshida I et al. (1989) Effects of drugs and fatty acids related to Reye syndrome on brain water content in rats. Acta Pediatr Jpn 312:115–119

Kundu RK, Tonsgard JH, Getz GS (1991) Induction of omega-oxidation of monocarboxylic acids in rats by acetylsalicylic acid. J Clin Invest 88:1865–1872

LaBrecque DR (1979) Heritable urea cycle enzyme deficiency – liver disease in 16 patients. J Pediatrics 94:580–587

Latham PS, LaBrecque DR, McReynolds JW et al. (1989) Liver ultrastructure in mitochondrial urea cycle enzyme deficiencies and comparison with Reye's syndrome. Hepatology 4:404–407

Lichtenstein PK, Heubi JE, Dougherty CC et al. (1983) Grade I Reye's syndrome; a frequent cause of vomiting and liver dysfunction after varicella and upper respiratory tract infection. N Engl J Med 309:133–139

Linneman CC Jr, Shea L, Partin JC et al. (1975) Reye's syndrome: epidemiologic and viral studies 1963–1974. Am J Epidemiol 101:517–526

Lovejoy FH, Smith AL, Bresman ML et al. (1974) Clinical staging of Reye's syndrome. Am J Dis Child 128:36–41

Martens ME, Lee CP (1984) Reye's syndrome: salicylates and mitochondrial function. Biochem Pharmacol 33:2869

Meythaler JM, Varma RR (1987) Reye's syndrome in adults: diagnostic considerations. Arch Intern Med 147:61–64

Mock DM (1986) Fatty acids in Reye's syndrome (editorial). Hepatology 8:1414–1415

Morse RS, Holmes AW, Levin S (1975) Reye's syndrome in an adult. Am J Dig Dis 20:1184–1190

Mortimer EA Jr, Lepow ML (1962) Varicella with hypoglycemia possibly due to salicylates. Am J Dis Child 103:583–590

Murphy MG, Jollimore C, Crocker JF et al. (1992) Beta oxidation of (1–14c) palmitic acid by mouse astrocytes in primary culture: effects of agents implicated in the encephalopathy of Reye's syndrome. J Neurolsci Res 33:445–454

Noda S, Umazaki H, Yamamoto K et al. (1988) Reye-like syndrome following treatment with the pantothenic acid antagonist, calcium hopantenate. J Neurol Neurosurg Psychiatry 51:582–585

Osterloh J, Cunningham W, Dixon A et al. (1989) Biochemical relationships between Reye's and Reye's-like metabolic and toxicologic syndromes. Med Toxicol Adverse Drug Exp 4:272–294

Partin JC, Schubert WK, Partin JS (1971) Mitochondrial ultrastructure in Reye's syndrome encephalopathy and fatty degeneration of the viscera. N Engl J Med 285:1339–1343
Partin JC, Partin JS, Schubert WK et al. (1975) Brain ultrastructure in Reye's syndrome (encephalopathy and fatty alteration of the viscera). J Neuropathol Exp Neurol 34:425–444
Partin JS, McAdams AJ, Partin JC et al. (1978) Brain ultrastructure in Reye's syndrome II. J Neuropathol Exp Neurol 37:796–819
Partin JS, Dougherty CC, McAdams J et al. (1984) A comparison of liver ultrastructure in salicylate intoxication and Reye's syndrome. Hepatology 4:687–690
Remington PL, Rowley D, McGee H et al. (1984) Decreasing trends in Reye syndrome and aspirin use in Michigan 1979–1984. Pediatrics 77:93
Remington PL, Shabino CL, McGee H et al. (1985) Reye syndrome and juvenile rheumatoid arthritis in Michigan. Am J Dis Child 139:870–872
Reye DRK, Morgan G, Baral J (1963) Encephalopathy and fatty degeneration of viscera: a disease entity in childhood. Lancet II:749–752
Robinson BH, Taylor J, Cutz E et al. (1978) Reye's syndrome: preservaion of mitochondrial enzymes in brain and muscle compared with liver. Pediatr Res 12:1045–1047
Roe CR, Coates PM (1989) Acyl-CoA dehydrogenase deficiencies. In: Scriver CR, Beaudet AL, Sly WS et al (eds). The metabolic basis of inherited disease, 6th edn. McGraw-Hill, New York, pp 889–914
Rognstad R (1991) Effects of salicylate on hepatocyte lactate metabolism. Biomed Biochim Acta 50:921–930
Rosenfeld RG, Liebhaber MI (1976) Acute encephalopathy in siblings; Reye's syndrome vs salicylate intoxication. JAMA 130:295–297
Rowe PC, Valle D, Brusilow SW (1988) Inborn errors of metabolism in children referred with Reye's syndrome: a changing pattern. JAMA 260:3167–3170
Rubin RJ, Gregg MD (1975) Influenza surveillance in the United States 1972–1974. Am J Epidem 102:225–232
Safe S, Hutzinger O, Crocker JFS et al. (1979) The role of chemicals in Reye's syndrome. In: Crocker JFS (ed) Reye's syndrome II. Grune and Stratton, New York, pp 3–12
Sakaida N, Senzaki H, Shikata N et al. (1990) Microvesicular fatty liver in rats with resembling Reye's syndrome induced by 4-pentanoc acid. Acta Pathol Jpn 40:635–642
Schoeman MN, Batey RG, Wilden B (1991) Recurrent acute fatty liver of pregnancy associated with a fatty acid oxidation defect in the offspring. Gastroenterology 100:544–548
Schubert WK, Partin JC, Partin JS (1972) Encephalopathy and fatty liver (Reye's syndrome). In: Popper H, Schaffner F (eds) Progress in liver disease, vol 4. Grune and Stratton, New York, pp 489–510
Seifter S, England S (1994) Energy metabolism. In: Arias IM, Boyer JL, Fausto N et al (eds) The liver: biology and pathobiology, 3rd edn. Raven, New York, pp 323–364
Sinniah R, Sinniah D, Chia LS et al. (1989) Animal model of margosa oil ingestion with Reye-like syndrome: pathogenesis of microvesicular fatty liver. J Pathol 159:255–264
Starko KM, Ray CG, Moninguez LB et al. (1980) Reye's syndrome and salicylate use. Pediatrics 66:859–864
Sweetman L (1989) Branched chain organic acidurias. In: Scriver CR, Beaudet AL, Sly WS et al (eds) The metabolic basis of inherited disease, 6th edn. McGraw-Hill, New York, pp 791–819
Sullivan-Bolyai JZ, Corey LE (1981) Epidemiology of Reye syndrome. Johns Hopkins University School of Hygiene Public Health 3:1–26
Sullivan-Bolyai JZ, Marks JS, Johnson D et al. (1980) Reye's syndrome in Ohio. Am J Epidemiol 112:629–638

Tang TT, Siegesmund KA, Sedmak GV et al. (1975) Reye's syndrome: a correlated electron microscopic, viral and biochemical observation. JAMA 232:1339–1346
Taylor JP, Gustafson MD, Johnson CC et al. (1985) Antipyretic use among children during the 1983 influenza season. Am J Dis Child 139:486–488
Tonsgard JH, Getz GS (1985) Effect of Reye's syndrome serum on isolated chinchilla liver mitochondria. J Clin Invest 76:816
Tonsgard JH, Mendelson SA, Meredith SC (1988) Binding of straight-chain saturated dicarboxylic acids to albumin. J Clin Invest 82:1567–1573
Touma EH, Charpentier C (1992) Medium chain acyl-CoA dehydrogenase deficiency. Arch Dis Childhood 67:142–145
Tracey BM, Cheng KN, Rosankiewicz J et al. (1988) Urinary C_6–C_{12} dicarboxylic acylcarnitines in Reye's syndrome. Clin Chim Acta 175:79–87
Treem WR, Piccoli DA, Hale DE et al. (1986) Medium chain and long chain acyl CoA dehydrogenase deficiency: clinical, pathologic and ultrastructural differentiation from Reye's syndrome. Hepatology 6:1270–1278
Varma RR, Cherayil GD, Casper JT et al. (1974) Short chain fatty acids in Reye's syndrome: dissimilarity to isovaleric and alfa methyl butyric acidemias. Clin Res 22:606A (abstract)
Varma RR, Casper JT, Lewis JD et al. (1976) Changing patterns of Reye's syndrome. In: Pollack JD (ed) Reye's syndrome. Grune and Stratton, New York, pp 416–417
Varma RR, Reidel DR, Komorowski RA et al. (1979) Reye's syndrome in nonpediatric age groups. JAMA 242:1373–1375
Vockley J, Vockley M, Lin SP et al. (1992) Normal N-acetylglutamate concentration measured in liver from a new patient with N-acetylglutamate synthetase deficiency: physiologic and biochemical implications. Biochem Med Metab Biol 47:38–46
Waldman RJ, Hall WN, McGee H et al. (1982) Aspirin as a risk factor in Reye's syndrome. JAMA 242:3089–3094
Yamashita F et al. (1979) Reye's syndrome in Japan. In: Crocker JFS (ed) Reye's syndrome II. Grune and Stratton, New York, pp 51–68
Yoshida Y, Fujii M, Brown FR et al. (1988) Effect of salicylic acid on mitochondrial-peroxisomal fatty acid catabolism. Pediatr Res 23:338
You K (1983) Salicylate and mitochondrial injury in Reye's syndrome. Science 221:163
Young RSK, Torrenti D, Williams RH et al. (1984) Reye's syndrome associated with long-term aspirin therapy. JAMA 251:754–756
Zimmerman HJ, Ishak KG (1982) Valproate-induced hepatic injury: analysis of 23 fatal cases. Hepatology 2:591–597

CHAPTER 15

Drug Hepatotoxicity in the Elderly

K. KITANI

A. Introduction

Hepatotoxicity of drugs is a consequence of many different processes occurring in the liver, including the sensitivity of the liver to drugs and the metabolism in the liver for the detoxification and activation of drugs (MITCHELL and JOLLOWS 1975), all of which may be affected by aging. Despite an earlier suggestion by clinicians that the elderly may be more susceptible to drug hepatotoxicity, there has been no conclusive data to confirm this hypothesis. In this chapter, past clinical information on this topic will be briefly reviewed first. This will be followed by a summary of past experimental studies on animals, in particular rodents in comparison to humans. Unfortunately, the results from experimental animals are often difficult to extrapolate to clinical situations for various reasons. However, a comprehensive but critical review of the past data in experimental animals may be of help for the proper interpretation of these data and for the future elucidation of this complicated but very important clinical and experimental problem.

B. Clinical Information

The information available on drug hepatotoxicity in elderly humans is quite limited. The impression of clinicians that elderly people may be more susceptible to drug reactions in the liver has not yet been proven.

I. Idiosyncratic Hepatotoxicity: The Swedish Experience

A study by WOODHOUSE et al. (1986) performed in Sweden is one of the very limited but valuable information sources on this subject. They examined all the hepatic adverse drug reactions reported to the Swedish Adverse Drug Reactions Advisory Committee from 1980 to 1984. It was considered that adverse drug reactions are most thoroughly reported in this country among the major developed countries in the world. Furthermore, the prescription information was monitored by the National Corporation of Swedish Pharmacies. From these data, the percentage of reports of hepatic adverse drug reactions and the percentage of prescriptions among patients over 65 years of age were calculated for individual drugs and these values were compared with those in patients under 65 years of age. Hepatic adverse drug reactions defined by these authors included: (1) abnormal liver function tests, (454 cases), (2) hepatitic reactions (201 cases), (3) intrahepatic cholestasis (61 cases), (4) jaundice (74 cases), (5) hypersensitivity (12 cases) and (6) hepatopathy (5 cases).

Table 1 summarizes these data. The total number of reports on hepatic drug reactions of the whole population was 807, of which 234 (29%) were in those over 65 years in age. Compared with 17%, which is the percentage of persons aged over 65 years relative to the whole population in this country, 29% appears to agree with the impression of clinicians that aged people are more susceptible to hepatic adverse reactions in general. However, when ratios of percentage of reports divided by percentage of prescriptions were calculated, ratio values were mostly distributed in the range close to unity. In fact, the average of ratios of 11 different drugs was 0.94 (Table 1). A ratio higher than 1.0 indicates that elderly people are more susceptible to a reaction from that particular drug. Among the 11 drugs thus monitored, only nitrofurantoin (1.43) and sulindac (1.32) gave ratios substantially exceeding 1.0. The average ratio of 0.94, however, clearly indicates that overall hepatic adverse drug reactions in the elderly do not have a higher incidence than those in the young population when numbers of reactions are corrected by numbers of prescriptions. Indeed, the seemingly higher incidence of hepatic adverse reactions in the elderly (29%) relative to the percentage of persons in the elderly population (17%) could be attributed almost totally to the higher incidence of prescriptions to the elderly (32%) among the whole population in this country.

The results of the study provide no support for the hypothesis that the elderly are at a higher risk from hepatic adverse drug reactions. These data, however, are based on reports to the Committee and results could be biased by a possibly lower report rate for the elderly. The authors, however, concluded that this possibility is not likely (Woodhouse et al. 1986).

Table 1. Hepatic ADR and the effect of age, corrected for age-related prescribing variables

Drug	% Reports >65 years	% Prescriptions >65 years	Ratio % reports >65 years to % prescriptions >65 years
Zimelidine	24	24	1.00
Cotrimoxazole	40	34	1.18
Cimetidine	32	27	1.18
Sulindac	50	37	1.32
Carbamazipine	18	17	1.05
Nitrofurantoin	43	30	1.43
Chlorpromazine	20	32	0.63
Hydralazine	37	55	0.67
Phenytoin	12	23	0.52
Naproxen	37	37	1.00
Piroxicam	20	44	0.45
Overall	30	32	0.94

II. Dose-Dependent Hepatotoxicity

Most of the hepatic adverse reactions reported in the above study are type B, i.e., idiosyncratic reactions and not of a dose-related type. It is possible therefore that certain subgroups of old patients are at a higher risk especially from those reactions of a dose-related type, because of malnutrition, diseases and/or frailty, which could result in lower drug clearances and eventually altered drug responsiveness.

It is at the moment extremely difficult to prove the above possibility, because of the general lack of data corrected for age-related prescription variables. Only a few studies which have examined this theory can be found in the past literature. NEUBERGER and WILLIAMS (1984) reported that the average age of 48 patients admitted to the King's College Hospital Liver Unit in London with halothane-associated fulminant hepatic failure was 57 years, which was considerably higher than the average age of patients undergoing general anesthesia (mostly receiving halothane).

A nonsteroidal anti-inflammatory drug, benoxaprofen, may be another example of this type of adverse drug reaction in the liver which could be more severe in the elderly. According to JAMES (1988), unpublished data from the DHSS in the United Kingdom suggest that, while the mean age of individuals receiving the drug was about 59 years, the mean age of those sustaining adverse drug reactions was about 66 years and, in individuals with severe reactions, fatal reactions occurred in those with an average age of 75 years. Of the total of nine patients with fatal hepatic failure associated with benoxaprofen reported by TAGGART and ALDERDYCE (1982) and GOUDIE et al. (1982), six were over 80 and the remainder were over the age of 70 years. Severe (often fatal) hepatic failure caused by acetaminophen could also be another example of a condition from which the elderly are at higher risk. No such conclusion, however, can be drawn for this drug from the literature. More discussion will follow later on this drug in the section dealing with experimental data.

For other drugs, practically no information is available except for only sporadic case reports describing hepatotoxicity caused by various drugs which occurred in elderly subjects. These case reports are meticulously summarized in a review by BAILLIE et al. (1989a). After reviewing available clinical information, BAILLIE et al. (1989a), however, concluded that there is no evidence for a higher risk for hepatotoxicity with these drugs in the elderly compared with the young.

C. Age-Related Alterations in Hepatic Detoxifying Functions: Discrepancies Between Human and Animal Data

As reviewed above, the information on humans in terms of hepatic adverse reactions in the elderly is extremely limited and no clear conclusion can be drawn. In order to complement the paucity of clinical information, data from experimental animals are critically needed; however, again studies in animals are also quite limited and the data quite discrepant.

Hepatic adverse drug reactions are heterogeneous in nature. As discussed earlier, the idiosyncratic type (type B) reactions are much more commonly observed in human populations. Unfortunately, there is no experimental counterpart for this type of drug reaction in animals. In humans, estradiol and chlorpromazine are known to cause this type of reaction, which is represented primarily by intrahepatic obstructive jaundice. Both of these drugs can cause cholestasis in experimental animals; however, the cholestasis in animals is represented by a rapid drop in bile flow rate without development of jaundice, and this experimental cholestasis is clearly dose dependent. Thus, cholestases in humans caused by these drugs are not reproduced in these experimental animal models. The use of experimental animals for elucidating the problem of hepatic drug reactions affected by aging, therefore, may be limited to the other category, i.e., dose-related drug reactions. For this type of reaction, several different factors are involved, all of which may be modified by aging. These include hepatic-drug-metabolizing systems such as the microsomal cytochrome monooxygenase system (phase I) and phase II conjugation reactions as well as the sensitivity of the liver to toxicants. It should be noted that, while many drugs are inactivated by the above reactions, some drugs are converted to more toxic materials by means of these biotransformations, especially the phase I reactions (MITCHEL and JOLLOWS 1975). The above reactions are regulated by enzyme activities, substrates for reactions such as glutathione (GSH) (for phase II reactions) and cofactors of reactions. Furthermore, there is increasing evidence that at least some hepatic adverse reactions from drugs involve oxidative tissue damage, and therefore antioxidant variables in the liver [i.e., reduced glutathione (GSH), vitamin C, E, etc., and antioxidant enzymes such as superoxide dismutase (SOD), catalase (CAT) and GSH peroxidase (GSH Px)] are also involved. All of these variables may (or may not) be affected by aging. The consequence is extremely complicated and it would be natural to conclude that no generalization can be made for drugs in general. First, some considerations will be made on these variables in relation to age in animals as well as in humans.

I. Phase I Drug Metabolism

The effect of age on the microsomal monooxygenase system has been studied most extensively in the past 3 decades using experimental animals. The earlier information that the function of this system generally declines with age was derived primarily from studies using male rats (KATO et al. 1964). These data have created a viewpoint that such a decline may also happen in human livers (for review, see KITANI 1988). Extensive studies in recent years, however, have revealed that the initial observation that the function of this system declines with age is limited to this sex of this particular species of animal. Even in female rat livers, such a decline cannot be reproduced (Fig. 1) (FUJITA et al. 1985a; KAMATAKI et al. 1985; KATO and TAKANAKA 1968). It is true that in some mouse strains the decline has also been observed (for review, see KITANI 1988). However, the decline cannot be generalized even in mouse species. It turned out that a drastic decline with age in some enzyme activities observed in male rat livers was nothing but a feminization of proportions of cytochrome P450 isozymes in male rat livers, while in female rat livers no alteration was observed in either enzyme activity or in isozyme proportions during aging (FUJITA et al. 1985a; KAMATAKI et al. 1985). In addition, subsequent studies in nonhuman primates (MALONEY et al. 1986; SUTTER et al. 1985) have agreed that the function of the hepatic microsomal P450 system never declines with aging per se. Human data are more difficult to obtain; however, available data on biopsied liver tissues in humans also agree with this contention (BOOBIS and DAVIES 1984; JAMES et al. 1982; WYNNE et al. 1988) (for review, see KITANI 1988). How can this information be reconciled with the bulk of data reporting lowered hepatic drug clearances in the elderly? This issue has been extensively discussed by the author in several published articles (KITANI 1986, 1988, 1990a,b). Here it will be only briefly discussed.

While it is true that many past clinical pharmacokinetic studies have shown significantly lower clearance values of drugs which are primarily me-

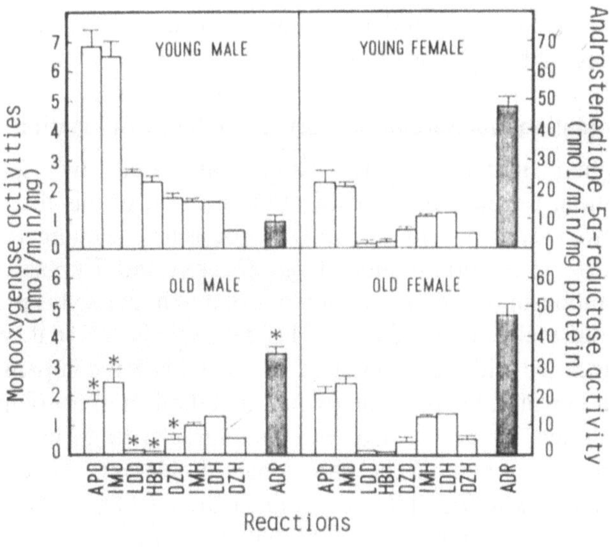

Fig. 1. Hepatic microsomal drug-metabolizing enzyme activities in young (6-month-old) and old (30-month-old) male and female rats. *Significantly different from corresponding activities in young male rats. *APD*, aminopyrine *N*-demethylase; *IMD*, imipramine *N*-demethylase; *LDD*, lidocaine *N*-deethylase; *HBH*, hexobarbital hydroxylase; *DZD*, diazepam *N*-demethylase; *IMH*, imipramine 3-hydroxylase; *LDH*, lidocaine 3-hydroxylase; *DZH*, diazepam 3-hydroxylase; *ADR*, androstenedione 5α-reductase. (Reproduced with the permission of the publisher, FUJITA et al. 1986)

tabolized by the liver in the elderly, many other studies have reached a conclusion that there are no significant differences in clearance values between young and old subjects (for review, see KITANI 1988). Since the liver weight steadily declines with age in humans, if clearance values are compared on the basis of unit liver weight, the apparent differences in clearance values between young and old subjects reported in many studies in the past may become even smaller (WYNNE et al. 1990). The criteria for the selection of subjects may also be another factor significantly contributing to differences among different studies. The health condition of subjects under study may affect the results considerably, especially in the elderly, since minor (often overlooked) undernutrition, frailty, morbidity and postmorbid conditions may affect the hepatic metabolism of drugs more profoundly in the elderly (WYNNE et al. 1990). This problem will be discussed in a later section.

II. Phase II Metabolism

In general, phase II reactions are more stable with aging in human livers than phase I reactions (for review, see KITANI 1988). In contrast with the phase I reactions, however, the phase II reactions have not been studied in relation to age very extensively in rodents, and review articles can scarcely be found in the literature. In order to properly interpret the results of pharmacodynamic studies such as those on hepatotoxicity of drugs affected by aging, it is extremely important to have a good knowledge of the underlying detoxifying functions in the liver affected by aging. Here a brief review of phase II reactions affected by aging is offered.

1. Glucuronidation and Sulfation: Acetaminophen Conjugation

Acetaminophen metabolism is mainly mediated by sulfation and glucuronidation. Because of the clinical implication of this drug in terms of drug hepatotoxicity in the elderly, several groups have examined the metabolism of the drug in relation to animal age. SWEENY and WEINER (1985) examined the metabolism of acetaminophen in isolated hepatocytes prepared from young and old male Fischer 344 (F-344) rats and found that, while sulfate formation declined with age, increased glucuronidation compensated for the decline of the former, keeping the overall metabolism of acetaminophen unchanged with age. These in vitro data also agree with an in vivo clearance study of acetaminophen in the same male F-344 rats by GALINSKY and CORCORAN (1986), who found that the total clearance of acetaminophen in old rats was similar to that in the young, but that the clearance of sulfate decreased while glucuronide formation increased with age. GALINSKY et al. (1986) further examined glucuronidation and sulfation reactions in vitro in the liver of young and old male F-344 rats. They found that the rates of some reactions that were higher in females at a young age increased with age in male rat livers, while some others that were lower in females at a young age tended to decrease with age in male rat livers. Thus, overall alterations of conjugation reactions caused by aging in male rat livers were again a feminization of male rat livers with age, the observation initially found for the cytochrome P450 isozyme population. Later the same group looked for changes in female rat livers with age but found little change (GALINSKEY et al. 1990). WOODHOUSE and HERD (1993), however, reported that, in Brown Norway (BN) rats, rates of formation of conjugated metabolites of acetaminophen did not change with age in either sex, although they observed that glucuronidation was more rapid in females than in males, while the sulfation reaction was more rapid in males when they were young. In agreement with their own data in BN rats, they also reported that both glucuronidation and sulfation of acetaminophen were unaffected in fit elderly humans compared with the young (WYNNE et al. 1990). This observation is also supported by a subsequent in vitro study by the same group on biopsied human liver tissues (HERD et al. 1991). This group has also found a reduction of morphine clearances due to glucuronidation in elderly humans, which, however, was in the range that could be explained by the reduction of liver volume in the aged (BAILLIE et al. 1989b).

2. Glutathione *S*-Transferases

Glutathione *S*-transferases (GSTs) are a group of multifunctional proteins serving several different roles in detoxifying endo- and xenobiotics including drugs. These proteins are known to bind to a number of hydrophobic compounds (MANNERVIK et al. 1985). Furthermore, they catalyze the conjugation of a number of substances with reduced GSH. These two different features of GSTs make these proteins unusually versatile agents against the damaging effects of various noxious agents. Alterations of enzyme activities and proportions of isozymes with aging, if they occur, would have a profound influence on the detoxifying capacity of the liver, leading to altered drug hepatotoxicity in the elderly. Isozymes of GSTs are known to be all dimeric proteins of about 50 kDa in molecular weight consisting of two subunits. These isozymes have overlapping substrate specificity. Accordingly, the determination of enzyme activities becomes complex and may differ depending on substrate concentration. Kinetic studies are also not easy to resolve since often more than two isozymes with different K_m values are involved in the conjugation of a single substrate (CARRILLO et al. 1990). Measurement of concentrations of each isozyme would be the best choice, especially for analyzing age-assoicated changes in these enzymes. However, technically, these measurements are not easy to perform since many isozymes have overlapping antigenicities. Keeping these limitations in mind, several past studies on rat livers which compared enzyme activities for different substrates are summarized in Table 2.

As is apparent, results are very controversial even for the same substrate in the same sex of rats. Despite these discrepancies, our own studies on F-344 rats indicated that changes (decrease) with age are more clearly seen in male rats (FUJITA et al. 1985b; CARRILLO et al. 1991), while in female rat livers changes are modest, if any (FUJITA et al. 1985b; CARRILLO et al. 1991).

Table 2. Age-related differences in GST activities in rat livers

Strain	Age	Sex	Substrates						Authors
			CDNB	DCNB	STOX	PBO	BSP	EA	
Wistar	4.5, 12, 24 months	M	–	↓					KITAHARA et al. 1982
F-344	3, 12, 24 months	M			↓				SPEARMAN et al. 1983
F-344	3, 12, 24 months	F			–				SPEARMAN and LEIBMAN 1983
F-344	3, 12, 24 months	M	–	↓					SPEARMAN and LEIBMAN 1984a,b
F-344	3, 12, 24 months	F	↑	–					SPEARMAN et al. 1983
F-344	1.5, 3, 6,	M	–	↓	↓	↓	↓		FUJITA et al. 1985b
	12, 24, 28 months	F							
F-344	12, 24, 28 months	F	–	–	–	–	–		FUJITA et al. 1985b
F-344	60 days vs. 22 months	F	↑	↓		↑		–	LEAKEY et al. 1989
SD	24–104 weeks	M	–						CHENGELIS 1988
SD	24–104 weeks	F	–						CHENGELIS 1988
BN	11–144 weeks	M	–	–					COECKE et al. 1990
BN	11–144 weeks	F	↑	–					COECKE et al. 1990
Wistar-Furth	4, 26, 31 months	M	↓						JI et al. 1990
SD	3 vs. 30 months	M	–						TARLOFF et al. 1991
F-344	6 vs. 26 months	M	–	↓	↓	–	↓		CARRILLO et al. 1991
F-344	6 vs. 26 months	F	–	↓	↓	–	–		CARRILLO et al. 1991

CDNB, 1-chloro-2,4-dinitrobenzene; DCNB, 1,2-dichloro-4-nitrobenzene; STOX, styrene oxide; PBO, *trans*-4-phenyl-3-buten-2-one; BSP, sulfobromophthalein sodium tetrahydrate; EA, ethacrinic acid; M, male; F, female.

In C57 BL female mouse livers, a significant decline in enzyme activities with age was found only toward 1,2-dichloro-4-nitro-benzene (DCNB), while activities toward four other substrates stayed unchanged (CARRILLO et al. 1989) (Fig. 2). When GST subunit proportions were investigated in F-344 rats (CARRILLO et al. 1991), we found, as expected, a clear difference in subunit proportion between young male and female rat livers (Fig. 3). As age advanced, the proportion pattern of male rat livers became close (if not identical) to that of young female rat livers (Fig. 3) due to an increase in subunit 2 and a decrease in subunit 4 concentrations with age. Unexpectedly, however, in female rat livers the subunit proportion also changed drastically with age, and the pattern in old female rat livers became different from those of both young male and female rats (Fig. 3). Thus, it appears that, while enzyme activities of GSTs in female F-344 rats remain fairly stable, the proportion of subunits (and eventually isozymes) drastically changes with age, perhaps keeping enzyme activities fairly stable during aging. It should be noted, however, that although the change of the subunit proportion with age in our study is very clear (Fig. 3), it cannot be generalized even for female rats, since in our study in female F-344 rats the decline in subunit 4 concentration was the most marked change with age, while in female BN rat livers this did not happen during aging (ROGIERS et al. 1991), although the pattern in young female rats looks rather similar for these two different strains. Similarly, in male rat livers, an increase in subunit 2 and decreases in subunit 3 and 4 concentrations were prominent changes with age in Fischer rats, while in BN rats the patterns were more or less comparable for young and old rats (ROGIERS et al. 1991).

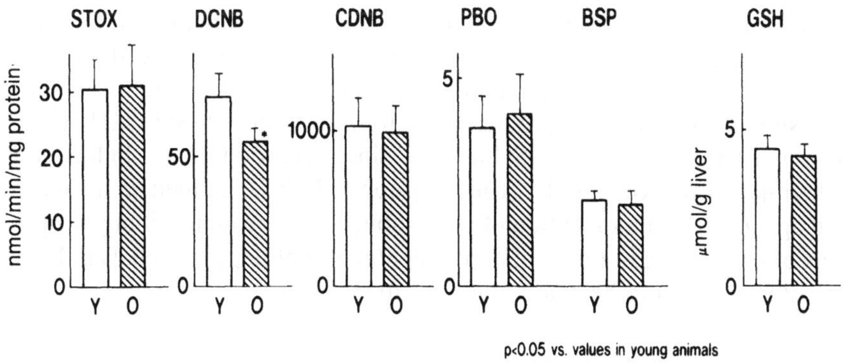

Fig. 2. Enzyme activities of GSTs toward five different substrates in liver cytosols obtained from young (*Y*, 8-month-old) and old (*O*, 27-month-old) female C57Bl mice. *Significantly different from the corresponding value in young mouse livers. *BSP*, sulfobromophthalein; *PBO*, benzalacetone; *STOX*, styrene oxide; *DCNB*, 1,2-dichloro-4-nitrobenzene; *CDNB*, 1-chloro-2,4-dinitrobenzene; *GSH*, total glutathione. (The figure was drawn based on the data reported previously by CARRILLO et al. 1989, with the permission of the publisher)

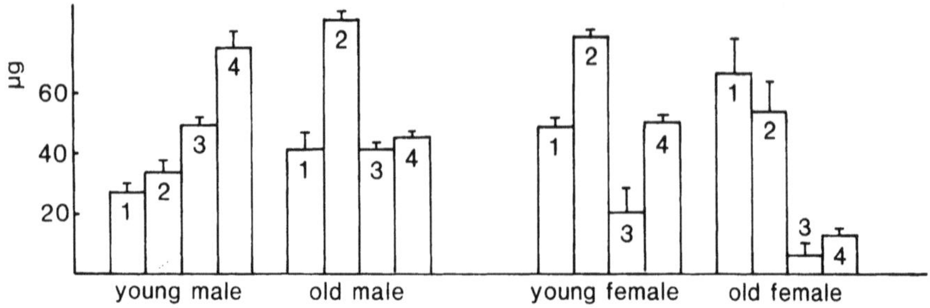

Fig. 3. Amounts of subunits in liver cytosol in young and old Fischer-344 rats of both sexes. The amount of each subunit is the sum of values in all subfractions by affinity column separation. *Significantly different from corresponding values in young rats ($P < 0.05$). (Reproduced from CARRILLO et al. 1991, with the permission of the publisher)

Changes in GST activities in rats may again follow to some extent the general rule (i.e., a feminization) originally formulated for phase I reactions (KITANI 1988). However, we should not be confused by the variability found in the past literature in experimental animals, when we try to extrapolate these animal data to humans. Judging from past studies, it appears that phase II reactions stay fairly stable with age in humans (HERD et al. 1991; KITANI 1988; WYNNE et al. 1990). Variability of results in studies using rodents should be taken to indicate caution that studies performed in a single animal model have limitations in terms of generalization of the data. It is well conceivable that the results in pharmacodynamic studies using aging rodents will also become quite variable.

Finally, we found that the subunit elution through affinity chromatography tended to be more rapid in old rat livers than in young ones. This was observed for all four subunits in male and for at least subunit 1 in female rat livers (CARRILLO et al. 1991). The change in elution pattern with age most probably suggests that some modification in chemical structure occurred for GST subunits during aging, changing their affinities to *S*-hexyl GSH (used as the eluent) and possibly to GSH as well. Since retention times of all subunits in high-performance liquid chromatography (HPLC) remained unchanged with aging, such a modification of each subunit may be minor, if any. Implications of this finding in terms of experimental gerontology as well as in human toxicology remain to be studied in the future.

III. Oxidant and Antioxidant Variables

Many hepatotoxicities (e.g., those caused by carbon tetrachloride and acetaminophen) are believed to be at least partially caused by oxidative metabolites. Antioxidant strategies in the liver may play a significant role in the prevention of such hepatotoxicities. Accordingly, antioxidant variables affected by aging may become a critical factor for some types of age-related drug hepatotoxicity, as discussed earlier.

1. Lipid Peroxidation

Lipid peroxidation as determined by the production of thiobarbiturate-reacting substrates (TBSs) was reported to increase with age in male rat livers by LEE and YU (1991), suggesting that the spontaneous lipid peroxidation is increased with age in the liver. However, RIKANS et al. (1991) clearly demonstrated that the formation of TBSs increases with age in male but decreases in female rat livers, indicating caution should be given to such a simplistic conclusion obtained from only male rat livers.

2. Glutathione

Although the protective role of GSH in the liver against drug-induced hepatotoxicity is well known (MITCHELL et al. 1973, 1974), the alteration with age in concentrations of GSH has been controversial. Earlier workers have shown a considerable reduction in GSH concentration in the liver with age in mice (STOHS et al. 1982); however, this reduction does not appear to be a general feature for this substance with aging. In C57BL female mice (RIKANS et al. 1992a,b; CARRILLO et al. 1989) as well as in F-344 male rats (RIKANS and KOSANKE 1984), both total and reduced GSH concentrations stayed essentially unchanged with age. Since in human livers GSH concentration was reported to barely decline with age (JAMES et al. 1982), animal models which show a drastic decline with age in GSH concentration may not be an appropriate model. This stability of GSH concentration with aging, however, does not indicate that GSH concentration is always the same in the elderly as in the young. When an acute ethanol challenge was given, GSH concentration stayed low for a longer period in old rat livers, despite comparable basal concentrations for young and old animal livers (RIKANS and SNOWDON 1989). Factors which potentially can modify GSH concentrations such as alcohol intake, malnuturition and morbidity may affect elderly individuals more profoundly than the young. In this regard, the turnover of GSH in the liver may be a better parameter than static GSH concentration, in order to uncover a potential age difference in the hepatic detoxifying functions. LAUTERBURG et al. (1980) have shown that hepatic GSH turnover declines in a linear fashion with age. Unfortunately, however, this study used rather young animals with increasing body weight. In fact, body weight of animals was used as an index of animal age, suggesting that the oldest animals studied are younger than 6 months of age. Apparently, the interpretation of the data is valid in terms of the development of animals, but not in terms of aging. In fact, the extrapolation of the line obtained from the linear regression between weights and turnover values of animals indicates that the turnover value will reach the zero value very soon, which is totally unlikely. This type of information on truly aged animals is very useful, however.

3. Antioxidant Enzymes

Superoxide dismutase (SOD), catalase (CAT) and GSH peroxidase (GSH Px) are all antioxidant enzymes present in the liver. These enzymes work efficiently to protect bodies (the liver tissue specifically) against oxidative stresses.

The reaction catalyzed by SOD yields H_2O_2, which is as toxic as oxygen free radicals. H_2O_2 can be quenched by CAT or GSH Px. If these enzyme activities decline with age, it may play a significant role in the hepatotoxicity related to oxidative damage. Indeed, Reiss and Gershon (1978) have provided evidence that SOD enzyme activities drastically decline with age in the liver. They have further shown that this decline is due to the formation of an enzymatically fragile (heat-susceptible) but immunologically stable isozyme (altered enzyme) during aging.

Similar alterations of enzyme molecules during aging have been suggested for different enzymes by different investigators in the past (Oliver et al. 1987; Wulf and Cutler 1979). Table 3 summarizes some of the past studies concerning the age-related alterations in SOD enzyme activities in the liver. It is apparent that the thesis of Gershon (Reiss and Gershon 1978) that SOD activities decline with age cannot be generalized. In many studies, unaltered, or even increased SOD activities with age can be found. At the moment, there is no clear explanation for these discrepancies among past studies on this important issue. Again, animal strains and sexes may play a role. Furthermore, the methodology used to determine SOD activities may also be another factor causing these discrepancies. We have found that SOD activities changed little with age in both male and female rat livers (Carrillo et al. 1992).

Catalase activities are another controversial subject. The group of Richardson (Semsei et al. 1989; Rao et al. 1990) has shown a definite decline in CAT activities with age as well as in the level of mRNA for CAT in the liver, suggesting that this may be an important factor in the age-induced deteriora-

Table 3. Reported changes in SOD activities in rat livers with age

	Cu Zn SOD		Mn SOD	
	Sex	Reference	Sex	Reference
Decrease	M	Reiss and Gershon 1976, 1978	M	Kellog and Fridovich 1976
	M	Semsei et al. 1989	M	Cao-Danh et al. 1983
	M	Rao et al. 1990	M	Carrillo et al. 1992
	F	Cand and Verdeth 1989	M	Ji et al. 1990
	M	Ji et al. 1990		
Increase	M	Carrillo et al. 1992	M and F	Rikans et al. 1992c
			F	Carrillo et al. 1992
No alteration	M	Kellog and Fridovich 1976		
	M	Cao-Danh et al. 1983		
	M	Lammi-Keefe et al. 1984		
	M and F	Rikans et al. 1991		
	F	Carrillo et al. 1992		

M, male rats; F, female rats.

tion of cellular function. We have found that the decline in CAT activity with age occurs in male rat livers, but that the CAT activity increases with age in female rat livers (CARRILLO et al. 1992). RIKANS et al. (1991) have also clearly shown that CAT activities decrease with age in male but increase in female rat livers. This is again a very important example showing how variable the results can be in terms of the effect of age on liver enzyme activities. To the knowledge of the author, nothing is known about human livers with regard to age-associated alterations in activities of antioxidant enzymes. However, it appears that there is no experimental basis in general terms to support the view that these enzyme activities decline in natural aging processes. Again it should be emphasized that this rule may not hold in pathological processes in the elderly as has been and will be once again discussed for GST levels below.

D. Morbidity and Frailty as Major Factors for Lowered Drug Clearances in the Elderly: A Possible Role in Hepatotoxicity

While it appears that basal (physiological) drug-metabolizing (and detoxifying) activities change little with aging in healthy human subjects, it does not mean that the risk of hepatic drug reactions in elderly subjects under medical care is the same as that in the young. WYNNE et al. (1990) have reported that while acetaminophen clearance values are not different between young and old healthy subjects when compared on the basis of unit liver weight, *frail elderly* subjects had significantly lower clearance values than both young and *old healthy* subjects. These frail subjects are not patients under medical care. It is conceivable that elderly *patients* under medical care suffering from morbidity and undernutrition are likely to have more pronounced lower clearance values and to be at a higher risk of adverse drug reactions. Figure 4 provides experimental support for the contention by WYNNE et al. (1990) that frailty

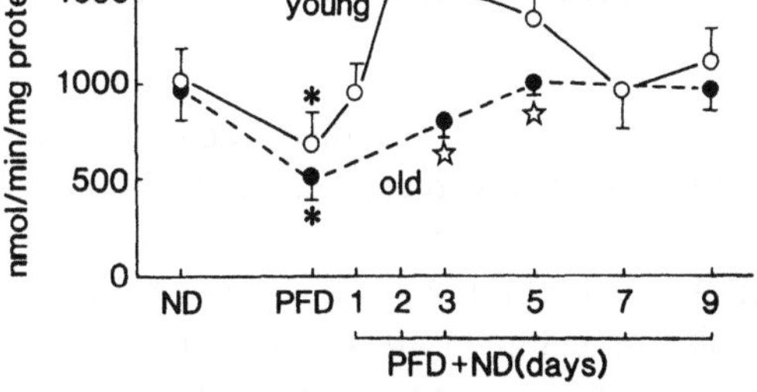

Fig. 4. Changes in activities of CSTs toward CDNB before and during diet manipulation in female C57 BL mice. *Significantly different from corresponding values in control mice on the ND only ($P < 0.05$). ☆Significantly different from corresponding values in young mouse livers ($P < 0.05$). (Reproduced from CARRILLO et al. 1989, with the permission of the publisher). PFD: Protein E free diet for 1 week

(and morbidity) may be the major potential factor for actual alterations of some of the pharmacokinetics encountered in the elderly.

When young and old C57BL female mice were compared in terms of GST activities and GSH content in the liver, the values were almost identical for both age groups, except for GST activities towards 1,2-dichloro-4-nitrobenzene (DCNB), which were significantly lower in old animal livers (Fig. 2). When these animals were fed with a protein-free diet (PFD) for 1 week, all the values became significantly lower than the respective control (physiological) values. However, differences between the two age groups were again very minor. A large difference in GST activities between young and old animal livers became manifest when animals began to eat a normal diet (ND) after 1 week of PFD. In young animal livers, GST activities began to increase immediately after ND refeeding, reaching values far exceeding their basal values (overshooting) in 2 days of ND. Then these high values started to return to basal levels, slowly coming *down* from their peak. In contrast, in old animal livers, such an overshooting phenomenon did not occur, with enzyme activities slowly returning to their basal levels by coming *up* from the bottom values (Fig. 4, CARRILLO et al. 1989). Thus, even if basal detoxifying systems are comparable for young and old animal livers, stress factors stemming from frailty and morbidity such as infections and malnutrition (and possibly alcohol abuse, etc.) may more strongly depress detoxifying functions in aged organisms, and, more importantly, the recovery from these stress-induced malfunctions may often be less efficient (and slower) in the elderly. Elderly subjects are more prone to various morbidities, malnutrition and frailty than are the young. If we assume that these stresses adversely modify hepatic detoxifying systems more severely in the elderly than in the young, then some of the sporadic but more severe (and often fatal) hepatic drug reactions in the elderly as discussed earlier (e.g., halothane, benoxaprofen and possibly acetaminophen) could be reasonably explained, even on the assumption that basal detoxifying functions in the liver are essentially unaltered with aging per se.

E. Adverse Drug Reactions in the Liver in Old Animals: Mini Review

As discussed earlier, the information on drug hepatotoxicity affected by aging is quite limited, even in studies with experimental animals. Although there is a definite advantage of using experimental animals to control many variables that are difficult in surveys on human data, the data from the past literature on experimental animals are again very discrepant, depending on the sex, strain and species of animals as well as on the kind of drugs examined, thus making the extrapolation of the data to humans even more difficult. Variability in the results, even with the same drug, is quite conceivable since changes in liver drug-metabolizing capacities caused by aging are so variable, depending on the animal model used as discussed earlier. Clearly, we must be very cautious about interpreting these animal data. Future studies must be designed based on a thorough understanding of the fact that these regulating factors are altered with age quite differently among the different animal models. Several examples will be discussed below.

I. Hepatocyte Susceptibility to Chlorpromazine and Erythromycin Estolate

Both of these drugs are known to occasionally cause rather severe cholestasis represented by intrahepatic obstructive jaundice. As discussed earlier, hepatic reactions clinically encountered with these drugs are primarily of type B. Thus, the data obtained from animal livers cannot be directly extrapolated to humans (see Sect. C). With these limitations in mind, ABERNATHY et al. (1980) compared susceptibility of isolated hepatocytes prepared from livers of male rats of different ages (1–24 months) with those of these drugs. By using leakages of lactate dehydrogenase (LDH) and other proteins into incubation media as criteria, they concluded that hepatocyte surface membranes of older animals were more resistant to these drugs, a conclusion opposite to that which had been suspected. One-month-old rats are still in their development period. However, even if young animals were properly selected for age (3, 10 months), a similar conclusion can be drawn from their study. This observation may not be surprising, since we are now obtaining more and more convincing evidence that the surface membranes of hepatocytes (more specifically protein movement) are becoming more rigid with age (ZS-NAGY et al. 1986, 1989). This result, however, cannot be interpreted as meaning that elderly humans are likely to be less susceptible to hepatocyte drug reactions caused by these drugs, since mechanisms for hepatotoxicities caused by these drugs are totally different between human and animal livers as discussed earlier.

II. Acetaminophen Hepatotoxicity: An Example of Variability of the Results in Studies Using Rodents

The impression of clinicians that acetaminophen hepatotoxicity may occur more frequently and/or become more severe in elderly subjects has been maintained for a long time without any clear validation. Experimental study, if possible, may help our understanding of this particular issue.

Based on the above hypothesis, RIKANS and her group (RIKANS and MOOER 1988; RIKANS 1989) compared hepatotoxicity caused by acetaminophen between young and old male rats, using excretion of enzymes into plasma and liver histology as criteria. Contrary to their expectation, they found that old rat livers were clearly less susceptible to acetaminophen challenge (Fig. 5). Microsomal glucuronidation and cytosolic sulfation are known to be major metabolic pathways for acetaminophen in the liver; however, some amounts of acetaminophen are believed to be metabolized by the mi-

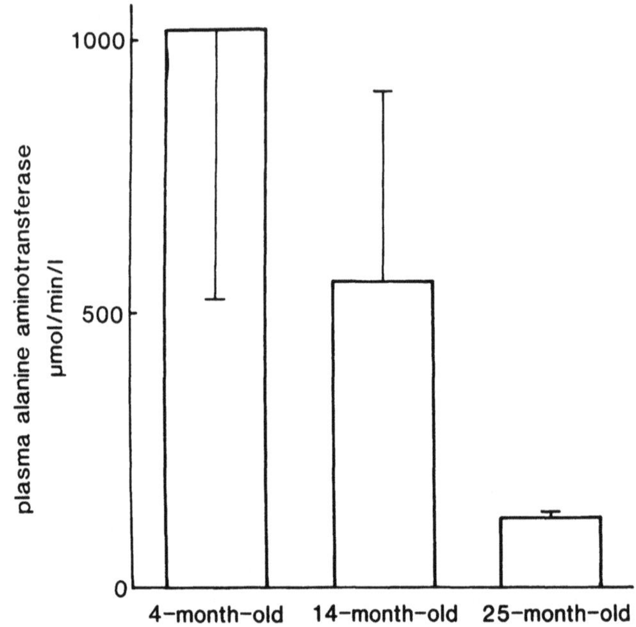

Fig. 5. Plasma alanine aminotransferase levels in male Fischer-344 rats of different ages 24h after i.p. injection of 800mg/kg acetaminophen. (Produced from data by RIKANS and MOORE 1988, with the permission of the publisher and authors)

crosomal monooxygenase system to be an active toxicant(s), leading to irreversible binding to proteins, and finally ending in hepatocyte damage, although mechanisms underlying acetaminophen-induced hepatotoxicity remain unelucidated (ROGEN et al. 1983). As discussed earlier, in general, activities of the microsomal monooxygenase system in male rat livers decline very drastically during aging (KITANI 1988). It is conceivable that the decrease in the formation of toxic metabolite(s) due to lowered enzyme activities in old age contributed to the lower hepatocyte susceptibility in old male rats to acetaminophen. Since such a drastic decline of the function of the system does not occur in human livers for either sex (for review, see KITANI 1988), it may not be appropriate to extrapolate these data in male rats directly to the human condition. In female rat livers, this system is known to stay essentially unchanged with aging as in human livers. Accordingly, we did a similar study in female rats (KITANI 1990a). As expected, the susceptibility of the liver to acetaminophen challenge was comparable for young and old female rats, but again there was no clear evidence that elderly subjects are more prone to this type of hepatotoxicity (Fig. 6). The problem of studying acetaminophen hepatotoxicity in this rat strain is that they die (possibly of systemic toxicity) before they develop severe hepatotoxicity. Unlike some specific mouse strains, where drastic changes in cytochrome P450 with age are known, in livers of C57BL mice of both sexes the monooxgenase system stays fairly stable with age as in female rat livers (FUJITA et al. 1986). When we examined C57BL mice

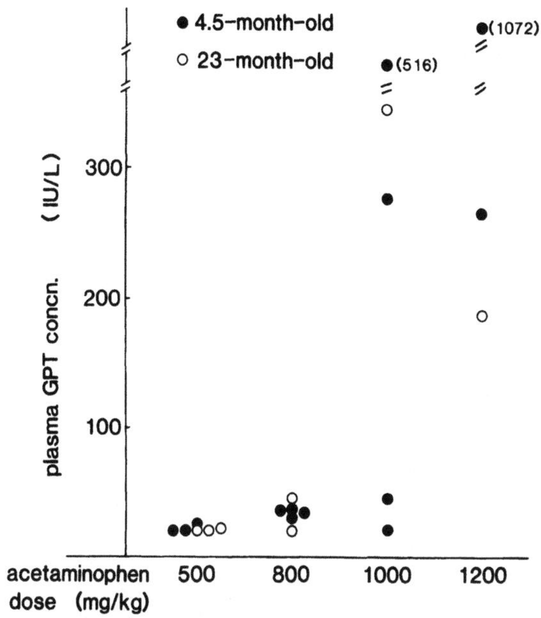

Fig. 6. Plasma alanine aminotransferase levels in young and old female Fischer-344 rats 24 h after i.p. injection of acetaminophen. (KITANI et al., unpublished data)

of both sexes, unexpectedly, we again found a lowered susceptibility in old male mice to acetaminophen as RIKANS and MOORE (1988) saw in male rat livers (Fig. 7). Since male C57BL mice do not exhibit such a drastic decline in cytochrome P450 enzyme activities as do male rats (FUJITA et al. 1986) seemingly similar results between male rats and mice must have different explanations. Our results are also not explainable by an earlier observation by SWEENY and WEINER (1985) who found no difference between young and old mouse hepatocytes in terms of the detoxification (sulfation and glucuronidation) or toxication [glutathione conjugation of toxic metabolite(s)] pathway for acetaminophen. At the moment, we have no plausible explanation for our observation in old male mice. When we looked at female mice, we saw some tendency of a higher susceptibility to the drug in old mice although the difference between the two age groups did not attain statistical significance (Fig. 7). Nevertheless, since in this figure (Fig. 7) some old animals showed considerably higher plasma GPT levels, while the majority had values in the normal range, it appears to suggest that the variability of susceptibility to acetaminophen challenge becomes greater with age in some female mice, a phenomenon which is likely to happen in humans of both sexes, although there is no evidence that female mice are an animal model that most closely resembles humans in this regard. However, the variability of the results [i.e., decreased (male rats and mice), increased (female mice) and unchanged (female rats) susceptibility to acetaminophen] depending on different animal models must be taken into serious consideration in future experimental studies, and we

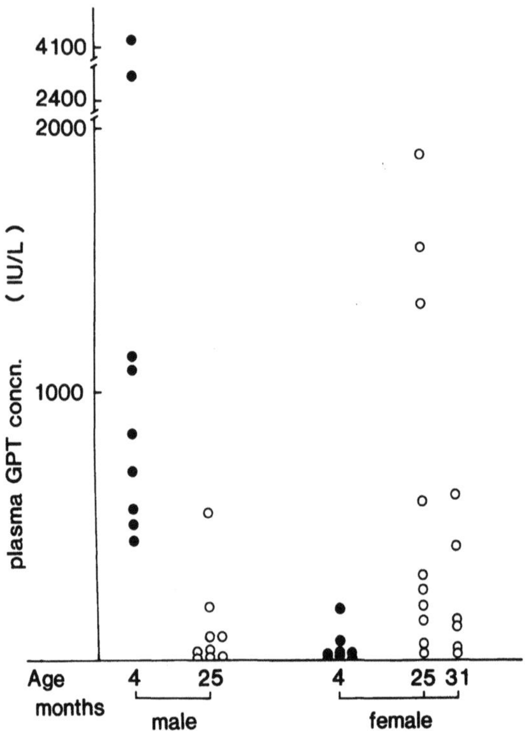

Fig. 7. Plasma alanine aminotransferase levels in young and old C57BL mice of both sexes 24 h after i.p. injection of acetaminophen at a dose of 500 mg/kg. (KITANI et al., unpublished data)

must realize how important the selection of animal model is for pursuing the problem of drug hepatotoxicity in elderly humans using experimental animals.

III. Ethanol Metabolism in the Liver and Its Hepatotoxicity: Another Controversy

Ethanol consumption is often increased in the elderly. If hepatocyte susceptibility to ethanol is increased with age, the overall problem of ethanol-induced hepatotoxicity will become even greater in the elderly. There have been several attempts to elucidate this problem. Alcohol hepatotoxicity is an example of the consequences of complex biochemical events in the liver. Ethanol is believed to have a major metabolic pathway by means of cytosolic alcohol dehydrogenase (ADH). Another pathway by means of the microsomal monooxygenase system [i.e., the microsomal ethanol elimination system (MEOS)] has been claimed (RUBIN and LIEBER 1972). Although the exact mechanism(s) for hepatotoxicity of ethanol is still under debate, at least several possibilities have been suggested. A direct hepatotoxicity of ethanol (or its metabolites) appears to still be a matter of debate. Although chronic ingestion of ethanol has been reported to cause fatty liver, leading to liver cirrhosis, an acute intoxication of ethanol may more directly involve the central nervous system (OTT et al. 1985). Thus, it is difficult to draw precise conclusions about the effect(s) of aging on acute hepatotoxicity caused by ethanol. However, the author has found scattered reports, mostly in terms of the effect of aging on ethanol metabolism in the liver. Only one report referred to an acute hepatotoxicity by ethanol in relation to age (RIKANS and SNOWDON 1989). These references will be briefly summarized and discussed.

SEITZ et al. (1989) examined the metabolism of ethanol in male rats up to 19 months of age. They found that ethanol metabolism (both in vivo and in vitro) becomes significantly lower in old (19 months) than in younger male animals. Furthermore, chronic feeding of ethanol led to the higher accumulation of fats in hepatocytes in old male rats than in young ones. However, there was no significant difference in ethanol metabolism in livers between young (4 months) and middle-aged (12 months) female rats (SEITZ et al. 1989). WIBERG et al. (1970) also reported that ethanol metabolism was lower but acetaldehyde formation higher in liver slices obtained from old male rats than in those from younger ones. Since there was a considerable decrease in ethanol metabolism in male rats of the middle-aged group (12 months) compared with younger ones, it appears that the observation made in male rats showing decreased ethanol metabolism in old animals does not appear to be justified for simple extrapolation to humans.

RIKANS and SNOWDON (1989) examined hepatotoxicities of ethanol in female rats in relation to animal age. Although they did not observe any decline in ethanol metabolism with age in female rats, as was shown in the above study by SEITZ et al. (1989), they did observe a distinct increase in plasma alanine aminotransferase and sorbitol levels 4h after the administration of ethanol in old female rats compared with young rats. These transient increases in plasma retention of enzymes returned to physiological levels at 16h and no differences were observed in these enzyme levels among different age groups at this time point. Interestingly, however, they did observe that GSH levels in the liver stayed at lower levels at 16h in older animals than in young animals (RIKANS and SNOWDEN 1989).

The reduction in GSH levels by ethanol intake may occur from an increased efflux from the liver (possibly caused by increased demand by extrahepatic organs) and reduced GSH synthesis (FERNANDEZ-CHECA et al. 1989). Slowed recovery of GSH levels in the liver after ethanol ingestion in old animals may play a significant role not only in ethanol hepatotoxicity but, more importantly, in drug hepatotoxicity in the elderly in broader terms, since this substance is believed to play an important role in the detoxification of so many toxicants (MITCHELL et al. 1973, 1974). In humans, GSH concentrations in plasma (and possibly the liver) were shown to be reduced in chronic alcoholics (LAUTERBERG and VELEZ 1988). Acetaminophen hepatotoxicity was reported to be more commonly seen in alcoholic subjects (DENISON et al. 1987). Although there is no direct proof that the elderly humans are more prone to ethanol-induced hepatotoxicity, the lowered GSH levels caused by ethanol intake appear to be a significant risk factor for potential drug hepatotoxicity in the elderly.

Except for this information, the author has been unable to collect any data on ethanol hepatotoxicity in relation to age. However, there are some reports examining ethanol metabolism both in vivo and in vitro in relation to animal age. Here a brief summay of these data will be discussed. In general, the decrease in MEOS activity with age in male rats, with no change in females, could be generalized from our knowledge on the effect of age on the microsomal monooxygenase system in rats. Cytosolic alcohol dehydrogenase (ADH) activities were reported to increase (RIKANS and KLING 1987; RIKANS and MOORE 1987; WIBERG et al. 1970) in male rats but to stay unchanged in female rats with age (RIKANS and SNOWDON 1989; SEITZ et al. 1989). There are some exceptions to this rule. SEITZ et al. (1989) did not observe a significant increase in ADH activities in male rats with age. GELLERT et al. (1988) reported that in female SD rats activities of both ADH and aldehyde dehydrogenase as well as MEOS activities all declined with age. GELLERT et al. (1988), however, used very young animals (2 and 8 weeks old) and compared values from these with those from 30-month-old rats. With today's standards of gerontology, 6- to 8-month-old rats must be used as young adults; otherwise it is not certain whether the age differences shown in the study by GELLERT et al. (1988) were caused by development as opposed to true aging processes.

At least in F-344 rats, the rule that aged males become feminized in terms of drug-metabolizing enzymes that was originally developed for cytochrome P450 enzymes (and later extended to phase II reactions) appears to be justified for cytosolic ADH, since in young animals activities in male rats, which are much lower than those in females, increased with age, approaching the values found in young (and old) female rats (RIKANS and KLING 1987; RIKANS and MOORE 1987). The overall consequences are that in old age ADH activities become very close for male and female rats (RIKANS and KLING 1987; RIKANS and MOORE 1987). The author has emphasized this rule in the past, with caution for the generalization of the results obtained from male rats (for review, see KITANI 1988). Looking at the past literature more extensively, however, the author has realized that he must retain some reservations about the above rule, since in some rat strains sex differences for microsomal monooxygenase activities do not appear to be as clear as they are for some other strains, such as F-344 rats. In terms of alcohol elimination capacities, F-344 rats had the most distinct difference between the two sexes, with clearance values in males far greater than in females. In contrast, in some other rat strains such a distinct sex difference could not be observed (ERICKSON 1984). More studies must be done to clarify this point using different strains of rats, since most of the observations in the past in terms of the age effect on cytochrome P450 enzyme activities have been made in F-344 rats. In humans, there is again no clear evidence that aging affects ethanol metabolism. WYNNE et al. (1988) have found no significant difference in ethanol elimination rate between young and old subjects, which agrees with the results of a previous study by VESTAL et al. (1977).

IV. Hepatotoxicities by Other Toxicants

RIKANS and her group also examined a variety of toxicants in terms of age-related hepatotoxicity both in vivo and in vitro. They found the hepatotoxicity of carbon tetrachloride remained unchanged with age in male F-344 rats (RIKANS and KOSANKE 1984). Since carbon tetrachrolide is believed to result in its hepatocyte toxicity through its biotransformation to the trichloromethyl free radical produced by means of cytochrome P450, it was expected that the hepatotoxicity may be reduced in old male rats. The mechanism(s) for this unexpected finding was extensively discussed by the authors (RIKANS and KOSANKE 1984). It appears most likely that the reduced formation of active metabolites of carbon tetrachloride with age was counterbalanced by a decrease in antioxidant enzyme activities such as SOD and especially CAT in old male rat livers which have since been proved (RIKANS et al. 1992c). It is also possible that the accelerated natural peroxidation process which was shown to occur in male rat livers was a contributing factor. As discussed earlier, it has been shown by the same authors that changes in CAT activities and lipid peroxidation with age in female rat livers are different from those in males (RIKANS et al. 1991, 1992c). They also found that diquat-induced liver damage as examined in isolated hepatocytes was accentuated several fold in hepatocytes obtained from old male F-344 rats compared with those from young rats (RIKANS and CAI 1992, 1993). On the other hand, the same group found that aged C57BL mice are more resistant to the hepatotoxic effects of endotoxin and galactosamine simultaneously administered intraperitoneally than are young mice (HORNBROOK et al. 1993). Similarly, the same authors previously reported that old male F-344 rats were more resistant to galactosamine challenge than young ones in terms of galactosamine- and bromobenzene-induced liver damage (RIKANS and KOSANKE 1984), while old animals were more vulnerable to allyl-alcohol-induced hepatic injury (RIKANS 1984, 1987; RIKANS and KOSANKE 1984) (for review, see RIKANS 1989). These results again suggest that the hepatotoxicity of drugs in elderly experimental animals is extremely variable, depending on the drug and the sex, strains and species of the animal. Clearly, more studies are needed to investigate this clinically important problem of drug hepatotoxicity in the elderly which remains mostly unelucidated.

F. Conclusions and Suggestions for Future Studies

As has been briefly reviewed, drug hepatotoxicity in the elderly is a complex phenomenon involving so many different factors, all of which can be functions of aging. Clinical studies are difficult to perform in a controlled and prospective way, and, with humans we mostly have to rely on sporadic case reports.

The results of animal experiments are difficult simply to extrapolate to humans, since they are quite variable, depending on the animal model selected. Despite these limitations, more work must be done using experimental animals. However, in this effort, the variability of factors regulating the results should be carefully considered. For example, animals that have rather stable liver detoxifying functions such as phase I and II reactions with age (e.g., female rats, female mice of some strains such as C57BL) should be preferred to other animal models where these systems decline drastically with age (e.g., F-344 male rats, Swiss Webster female mice), since the former appears to more closely mimic human situations. Some other mouse strains are also known to show a drastic change with age. Results obtained from such animal models are not appropriate for the purpose of projecting the data to human situations. Despite these limitations, the use of experimental animals, if properly selected and interpreted, is expected to help our further understanding of this barely elucidated problem. The author, however, also wants to issue the caution that there is no ideal animal model for pursuing this problem. The above-mentioned female rats and C57BL female mouse models are only better choices than singular male rats, and there is no assurance that the results obtained from female rats can be interpreted clearly in clinical terms. It is the belief of the author, however, that the problem of drug hepatotoxicity in the elderly should be studied with a full awareness of the possibility that stress-induced deterioration of liver functions may elucidate potential differences between young and old animals in both liver functions and hepatotoxicities.

References

Abernathy CO, Lukacs L, Zimmerman HJ (1980) Cytotoxic effects of erythromycin estolate and chlorpromazine on hepatocytes isolated from rats of varying ages: a brief note. Mech Ageing Dev 12:1–6

Baillie SP, Yelland C, Woodhouse KW (1989a) Hepatic adverse drug reactions in the elderly. Adverse Drug React Acute Pois Rev 8:153–163

Baillie SP, Bateman DN, Coates PE, Woodhouse KW (1989b) Age and the pharmacokinetics of morphine. Age Ageing 18:258–262

Boobis AR, Davies DS (1984) Human cytochrome P-450. Xenobiotica 14:151–185

Cand F, Verdetti W (1989) Superoxide dismutase, glutathione peroxidase, catalase, and lipid peroxidase, in major organs of the aging rats. Free Rad Biol Med 7:59–63

Cao-Danh H, Benedetti MS, Dostert P (1983) Differential changes in superoxide dismutase activity in brain and liver of old rats and mice. J Neurochem 40:1003–1007

Carrillo MC, Kitani K, Kanai S, Sato Y, Nokubo M, Ohta M, Otsubo K (1989) Differences in the influence of diet on hepatic glutathione S-transferase activity and glutathione content between young and old C57 black female mice. Mech Ageing Dev 47:1–15

Carrillo MC, Nokubo M, Sato Y, Kanai S, Ohta M, Kitani K (1990) Effect of protein-free diet on activities and subunits of glutathione S-transferase in livers of young and aged female rats. Mech Ageing Dev 56:237–251

Carrillo MC, Nokubo M, Kitani K, Satoh K, Sato K (1991) Age-related alterations of enzyme activities and subunits of hepatic glutathione S-transferases in male and female Fischer-344 rats. Biochim Biophys Acta 1077:325–331

Carrillo MC, Kanai S, Sato Y, Kitani K (1992) Age-related changes in antioxidant enzyme activities are region and organ selective as well as sex in the rat. Mech Ageing Dev 65:187–198
Chengelis CP (1988) Age- and sex-related changes in epoxide hydrolase, UDP-glucuronosyl transferase, glutathione S-transferase, and PAPS sulphotransferase in Sprague-Dawley rats. Xenobiotica 18:1225–1237
Coecke S, Vandenberghe Y, Callaerts A, Sonck W, Verleye G, Van Bezooijen CFA, Vercruysse A, Rogiers V (1990) Hepatic cytosolic glutathione S-transferase activities in ageing Brown Norway rats – importance of sex differences and phenobarbital treatment for studies of ageing. Mech Ageing Dev 55:189–198
Denison H, Kaczynski J, Wallerstedt S (1987) Paracetamol medication and alcohol abuse: a dangerous combination for the liver and the kidney. Scand J Gastroenterol 22:701–704
Erickson CK (1984) Ethanol clearance in nine inbred rat strains. Alcohol Clin Exp Res 8:491–494
Fernandez-Checa JC, Ookhtens M, Kaplowitz N (1989) Effects of chronic ethanol feeding on rat hepatocytic glutathione. Relationship of cytosolic glutathione to efflux and mitochondrial sequestration. J Clin Invest 83:1247–1252
Fujita S, Kitagawa H, Chiba M, Suzuki T, Ohta M, Kitani K (1985a) Age and sex associated differences in the relative abundance of multiple species of cytochrome P-450 in rat liver microsomes – a separation by HPLC of hepatic microsomal cytochrome P-450 species. Biochem Pharmacol 34:1861–1864
Fujita S, Kitagawa H, Ishizawa H, Suzuki T, Kitani K (1985b) Age associated alterations in hepatic glutathione-S-transferase activities. Biochem Pharmacol 34:3891–3894
Fujita S, Chiba M, Suzuki T, Kitani K (1986) Effect of senescence on the hepatic metabolism of drgus affecting the central nervous system in rats and mice. In: Kitani K (ed) Liver and aging – 1986, liver and brain. Elsevier Science, Amsterdam, pp 103–112
Galinsky RE, Corcoran GB (1986) Influence of advanced age on the formation and elimination of acetaminophen metabolites by male rats. Pharmacology 32:312–320
Galinsky RE, Kane RE, Franklin MK (1986) Effect of aging on drug metabolizing enzymes important in acetaminophen elimination. J Pharmacol Exp Ther 237:107–113
Galinsky RE, Johnson DH, Kane RE, Franklin MR (1990) Effect of aging on hepatic biotransformation in female Fischer 344 rats: changes in sulfotransferase activities are consistent with known gender related changes in pituitary growth hormone secretion in aging animals. J Pharmacol Exp Ther 255:577–583
Gellert J, Geisbüsch B, Teschke R (1988) Impaired ethanol metabolism with advancing age in female rats: studies on its mechanism. Adv Biosci 71:225–229
Goudie BM, Birnie GF, Watkinson G et al. (1982) Jaundice associated with the use of benoxaprofen. Lancet I:959–961
Herd B, Wynne H, Wright P, Lames O, Woodhouse K (1991) The effect of age on glucuronidation and sulphation of paracetamol by human liver fractions. Br J Clin Pharmacol 32:768–770
Hornbrook KR, Kosanke SD, Rikans LE (1993) Aged mice are resistant to the hepatotoxic effects of endotoxin and galactosamine. Exp Mol Pathol 59:27–37
James OFW (1988) Parenchymal liver disease in the elderly. In: Bianchi L, Holt P, James OFW (eds) Aging in liver and gastrointestinal tract. MTP Press, Lancaster, pp 359–369
James OFW, Rawlins MD, Woodhouse K (1982) Lack of ageing effect on human microsomal monooxygenase enzyme activities and on inactivation pathways for reactive metabolic intermediates. In: Kitani K (ed) Liver and aging—1982. Elsevier Biomedical, Amsterdam, pp 395–408
Ji LL, Dillon D, Wu E (1990) Alteration of antioxidant enzymes with aging in rat skeletal muscle and liver. Am J Physiol 27:R918–923

Kamataki T, Maeda K, Shimada M, Kitani K, Nagai T, Kato R (1985) Age-related alteration in the activities of drug-metabolizing enzymes and contents of sex-specific forms of cytochrome P-450 in liver microsomes from male and female rats. J Pharmacol Exp Ther 233:222–228

Kato R, Takanaka A (1968) Metabolism of drugs in old rats. I. Activities of NADPH linked electron transport and drug-metabo-lizing enzyme systems in liver microsomes of old rats. Jpn J Pharmacol 18:381–388

Kato R, Vassanelli P, Frontino G, Chiesara E (1964) Variation in the activity of liver microsomal drug metabolizing enzymes in rats in relation to the age. Biochem Pharmacol 13:1037–1051

Kellogg EW, Fridovich J (1976) Superoxide dismutase in the rat and mouse as a function of age and longevity. J Gerontol 31:405–408

Kitahara A, Ebina T, Ishikawa T, Soma Y, Sato K, Kanai S (1982) Changes in activities and molecular forms of rat hepatic drug metabolizing enzymes during aging. In: Kitani K (ed) Liver and aging—1982, liver and drugs. Elsevier Biomedical, Amsterdam, pp 135–143

Kitani K (1986) Does the liver age in man? (Editorial) Hepatol Rapid Rev 16:V–XIX

Kitani K (1988) Drugs and the ageing liver. Life Chem Rep 6:143–230

Kitani K (1990a) Evaluation of rodent models for the study of age-related modifications in toxic response. In: Volans GN, Sims J, Sullivan FM, Turner P (eds) Basic science in toxicology. Proceedings of the 5th international congress on toxicology. Taylor and Francis, London, pp 422–431

Kitani K (1990b) Aging and the liver. In: Popper H, Schaffner F (eds) Progress in liver diseases, vol IX. Saunders, Philadelphia, pp 603–623

Lammi-Keefe CJ, Swan PB, Hegarty PVJ (1984) Copper-zinc and manganese superoxide dismutase activity in brain and liver of old rats and mice. J Neurochem 40:1003–1007

Lauterburg BH, Velez ME (1988) Glutathione deficiency in alcoholics: risk factor for paracetamol hepatotoxicity. Gut 29:1153–1157

Lauterburg BH, Vaishnav Y, Stillwell WG, Mitchell JR (1980) The effects of age and glutathione depletion on hepatic glutathione turnover in vivo determined by acetaminophen probe analysis. J Pharmacol Exp Ther 213:54–58

Leakey JA, Cunny HC, Bazare J Jr, Webb PJ, Lipscomb JC, Slikker W Jr, Feuers RJ, Duffy PH, Hart RW (1989) Effects of aging and caloric restriction on hepatic drug metabolizing enzymes in the Fischer 344 rats. II: effects on conjugating enzymes. Mech Ageing Dev 48:157–166

Lee DW, Yu BP (1991) The age-related alterations in liver microsomal membranes: the effect of lipid peroxidation and dietary restriction. In: Kitani K (ed) Liver and aging—1990. Excerpta Medica, Amsterdam, pp 17–29

Maloney AG, Schmucker DL, Vessey DS, Wang RK (1986) The effects of aging on the hepatic microsomal mixed function oxidase system of male and female monkeys. Hepatology 6:282–287

Mannervik B, Alin P, Guthenberg C, Jensson H, Tahir MK, Warholm M, Jörnvall H (1985) Identification of three classes of cytosolic glutathione transferase common to several mammalian species: correlation between structural data and enzymatic properties. Proc Natl Acad Sci USA 82:7202–7206

Mitchell JR, Jollows DJ (1975) Metabolic activation of drugs to toxic substances. Gastroenterology 68:392–410

Mitchell JR, Jollow J, Potter WZ, Gillette JR, Brodie BB (1973) Acetaminophen-induced hepatic necrosis. IV. Protective role of glutathione. J Pharmacol Exp Ther 187:211–217

Mitchell JR, Thorgeirsson SS, Potter WZ, Jollow DJ, Keiser H (1974) Acetaminophen-induced hepatic injury: protective role of glutathione in man and rationale for therapy. Clin Pharmacol Ther 16:676–684

Neuberger J, Williams R (1984) Halothane anaesthesia and liver damage. Br Med J 289:1136–1139

Oliver CN, Levine RL, Stadtman ER (1987) A role of mixed function oxidation reactions in the accumulation of altered enzyme forms during aging. J Geriatr Soc 947–956
Ott JF, Hunter BE, Walker DW (1985) The effect of age on ethanol metabolism and on the hypothermic and hypnotic responses to ethanol in the Fischer 344 rat. Alcohol Clin Exp Res 9:59–65
Rao G, Xia E, Richardson A (1990) Effect of age on the expression of antioxidant enzymes in male Fischer F-344 rats. Mech Ageing Dev 53:49–60
Reiss U, Gershon D (1976) Comparison of cytoplasmic superoxide dismutase in liver, heart and brain of aging rats and mice. Biochem Biophys Res Commun 73:255–261
Reiss U, Gershon D (1978) Methionine sulfoxide reductase: a novel protective enzyme in liver and its potentially significant role in aging. In: Kitani K (ed) Liver and aging – 1978. Elsevier/North-Holland Biomedical, Amsterdam, pp 55–61
Rikans LE (1984) Influence of aging on the susceptibility of rats to hepatotoxic injury. Toxicol Appl Pharmacol 73:243–249
Rikans LE (1987) The oxidation of acrolein by rat liver aldehyde dehydrogenases. Relation to allyl alcohol hepatotoxicity. Drug Metab Dispos 15:356–362
Rikans LE (1989) Influence of aging on chemically induced hepatotoxicity: role of age-related changes in metabolism. Drug Metab Rev 20:87–110
Rikans LE, Cai Y (1992) Age-associated enhancement of diquat-induced lipid peroxidation and cytotoxicity in isolated rat hepatocytes. J Pharmacol Exp Ther 262:271–278
Rikans LE, Cai Y (1993) Diquat-induced oxidative damage in BCNU-pretreated hepatocytes of mature and old rats. Toxicol Appl Pharmacol 118:263–270
Rikans LE, Kling R (1987) Effects of aging and testosterone administration on liver alcohol dehydrogenase activity in male Fischer 344 rats. Alcohol Clin Exp Res 11:562–566
Rikans LE, Kosanke SD (1984) Effect of aging on liver glutathione levels and hepatocellular injury from carbon tetrachloride, allyl alcohol or galactosamine. Drug Chem Toxicol 7:595–604
Rikans LE, Moore DR (1987) Effect of age and sex on allyl alcohol hepatotoxicity in rats: role of liver alcohol and aldehyde dehydrogenase activities. J Pharmacol Exp Ther 243:20–26
Rikans LE, Moore DR (1988) Acetaminophen hepatotoxicity in aging rats. Drug Chem Toxicol 11:237–247
Rikans LE, Snowden CD (1989) Effects of acute ethanol administration on female rat liver as a function of aging. Life Sci 45:1373–1379
Rikans LE, Moore DR, Snowden CD (1991) Sex-dependent differences in the effects of aging on antioxidant defense mechanisms of rat liver. Biochim Biophys Acta 1074:195–200
Rikans LE, Kitani K, Nokubo M, Kanai S (1992a) Hepatic glutathione (GSH) regulation in young and old C57BL mice. Toxicologist 12:418 (abstract)
Rikans LE, Nokubo M, Kanai S, Kitani K (1992b) Diurnal variation in hepatic glutathione content as a function of age. Drug Dev Res 26:461–465
Rikans LE, Snowden CD, Moore D (1992c) Effect of aging on enzymatic antioxidant defenses in rat liver mitochondria. Gerontology 38:133–138
Rogen GM, Singletary WV Jr, Rauckman EJ, Killenberg PG (1983) Acetaminophen hepatotoxicity. An alternative mechanism. Biochem Pharmacol 32:2053–2059
Rogiers V, Coecke S, Vandenberghe Y, Morel F, Callaerts A, Verleye G, Van Bezooijen CFA, Guillouzo A, Vercruysse A (1991) Effect of the aging process on the gender and phenobarbital dependent expression of glutathione S-transferase subunits in Brown Norway rat liver. Biochem Pharmacol 42:491–498
Rubin E, Lieber CS (1972) Ethanol metabolism in the liver. In: Popper H, Schaffner F (eds) Progress in liver diseases, vol IV. Grune and Stratton, New York, pp 549–566

Seitz HK, Meydani M, Ferschke I, Simanowski UA, Boesche J, Bogusz M, Hoepker W, Blumberg JB, Russell RM (1989) Effect of aging on in vivo and in vitro ethanol metabolism and its toxicity in F344 rats. Gastroenterology 97:446–456

Semsei I, Rao G, Richardson A (1989) Changes in the expression of superoxide dismutase and catalase as a function of age and dietary restriction. Biochem Biophys Res Commun 164:620–625

Spearman ME, Leibman KC (1983) Hepatic and pulmonary cytosolic metabolism of epoxides effects of aging on conjugation with glutathione. Life Sci 33:2615–2625

Spearman ME, Leibman KC (1984a) The effects of aging on hepatic and pulmonary glutathione S-transferase activities in male and female Fischer 344 rats. Biochem Pharmacol 33:1309–1313

Spearman ME, Leibman KC (1984b) Aging selectively alters glutathione S-transferase isozyme concentrations in liver and lung cytosol. Drug Metab Dispos 12:661–671

Stohs SJ, Al-Turk WA, Angle CR (1982) Glutathione *S*-transferase and glutathione reductase activities in hepatic and extrahepatic tissues of female mice as a function of age. Biochem Pharmacol 31:2113–2116

Sutter MA, Gibson G Williams LS, Wang RK, Schmucker DL (1985) Comparison of the hepatic mixed function oxidase systems of young, adult and old non-human primates (Macaca nemestrina). Biochem Pharmacol 34:2983–2987

Sweeny DJ, Weiner M (1985) Metabolism of acetaminophen in hepatocytes isolated from mice and rats of various ages. Drug Metab Dispos 13:377–379

Taggart HM, Alderdyce JM (1982) Fatal cholestatic jaundice in elderly patients taking benoxaprofen. Br Med J 284:1372

Tarloff JB, Goldstein RS, Sozio RS, Hook JB (1991) Hepatic and renal conjugation (phase II) enzyme activities in young adult, middle-aged, and senescent male Sprague-Dawley rats. Proc Soc Exp Biol Med 197:297–303

Vestal RE, McGuire EA, Tobin JD, Andres R, Norris AH, Mezey E (1977) Aging and ethanol metabolism. Clin Pharmacol Ther 21:343–354

Wiberg GS, Trenholm HL, Coldwell BB (1970) Increased ethanol toxicity in old rats: changes in LD_{50}, in vivo and in vitro metabolism, and liver alcohol dehydrogenase activity. Toxicol Appl Pharmacol 16:718–727

Woodhouse K, Herd B (1993) The effect of age and gender on glucuronidation and sulphation in rat liver: a study using paracetamol as a model substrate. Arch Gerontol Geriatr 16:111–115

Woodhouse KW, Mortimer O, Wiholm BE (1986) Hepatic adverse drug reactions: the influence of age. In: Kitani K (ed) Liver and aging—1986, liver and brain. Elsevier Science, Amsterdam, pp 75–80

Wulf JH, Cutler RG (1979) Altered protein hypothesis of mammalian aging process I, thermal stability of glucose-6-phosphate dehydrogenase in C57BL/6J mouse tissues. Exp Gerontol 9:189–196

Wynne HA, Mutch E, James OFW, Rawlins MD, Woodhouse KW (1987) The effect of age on mono-oxygenase enzyme kinetics in rat liver microsomes. Age Ageing 16:153–158

Wynne HA, Mutch E, James OFW, Wright P, Rawlins MD, Woodhouse KW (1988) The effect of age upon the affinity of microsomal mono-oxygenase enzymes for substrate in human liver. Age Ageing 17:401–405

Wynne HA, Cope LH, Herd B, Rawlins MD, James OFW, Woodhouse KW (1990) The association of age and frailty with paracetamol conjugation in man. Age Ageing 19:419–424

Zs.-Nagy I, Kitani K, Ohta M, Imahori K (1986) Age-dependent decrease of the lateral diffusion constant of proteins in the plasma membrane of hepatocytes as revealed by fluorescence recovery after photobleaching in tissue smears. Arch Gerontol Geriatr 5:131–146

Zs.-Nagy I, Kitani K, Ohta M (1989) Age-dependence of the lateral mobility of proteins in the plasma membrane of hepatocytes of C57/BL/6 mice: FRAP studies on liver smears. J Gerontol Biol Sci 44:B83–B87

CHAPTER 16

Effect of Liver Disease on Drug Metabolism and Pharmacokinetics

P.G. WELLING and W.F. POOL

A. Introduction

The processes of drug absorption, distribution, metabolism and excretion, and the rates at which they occur, are recognized as critical factors influencing the degree and time course of drug pharmacologic action in the body. Disease states affecting different organs may have a variety of effects on drug disposition and also on pharmacologic and pharmacodynamic effects. The two organs that are recognized as having the greatest influence on drug disposition, either directly or indirectly, are the kidney and the liver. While most clinical studies carried out early in drug development are conducted in healthy subjects, renal or hepatic impairment may exert a considerable influence on both the disposition and the pharmacodynamic consequences of an administered drug.

The influence of renal insufficiency on drug disposition is well characterized in terms of markers of renal function, for example, creatinine clearance, serum creatinine, and inulin clearance. The impact of renal impairment on drug pharmacokinetics can generally be accurately predicted based on the relative contributions of metabolism and renal excretion to overall drug clearance from the body and, with few exceptions, the influence of renal failure on drug pharmacokinetics and pharmacodynamics is predictable and manageable in the clinical situation.

Such is unfortunately not the case with liver disease. Despite a large number of studies and attempts to establish guidelines for drug administration in patients with liver disease, it is still not possible to predict with any accuracy the effect of liver disease on the pharmacokinetics or pharmacodynamics of a particular drug. This is no doubt due both to the overall structure and unique position of the liver in the cardiovascular system and also to the heterogeneous nature of liver disease and the different effects that liver disease may have on metabolism and distribution of particular drugs.

The purpose of this chapter is to review various approaches that have been used to better understand how liver impairment may affect drug disposition, to describe the effects of liver impairment on various therapeutic classes of drugs, and to suggest guidelines for drug use in patients with liver failure.

B. Function and Structure of the Liver

Unlike the kidneys, which derive their blood supply exclusively via the renal arteries, the liver receives blood both from the hepatic arteries and also from the splanchnic portal circulation. It is this dual blood supply, one arising from the systemic circulation and the other carrying absorbed substances from the gastrointestinal (GI) tract, that places the liver in a unique position as an eliminating organ. By receiving portal blood the liver "sees" substances before they enter the systemic circulation and can thus metabolize drugs with variable efficiency, thereby influencing drug systemic availability. Blood reaching the liver via the hepatic arteries, on the other hand, carries substances that have already entered and have been diluted into the systemic circulation so that, for those substances that reach the liver by this route and are metabolized in the liver, this organ acts purely as an eliminating organ.

Regardless of the source of the hepatic blood supply, vascular exchange occurs through the sinusoids to the hepatic vein. While red blood cells and other formed elements are confined to the inner axial core of the sinusoid, dissolved substances can freely exchange with the liver parenchymal cells via the fluids in the outer space of the sinusoid, the space of Disse.

The location of the liver between the splanchnic and systemic circulations is well suited to its many functions. These include the synthesis of most plasma proteins including albumin, α-1-acid glycoproteins and clotting factors, regulation and synthesis of amino acids, fatty acids, cholesterol and glucose, synthesis of bile acid urea, and removal from blood of ammonia, endotoxins, bilirubin, endogenous hormones, and other waste products, and also the metabolism of drugs, usually to more hydrophilic substances that can subsequently be removed from the circulation by the kidneys or excreted in bile (ARNS et al. 1988).

Drug metabolism reactions are conveniently differentiated into phase 1, which involves oxidation, reduction, or hydrolysis, and phase 2, which involves conjugation reactions. Phase 1 reactions are controlled predominantly by the cytochrome P450 enzyme systems in the smooth endoplasmic reticulum located predominantly in the pericentral region of the liver. Reduction and hydrolysis reactions occur mainly in the cell cytoplasm. Phase 2 conjugation reactions occur in various sites of the liver. Glucuronidation, which is mediated by uridine diphosphate (UDP)-glucuronyl transferase enzymes, occurs in the rough endoplasmic reticulum (SECOR and SCHENKER 1987). These enzymes occur throughout the liver with highest concentrations in the periportal region. Other reactions, including sulfation, acetylation, and conjugation with glycine, glutamine, or glutathione are generally thought to occur in the cytosolic fraction. Location of these various enzymes within the cell, and generally throughout the liver, plays an important role in the degree to which various types of liver disease affect their activity and hence on drug metabolism and pharmacokinetics.

C. Types and Severity of Liver Disease

The function of the liver may be impaired by various conditions, for example, nutritional status (HATHCOCK 1985), environmental factors (O'MAHONY and WOODHOUSE 1994), and many disease states such as acquired immunodeficiency syndrome (LEE et al. 1993), cirrhosis, acute hepatitis, biliary status, hepatic neoplasm, and drug-induced liver disease, and may range from acute effects (LEWIS and ZIMMERMAN 1989) to chronic changes associated with ageing (MOONEY et al. 1985; WOODHOUSE 1985; O'MAHONY and WOODHOUSE 1994). The liver has marked excess capacity of most of its enzyme systems (EAGLE and STRUNIN 1990). For example, bilirubin elimination must fall below 10% of normal before jaundice develops. Similarly, in the normal liver urea formation occurs at 60% capacity, while glucose maintenance requires only 20% of liver function and albumin and clotting factors are synthesized by only a small percentage of liver cells at any one time (ARNS et al. 1988). The excess liver capacity, together with the possible influence of a variety of enzyme inducing substances such as alcohol and agricultural and industrial chemicals, make it difficult to determine the precise extent of liver injury. Liver injury may be manifest and described in terms of both hepatic function and vascular changes.

I. Changes in Hepatic Function

Changes in hepatocyte function have been reported in liver disease and such changes have been associated with the sick-cell hypothesis (MCLEAN and MORGAN 1991). Hepatic enzyme levels are affected by liver cirrhosis but changes are not uniform among enzyme classes (BROSEN 1990; MURRAY et al. 1986; MURRAY 1992). Liver disease is associated with changes in the hepatic sinusoids, with changes in the endothelial lining and deposition of mucopolysaccharides, collagen, and fibrin. These changes have been associated with an increased blood-hepatocyte barrier leading to hepatocellular necrosis (HORN et al. 1987; SOTANIEMI et al. 1986). Other changes associated with hepatocyte function include development of diffuse fibrosis leading to resistance to blood flow.

II. Changes in Hepatic Vasculature

An alternative to the sick-cell hypothesis for liver failure is the intact hepatocyte hypothesis (BRANCH 1982; BRANCH and SHAND 1976). This hypothesis, similar to the intact nephron hypothesis associated with renal failure, assumes that the diseased liver consists of regions of nonfunctional cells and other regions that are not involved at all in the disease process and are morphologically normal. As liver disease progresses, with associated fibrotic infiltration, there is altered vascular distribution with loss of tributaries of the portal vein, leading to diversion of blood flow within the liver. As a consequence of the resulting hepatic resistance, portal venous pressure increases and extrahepatic collateral veins between portal and systemic circulations dilate and may divert up to 60% of blood flow in the splanchnic and mesenteric veins from the liver (BRANCH and SHAND 1976).

While both the sick-cell and intact hepatocyte theories are interesting alternatives to characterize the nature and extent of liver failure and its impact on metabolism and pharmacokinetics of drugs, neither one alone accurately predicts the impact of impaired liver function on individual drugs. This reflects the complex nature of liver failure and its relationship to drug disposition.

III. Changes in Renal Function

Renal blood flow may be reduced in cirrhosis. Glomerular function is variable in early cirrhosis but is usually decreased when ascites develops (KLINGER et al. 1970). Renal sodium retention is an important factor in development of ascites. With progression of liver disease these factors can lead to renal failure (SHEAR et al. 1965). Reduced renal clearance in patients with impaired liver function has been reported for a number of drugs including furosemide (GONZALEZ et al. 1982), bumetanide (MARCANTONIO et al. 1983), cimetidine and ranitidine (CELLO and ØIE 1983; SMITH et al. 1984). However, renal elimination of drugs is not influenced by liver disease unless renal function itself is also impaired (MCLEAN and MORGAN 1991).

IV. Ascites

Increased fluid retention by the kidneys and increased production of lymph both lead to formulation of ascites (ARNS et al. 1988). Increased production of lymph in the liver is related to changes in pressure within the sinusoidal spaces. When increased lymph production exceeds the capacity of lymph channels, lymph may enter the peritoneal cavity. This, together with sodium-related water retention by the kidneys, leads to the condition of peritoneal ascites. From a pharmacokinetic viewpoint, the condition of ascites may change drug disposition by increasing the overall distribution volume, which may be exacerbated by simultaneous reduction in drug binding to plasma proteins.

D. Pharmacodynamic Factors

While drug metabolism and pharmacokinetics may be altered in liver disease, the degree of alteration depending on the type and extent of liver injury, pharmacodynamic changes may also occur that may or may not be related directly to drug or metabolite dispositional changes. Due to the complexity and often competing nature of factors affecting drug disposition in liver failure, changes in pharmacodynamic response may occur at what appear to be "normal" therapeutic drug levels. Increased cerebral sensitivity to a number of compounds including morphine, chlorpromazine, and also the diazepines

(BRANCH et al. 1976b) has been demonstrated in patients with liver disease, particularly in patients with prior hepatic encephalopathy (SECOR and SCHENKER 1987; FOWLER and SCHAFER 1981).

The three major mechanisms postulated to cause altered pharmacodynamic response, particularly those associated with the central nervous system, are altered drug access to the site of action due to reduced binding to plasma proteins (ROWLAND and TOZER 1989), altered blood-brain barrier permeability (SCHENTAG et al. 1981), and altered receptor response (BRANCH et al. 1976b; MCCONNELL et al. 1982). Although increased response to benzodiazepines was attributed to increased γ-aminobutyric acid (GABA) and benzodiazepine-binding sites in hepatic encephalopathy (SCHAFER et al. 1983; ZENEROLI 1985; FOWLER and SCHAFER 1981), other studies have not confirmed these changes (BUTTERWORTH et al. 1988; MADDISON et al. 1987).

E. Pharmacokinetic Factors

Before discussing the influence of liver disease on drug pharmacokinetics it is pertinent to review briefly some of the basic aspects of pharmacokinetic modeling (WELLING 1993).

I. Linear Pharmacokinetic Models

1. One-Compartment Model, Intravenous Dosing

For most compounds the simple one-compartment pharmacokinetic model is adequate to describe drug disposition. This model assumes that drug rapidly and homogeneously equilibrates into certain body fluids and tissues, and that relative drug concentrations in various tissues remain constant as long as there is drug in the body. Compartment models may be concerned with spatial changes, that is transfer of drug from one place to another, or with chemical changes, for example, metabolism of drug to a different chemical form. Following are some examples and uses of the one-compartment model. This model is shown in Fig. 1, in which D is the dose, A is the amount of drug in the body at any time, t, after dosing, C is the drug concentration, V is the drug distribution volume, and the three ks are first-order rate constants for urinary excretion, k_e, metabolism, k_m, and overall excretion, k_{el}, where $k_{el} = k_e + k_m$.

From Fig. 1, the standard expression for drug concentration at any time t after intravenous injection, expressed in exponential and logarithmic forms, is given by Eqs. 1 and 2.

$$C = C_0 e^{-k_{el} t} \quad (1)$$

$$\text{Log}\, C = \text{Log}\, C_0 - \frac{k_{el} \cdot t}{2 \cdot 3} \quad (2)$$

From these expressions a plot of the logarithm of drug concentration against time is linear, as in Fig. 2. The slope yields the elimination-rate constant k_{el} and the elimination half-life, $t_{1/2}$. Dividing the dose D by the extrapolated value C_0 at zero time yields the distribution volume V. Multiplying V by k_{el} yields the plasma clearance Cl_p. Cl_p can also be obtained by dividing dose D by the area under the plasma curve, as in Eqs. 3 and 4.

$$\mathrm{AUC}^{(0-\infty)} = C_0 \int_0^{\infty} e^{-k_{el}t} \cdot \mathrm{d}t = \frac{C_0}{k_{el}} \tag{3}$$

Thus

$$\frac{D}{C_0 / k_{el}} = \frac{DVk_{el}}{D} = Vk_{el} = Cl_p \tag{4}$$

If the quantity of unchanged drug cleared in urine, A_u^{∞}, is known then the renal clearance Cl_r can be calculated from Eq. 5:

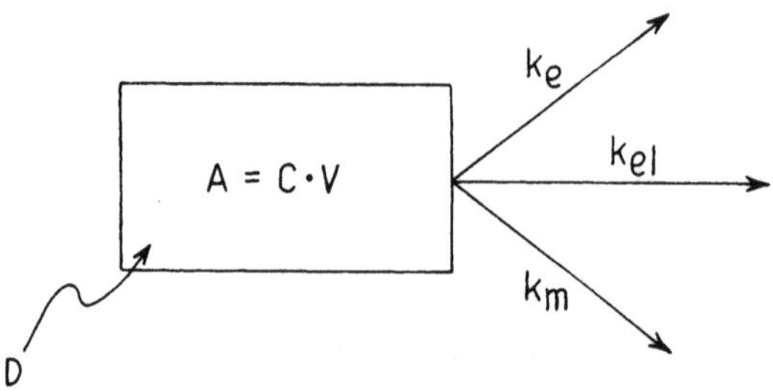

Fig. 1. One-compartment open model with bolus intravenous injection: D is the dose, A is the amount of drug in the body, and C is the concentration of drug in body fluids. (Reproduced with permission from WELLING 1986a)

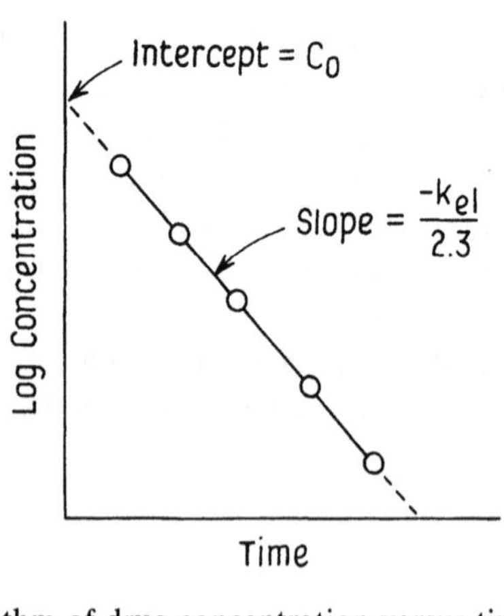

Fig. 2. Plot of the logarithm of drug concentration versus time following intravenous bolus injection. (Reproduced with permission from WELLING 1986b)

$$Cl_r = \frac{A_u^{\infty}}{AUC^{(0-\infty)}} \tag{5}$$

or from Eq. 6:

$$Cl_r = \frac{A_u^{t}}{AUC^{(0-t)}} \tag{6}$$

One can then obtain k_e from Eq. 7:

$$k_e = \frac{Cl_r k_{el}}{Cl_p} \tag{7}$$

and k_m from $k_m = k_{el} - k_e$. Metabolic clearance is then obtained from Eq. 8.

$$Cl_m = k_m V \tag{8}$$

Thus, values of many pharmacokinetic parameters can be obtained from a relatively small amount of blood level or urinary excretion data.

2. First-Order Absorption and Elimination

This model differs from the intravenous bolus model and is necessarily more complex in that both drug absorption and elimination are controlled by first-order kinetics. There are many forms of this model depending on the type of drug, its intrinsic release and absorption characteristics, and its overall pharmacokinetic profiles. The treatment here is limited only to a simple general model as described in Fig. 3. The basic expression to describe plasma drug levels following a single oral dose of a drug when absorption and elimination are both controlled by first-order processes is given by Eq. 9.

$$C = \frac{FD}{V}\left(\frac{k_a}{k_a - k_{el}}\right)\left(e^{-k_{el}t} - e^{k_a t}\right) \tag{9}$$

This equation incorporates first-order rate constants for both absorption and elimination. It incorporates also the function F, the fraction of dose that is absorbed from the dosage form into the systemic circulation. After intravenous administration the parameter F does not appear in kinetic models because all of the drug is available to the systemic circulation, $F = 1$. However, after oral doses, F is generally less than 1 and complete absorption cannot be assumed. Incomplete drug availability to the systemic circulation may result from a number of factors including low or slow solubility, degradation of drug in the GI tract, poor membrane penetration, and presystemic intestinal or hepatic metabolism or biliary excretion. The uncertain value of F makes it impossible to calculate a drug distribution volume after oral dosing because, while all other parameters in Eq. 9 can be resolved by standard procedures, the parameters F and V cannot be resolved without additional information such as intravenous data or urinary excretion. A low plasma drug level after oral dosing may be due to poor bioavailability, a large distribution volume, or a combination of these. The standard procedure for obtaining parameter values for this model is illustrated in Fig. 4.

Whether analysis is by one of a number of available computer programs, or by simple graphic analysis, the principle is the same. When plotted on semilogarithmic graph paper the absorption phase of a drug profile is curved because this portion of the profile is biexponential. After absorption is complete, the exponential term $e^{-k_a t}$ in Eq. 9 reduces to zero and the elimination phase is then monoexponential and is described by a straight line governed by the rate constant k_{el}, with a zero-time intercept of $(FD/V)(k_a/(k_a - k_{el}))$. The absorption rate constant can then be obtained by the method of residuals. The value of FD/V is obtained from the known value of the intercept $(FD/V)(k_a/(k_a\ k_{el}))$ and also known values of k_a and k_{el}. As stated above the value of FD/V cannot be further resolved because both F and V are unknown. The area under the plasma curve from zero to infinity is given by Eq. 10.

$$\mathrm{AUC}^{(0-\infty)} = \frac{FD}{Vk_{el}} \tag{10}$$

Dividing this expression by the equivalent expression for the $\mathrm{AUC}^{(0-\infty)}$ after intravenous administration, D/Vk_{el}, yields Eq. 11, where F is the absolute bioavailability to the systemic circulation. Thus, if intravenous data are available, absolute drug bioavailability can be obtained through the relationship shown in Eq. 11.

$$\frac{\mathrm{AUC}^{(0-\infty)}\mathrm{p.o.}}{\mathrm{AUC}^{(0-\infty)}\mathrm{i.v.}} = \frac{FD/Vk_{el}}{D/Vk_{el}} = F \tag{11}$$

3. Repeated Dosing with Linear Pharmacokinetics

Almost all therapeutic drug doses are given as repeated dosage regimens. It is important during any such regimen to understand the rate and extent of

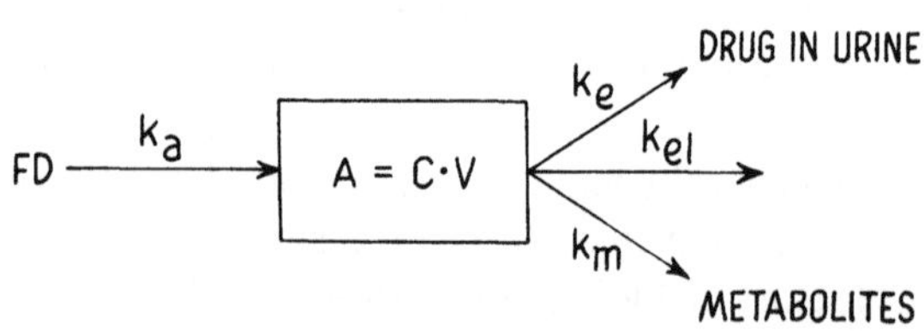

Fig. 3. One-compartment open model with first-order absorption and elimination, where F is the fraction of the dose, D, absorbed from the dosage site into the systemic circulation, and k_a is the first-order rate constant for drug absorption. (Reproduced with permission from WELLING 1986c)

drug accumulation and how accumulation can be predicted from single-dose data.

Regardless of the rate or frequency of administration, the rate of drug accumulation is controlled solely by the drug elimination rate. A reasonable estimate of the time taken for drug accumulation to be complete is the time to reach 95% of steady-state conditions. This is approximately 4.5 drug elimination drug half-lives. For example, if a drug has an elimination $t_{1/2}$ of 12 h, and is dosed twice daily, then circulating drug levels will have reached 95% of those to be expected at steady state by the fifth dose, that is by approximately 60 h. If, on the other hand, the drug with the same $t_{1/2}$ is dosed once daily, then steady-state levels will be achieved by the third dose. If the same drug were dosed q6h, then 11–12 doses would be required to reach 95% of steady-state levels.

Thus, provided the same amount of drug is given with each dose, regardless of the frequency of dosing, then four times as much drug would have been administered in the q6h regimen compared to the once daily regimen. It would take the same length of time to reach steady-state conditions with all three regimens but, dependent on the dosage frequency, the actual amount of drug administered during that time period and therefore the steady-state level reached would be different.

This introduces the concept of accumulation factor. How much higher will steady-state circulating drug levels be than those following the first dose? This

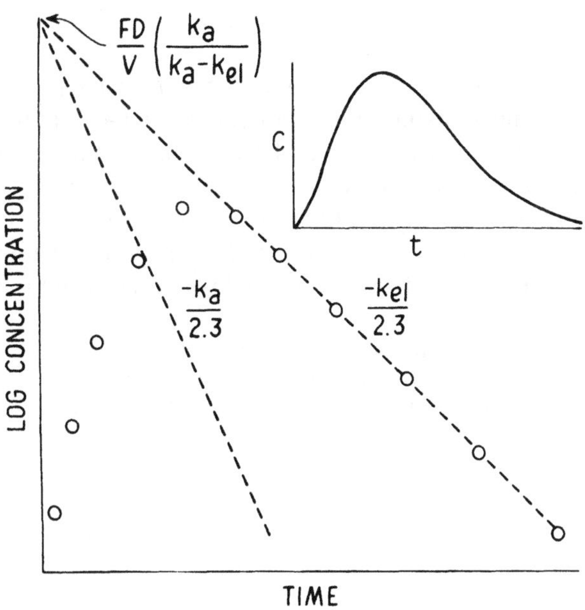

Fig. 4. Plot of the logarithm of drug concentration versus time for a drug that obeys one-compartment model kinetics with first-order absorption and elimination. The concentration is plotted on a linear scale *in the inset.* (Reproduced with permission from WELLING 1986d)

can readily be calculated provided the drug kinetics are linear. One approach is by means of Eq. 12.

$$R = \frac{1}{1 - 2^{-\varepsilon}} \tag{12}$$

where R is the accumulation factor and ε is the ratio of the dosing interval τ divided by the drug elimination $t_{1/2}$, $\varepsilon = \tau/t_{1/2}$. Typically, if a drug is administered at dosage intervals approximately equal to its $t_{1/2}$, then $\varepsilon = 1$ and $R = 2$. If, on the other hand, the drug is given at a dosage interval only one-fourth of the $t_{1/2}$, then $\varepsilon = 0.25$ and $R = 6.3$. If the dosage interval is fourfold longer than the $t_{1/2}$, then $\varepsilon = 4$ and $R = 1.1$. The range of R values that are obtained with different ε values is given in Table 1.

II. Nonlinear Pharmacokinetic Models

Many drugs exhibit nonlinear pharmacokinetics, usually as a result of saturable hepatic metabolism. All drug-metabolizing enzymes are saturable and some metabolism pathways are more readily saturable than others. For a drug that is eliminated from the body by a single, saturable metabolic pathway, an appropriate kinetic model is shown in Fig. 5, in which V_m is the maximum rate of drug elimination and K_m is the Michaelis constant for a particular enzyme system. For this saturable system, elimination is apparently first order when C is small relative to K_m but approaches zero order as C increases relative to K_m.

Figure 6 shows how the apparent elimination $t_{1/2}$ can change with increasing dose for a drug metabolized by nonsaturable (A), saturable (B), and parallel saturable and nonsaturable pathways (C). If a single, saturable pathway is involved, case B, the apparent elimination $t_{1/2}$ will increase with increasing drug concentration, giving rise to marked nonlinearity in dose-plasma level relationships. Coexistence of saturable and nonsaturable pathways, case C, gives rise to less profound effects because at high doses the nonsaturable (first-

Table 1. Changes in the accumulation factor R with changing values of ϵ (Reproduced with permission from WELLING 1986e)

ϵ	R
0.25	6.3
0.5	3.4
1	2.0
2	1.33
3	1.14
4	1.07

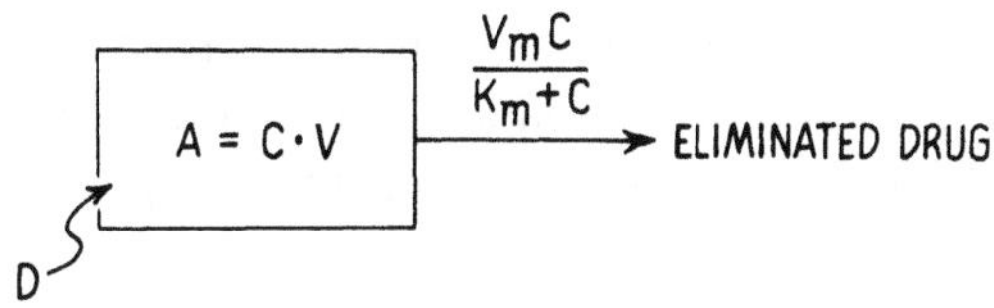

Fig. 5. One-compartment model with saturable elimination after bolus intravenous injection. (Reproduced with permission from WELLING 1986f)

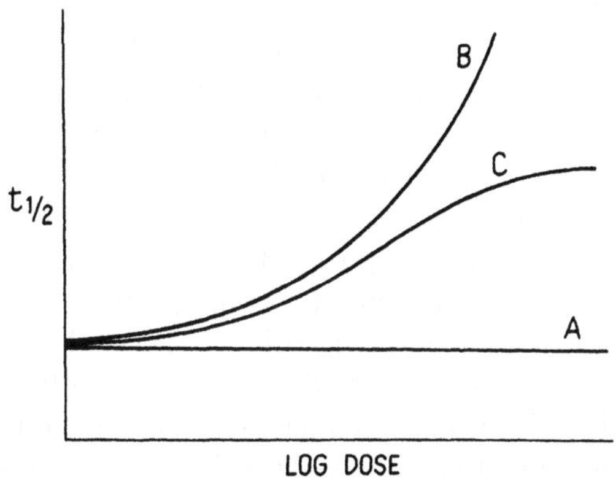

Fig. 6. Changes in apparent elimination half-life with increasing dose for drugs that are cleared from the body by *A*, nonsaturable; *B*, saturable; and *C*, parallel saturable and nonsaturable pathways. (Reproduced with permission from WELLING 1986g)

order) pathway predominates and the dose-related increase in $t_{1/2}$ tends to flatten out. In case A there is no change in $t_{1/2}$ with increasing dose size.

The problem of disproportionate increases in drug levels with increasing doses of a drug whose elimination is saturable can be best illustrated by Eq. 13. This equation, while containing some assumptions, relates $AUC^{(0-\infty)}$ to dose, distribution volume, and V_m for the situation when $C >> K_m$.

$$AUC^{(0-\infty)} = \frac{D^2}{(2 \cdot V^2 \cdot V_m)} \tag{13}$$

In this equation the area under the drug concentration curve is proportional to the square of the dose rather than the dose. Thus doubling the dose would increase the AUC, and hence organ and tissue exposure, fourfold, provided the distribution volume V remains relatively constant.

III. Impact of Liver Disease

The pharmacokinetic parameters most likely to be affected by impaired liver function are distribution, clearance, and elimination half-life. For drugs that are eliminated only by metabolism, a quantitative relationship between hepatic clearance (Cl_H) and intrinsic clearance of unbound or protein free drug Cl'_{int}, hepatic blood flow Q, and drug free fraction f_B is given by Eq. 14 (ARNS et al. 1988).

$$Cl_H = Q \cdot \frac{f_B Cl'_{int}}{Q + f_B Cl'_{int}} \tag{14}$$

This relationship has been used to attempt to predict the outcome of liver impairment when the determinants are modified. In particular, Eq. 14 may differentiate between those drugs that are highly or poorly extracted by the liver. From the equation, the hepatic clearance of highly extracted drugs ($Q << f_B Cl'_{int}$) approaches and becomes limited by hepatic blood flow. The metabolism of such drugs is said to be hepatic blood flow-limited and clearance is relatively insensitive to changes in protein binding. On the other hand, hepatic clearance of poorly extracted drugs ($Q >> f_B Cl'_{int}$) may be approximated by $f_B Cl'_{int}$ and for these drugs not only is hepatic clearance relatively inefficient but it is also dependent on any changes of protein binding that may occur as a result of impaired liver function. The metabolism of such drugs is said to be enzyme capacity limited. Traditionally, those drugs whose hepatic extraction is greater than 70% are defined as flow limited, while those whose hepatic extraction is less than 30% are considered to be enzyme capacity limited. Many drugs have intermediate values and do not clearly fit into either of these two categories.

Enzyme-capacity-limited drugs are further defined as those which are protein binding-sensitive and those which are protein binding-insensitive. The hepatic clearance for capacity-limited drugs that are extensively (>85%) bound to plasma proteins is likely to be significantly affected by alterations in protein binding. The clearance of drugs that are only moderately bound, on the other hand, is likely to be relatively insensitive to changes in protein binding. As with the flow rate and capacity-limited classifications, many drugs have intermediate protein-binding values and are likely to exhibit moderate sensitivity to changes in protein binding. Some drugs that fall into the flow-limited, capacity-limited binding-sensitive, and capacity-limited binding-insensitive categories are given in Table 2.

While it is intellectually satisfying to classify drugs as in Table 2, the variable nature of liver failure, and also possible extrahepatic involvement, make prediction from such classifications to individual drugs and patient situations extremely tenuous. For example, hepatic blood flow is likely to progressively decrease in moderate and severe cirrhosis but is likely to be unchanged or may even increase in viral hepatitis. Similarly, hepatic cell mass is generally not affected in moderate cirrhosis, is decreased in severe cirrhosis and may be unaffected, increased, or decreased in hepatitis. Intrinsic hepatocyte function, on the other hand, uniformly decreases in severe cirrhosis and in viral and alcoholic hepatitis (BLASCHKE 1977).

1. Distribution Volume

The distribution volume relates the amount of drug in the body to the concentration of drug in plasma or serum. Most distribution volumes described in the literature are "apparent" in that they are calculated based on total (free plus protein-bound) drug rather than drug that is unbound and therefore free to equilibrate between plasma or serum and other body tissues and fluids. The fraction of drug that can penetrate into tissues and ultimately to the site of action, provided this site is outside the cardiovascular system, is sensitive both to plasma protein and tissue binding, and also to body composition, all of which are likely to change in liver disease.

2. Elimination Half-Life

The distribution volume (V) of a drug is related to plasma clearance (Cl_{p}) as in Eq. 15, where k_{el} is the first-order elimination rate constant for a drug that obeys first-order elimination kinetics, and $t_{1/2}$ is the associated elimination half-life.

$$V = \frac{Cl_p}{k_{\text{el}}} = \frac{Cl_{\text{p}} \cdot t_{1/2}}{\ln 2} \tag{15}$$

Equation 15 rearranges to Eq. 16:

$$t_{1/2} = \frac{V \cdot \ln 2}{Cl_{\text{p}}} \tag{16}$$

Table 2. Examples of flow-limited, capacity-limited binding-sensitive, and capacity-limited binding-insensitive drugs (Reproduced with permission from ARNS et al. 1988)

Flow limited	Capacity limited	
	Binding sensitive	Binding insensitive
Acebutolol	Carbamazepine	Adriamycin
Chlormethiazole	Cefoperazone	Aminopyrine
Ketoconazole	Chloramphenicol	Amylobarbital
Labetolol	Chlordiazepoxide	Antipyrine
Lidocaine	Diazepam	Caffeine
Meperidine	Digitoxin	Cyclophosphamide
Metoprolol	Diphenylhydantoin	Hetobarbital
Morphine	Fenprofen	Isoniazid
Pentazocine	Ibuprofen	Phenacetin
Pethidine	Nafcillin	Phenobarbital
Propranolol	Prednisone	Pindolol
Propoxyphene	Tolbutamide	Theophylline
Tricyclic antidepressants	Valproic acid	
Verapamil	Warfarin	

Equation 16 particularly explains the complex relationship between liver function and pharmacokinetics. Reduced intrinsic hepatic clearance is likely to prolong drug half-life. On the other hand, particularly for capacity-limited–protein binding-sensitive drugs, reduced binding in liver disease would tend to increase hepatic extraction efficiency and may reduce the elimination half-life. Reduced binding may also increase the drug distribution volume and hence also the amount of drug that is free to distribute into tissues. This, in turn, will tend to increase the elimination half-life. The importance of considering these different factors when interpreting blood level data has been emphasized by BLASCHKE (1977) in the analysis of two studies. AZZOLLINI et al. (1972) reported increased elimination half-life of chloramphenicol in cirrhosis. However, further analysis of the data showed that clearance of the drug was similar in cirrhotic patients and healthy controls, clearly indicating a change in distribution volume. In a second study, HINTHORN et al. (1976) reported no change in the half-life of clindamycin in cirrhosis, although further analysis showed that clearance of the drug was actually substantially reduced in cirrhosis compared to controls.

3. Protein Binding

The majority of acidic drugs bind specifically to albumin whereas basic drugs tend to bind to both albumin and α_1-acid glycoproteins. While synthesis of albumin is commonly decreased in liver disease, giving rise to possibly increased intrinsic hepatic extraction and also increased distribution volume, many acute conditions affecting the liver give rise to increased synthesis of acute-phase α_1-acid glycoproteins, which would have the opposite effect to that from decreased synthesis of plasma albumin (PIAFSKY et al. 1978; PIAFSKY 1980). Reduced levels of α_1-acid glycoprotein have also been demonstrated in cirrhosis, however, giving rise to increased fractions of free drug (BARRE et al. 1983).

4. Presystemic Clearance

As a consequence of its location in the cardiovascular system, the liver receives blood from the regions of the upper and middle GI tract via the portal system. Any drug absorbed from this region is exposed to the metabolizing enzymes and biliary excretion mechanisms of the liver before reaching the systemic circulation and is liable to undergo first-pass hepatic clearance, or the first-pass effect. Drugs that undergo extensive first-pass metabolism often exhibit low and variable bioavailability. The major cause of frequently observed interindividual differences in kinetics is variability in drug metabolic activity (BREIMER 1983; TAM 1993). Factors influencing interindividual variability in first-pass metabolism include genetic factors, age, and gender, as well as disease states and environmental factors such as diet, smoking, chemical exposure, and concurrent medications. Enzyme saturation may also play a significant role in variable first-pass metabolism. The fraction of an absorbed oral dose that escapes first-pass hepatic clearance has been described by Eq. 17 (WILKINSON 1980).

$$F = 1 - f_{\mathrm{H}}E = \frac{Q + f_{\mathrm{B}}Cl'_{\mathrm{int}}\left(1 - f_{\mathrm{H}}\right)}{Q + f_{\mathrm{B}}Cl'_{\mathrm{int}}} \tag{17}$$

where F is the fraction of the absorbed dose which escapes presystemic elimination, E is the hepatic extraction ratio, and f_{H} is the fraction of mesenteric blood flow passing through the functioning liver. In the case of a high-extraction, flow-limited drug, only a small fraction of absorbed compound will reach the systemic circulation. On the other hand, for a capacity-limited drug with low intrinsic clearance a relatively large fraction will reach the systemic circulation. Regardless of whether a drug is high or low clearance, any reduction in intrinsic clearance will decrease the first-pass effect and the extent of change will likely be greater with increasing initial intrinsic clearance values. The presence of extrahepatic, and possibly also intrahepatic, vascular shunts will also diminish the first-pass effect, resulting in increased oral systemic bioavailability. The phenomenon of increased systemic bioavailability of orally administered drugs in cirrhotic patients has been demonstrated for a number of compounds including meperidine, pentazocine (NEAL et al. 1979), propranolol (WOOD et al. 1978), and chlormethiazole (PENTIKÄINEN et al. 1978).

F. Markers of Liver Disease Relevant to Drug Metabolism and Pharmacokinetics

Consistent with the complex structure and function of the liver, no single diagnostic test has been identified that can be used to adequately characterize liver function and its relationship to drug pharmacokinetics. Among the original diagnostic tests, Pugh's modification of Child's classification has been used extensively in clinical practice (PUGH et al. 1973). As shown in Table 3, this scale uses both clinical and biochemical parameters to generate a single number relating to severity of liver disease.

Table 3. Grading of severity of liver disease (Reproduced with permission from PUGH et al. 1973)

Clinical and biochemical measurement	Points scored for increasing abnormalities		
	1	2	3
Encephalopathy (grade)	None	1 and 2	3 and 4
Bilirubin (μmol/l)	<25	24–40	>40
Albumin (g/l)	35	28–35	<28
Prothrombin time (seconds prolonged)	1–4	4–6	>6

Other diagnostic tests involve monitoring bile pigments, serum bile acids, bilirubin, albumin, α-fetoprotein, ferritin, lipids, ceruloplasmin, ammonia, and the enzymes alkaline phosphatase (ALP), aspartate aminotransferase (AST), alanine aminotransferase (ALT), lactate dehydrogenase, and γ-glutamyltr-ansferase (GGT) (CHOPRA and GRIFFIN 1985).

Other tests have utilized advances in contrast cholangiography, radiology, and nuclear medicine (CHOPRA and GRIFFIN 1985; HATTNER and ENGELSTAD 1983; MAY 1986). Although all of these tests provide information regarding cellular function or intra-, or extrahepatic vascular status, they have not proven to be generally useful in predicting the way in which impaired liver function may affect metabolism or pharmacokinetics of particular drugs in patients. Some studies have demonstrated significant correlations between liver function tests and drug metabolism (BRANCH et al. 1973; ANDREASEN et al. 1974; HEPNER and VESELL 1975) while others have found no relationships (KLOTZ et al. 1974, 1975; THOMSON et al. 1973).

Good correlations were obtained between the elimination rate of amylobarbital (MAWER et al. 1972), procainamide (DUSOUICH and ERILL 1977), and phenylbutazone (WALLACE and BRODIE 1976) and serum albumin levels. Similarly, procainamide (DUSOUICH and ERILL 1977) and antipyrine elimination half-lives varied directly with prothrombin activity, and negative correlations were obtained between clearance of a number of compounds including antipyrine (BURNETT et al. 1976) and clindamycin (AVANT et al. 1975) and serum bilirubin and also between clindamycin clearance and serum glutamic oxalo-acetic transaminase (SGOT) values (AVANT et al. 1975). On the other hand, no correlations were obtained between clearance of diazepam (KLOTZ et al. 1975), chlordiazepoxide (ROBERTS et al. 1978), and meperidine (MCHORSE et al. 1975) with conventional liver function tests. Thus, correlations between conventional liver tests and drug metabolism and pharmacokinetics tend to be unreliable (HOYUMPA and SCHENKER 1982).

The clearance of compounds such as antipyrine, aminopyrine, phenacetin, and caffeine has been examined as indices of drug metabolism capacity. With antipyrine, the rate of metabolism is monitored from disappearance of drug from plasma as a result of multiple metabolic pathways. With aminopyrine, phenacetin, and caffeine, on the other hand, procedures are available to determine metabolism efficiency by measuring exhaled ^{13}C-CO_2 or ^{14}C-CO_2 in breath resulting from metabolic demethylation of administered labeled compound. The use of noninvasive tests as measures of liver function, and their use as predictors of drug metabolism, has been reviewed by VESELL (1984) and GOLDBERG and BROWN (1987).

G. Examples of Effects of Liver Disease on the Pharmacokinetics of Some Drug Therapeutic Classes

For all drug classes, drug must be administered to patients with liver impairment with knowledge of the extent to which hepatic metabolism contributes to systemic clearance and also a knowledge of pharmacodynamic sequelae of impaired liver function.

I. Cardiovascular Agents

Digitoxin is cleared from the body mainly by hepatic metabolism while digoxin is cleared principally unchanged in the urine. Consistent with this, clinical data suggest that digitoxin elimination is impaired in liver failure but that of digoxin is unchanged (STORSTEIN and AMLIE 1975). Substantial reduction is reported in the clearance of lidocaine in chronic liver disease (WILLIAMS et al. 1976) and of *d*-propranolol in cirrhosis (BRANCH et al. 1976). Both of these drugs are highly extracted by the liver so that reduced clearances may be associated with reduction in hepatic blood flow in hepatic disease, although reduced intrinsic clearance may also play a role (PESSAYRE et al. 1978). The free fraction of circulating *d*-propranolol increases in liver cirrhosis (BRANCH et al. 1976a), which may not only partly compensate for decreased intrinsic clearance but may also give rise to increased central nervous system activity for a given systemic total drug concentration in cirrhotic patients. The oral bioavailability of *d*-propranolol, and also pethidine, is increased approximately 40% in cirrhotic patients, compared to normal controls (WOOD et al. 1978). Because of decreased clearance, doses of lidocaine and *d*-propranolol should be reduced in patients with liver impairment. This is important because of the low therapeutic index of lidocaine, on the one hand, and of the exacerbation of the effect of increased circulating propranolol due to the increased free fraction on the other.

Disopyramide clearance is decreased in cirrhosis, leading to a recommendation for dose reduction, and the elimination half-life of procainamide is increased (SECOR and SCHENKER 1987). Quinidine elimination half-life is also increased and protein binding is decreased in cirrhosis, leading to a recommendation that the drug dose should be lowered by 70%, with drug level monitoring, in severe liver disease (POWELL et al. 1982).

Elimination of encainide, lorcainide, and flecainide, all extensively metabolized by the liver, is reduced in liver impairment. While doses of lorcainide and flecainide should be reduced in liver impairment (KLOTZ et al. 1979; MCQUINN et al. 1988), dose adjustment of encainide is probably not necessary because circulating concentrations of the active metabolite are correspondingly lower (QUART et al. 1986). The clearance of mexiletine is markedly reduced in cirrhosis (PENTIKÄINEN 1986).

Among the β-receptor antagonists, propranolol, metoprolol, and labetol undergo extensive hepatic metabolism and their clearance is decreased in cirrhosis (WATSON et al. 1987; REGÅRDH et al. 1981; HOMEIDA et al. 1978). Pindolol and bisoprolol are metabolized in the liver and also the kidneys so that dose adjustment in patients with liver impairment is probably not required (KIRCH et al. 1987; OHNHAUS et al. 1982). Atenolol and sotalol are metabolized predominantly in the kidneys so that dose adjustment for these agents in liver impairment is probably also unnecessary. However, atenolol has been reported to cause renal insufficiency in patients with chronic liver disease (KIRCH et al. 1983).

The calcium channel blocking agents appear to be uniformly affected by liver impairment. Clearance of verapamil (FINUCCI et al. 1988), nifedipine (KLEINBLOESEM et al. 1986), diltiazem (ECHIZEN and EICHELBAUM 1986), nicardipine (RAZAK et al. 1990), nisoldipine (BREIMER et al. 1986), nitrendipine (EICHELBAUM et al. 1988), isradipine (COTTING et al. 1990), amlodipine (ABERNETHY 1989), and felodipine (REGÅDH et al. 1989) is reduced in liver impairment and dose reduction of these drugs is warranted (SIERSEMA and WILSON 1992). The angiotensin-converting enzyme inhibitors, on the other hand, are relatively unaffected by impaired liver function. Only small pharmacokinetic changes with little or no clinical significance have been reported for captropril (DASKALOPOULOS et al. 1987), enalopril (OHNISHI et al. 1989), and lisinopril (HAYES et al. 1989). In cases of ascites, captopril has been claimed to impair rather than promote sodium excretion, thus contraindicating this agent in patients with cirrhosis and ascites (DASKALOPOULOS et al. 1987).

Liver impairment has complex effects on the pharmacokinetics and pharmacodynamics of the loop diuretic furosemide. While the pharmacokinetics of furosemide are not significantly altered in compensated cirrhosis, the circulating free fraction may increase in ascites, leading to toxicity (KELLER et al. 1981). Similarly with high doses of furosemide, reduced natriuretic effect, increased sensitivity to hypokalemia, and increased risk of encephalopathy has been reported (KELLER et al. 1981). Among the other diuretics, clearance of bumetanide (MARCANTONIO et al. 1983) and triamterine (VILLENEUVE et al. 1984) is reduced in cirrhosis, the elimination half-life of amiloride is increased in hepatitis (SPAHN et al. 1987), while spironolactone appears to be relatively unaffected by liver disease at therapeutic levels (ABSHAGEN et al. 1977).

II. Drugs Acting on the Central Nervous System

Among the benzodiazepines, the presence of acute viral hepatitis or cirrhosis reduces drug clearance of diazepam and chlordiazepoxide by approximately 50%. These changes may be accompanied by changes in distribution volume, but are nonetheless associated with increased elimination half-lives (KLOTZ et al. 1977; ROBERTS et al. 1978). The influence of liver impairment on clearance and elimination half-life of lorazepam is variable (KRAUS et al. 1978), while the clearance and half-life of oxazepam is unaffected by either cirrhosis or viral acute hepatitis (SHULL et al. 1976). It is thus recommended that oxazepam be the benzodiazepine of choice in patients with hepatic impairment (WILLIAMS and MAMELOK 1980).

Hepatic impairment may substantially reduce the capacity of the liver to eliminate barbiturates and narcotic analgesics. In patients with compensated or decompensated cirrhosis, or with acute viral hepatitis, the clearance of hexobarbital is reduced by 50% (BREIMER et al. 1975; ZILLY et al. 1978), while pentobarbital half-life was increased moderately in patients with cirrhosis and hepatic neoplasma but was not affected in patients with acute viral hepatitis (SINGH et al. 1977). Clearance of both phenobarbital and amylobarbital is reduced in cirrhosis (ALVIN et al. 1975).

Narcotic analgesics may cause excessive sedation in cirrhosis and may also induce or exacerbate encephalopathy (SIERSEMA and WILSON 1992). Oral bioavailability of pethidine and pentazocine is increased in cirrhosis (POND et al. 1980), while systemic clearance of pethidine is decreased by 50% in acute or chronic hepatic disease (POND et al. 1979; MCHORSE et al. 1975). Both oral and parenteral doses of these agents should be reduced in liver impairment (NEAL et al. 1979). While morphine pharmacokinetics are unchanged in mild liver disease because of extensive extrahepatic metabolism, excessive sedation nonetheless occurs in cirrhosis (MAZOIT et al. 1990). Morphine is inactivated in man primarily by glucuronidation with most of the gluronide being excreted in urine. The drug has a high extraction ratio and undergoes extensive first-pass metabolism after oral doses. In a study in cirrhotic patients, systemic clearance of morphine was unchanged relative to controls, probably due to extrahepatic conjugation or to protected intrahepatic conjugation (PATWARDHAN et al. 1981).

Accumulation of phenytoin levels occurs in patients with cirrhosis and acute viral hepatitis (KUTT et al. 1964). Valproate clearance is decreased and its distribution volume increased in cirrhosis and hepatitis (KLOTZ et al. 1978), while the pharmacokinetics of primidone are unaffected in viral hepatitis (PISANI et al. 1984).

III. Antimicrobial Agents

Studies on the pharmacokinetics of antimicrobial agents have been carried out in only a small number of patients with liver impairment. Many antibiotics are water soluble and are excreted for the most part unchanged in urine. They are thus not susceptible to changes in liver function impairment unless it is associated with secondary changes in renal function. For example, the penicillins ampicillin and carbenicillin require no dose adjustment in liver disease unless there is associated renal impairment (HOFFMAN et al. 1970). On the other hand, the broad-spectrum penicillin, mezlocillin, and probably also azlocillin require dose reduction in cirrhosis (BUNKE et al. 1983).

Many of the first- and second-generation cephalosporins are excreted mainly unchanged in urine and, except in cases of renal involvement secondary to hepatic impairment, can be dosed regardless of hepatic function. Among the third-generation cephalosporins, ceftriaxone (STOECKEL et al. 1984), cefotaxime (HÖFFKEN et al. 1984; VINCENT et al. 1988), and cefoperazone (SAUDEK et al. 1989) elimination involves liver function and clearance of these agents may be reduced in patients with liver disease.

As mentioned earlier in this chapter, although no change was reported in elimination half-life of clindamycin in liver impairment (AZZOLLINI et al. 1972), reanalysis of these data demonstrated substantial alterations in plasma clearance and distribution clearance (BLASCHKE 1977). On the other hand, doubling of the elimination half-life of chloramphenicol in patients with cirrhosis was attributed to altered drug distribution rather than a change in clearance (BLASCHKE 1977). The possibility of hematological toxicity was postulated for patients with cirrhosis with increased chloramphenicol levels due to saturation of iron-binding capacity (SUHRLAND and WEISBERGER 1963).

The macrolide antibiotics erythromycin and roxithromycin do not require dose adjustment in compensated liver disease (HALL et al. 1982; PERITI and MAZZEI 1987), but changes in binding of erythromycin to serum α-1-acid glycoprotein may influence its pharmacokinetics in liver impairment (BARRE et al. 1987). Elimination of the macrolide antibiotic miocamycin is delayed in compensated cirrhosis and dose reduction is recommended (MIGLIOLI et al. 1989). Vancoymcin clearance is reduced and its elimination half-life is prolonged in liver disease (BROWN et al. 1983). A 50% dose reduction is recommended.

The pharmacokinetics of the antituberculosis agents ethambutol, streptomycin, cycloserine (SECOR and SCHENKER 1987), and *p*-aminosalicylic acid (HELD and FRIED 1977) is unaffected by liver disease in the absence of renal involvement. Isoniazid actylation, which is genetically determined as "slow" or "fast," is affected only in cases of severe liver impairment (ACOCELLA et al. 1972).

IV. Other Drugs

The impact of liver disease on drugs in other therapeutic areas is similarly variable and inconsistent. Liver disease diminishes the clearance or prolongs the elimination half-life of antipyrine, paracetamol, theophylline, and heparin (WILLIAMS and MAMELOK 1980). The half-life of theophylline may increase to up to 25 h in hepatic disease (MANGIONE et al. 1978) and careful monitoring of serum theophylline levels is recommended.

Among the antiinflammatory agents, liver disease has been shown to have little effect on conversion of prednisone to the active form prednisolone (SCHALM et al. 1977; RENNER et al. 1986). However, increased side effects have been reported for both prednisolone and prednisone in liver failure and dose reduction is recommended (RENNER et al. 1986). However, dose reduction is not recommended in patients with portosystemic shunts and liver disease (BERGREM et al. 1983). Cyclosporine elimination is delayed in moderate liver impairment (YEE et al. 1984), but its elimination is variable in primary biliary cirrhosis (DE GROEN et al. 1988). Frequent monitoring of cyclosporine blood levels is recommended in patients with liver disease. Tolbutamide metabolism is not altered in acute viral hepatitis. It has been suggested that acute hepatic disease may in fact accelerate elimination of tolbutamide due to reduced protein binding (WILLIAMS et al. 1977). However, in another report the elimination half-life of tolbutamide was doubled in patients with liver cirrhosis

(UEDA et al. 1963). There appear to have been no further reports on the effect of liver disease on the pharmacokinetics of other hypoglycemic agents.

H. Conclusions

The relationships between impaired liver function and pharmacokinetic and pharmacodynamic activity of therapeutic agents are complex. The degree of complexity results from many contributing factors including the unique position of the liver in the cardiovascular system, different types and severity of liver disease, the degree of involvement of hepatic metabolism and/or biliary excretion in drug elimination, the degree of first-pass hepatic clearance of orally administered compounds, the precise way in which a therapeutic agent is metabolized, particularly the relative contributions of phase 1 and phase 2 metabolic pathways, the degree of extrahepatic involvement, and also pharmacodynamic contributions. It is perhaps not surprising that, after so many years of study, construction of sophisticated clearance models, characterization of drugs into those whose metabolism is flow rate or enzyme capacity limited, and also detailed investigation of clearance of particular compounds, it is still extremely difficult to predict the effect of liver impairment on the disposition of a particular drug in a patient or patient population. Too little is known regarding the relative contributions of altered hepatic blood flow due to shunting and reduced intrinsic cellular metabolism activity, and also of the relative contributions of reduced clearance, decreased or increased binding to plasma proteins, and altered distribution volume to permit accurate prediction of pharmacokinetic and pharmacodynamic consequences, together with appropriate dosage regimen changes.

The wealth of information that has been obtained on this topic does nonetheless permit some generalizations. If a drug is cleared from the body by metabolism, then its clearance is likely to be reduced in liver disease and the effect will increase with increasing impairment of liver function. Oral availability of drugs that are subject to high hepatic clearance is likely to be increased in patients with cirrhosis and also in cases of portacaval shunting (NEAL et al. 1979). Similarly the binding of highly protein bound drugs will tend to decrease, which may compensate for reduced clearance, thus modulating any effect on drug elimination half-life. However, increased distribution volume associated with decreased protein binding may have the opposit effect. The presence of ascites, and possibly also encephalopathy, in liver failure further complicates prediction of pharmacokinetic changes and also pharmacokinetic-pharmacodynamic relationships. The use of exogenous substances as markers has to date been only moderately successful in predicting the effect of liver impairment on drug metabolism and pharmacokinetics. However, the high current interest in developing noninvasive tests using probe substrates may improve pharmacokinetic prediction in the future.

The above constraints, and also the compounding problems of drug-drug interactions in severely ill, often ageing, patients demonstrate the difficulties of administering essential drugs to patients with liver disease. It has been pointed out, however, that even in cases of severe liver impairment, changes in drug clearances or elimination half-lives are seldom greater than two- or threefold (WILKINSON 1980). This is in stark contrast to renal failure, which can have profound effects on drug distribution and elimination. However, some individuals with marked liver impairment may exhibit far greater changes than others so that attempts to generalize pharmacokinetic changes in a particular individual are tenuous. Because of the potential impact of liver impairment on the pharmacokinetics of highly metabolized drugs, the use of agents which are cleared predominately by extrahepatic routes is preferred. Drugs which rely on metabolic activation to a pharmacologically active metabolite should be avoided. When these alternatives are not available, careful drug blood level and biochemical monitoring is essential.

Thus, while considerable progress has been made toward understanding the mechanisms and clinical implications of altered drug metabolism and pharmacokinetics in liver impairment, the science has a way to go before accurate pharmacokinetic prediction in a particular patient is feasible. Until this goal is realized, drug treatment for patients with liver impairment has to be adjusted on an individual basis depending on observed pharmacokinetic and clinical outcomes.

References

Abernethy DR (1989) The pharmacokinetic profile of amlodipine. Am Heart J 118 (pt2):1100–1103

Abshagen U, Rennekamp H, Luszpinski G (1977) Disposition kinetics of spironolactone in hepatic failure after single doses and prolonged treatment. Eur J Clin Pharmacol 11:169–176

Acocella G, Bonollo L, Garimoldi M, Mainardi M, Tenconi LT, Nicoli FB (1972) Kinetics of rafampicin and isoniazid administered alone and in combination to normal subjects and in patients with liver disease. Gut 13:47–53

Alvin J, McHorse T, Hoyumpa A, Bush MT, Schenker S (1975) The effect of liver disease in man on the disposition of phenobarbital. J Pharmacol Exp Ther 192:224–235

Andreasen PB, Ranek L, Statland RE, Tygstrup N (1974) Clearance of antipyrine-dependence of quantitative liver function. Eur J Clin Invest 4:129

Arns PA, Wedlund PJ, Branch RA (1988) Adjustment of medications in liver failure. In: Chernow B (ed) The pharmacologic approach to the critically ill patient. Williams and Wilkins, Baltimore, pp 85–111

Avant GR, Schenker S, Alford RH (1975) The effect of cirrhosis on the disposition and elimination of clindamycin. Am J Dig Dis 20:223–229

Azzollini F, Gazzaniga A, Lodola E, Natangelo R (1972) Elimination of chloramphenicol and thiamphenicol in subjects with cirrhosis of the liver. Int J Clin Pharmacol 6:130–134

Barre J, Houin G, Brunner F, Bree F, Tillement J-P (1983) Disease-induced modifications of drug pharmacokinetics. Int J Clin Pharmacol Res 3:215–226

Barre J, Mallat A, Rosenbaum J, Deforges L, Houin G, Dhumeaux D, Tillement J-P (1987) Pharmacokinetics of erythromycin in patients with severe cirrhosis. Re-

spective influence of decreased serum binding and impaired liver metabolic capacity. Br J Clin Pharmacol 23:753–757
Bergrem H, Ritland S, Opedal I, Bergan A (1983) Prednisolone pharmacokinetics and protein binding in patients with portosystemic shunt. Scand J Gastroenterol 18:273–276
Blaschke TF (1977) Protein binding and kinetics of drugs in liver diseases. Clin Pharmacokinet 2:32–44
Branch RA (1982) Drugs as indicators of hepatic function. Hepatology 2:97–105
Branch RA, Shand DG (1976) Propranolol disposition in chronic liver disease: a physiological approach. Clin Pharmacokinet 1:264–279
Branch RA, Herbert CM, Read AF (1973) Determinants of serum antipyrine half-lives in patients with liver disease. Gut 14:569–573
Branch RA, James J, Read AE (1976a) A study of factors influencing drug disposition in chronic liver disease using the model drug (+)-propranolol. Br J Clin Pharmacol 3:243–249
Branch RA, Morgan MH, James J, Read AE (1976b) Intravenous administration of diazepam in patients with chronic liver disease. Gut 17:975–983
Breimer DD (1983) Variability in human drug metabolism and its implications. Int J Clin Pharmacol Res 3:399–413
Breimer DD, Zilly W, Richter E (1975) Pharmacokinetics of hexobarbital in acute hepatitis and after apparent recovery. Clin Pharmacol Ther 18:433–440
Breimer DD, Lodewijks MThM, van Brummelen P, van Harten J, Wilson JHP (1986) Pharmacokinetics and haemodynamic effects of nisoldipine in patients with liver cirrhosis. Br J Pharmacol 89:482P
Brosen K (1990) Recent developments in hepatic drug oxidation. Implications for clinical pharmacokinetics. Clin Pharmacokinet 18:220–239
Brown N, Ho DHW, Fong KL, Bogerd L, Maksymiuk A, Bolivar R, Fainstein V, Bodey GP (1983) Effects of hepatic function on vancomycin clinical pharmacology. Antimicrob Agents Chemother 23:603–609
Bunke CM, Aronoff GR, Brier ME, Sloan RS, Luft FC (1983) Mezlocillin kinetics in hepatic insufficiency. Clin Pharmacol Ther 33:73–76
Burnett DA, Barak AJ, Tuma DJ, Sorrell MF (1976) Altered elimination of antipyrine in patients with acute viral hepatitis. Gut 17:341–344
Butterworth RF, Lovoie J, Giguere JF, Pomier-Layrargues G (1988) Affinities and densities of high affinity [^{3}H]muscimol (GABA-A) binding sites and of central benzodiazepine receptors are unchanged in autopsied brain tissue from cirrhotic patients with hepatic encephalopathy. Hepatology 8:1084–1088
Cello JP, Øie S (1983) Cimetidine disposition in patients with Laennec's cirrhosis during multiple dosing therapy. Eur J Clin Pharmacol 25:223–229
Chopra S, Griffin PH (1985) Laboratory tests and diagnostic procedures in evaluation of liver disease. Am J Med 79:221–230
Cotting J, Reichen J, Kutz K, Laplanche R, Nuesch E (1990) Pharmacokinetics of isradipine in patients with chronic liver disease. Eur J Clin Pharmacol 38:599–603
Daskalopoulos G, Pinzani M, Murray N, Hirschberg R, Zipser RD (1987) Effects of captopril on renal function in patients with cirrhosis and ascites. J Hepatol 4:330–336
DeGroen PC, McCallum DK, Moyer TP, Wiesner RH (1988) Pharmacokinetics of cyclosporine in patients with primary biliary cirrhosis. Transplant Proc 20 [Suppl 2]:509–511
DuSouich P, Erill S (1977) Metabolism of procainamide and p-aminobenzoic acid in patients with chronic liver disease. Clin Pharmacol Ther 22:588–595
Eagle CJ, Strunin L (1990) Drug metabolism in liver disease. Curr Anaesth Crit Care 1:204–212
Echizen H, Eichelbaum M (1986) Clinical pharmacokinetics of verapamil, nifedipine, and diltiazem. Clin Pharmacokinet 11:425–429
Eichelbaum M, Mikus G, Mast V, Fischer C, Kuhlmann U, Machleidt C (1988) Pharmacokinetics and pharmacodynamics of nitrendipine in healthy subjects and pa-

tients with kidney and liver disease. J Cardiovasc Pharmacol 12 [Suppl 4]:S6–S10
Finucci GF, Padrini R, Piovan D, Melica E, Merkel C, Gatta A, Zuin R (1988) Verapamil pharmacokinetics and liver function in patients with cirrhosis. Int J Clin Pharmacol Res 8:123–126
Fowler JM, Schafer DM (1981) A mechanism for the increased sensitivity to benzodiazepines in hepatocellular failure: evidence from an animal model. Gastroenterology 80:1359
Goldberg DM, Brown D (1987) Advances in the application of biochemical tests to diseases of the liver and biliary tract: their role in diagnosis, prognosis, and elucidation of pathogenic mechanisms. Clin Biochem 20:127–148
Gonzalez G, Aransibia A, Rivas MI, Caro P, Antezana C (1982) Pharmacokinetics of frusemide in patients with hepatic cirrhosis. Eur J Clin Pharmacol 22:315–320
Hall KW, Nightingale CH, Gibaldi M, Nelson E, Bates TR, DiSanto AR (1982) Pharmacokinetics of erythromycin in normal and alcoholic liver disease subjects. J Clin Pharmacol 22:321–325
Hathcock JN (1985) Nutrient and non-nutrient effects on drug metabolism. Drug Nutr Interactions 4:217–234
Hattner RS, Engelstad BL (1983) Diagnostic imaging and quantitating physiologic function using radionuclide techniques in gastrointestinal disease. In: Sleisinger MH, Fordtran JS (eds) Gastrointestinal disease: pathophysiology, diagnosis, management, 3rd edn, vol 2. Saunders, Philadelphia, pp 1667–1688
Hayes PC, Plevris JN, Bouchier IA (1989) Pharmacokinetics of enalapril and lisinopril in subjects with normal and impaired hepatic function. J Hum Hypertens 3 [Suppl 1]:153–158
Held H, Fried F (1977) Elimination of para-aminosalicylic acid in patients with liver disease and renal insufficency. Chemotherapy 23:405–415
Hepner GW, Vesell ES (1975) Quantitative assessment of hepatic function by breath analysis after oral administration of [^{14}C]aminopyrine. Ann Intern Med 83:632–638
Hinthorn DR, Baker LH, Romig DA, Hassanein K, Liu C (1976) Use of clindamycin in patients with liver disease. Antimicrob Agents Chemother 9:495–501
Höffken G, Lode H, Koeppe P, Ruhnke M, Borner K (1984) Pharmacokinetics of cefotaxime and desacetyl-cefotaxime in cirrhosis of the liver. Chemotherapy 30:7–17
Hoffman TA, Cestero R, Bullock WE (1970) Pharmacodynamics of carbenicillin in hepatic and renal failure. Ann Intern Med 73:173–178
Homeida A, Jackson L, Roberts CJC (1978) Decreased first-pass metabolism of labetolol in chronic liver disease. Br Med J 2:1048–1050
Horn T, Christoffersen P, Henriksen JH (1987) Alcoholic liver injury: defenestration in noncirrhotic liver – a scanning electron microscope study. Hepatology 7:77–82
Hoyumpa AM, Schenker S (1982) Major drug interactions: effect of liver disease, alcohol and malnutrition. Annu Rev Med 33:113–149
Keller E, Hoppe-Seyler G, Mumm R, Schollmeyer P (1981) Influence of hepatic cirrhosis and end-stage renal disease on pharmacokinetics and pharmacodynamics of furosemide. Eur J Clin Pharmacol 20:27–33
Kirch W, Schäfer-Korting M, Mutschler E, Ohnhaus EE, Braun W (1983) Clinical experience with atenolol in patients with chronic liver disease. J Clin Pharmcol 23:171–177
Kirch W, Rose I, Demers HG, Leopold G, Pabst J, Ohnhaus EE (1987) Pharmacokinetics of bisoprolol during repeated oral administration to healthy volunteers and patients with kidney or liver disease. Clin Pharmacokinet 13:110–117
Kleinbloesem CH, van Harten J, Wilson JHP, Danhof M, van Brummele P, Breimer DD (1986) Nifedipine: kinetics and hemodynamic effects in patients with cirrhosis after intravenous and oral administration. Clin Pharmacol Ther 40:21–28
Klinger EL, Vaamonde CA, Vaamonde LS, Lancestremere RG, Morosi HJ, Frisch E, Papper S (1970) Renal function changes in cirrhosis of the liver. Arch Intern Med 125:1010–1015

Klotz U, Antonin KH, Brugel H, Bieck PR (1977) Disposition of diazepam and its major metabolite desmethyldiazepam in patients with liver disease. Clin Pharmacol Ther 21:430–436

Klotz U, Avant GR, Hoyumpa A, Schenker S, Wilkinson GR (1975) The effects of age and liver disease on the disposition and elimination of diazepam in adult man. J Clin Invest 55:347–359

Klotz U, Fischer C, Müller-Seydlitz P, Schulz J, Müller WA (1979) Alterations in the disposition of differently cleared drugs in patients with cirrhosis. Clin Pharmacol Ther 26:221–227

Klotz U, McHorse TS, Wilkinson GR (1974) The effect of cirrhosis on the disposition and elimination of meperidine (pethidine) in man. Clin Pharmacol Ther 16:667–675

Klotz U, Rapp T, Müller WA (1978) Disposition of valproic acid in patients with liver disease. Eur J Clin Pharmacol 13:55–60

Kraus JW, Desmond PV, Marshall JP, Johnson RF, Schenker S, Wilkinson GR (1978) Effects of aging and liver disease on disposition of lorazepam. Clin Pharmacol Ther 24:411–419

Kutt H, Winters W, Scherman R, McDowell F (1964) Diphenylhydantoin and phenobarbital toxicity. Arch Neurol 11:649–656

Lee BL, Wong D, Benowitz NL, Sullam PM (1993) Altered patterns of drug metabolism in patients with acquired immunodeficiency syndrome. Clin Pharmacol Ther 53:529–535

Lewis JH, Zimmerman HJ (1989) Drug-induced liver disease. Med Clin N Am 73:775–792

Maddison JE, Dodd PR, Morrison M, Johnston GA, Farrell GC (1987) Plasma GABA, GABA-like activity and the brain GABA-benzodiazepine receptor complex in rats with chronic hepatic encephalopathy. Hepatology 7:621–628

Mangioni A, Imhoff TE, Lee RV, Shum LY, Jusko WJ (1978) Pharmacokinetics of theophylline in hepatic disease. Chest 73:616–622

Marcantonio LA, Auld WHR, Murdoch WR, Purohit R, Skellern GG, Howes CA (1983) The pharmacokinetics and pharmacodynamics of the diuretic bumetanide in hepatic and renal disease. Br J Clin Pharmacol 25:245–252

Mawer GE, Miller NE, Turnberg LA (1972) Metabolism of amylobarbitone in patients with chronic liver disease. Br J Pharmacol 4:549–560

May GR (1986) Hepatobiliary imaging. In: Gitnick G (ed) Current hepatology. Year Book Medical Publishers, Chicago, pp 361–379

Mazoit JX, Sandouk P, Scherrmann J-M, Roche A (1990) Extrahepatic metabolism of morphine occurs in humans. Clin Pharmacol Ther 48:613–618

McConnell JB, Curry SH, Davies M, Williams R (1982) Clinical effects and metabolism of diazepam in patients with chronic liver disease. Clin Sci 63:75–80

McHorse TS, Wilkinson GR, Johnson RF, Schenker S (1975) Effect of acute viral hepatitis in man on the disposition and elimination of meperidine. Gastroenterology 68:775–780

McLean AJ, Morgan DJ (1991) Clinical pharmacokinetics in patients with liver disease. Clin Pharmacokinet 21:42–69

McQuinn RL, Pentikäinen PJ, Chang SF, Conrad GJ (1988) Pharmacokinetics of flecainide in patients with cirrhosis of the liver. Clin Pharmacol Ther 44:566–572

Miglioli PA, Pivetta P, Orlando R, Palatini P, Varotto A, Okolicsanyi L (1989) Pharmacokinetics in patients with liver cirrhosis. Chemotherapy 35:330–332

Mooney H, Roberts R, Cooksley WGE, Halliday JW, Powell LW (1985) Alterations in the liver with ageing. Clin Gastroenterol 14:757–771

Murray M (1992) P450 enzymes: inhibition mechanisms, genetic regulation and effects of liver disease. Clin Pharmacokinet 23:132–146

Murray M, Zaluzny L, Farrell GC (1986) Drug metabolism in cirrhosis. Selective changes in cytochrome P450 isozymes in the choline-deficient rat model. Biochem Pharmacol 35:1817–1824

Neal EA, Meffin PJ, Gregory PB, Blascke TF (1979) Enhanced bioavailability and decreased clearance of analgesics in patients with cirrhosis. Gastroenterology 77:96–102
Ohnhaus EE, Münch U, Meier J (1982) Elimination of pindolol in liver disease. Eur J Clin Pharmacol 22:247–251
Ohnishi A, Tsuboi Y, Ishizaki T, Kubota K, Ohno T, Yoshida H, Kanezaki A, Tanaka T (1989) Kinetics and dynamics of enalapril in patients with liver cirrhosis. Clin Pharmacol Ther 45:657–665
O'Mahony MS, Woodhouse KW (1994) Age, environmental factors and drug metabolism. Pharmacol Ther 61:279–287
Patwardhan R, Johnson R, Sheehan J, Desmond P, Wilkinson G, Hoyumpa A, Branch R, Schenker S (1981) Morphine metabolism in cirrhosis. Gastroenterology 8:1344
Pentikäinen PJ, Hietakorpi S, Hainen MO, Lampinen LM (1986) Cirrhosis of the liver markedly impairs the elimination of mexiletine. Eur J Clin Pharmacol 30:83–88
Pentikäinen PJ, Neuvonen PJ, Tarpila S, Syvälahti E (1978) Effect of cirrhosis of the liver on the pharmacokinetics of chlormethiazole. Br J Med 2:861–863
Periti P, Mazzei T (1987) Pharmacokinetics of roxithromycin in renal and hepatic failure and drug interactions. J Antimicrob Chemother 20 [Suppl B]:107–112
Pessayre D, Lebrec D, Descatoire V, Peignoux M, Benhamou JP (1978) Mechanism for reduced drug clearance in patients with cirrhosis. Gastroenterology 74:566–571
Piafsky KM (1980) Disease-induced changes in the plasma binding of basic drugs. Clin pharmacokinet 5:246–262
Piafsky KM, Borga O, Odar-Cederlof I, Johansson C, Sjoqvist F (1978) Increased plasma protein binding of propranolol and chlorpromazine mediated by disease-induced elevations of plasma α_1-acid glycoprotein. N Engl J Med 299:1435–1439
Pisani F, Perucca E, Primerano G, D'Agostino AA, Petrelli RM, Fazio A, Oteri G, Di Perri R (1984) Single-dose kinetics of primidone in acute viral hepatitis. Eur J Clin Pharmacol 27:4165–4169
Pond SM, Tong T, Benowitz NL, Jacob P (1979) Bioavailability and clearance of meperidine in patients with chronic liver disease. Clin Pharmacol Ther 25:242
Pond SM, Tong T, Benowitz NL, Jacob P (1980) Enchanced bioiavailability of pethidine and pentozocine in patients with cirrhosis of the liver. Aust NZJ Med 10:515–519
Powell JR, Okada R, Conrad KA, Guentert TW, Riegelman S (1982) Altered quinidine disposition in a patient with chronic active hepatitis. Postgrad Med J 58:82–84
Pugh RNH, Murray-Lyon JM, Dawson JL, Pietroni MC, Williams R (1973) Transection of the oesophagus for bleeding oesophageal varices. Br J Surg 60:646–649
Quart BD, Gallo DG, Sami MH, Wood AJJ (1986) Drug interaction studies and encainide use in renal and hepatic impairment. Am J Cardiol 58:104c–113c
Razak TA, McNeil JJ, Sewell RB, Drummer OH, Smallwood RA, Conway EL, Lewis WJ (1990) The effect of hepatic cirrhosis on the pharmacokinetics and blood pressure response to nicardipine. Clin Pharmacol Ther 47:463–469
Regårdh CG, Edgar B, Olsson R, Kendall M, Collste P, Shansky C (1989) Pharmacokinetics of felodipine in patients with liver disease. Eur J Clin Pharmacol 36:473–479
Regårdh CG, Jordö L, Ervik M, Lundborg R, Olsson R, Rönn O (1981) Pharmacokinetics of metoprolol in patients with hepatic cirrhosis. Clin Pharmacokinet 6:375–388
Renner E, Horber FF, Jost G, Frey BM, Frey FJ (1986) Effect of liver function on the metabolism of prednisone and prednisolone in humans. Gastroenterology 90:819–828
Roberts RK, Wilkinson GR, Branch RA, Schenker S (1978) Effect of age and parenchymal liver disease on the disposition and elimination of chlordiazepoxide (librium). Gastroenterology 75:479–485
Rowland M, Tozer TN (1989) Clinical pharmacokinetics: concepts and applications. Lea and Febiger, Philadelphia, pp 189–190

Saudek F, Moravek J, Modr Z (1989) Cefoperozone pharmacokinetics in patients with liver cirrhosis, a predictive value of the ujoviridin test. Int J Clin Pharmacol Ther Toxicol 27:82–87

Schafer DF, Fowler JM, Munson PJ, Thakur AK, Waggoner JG, Jones EA (1983) Gamma-aminobutyric acid and benzodiazepine receptors in an animal model of fulminant hepatic failure. J Lab Clin Med 102:870–880

Schalm SW, Summerskill WHJ, Go VLW (1977) Prednisone for chronic active liver disease: pharmacokinetics including conversion to prednisolone. Gastroenterology 72:910–913

Schentag JJ, Cerra FB, Calleri GM, Rose JQ, Leising ME, French MA, Bernhard H (1981) Age, disease and cimetidine disposition in healthy subjects and chronically ill patients. Clin Pharmacol Ther 29:737–743

Secor JW, Schenker S (1987) Drug metabolism in patients with liver disease. Adv Intern Med 32:379–406

Shear L, Kleinerman J, Gabuzda GJ (1965) Renal failure in patients with cirrhosis of the liver. Am J Med 39:184–198

Shull HJ, Wilkinson GR, Johnson R, Schenker S (1976) Normal disposition of oxazepam in acute viral hepatitis and cirrhosis. Ann Intern Med 84:420–425

Siersema PD, Wilson JHP (1992) The effect of liver disease on drug metabolism. Eur J Intern Med 3:197–212

Singh D, Vijayvargiya, Kakrani AL (1977) Activity and inducibility of hepatic microsomal enzymes in liver diseases. Indian J Med Res 66:832–839

Smith IL, Ziemniak JA, Bernhard H, Eshelman FN, Martin LE, Schentag JJ (1984) Ranitidine disposition and systemic availability in hepatic cirrhosis. Clin Pharmacol Ther 35:487–494

Sotaniemi EA, Niemelä O, Risteli L, Stenbäck F, Pelkonen RO, Lahtela JT, Risteli J (1986) Fibrotic process and drug metabolism in alcoholic liver disease. Clin Pharmacol Ther 40:46–55

Spahn H, Reuter K, Mutschler E, Gerok W, Knauf H (1987) Pharmacokinetics of amiloride in renal and hepatic disease. Eur J Clin Pharmacol 33:493–498

Stoeckel K, Tuerk H, Trueb V, McNamara PJ (1984) Single-dose ceftriaxone kinetics in liver insufficiency. Clin Pharmacol Ther 36:500–509

Storstein L, Amlie J (1975) Digitoxin pharmacokinetics in chronic active hepatitis. Digestion 12:353

Suhrland LG, Weisberger AS (1963) Chloramphenicol toxicity in liver and renal disease. Arch Intern Med 112:161–168

Tam YK (1993) Individual variation in first-pass metabolism. Clin Pharmacokinet 25:300–328

Thomson PD, Melmon KL, Richardson JA, Cohn K, Steinbrunn W, Cudihee R, Rowland M (1973) Lidocaine pharmacokinetics in advanced heart failure, liver disease, and renal failure in humans. Ann Intern Med 78:99–508

Ueda H, Sakurai T, Ota M, Nakajima A, Kamii K, Maezawa H (1963) Disappearance rate of tolbutamide in normal subjects and in diabetes mellitus, liver cirrhosis, and renal disease. Diabetes 12:414–419

Vesell ES (1984) Noninvasive assessment in vivo of hepatic drug metabolism in health and disease. Ann NY Acad Sci 428:293–307

Villeneuve JP, Rocheleau F, Raymond G (1984) Triamterine kinetics and dynamics in cirrhosis. Clin Pharmacol Ther 35:831–837

Vincent P, Colombel JF, Husson MO, Izard D, Paris JC, Leclerc H (1988) Pharmacokinetics of cefotoxime in cirrhotic pateints with or without ascites. Presse Med 17:2331–2334

Wallace S, Brodie MJ (1976) Decreased drug binding in serum from patients with chronic hepatic disease. Eur J Clin Pharmacol 9:429–432

Watson RGP, Bastain W, Larkin KA, Hayes JR, McAinsh JA, Shanks RG (1987) A comparative pharmacokinetic study of conventional propranolol and long acting preparation of propranolol in patients with cirrhosis and normal controls. Br J Clin Pharmacol 24:527–535

Welling PG (1986) Pharmacokinetics: processes and mathematics ACS monograph 185, American Chemical Society, Washington DC, pp a: 141, b: 142, c: 164, d: 166, e: 196, f: 258, g: 264
Welling PG (1993) Pharmacokinetic principles: linear and nonlinear. In: Welling PG, de la Iglesia FA (eds) Drug toxicokinetics. Marcel Dekker, New York, pp 19–41
Wilkinson GR (1980) Influence of liver disease on pharmacokinetics. In: Evans WE, Schentag JJ, Jusko WJ (eds) Applied pharmacokinetics, principles of therapeutic drug monitoring. Applied Therapeutics, San Francisco, pp 57–75
Williams RL, Blaschke TF, Meffin PJ, Melmon KI, Rowland MR (1976) Influence of viral hepatitis on the disposition of two compounds with high hepatic clearance: lidocaine and idocyamine green. Clin Pharmacol Ther 200:290–299
Williams RL, Blaschke TF, Meffin PJ, Melmon KL, Rowland M (1977) Influence of acute viral hepatitis on disposition and plasma binding of tolbutamide. Clin Pharmacol Ther 21:301–309
Williams RL, Mamelok RD (1980) Hepatic disease and drug pharmacokinetics. Clin Pharmacokinet 5:528–547
Wood AJJ, Kornhauser DM, Wilkinson GR, Shand DG, Branch RA (1978) The influence of cirrhosis on steady-state blood concentrations of unbound propranolol after oral administration. Clin Pharmacokin 3:478–487
Woodhouse KW (1985) Drugs and the ageing gut, liver and pancreas. Clin Gastroenterol 14:863–881
Yee GC, Kennedy MS, Storb R, Thomas ED (1984) Effect of hepatic dysfunction on oral cyclosporine pharmacokinetics in marrow transplant patients. Blood 64:1277–1279
Zeneroli ML (1985) Hepatic encephalopathy. Experimental studies in a rat model of fulminant hepatic failure. J Hepatol 1:301–312
Zilly W, Breimer DD, Richter E (1978) Hexobarbital disposition in compensated and decompensated cirrhosis of the liver. Clin Pharmacol Ther 23:525–534

CHAPTER 17

Liver Reactions to Tacrine

T.F. WOOLF, W.F. POOL, R.M. WALKER, and D.K. MONTEITH

A. Introduction

Alzheimer's disease (AD) is a clinically debilitating dementia associated with various stages of memory dysfunction leading ultimately over a period of years to death. Extensive research is ongoing to determine the underlying etiology of the disease process as well as potential biochemical markers (AMADUCCI et al. 1993; WISNIEWSKI et al. 1993). Commonly associated with a decline in cognitive function is a decrease in central cholinergic transmission (DE SOUZA 1993). This cholinergic deficit theory has led to several approaches for treating the symptoms of AD involving acetylcholine esterase (AChE) inhibitors or muscarinic agonists. In the early to mid-1980s, SUMMERS and colleagues (1981, 1986, 1989) experimented with the use of the tetrahydroacridine derivative tacrine (1,2,3,4-tetrahydro-9-acridinamine monohydrochloride monohydrate, THA, Cognex) for the treatment of AD. After extensive clinical trials, tacrine administration was shown to produce statistically significant improvements in several measures of cognitive function (FARLOW et al. 1992; KNAPP et al. 1994). As a result of these clinical trials, tacrine has been approved by the United States Food and Drug Administration for the treatment of mild to moderate AD. Side effects commonly associated with tacrine treatment are cholinergic in nature involving gastrointestinal discomfort (KNAPP et al. 1994). Of more concern was the relatively high incidence (up to 50% of patients treated) of asymptomatic elevations in serum alanine aminotransferase (ALT) activity (KNAPP et al. 1994; NYBACK et al. 1993; O'BRIEN et al. 1991; ROBERTS et al. 1990; WATKINS et al. 1994).

The aim of this chapter is to present metabolic and toxicological studies encompassing animal, whole organ, cellular, subcellular, and chemical approaches designed to understand the underlying mechanism(s) responsible for tacrine-induced hepatotoxicity.

B. Clinical Experience

An adverse effect of tacrine in AD patients has been asymptomatic elevations in serum ALT activity (KNAPP et al. 1994; NYBACK et al. 1993; O'BRIEN et al. 1991; ROBERTS et al. 1990; WATKINS et al. 1994). WATKINS et al. (1994) recently summarized data obtained from 2446 patients treated with tacrine in clinical trials. Approximately 50% of patients developed serum ALT elevations greater than the upper limit of normal, while approximately half of those patients, or 25% of the total study population, developed greater than three times of the upper limit of normal.

Tacrine-induced elevations in serum ALT are not clearly dose related and are characteristically delayed in onset to between 4 and 8 weeks, in most patients, after initiation of treatment (Watkins et al. 1994). Serum aspartate aminotransferase activity was also elevated; although the magnitude of this elevation was generally less than that for ALT. Further, the increases in ALT were not accompanied by increases in alkaline phosphatase activity or bilirubin levels. Following cessation or reduction of tacrine administration, serum ALT activities return to a normal range. Interestingly, a greater incidence of ALT elevations has been observed in women than men. Age, body weight, and creatinine clearance did not seem to affect the incidence. Although smokers tend to have lower tacrine concentrations in plasma, smoking and alcohol history appeared not to significantly alter the incidence. A prospective study examining the effect of cigarette smoking on ALT elevations has not been conducted to clearly address the risk potential.

In most instances, patients with previous ALT elevations have been successfully readministered tacrine and most are titrated to higher doses without ALT elevations (Knapp et al. 1994; Watkins et al. 1994). Where readministration of tacrine did elicit a threefold or higher increase in serum ALT levels (approximately 25% of patients that restarted therapy), the increase occurred more rapidly with a mean of 22 days, as opposed to a mean of 48 days for initial exposure (Knapp et al. 1994; Watkins et al. 1994). However, the response is not exaggerated and ALT elevations were frequently lower than those which occurred initially.

A report by Ford et al. (1993) suggests that a correlation may exist with ALT elevations and tacrine or tacrine to metabolite (1-hydroxytacrine) plasma ratios. These findings are not definitive as 1-hydroxytacrine (velnacrine) administration is also known to produce ALT elevations (Schneider 1993; Murphy et al. 1991; Cutler et al. 1990a).

A limited number of liver biopsies have been reported in patients undergoing tacrine therapy (Roberts et al. 1990; Watkins et al. 1994). In one study (Roberts et al. 1990), four patients with abnormal ALT levels underwent liver biopsy. One patient had granulomatous hepatitis. Three patients had hepatocellular necrosis and mild fatty changes, primarily in the centrilobular region. One of these patients also had peripheral and hepatic eosinophilia. A second report of liver biopsies from a clinical study conducted in France (Watkins et al. 1994) includes two patients with hepatotoxicity attributed to treatment with tacrine. These pathologic findings were described as "lobular hepatitis" and included one patient with "focally confluent perivenular cell loss."

The extensive metabolism of tacrine and the potential for tacrine to form chemically reactive metabolite(s), as described later, suggested a relationship may exist between ALT elevations and ability to detoxify tacrine-derived reactive metabolite(s) (OESCH 1987; PARK et al. 1993). Glutathione-*S*-transferase μ (GSTμ), a detoxication enzyme (OESCH 1987), is polymorphically expressed in humans, with approximately 50% of the general population lacking the enzyme (LAFUENTE et al. 1993; HAEFELI et al. 1993). In a study conducted by PARK and colleagues (GREEN et al. 1995), polymerase chain reaction (PCR) methodology was used to assess GSTμ genotype status in 79 AD patients maintained on tacrine therapy. This study failed to demonstrate an association between GSTμ status and incidence of ALT elevations.

FONTANA et al. (1995) found a marked correlation between tacrine plasma concentrations and ability to metabolize caffeine, a marker substrate used to assess cytochrome P4501A2 (CYP1A2) activity (KALOW and TANG 1991, 1993). Phenotyping of individuals was performed prior to the study. However, no clear association was found with either the incidence or magnitude of ALT elevations. Thus, the delay in onset, lack of dose response, and low incidence of ALT elevations upon rechallenge are consistent with multiple mechanisms for tacrine-induced hepatotoxicity including an immune-mediated toxicity, metabolic idiosyncrasy, or direct toxicity.

C. Metabolism of Tacrine in Humans

Initial efforts to characterize metabolic fate of tacrine in humans were made in the early 1960s by KAUL (1962) with limited success. Originally the human metabolite, 1-hydroxytacrine, was discovered (EKMAN et al. 1989; HAUGHEY et al. 1994; HOOPER et al. 1994). However, more recently, the human disposition of tacrine has identified several additional mono- and dihydroxylated metabolites as well as at least two phenol glucuronides (Fig. 1) using carbon-14 radiolabeled substrate (POOL et al. 1992b). Quantitatively, no single urinary metabolite was found to account for more than 10% of the administered dose. Results from this study failed to show evidence for any potentially toxic N-acetylated or N-hydroxylated products as might be expected based on tacrine's heterocyclic aromatic amine structure (BUDINSKY et al. 1987; SIM et al. 1992; ORZECHOWSKI et al. 1992; HEIN et al. 1993).

The primary enzyme involved in human tacrine metabolism is CYP1A2 (MADDEN et al. 1993, 1994; SPALDIN et al. 1994; WOOLF et al. 1993a,b). This enzyme is known to be inducible by cigarette smoking (KALOW and TANG 1991; WANWIMOLRUK et al. 1993) and clearly smoking enhances tacrine metabolic clearance (WELTY et al. 1993). Several investigators have reported large intersubject variability in expression of CYP1A2 (BUTLER et al. 1992; KADLUBAR 1994). Recently, levels of this P450 were shown to differ between females and males, with females having markedly lower activities (RELLING et al. 1992). Ethnic differences have also been noted (RELLING et al. 1992). Higher CYP1A2 levels in the male population, however, do not appear to correlate with the higher incidence of ALT elevations which is found in

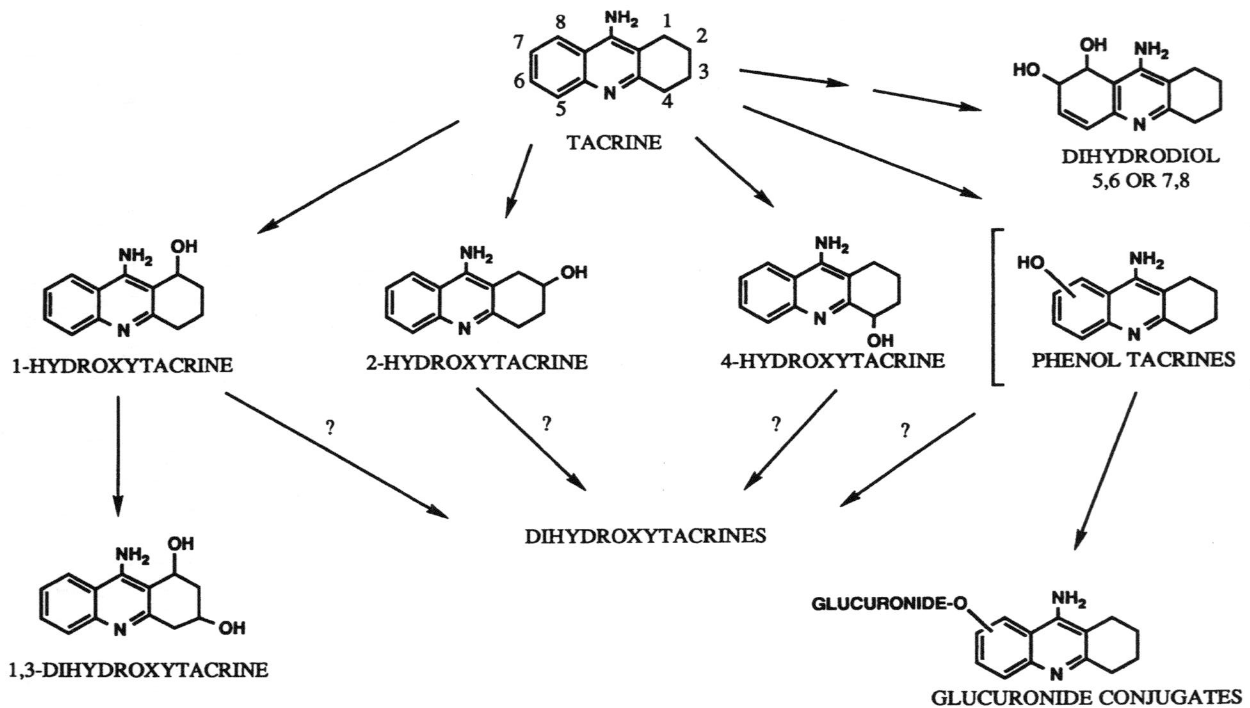

Fig. 1. Tacrine metabolic profile

females on tacrine therapy. Potential explanations include age effects and gender differences in detoxification enzymes.

D. Preclinical Toxicology

Preclinical safety evaluation studies of tacrine were conducted at doses of 0, 5, 10, 20, and 40 mg/kg per day for 4 weeks and 0, 5, 15, and 30 mg/kg per day for 26 and 52 weeks in Wistar rats and at 0, 3, 6, and 10 mg/kg per day for 4 weeks and 0, 1.5, 3, and 6 mg/kg per day for 26 and 52 weeks in beagle dogs. Tacrine was administered in the diet to groups of 15 or 25 rats/sex per dose level in the 4- or 26- and 52-week-long studies, respectively, and given in gelatin capsules to groups of three or four dogs/sex per dose level in the 4- or 26- and 52-week-long studies, respectively. There was no clear evidence of tacrine-induced hepatic injury as determined from the absence of increases in aminotransferase activities and changes in other clinical laboratory determinations as well as from the lack of histopathologic findings (WALKER et al. 1989). Clinical laboratory analyses were conducted every 3 months in the chronic dog studies and at termination in the rat studies. Occasional mild elevations in alanine and aspartate aminotransferase activities in individual control and treated animals were considered incidental or secondary to poor clinical condition, were not accompanied by histopathologic changes, and were therefore not considered a manifestation of primary tacrine-induced hepatotoxicity. Hepatocellular eosinophilia, correlating with glycogen depletion, was seen at all dose levels in the 52-week-long study in dogs. However, there were no additional hepatic degenerative or other inflammatory changes or elevations in aminotransferase activities, and hepatocellular eosinophilia was not observed in the previous 4- and 26-week-long studies in dogs. In the 52-week study in rats, mean plasma tacrine concentrations were highest at the end of the study, compared to earlier times (weeks 6 and 26), reaching approximately 1000 and 500 ng/ml in males and females, respectively, at the 30-mg/kg dose level. In the 52-week study in dogs, mean plasma tacrine concentrations at 2 h postdose were higher during the latter half of the study than after 13 weeks of dosing and ranged from approximately 120–200 ng/ml in males, and approximately 250–400 ng/ml in females at the high dose level (6 mg/kg). In comparison, tacrine concentrations in humans are much lower (CUTLER et al. 1990b). The mean C_{max} after nine doses of 10–30 mg given every 6 h ranged from 5.1 to 33.9 ng/ml in Alzheimer's patients.

In a chronic study in C57BL/6Nnia mice, tacrine was given in the drinking fluid, containing 0.02% sodium saccharin and 0.0015% methylsalicylate in distilled water, at resulting doses of 41.3 and 28.8 mg/kg per day after 4 and 6 months, respectively (FITTEN et al. 1987). There were up to 65% increases in ornithine carbamoyltransferase activity in the tacrine-treated groups compared to the vehicle controls; however, their significance is uncertain. While ornithine carbamoyl transferase is considered a relatively specific marker for hepatic toxicity (Zimmerman 1978), the changes were of small magnitude, and there were no accompanying aminotransferase determinations or histopathologic changes in the liver.

Single-dose studies in which tacrine was given by gavage (30 mg/kg) in an aqueous vehicle containing 0.5% methylcellulose were conducted in rodents (Walker et al. 1989, 1994, unpublished). In the initial study in 12-week-old male and female Wistar rats, mild to moderate elevations in ALT (three to five times controls) and aspartate aminotransferase (six to ten times controls) activities were measured at approximately 30 h postdose. Other clinical biochemistry measurements, including ornithine carbamoyltransferase, alkaline phosphatase, γ-glutamyltransferase, and creatine kinase, were unaffected. Light and electron microscopic evaluation of the livers showed increased periportal and midzonal hepatocellular fat in the tacrine-treated animals compared to controls, but no evidence of overt hepatic injury. Similar potential hepatic changes could not be elicited in 6-week-old Wistar rats or in B6C3F1 mice given the same 30-mg/kg dose level.

Modulation of the potential hepatic effects of a 30-mg/kg dose of tacrine in 6-month-old female Wistar rats was studied by inducing hepatic microsomal cytochrome P450 with phenobarbital, inhibiting hepatic microsomal cytochrome P450 with piperonyl butoxide, and depleting hepatic glutathione stores with diethyl maleate (Walker et al. 1994). Phenobarbital was given orally at a dose of 75 mg/kg per day for 4 days and tacrine administered 24 h after the last phenobarbital dose. Piperonyl butoxide and diethyl maleate were given intraperitoneally, at doses of 400 and 800 mg/kg, respectively, 30 min before tacrine administration. All animals were put to death approximately 24 h after tacrine dosing. Mortality, cholinergic clinical signs, and hepatic effects consisting of mild to moderate elevations in aminotransferase activities, similar to those seen in the initial acute hepatotoxicity study, and increased hepatocellular fat content occurred in animals given tacrine without pretreatment, compared to controls. The clinical indicators and potential hepatic effects of tacrine were generally reduced in phenobarbital-pretreated animals, but remained unaltered after piperonyl butoxide pretreatment. The mechanism by which phenobarbital confers protection is unknown since tacrine metabolism appears to be mediated mainly by CYP1A2. In contrast to the initial hepatotoxicity study, creatine kinase activity was elevated in untreated and pretreated groups given tacrine suggestive of cholinergic effects (particularly tremors). To what extent the clinical condition of the animals might be responsible for the aminotransferase elevations is not known, although aminotransferase elevations occurred without increases in creatine kinase activity in the initial tacrine hepatotoxicity study. Tacrine had no effect on the amount of hepatic microsomal cytochrome P450 as determined by carbon monoxide binding or mixed function oxidase activity as determined by aminopyrine *N*-demethylase and aniline hydroxylase in untreated or phenobarbital-pretreated animals. However, tacrine did appear to block the mild induction elicited by piperonyl butoxide 24 h post dose, which presumably occurs subsequent to the initial and intended inhibition of mixed function oxidase activity. Pretreatment with diethyl maleate did not exacerbate the effects of tacrine; however, the high mortality in this group limits interpretation. Consistent with previous studies, no overt light or electron microscopic evidence of tacrine-induced hepatocellular damage was observed.

Attempts to elicit an animal model for hepatotoxicity by increasing the tolerance of rats to higher acute doses of tacrine using atropine pretreatment/posttreatment regimens were not successful, due, at least in part, to aminotransferase elevations caused by atropine itself (WALKER et al. 1994).

In summary, tacrine may elicit hepatic effects in vivo, particularly in acute studies in rats, aminotransferase elevations are of small magnitude, and in the absence of overt microscopic evidence of degeneration, necrosis, or inflammation, are probably not, by themselves, indicative of significant toxicity. There was no clear evidence of hepatotoxicity in the repeated dose toxicity studies in mice, rats, or dogs.

E. Metabolism of Tacrine in Animals

The metabolic fate of tacrine was investigated in rat and dog (HSU et al. 1990a,b, 1991). Major metabolites identified were the 1-hydroxy and 2-hydroxy derivatives with lesser amounts of 4-hydroxytacrine. More recently, several additional hydroxylated metabolites of tacrine have been found that have similar chromatographic retention properties to those observed in human disposition studies (POOL et al. 1991, 1992c; MCNALLY et al. 1993). Nevertheless, major quantitative differences are apparent between rat, dog, and man, with rat and dog primarily excreting 1-hydroxytacrine in urine (Fig. 1). In an ancillary study, rats were pretreated with 3-methylcholanthrene (3-MC), a known inducer of both CYP1A1 and CYP1A2 (IWATA et al. 1993; ORZECHOWSKI et al. 1994). A marked effect was observed on the route of tacrine-derived radioactivity excretion as well as on the metabolic profile with enhanced levels of polar metabolites (POOL et al. 1992a).

The potential for irreversible binding of tacrine-derived radioactivity in vivo was assessed in both noninduced and 3-MC-pretreated rats. Autoradiographic results showed that, 96 h postdose, retention of tacrine-derived radioactivity in the liver was markedly increased in 3-MC-pretreated animals (unpublished data). Livers from a separate set of 3-MC-pretreated animals given tacrine were removed and homogenized prior to subcellular fractionation. Extraction of protein in the cytosolic and microsomal fractions showed higher total amounts of tacrine-derived binding in 3-MC-treated animals compared to control animals. In both control and 3-MC-treated animals, a larger fraction of bound tacrine-derived radioactivity was found in the cytosol. Thus, in vivo, tacrine is metabolically activated to species capable of irreversible binding to microsomal and cytosolic protein.

F. Cytotoxicity Studies

Determining the mechanism of tacrine-induced hepatotoxicity is difficult due to the lack of an animal model with clearly defined liver injury and histological lesions. Several in vitro studies have been published that investigate the mechanism of tacrine-induced hepatotoxicity using isolated hepatocytes and other cell systems (LOCKWOOD et al. 1988; MONTEITH and THEISS 1993; WALKER et al. 1989; MADDEN et al. 1993). Overt cytotoxicity in cultured hepatocytes occurs at relatively high tacrine concentrations [25 μg/ml (100 μM) for 24 h] when compared to circulating plasma concentrations in humans (up to approximately 40 ng/ml). Autoradiography studies in rats indicate approximately six- to tenfold higher total tacrine-derived radioequivalents in liver tissue than in blood (MCNALLY et al. 1989). Thus, tissue or cell concentrations of tacrine may be higher than plasma; however, the magnitude of the difference in the actual tacrine concentrations between plasma and liver can not be ascertained and can only be speculated upon. In the absence of other suitable models, the isolated hepatocyte is a reasonable model to study the toxicity of tacrine because it maintains metabolic and differentiated function in culture and historically has been used to demonstrate mechanisms of hepatocellular metabolism and toxicity (ACOSTA et al. 1987; BERRY 1988).

Specific cellular targets of toxicity have been investigated using suspension cultures of rat hepatocytes and monolayer cultures of rat and human hepatocytes and electron microscopic examination. Electron microscopic findings evident in endoplasmic reticulum, ribosomes, and mitochondria were demonstrated in monolayer cultures of rat and human hepatocytes (MONTEITH et al. 1995a). In addition, FARISS et al. (1994) demonstrated aggregation of ribosomes and ribosomal dysfunction and inhibition of protein synthesis in suspension cultures of rat hepatocytes. Decreased mitochondrial membrane potential and increased lysosomal/endosomal staining have been demonstrated using fluorescent microscopy and rhodamine-123 and fluoroescein isothiocyanate (FITC)-dextran, respectively (MONTEITH et al. 1995a). These studies identified cellular lesions at concentrations between 0.5 and 1.5 mM (125–375 μg/ml), substantially greater than circulating plasma drug concentrations; however, these high concentrations were required to induce cellular effects with short-term hepatocyte cultures.

The potential role of metabolism in cytotoxicity was investigated in primary cultures of rat hepatocytes (LOCKWOOD et al. 1988; MONTEITH and THEISS 1933; WALKER et al. 1989). DOGTEROM et al. (1988) demonstrated that ascorbate and tocopherol inhibited toxicity, while depletion of reduced glutathione (GSH) by diethyl maleate did not affect cytotoxicity as expressed by leakage of cytoplasmic enzymes. Tacrine decreased cellular GSH, which was not associated with cytotoxicity. Rat hepatocytes treated with P450 inducers including phenobarbital, β-napthoflavone, and benzanthracene (MONTEITH and THEISS 1933; WALKER et al. 1989), or the P450 inhibitor metyrapone (MONTEITH and THEISS 1933), resulted in only minor alterations in cytotoxicity, while the P450 inhibitor α-naphthoflavone increased cytotoxicity approximately fourfold.

The cytotoxic potency of tacrine in cultured hepatocytes from human, dog, mouse, and rat was not significantly different as assessed by leakage of cytoplasmic enzymes (MONTEITH and THEISS 1995). Monkey hepatocytes were approximately two-fold more sensitive than human hepatocytes while rabbit hepatocytes were approximately two-fold less sensitive (MONTEITH and THEISS 1995). In a separate study comparing monkey, dog, and rat hepatocytes, dog hepatocytes were approximately two-fold more sensitive than rat or monkey hepatocytes (SMOLAREK et al. 1990). In a study using neutral red as an indicator of cell viability (VIAU et al. 1993), primary cultures of rat hepatocytes were approximately eight-fold more sensitive to tacrine than primary cultures of dog hepatocytes. Rat hepatocytes had a similar sensitivity to tacrine as H4 and HepG2 cell lines (VIAU et al. 1993). These in vitro models suggest only minimal differences in sensitivity to tacrine-induced cytotoxicity in cultured hepatocytes, which may be reflective of a common mechanism(s) of cellular injury. Further, the mechanism of cytotoxicity appears related to chemical structure, rather than to cholinesterase inhibitory activity (MONTEITH et al. 1995b).

Tacrine-derived irreversible binding to hepatocellular protein was assessed in primary monolayer cultures and suspensions of rat hepatocytes. Tacrine-derived irreversible binding was observed in concentrations of picomoles bound per milligram intracellular protein (MONTEITH and THEISS 1993). α-Napthoflavone enhanced binding in rat hepatocytes, which was also associated with increased cytotoxicity (MONTEITH and THEISS 1993).

In vitro systems using human and rat liver microsomal preparations and human peripheral blood lymphocytes as target cells have also been used to assess tacrine-induced cytotoxic potential (MADDEN et al. 1993; PARK et al. 1993). Tacrine at approximately 50-μM concentrations required metabolic activation in order to effect a cytotoxic response. Addition of GSH to the incubation medium resulted in a marked decrease in cytotoxicity and irreversible binding. Addition of the CYP1A2 inhibitor enoxacin also protected against cytotoxicity and decreased irreversible binding (MADDEN et al. 1993). These results suggest, as with the previously described hepatocyte studies, an association between irreversible binding and cytotoxicity.

G. In Vitro Metabolism Studies

A series of in vitro human liver microsomal studies were conducted with $\leq 50\,\mu M$ tacrine concentrations to characterize the enzymology, major oxidative routes, and potential for tacrine-derived irreversible binding (WOOLF et al. 1993a,b; MADDEN et al. 1993; SPALDIN et al. 1994; PARK et al. 1993). Stable metabolites detected were the 1-, 2-, 4-, and 7-hydroxylated derivatives of tacrine (WOOLF et al. 1993a; MADDEN et al. 1993). A time course study in microsomes showed 1-hydroxytacrine to increase rapidly while 7-hydroxytacrine increased and then decreased with time suggestive of sequential metabolism. Both 2- and 4-hydroxytacrine were present in trace quantities. No additional stable metabolites were detected. Irreversible binding was delayed and then followed a near linear increase. Addition of human epoxide hydrase or coincubations with specific inhibitors of epoxide hydrase, namely trichloropropene oxide and cyclohexene oxide, did not significantly alter the extent of tacrine-derived irreversible binding (Woolf et al. 1993a; Madden et al. 1993). In these studies there was no evidence for N-hydroxylation of tacrine (Woolf et al. 1993a). Coincubations with GSH inhibited the binding of tacrine-derived radioactivity to microsomal protein; however, there was no evidence for adduct formation (Woolf et al. 1993a; Madden et al. 1993). This would suggest that GSH decreased binding by reducing a reactive electrophilic intermediate in a "futile cycle" type process (Park et al. 1993; Vermeulen et al. 1992). Incubations with 1-hydroxytacrine also resulted in irreversible binding, although to a lesser extent than with tacrine (Woolf et al. 1993a). Thus, results from these studies suggest involvement of a quinone-methide type pathway(s) in tacrine bioactivation (Fig. 2).

Attempts to trap a reactive quinone methide intermediate have met with limited success (Madden et al. 1994; Park et al. 1993). Coincubations of both tacrine and 7-hydroxytacrine with mercaptoethanol as a trapping reagent and human liver microsomes resulted in detectable adduct formation, although in trace amounts (Madden et al. 1994). Analysis of the isolated thioether adduct by mass spectrometry gave a molecular weight consistent with a 1:1 molar ratio of mercaptoethanol to 7-hydroxytacrine. Problems associated with adduct formation and their isolation have precluded efforts to develop ELISA-type assays to assess the potential for an immunological component to the hepatotoxicity process (Beaune and Bourdi 1993).

Studies using specific inhibitors of CYP1A2, CYP2C, CYP2D6, CYP2E1, and CYP3A4 showed nearly all of tacrine metabolism to be mediated by CYP1A2 at the 25 μM tacrine concentration studied. Heterologous expressed CYP1A2 was also found to readily turn over tacrine (Woolf et al. 1993b).

Similar stable metabolic profiles were observed in both human and rat microsomal incubations at tacrine concentrations of 1 μM; nevertheless a marked difference was observed in the overall rate of metabolism. In addition, a significant difference was observed in the extent of tacrine-derived irreversible binding (Woolf et al. 1993a). 3-MC-pretreated rat liver microsomes were found to produce a similar level of tacrine-derived irreversible binding as observed with human liver microsomes (Woolf et al. 1993a).

Metabolism and bioactivation of tacrine was investigated in microsomal preparations from mouse, dog, rabbit, rat, hamster, and human liver (Madden et al. 1994). In microsomes from all six species, tacrine underwent NADPH-dependent metabolism to stable and irreversibly bound metabolites. There was a 35-fold variation between species in the generation of reactive metabolites and a 17-fold variation in stable metabolite formation (Madden et al. 1994). Comparison of irreversible binding to stable metabolite formation for the various animal species would suggest that less tacrine is directed toward bioactivation pathway(s) than with human microsomes. Rabbit and mouse microsomes gave results comparable to human microsomes. The observed difference in metabolism and bioactivation of tacrine may be reflective of species difference in CYP1A2 (Soucek and Gut 1992).

H. Conclusions

Of the approximately 50% of patients receiving tacrine who have an increase in serum ALT, only 6% demonstrate increases greater than ten times the upper limit of normal. These elevations of serum ALT are relatively low when compared to compounds that induce cellular necrosis (Desmet 1993).

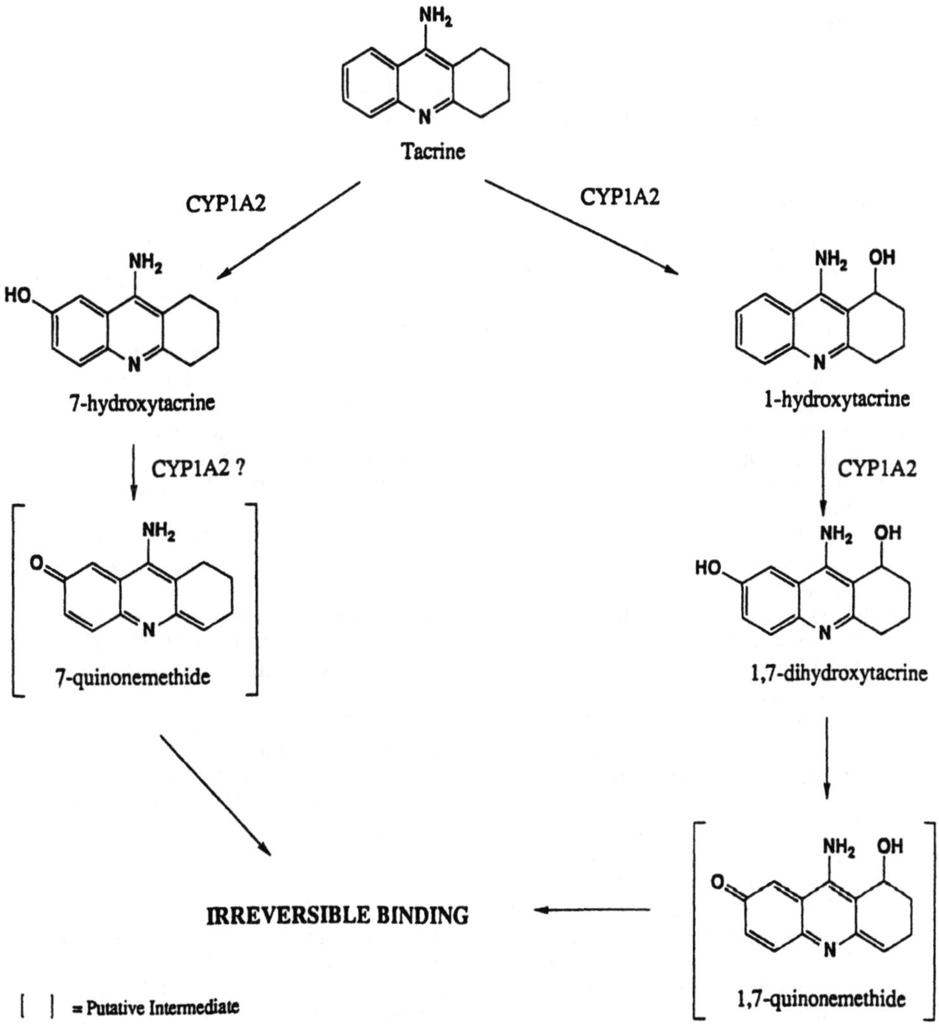

Fig. 2. Metabolic pathway for formation of reactive metabolite

While hepatocellular eosinophilia was observed in the 52-week dog study and was noted in a single human biopsy, no clear histological evidence of additional hepatic degeneration or correlation with increase in ALT levels was apparent in the dog or other animal models. However, only limited blood monitoring was conducted in chronic toxicology studies, while patient monitoring occurs weekly. Approximately three- to five-fold higher ALT activities than controls occurred in acute studies but were concurrent with neuromuscular effects, potentially confounding determination of hepatotoxicity.

The use of in vitro models has provided insight into the cellular organelles affected; however, these events occur at concentrations higher than the plasma concentrations attained following therapeutic dosing. Molecular evidence for reactive metabolite formation and irreversible protein binding would be supportive of both immunological and idiosyncratic drug-induced hepatotoxicity mechanisms. The pathologic findings from humans are suggestive of multiple mechanisms for toxicity. Further work is clearly needed to define the molecular and mechanistic events that may potentially contribute to tacrine-induced hepatotoxicity and to better characterize the subpopulations at risk.

References

Acosta D, Mitchell DB, Sorensen EMB et al. (1987) The metabolism and toxicity of xenobiotics in a primary culture system of postnatal rat hepatocytes. In: Rauckman EJ, Padilla G (eds) The isolated hepatocyte: use in toxicology and xenobiotic transformation. Academic, New York, pp 265–280

Amaducci L, Falcini M, Lippi A (1993) Descriptive epidemiology and risk factors for Alzheimer's disease. In: Corain B, Iqbal K, Nicolini M et al. (eds) Alzheimer's disease: advances in clinical and basic research. Wiley, New York, pp 105–111

Beaune PH, Bourdi M (1993) Autoantibodies against cytochromes P-450 in drug-induced autoimmune hepatitis. Ann NY Acad Sci 685:641–645

Berry CL (1988) The no-effect level and optimal use of toxicity data. Regul Toxicol Pharmacol 8:385–388

Budinsky RA, Roberts SM, Coats EA, Adams L, Hess EV (1978) The formation of procainamide hydroxylamine by rat and human liver microsomes. Drug Metab Dispos 1537:37–43

Butler MA, Lang NP, Young JF, Caporaso NE, Vineis P, Hayes RB, Teitel CH, Massengill JP, Lawsen MF, Kadlubar FF (1992) Determination of CYP1A2 and NAT2 phenotypes in human populations by analysis of caffeine urinary metabolites. Pharmacogenetics 2:116–127

Clement B, Schultze-Mosgau MH, Richter PH, Besch A (1994) Cytochrome P450-dependent N-hydroxylation of an aminoguanidine (amidinohydrazone) and microsomal retroreduction of the N-hydroxylated product. Xenbiotica 24:671–688

Cutler NR, Murphy MF, Nash RJ, Prior PL, De-Luna DM (1990a) Clinical safety, tolerance, and plasma levels of the oral anticholinesterase 1,2,3,4-tetrahydro-9-aminoacridin-1-ol-maleate (HP 029) in Alzheimer's disease: preliminary findings. J Clin Pharmacol 30:556–561

Cutler NR, Sedman AJ, Prior P, Underwoob BA, Selen A, Balough L, Kinkel AW, Gracon SI, Gamzu ER (1990b) Steady state pharmacokinetics of tacrine in patients with Alzheimer's disease. Psychopharmacol Bull 28:231–234

De Souza E (1993) Preclinical strategies for symptomatic treatment of cognitive deficits seen in Alzheimer's disease: focus on cholinergic mechanisms. In: Corain B, Iqbal K, Nicolini M et al. (eds) Alzheimer's disease: advances in clinical and basic research. Wiley, New York, pp 539–548

Desmet VJ (1993) Drug-induced liver disease: pathogenetic mechanism and histopathological lesions. Eur J Med 2:36–47

Dogterom P, Nagelkerke JF, Mulder GJ (1988) Hepatotoxicity of tetrahydroaminoacridine in isolated rat hepatocytes: effect of glutathione and vitamin E. Biochem Pharmacol 7:2311–2313

Ekman L, Lindström B, Roxin P (1989) Determination of tacrine and its 1-hydroxy metabolite in plasma using column liquid chromatography with ultraviolet detection. J Chromatogr 494:397–402

Fariss MW, Johnsen SA, Walton LP, Mumaw VR, Ray SD (1994) Tetrahydroaminoacridine-induced ribosomal changes and inhibition of protein synthesis in rat hepatocyte suspensions. Hepatology 20:240–246

Farlow M, Gracon SI, Hershey LA, Lewis KW, Sadowsky CH, Dolan-Ureno J (1992) A controlled trial of tacrine in Alzheimer's disease. J Am Med Assoc 268:2523–2529

Fitten LJ, Flood JF, Baxter CF, Tachiki KH, Perryman K (1987) Long-term oral adminstration of the memory-enhancing doses of tacrine in mice: a study of potential toxicity and side effects. J Gerontol 42:681–685

Fontana RJ, Turgeon DK, Woolf TF, Knapp MA, Foster NL, Watkins PB (1995) Tacrine hepatotoxicity: the prospective use of in vivo metabolic probes to identify potential susceptibility factors. Hepatology (in press)

Ford JM, Truman CA, Wilcock GK, Roberts CJC (1993) Serum concentrations of tacrine hydrochloride predict its adverse effects in Alzheimer's disease. Clin Pharmacol Ther 53:691–695

Green VJ, Pirmohamed M, Kitteringham NR, Knapp MJ, Park BK (1995) Glutathione S-transferase mu genotype (GSTM1*0) in Alzheimer's patients with tacrine transaminitis. Br J Clin Pharmacol 39:411–415

Haefeli WE, Srivastava N, Kelsey KT, Wiencke JK, Hoffman BB, Blaschke TF (1993) Glutathione S-transferase μ polymorphism does not explain variation in nitroglycerin responsiveness. Clin Pharmacol Ther 53:463–468

Haughey DB, McNaney CA, Collis MS, Brown RR, Siedlik PH, Balogh L, Klockowski PM (1994) Simultaneous determination of tacrine and 1-hydroxy-, 2-hydroxy-, and 4-hydroxytacrine in human plasma by high-performance liquid chromatography with fluorescence detection. J Pharm Sci 83:1582–1585

Hein DW, Doll MA, Rustan TD, Gray K, Feng Y, Ferguson RJ, Grant DM (1993) Metabolic activation and deactivation of arylamine carcinogens by recombinant human NAT1 and polymorphic NAT2 acetyltransferases. Carcinogenesis 14:1633–1638

Hooper WD, Pool WF, Woolf TF, Gal J (1994) Stereoselective hydroxylation of tacrine in rats and humans. Drug Metab Dispos 22:719–724

Hsu RS, Dileo EM, Chesson SM (1990a) High-performance liquid chormatography for the determination of tacrine and its metabolites in plasma. J Chromatogr 530:170–176

Hsu RS, Shutske GM, Dileo EM, Chesson SM, Linville R, Allen RC (1990b) Identification of the urinary metabolites of tacrine in the rat. Drug Metab Dispos 18:779–783

Hsu RS, Dileo EM, Chesson SM, Wong GS, Viau CJ (1991) Pharmacokinetics of tacrine in rats and dogs. Pharm Res 8:S–268 (PPDM8169)

Iwata N, Suzuki K, Minegishi K, Kawanishi T, Hara S, Endo T, Takahashi A (1993) Induction of cytochrome P450 1A2 by musk analogues and other inducing agents in rat liver. Eur J Pharmacol Environ Toxicol Pharmacol 248:243–250

Kadlubar FF (1994) Biochemical individuality and its implications for drug and carcinogen metabolism: recent insights from acetyltransferase and cytochrome P451A2 phenotyping and genotyping in humans. Drug Metab Rev 26:37–46

Kalow W, Tang B-K (1991) Caffeine as a metabolic probe: exploration of the enzyme-inducing effect of cigarette smoking. Clin Pharmacol Ther 49:44–48

Kalow W, Tang B-K (1993) The use of caffeine for enzyme assays: a critical appraisal. Clin Pharmacol Ther 53:503–514

Kaul PN (1962) Estimation and urinary excretion of tetrahydroaminoacridine. J Pharm Pharmacol 14:237–242
Knapp MJ, Knopman DS, Soloman PR, Pendlebury WW, Davis CS, Gracon SI (1994) A 30-week randomized controlled trial of high-dose tacrine in patients with Alzheimer's disease. J Am Med Assoc 271:985–991
Lafuente A, Pujol F, Carretero P, Villa JP, Cuchi A (1993) Human glutathione S-transferase μ (GSTμ) deficiency as a marker for the susceptibility to bladder and larynx cancer among smokers. Cancer Lett 68:49–54
Lockwood GF, Chenery RJ, Oldhanm HG, Standring P, Norman SJ (1988) The antipyrine breath test in the rat: a pharmacokinetic model. Eur J Drug Metab Pharmacokinet 13:207–214
Madden S, Woolf TF, Pool WF, Park BK (1993) An investigation into the formation of stable, protein-reactive and cytotoxic metabolites from tacrine in vitro: studies with human and rat liver microsomes. Biochem Pharmacol 46:13–20
Madden S, Spaldin V, Hayes RN, Woolf TF, Pool WF, Park BK (1994b) Species variation in the bioactivation of tacrine by hepatic microsomes. Xenobiotica 25:103–116
McNally W, Roth M, Young R, Bockbrader M, Chang T (1989) Quantitative whole-body autoradiographic determination of tacrine tissue distribution in rats following intravenous or oral dose. Pharm Res 6:924–930
McNally WP, Pool WF, DeHart P, Hanson B, Woolf TF (1993) Effect of multiple dose administration on distribution of [^{14}C] tacrine in rats: quantitative autoradiographic (QAR) and metabolic analysis. Proceedings of the 5th North American ISSX meeting, Tucson AZ
Monteith DK, Theiss JC (1993) The role of metabolism in the cytotoxicity of tetrahydroaminoacridine (THA) in hepatocytes. Toxicologist 13:139
Monteith DK, Theiss JC (1995) Comparison of tacrine-induced cytotoxicity in primary cultures of rat, mouse, monkey, dog, rabbit, and human hepatocytes. Drug Chem Toxicol (in press)
Monteith DK, Theiss JC, de la Iglesia FA (1995a) Tacrine hepatotoxicity mechanism. Am J Pathol (in press)
Monteith DK, Emmerling MR, Garvin J, Theiss JC (1995b) Cytotoxicity study of tacrine, structurally and pharmacologically related compounds using rat hepatocytes. Drug Chem Toxicol (in press)
Murphy MF, Hardiman ST, Nash RJ, Hugg FJ, Demkovich JJ, Dobson C, Knappe UE (1991) Evaluation of HP 029 (velnacrine maleate) in Alzheimer's disease. Ann N Y Acad Sci 640:P253–P262
Nyback H, Hassan M, Junthe T, Ahlin A (1993) Clinical experiences and biochemical findings with tacrine (THA). Acta Neurol Scand [Suppl] 88:36–38
O'Brien JT, Eagger S, Levy R (1991) Effects of tetrahydroaminoacridine on liver function in patients with Alzheimer's disease. Age Ageing 20:129–131
Oesch F (1987) Significance of various enzymes in the control of reactive metabolites. Arch Toxicol 60:174–178
Orzechowski A, Schrenk D, Bock KW (1992) Metabolism of 1- and 2-naphthylamine in isolated rat hepatocytes. Carcinogenesis 13:2227–2232
Orzechowski A, Schrenk D, Schut HAJ, Bock KW (1994) Consequences of 3-methylcholanthrene-type induction for the metabolism of 4-aminobiphenyl in isolated rat hepatocytes. Carcinogenesis 15:489–494
Park BK, Madden S, Spaldin V, Woolf TF, Pool WF (1993) Tacrine transaminitis: potential mechanisms. Alzheimer Dis Assoc Disord 8 [Suppl 2]:S39–S49
Pool WF, Bjorge SM, Windsor B, Black A, Change T, Woolf TF (1991) Comparison of brain to plasma metabolic distributions of tacrine and 1-hydroxytacrine in rat. Soc Neurosci 17:700
Pool WF, Bjorge SM, Change T, Woolf TF (1992a) Effect of 3-methylcholanthrene induction on the disposition of the cognition activator tacrine in rat. ISSX proceedings of the 4th North American ISSX meeting, vol 2, p 163

Pool WF, Bjorge SM, Chang T, Woolf TF (1992b) Metabolic disposition of the cognition activator tacrine in man: identification of phenol glucuronide metabolites in urine. ISSX proceedings of the 4th North American ISSX meeting, vol 2, p 164
Pool WF, Bjorge SM, Reily MD, Chang T, Woolf TF (1992c) Metabolic disposition of the cognition activator tacrine in dog: identification of dihydroxy metabolites including a dihydrodiol. ISSX proceedings of the 4th North American ISSX meeting, vol 2, p 162
Relling MV, Lin J-S, Ayers GD, Evans WE (1992) Racial and gender differences in N-acetyltransferase, xanthine oxidase, and CYP1A2 activities. Clin Pharmacol Ther 52:643–658
Roberts SK, Gibson PR, Bhathal PS, Ames DJ, Davies B, Fraser JRE (1990) Heterogeneity of hepatic adverse reactions to tetrahydroaminoacridine. Aust N Z J 20 [Suppl 1]:361
Schneider LS (1993) Clinical pharmacology of aminoacridines in Alzheimer's disease. Neurology 43 [Suppl 4]:S64–S79
Sim E, Hickman D, Coroneos E, Kelly SL (1992) Arylamine N-acetyltransferase. Biochem Soc Trans 20:304–309
Smolarek TA, Higgins CV, Amacher DE (1990) The biotransformation of tetrahydroaminoacridine (THA) in cultured hepatocytes as the cause of relative cytotoxicity in 3 species. Toxicologist 10:329
Soucek P, Gut I (1992) Cytochromes P-450 in rats: structures, functions, properties and relevant human forms. Xenobiotica 22:83–103
Spaldin V, Madden S, Pool WF, Woolf TF, Park BK (1994) The effect of enzyme inhibition on the metabolic activation of tacrine by human liver microsomes. Br J Clin Pharmacol 38:15–22
Summers WK, Viesselman JO, Marsh GM, Candelora K (1981) Use of THA in treatment of Alzheimer-like dementia: pilot study in twelve patients. Biol Psychiatry 16:145
Summers WK, Majovski LV, Marsh GM, Tachiki K, Kling A (1986) Oral tetrahydroaminoacridine in long-term treatment of senile dementia, Alzheimer type. N Engl J Med 315:1241–1245
Summers WK, Tachiki K, Kling A (1989) Tacrine in the treatment of Alzheimer's disease. Eur Neurol 29 [Suppl 3]:28–32
Vermeulen NPE, Bessems JGM, Van De Straat R (1992) Molecular aspects of paracetamol-induced hepatotoxicity and its mechanism-based prevention. Drug Metab Rev 24:367–407
Viau CJ, Curren RD, Wallace K (1993) Cytotoxicity of tacrine and velnacrine metabolites in cultured rat, dog and human hepatocytes. Drug Chem Toxicol 16:227–239
Walker RM, Clarke DW, Smith GS, Macallum GE, Barsoum NJ, Greaves P (1989) Hepatotoxicity of tacrine in animal models. Toxicologist 9:197 (787)
Walker RM, King LM, Clarke DW, Wojinski ZW, Houston BJ, Smith GS (1994) Hepatotoxicity studies of tacrine in female rats. Proceedings of the VIth congress of the International Society for Animal Clinical Biochemistry, p 154
Wanwimolruk S, Wong SM, Coville PF, Viriyayudhakorn S, Thitiarchakul S (1993) Cigarette smoking enhances the elimination of quinine. Br J Clin Pharmacol 36:610–614
Watkins PB, Zimmerman HJ, Knapp MJ, Gracon SI, Lewis KW (1994) Hepatotoxic effects of tacrine administration in patients with Alzheimer's disease. J Am Med Assoc 271:992–998
Welty D, Pool W, Woolf T, Posvar E, Sedman A (1993) The effect of smoking on the pharmacokinetics and metabolism of cognex in healthy volunteers. Pharm Res 10 [Suppl 10]:S334
Wisniewski HM, Wegiel J, Curie JR et al. (1993) β-Protein amyloidosis in Alzheimer's disease. In: Corain B, Iqbal K, Nicolini M et al. (eds) Alzheimer's disease: advances in clinical and basic research. Wiley, New York, pp 379–385

Woolf TF, Pool WF, Bjorge SM, Chang T, Goel OP, Purchase CFI, Schroeder MC, Kunze KL, Trager WF (1993a) Bioactivation and irreversible binding of the cognition activator tacrine using human and rat liver microsomal preparations: species difference. Drug Metab Dispos 21:874–882
Woolf TF, Pool WF, Kukan M, Bezek S, Kunze KL, Trager WF (1993b) Characterization of tacrine metabolism and bioactivation using heterologous expression systems and inhibition studies: evidence for CYP1A2 involvement. ISSX proceedings of the 5th North American Meeting
Zimmerman HJ (1978) Hepatotoxicity. Appleton-Centrury-Crofts, New York

CHAPTER 18

Mechanisms of Hypertransaminemia

M. PIRMOHAMED and B.K. PARK

A. Introduction

Drugs are a frequent cause of hepatic injury. Most drugs used in clinical practice at some time have been reported to cause hepatotoxicity, a recent textbook listing over 600 such drugs (STRICKER 1992). Thus, immediate recognition of drug-induced hepatic injury and appropriate action is of prime importance for all practising clinicians.

The severity of hepatic injury is widely variable not only with regard to the different drugs but also in different patients. The patient may present with clinical symptoms suggestive of hepatotoxicity, although often the hepatic injury is detected by monitoring of "liver function tests." It is important for the physician to be able to interpret such tests and relate them to the different forms of hepatic injury which can occur so that an appropriate management plan can be instituted.

The purpose of this chapter is to consider one form of liver function test monitoring, the transaminases, and the mechanisms by which hypertransaminemia can occur. There are no accurate data to indicate the overall frequency of drug-induced hypertransaminemia. The frequency tends to vary with different drugs; this is discussed later in the chapter.

B. Overview of Liver Transaminase Monitoring

I. Significance of the Different Tests Used to Monitor Liver Function

Although the purpose of this chapter is to discuss the mechanisms of hypertransaminemia, it is important to realize that in clinical practice the measurement of transaminase levels forms one facet of the monitoring of liver function, which, with the other tests used, gives an overall picture of the type of hepatic injury which may have occurred (WHITBY et al. 1984; STOLZ and KAPLOWITZ 1990). For this reason, all the tests used to monitor liver function are briefly discussed here. They can broadly be divided into three categories (STOLZ and KAPLOWITZ 1990):

1. A measurement of the hepatic elimination of exogenous and endogenous substances; excretion tests such as the sulfobromophthalein excretion test and the administration of probe substances such as antipyrine fall into this category. These tests are often only performed in specialized centers and are not routinely available. On the other hand, the determination of serum bilirubin concentration, which is routinely available, also falls into this category. A rise in the serum bilirubin concentration generally indicates an impairment of the ability of the biliary tree to excrete conjugated bilirubin, and usually allows the detection of hepatic injury prior to the development of overt jaundice. Hyperbilirubinemia is of serious concern when the injury is predominantly hepatocellular since it often reflects extensive damage, while it is of less concern when the injury is mainly cholestatic.
2. Tests which measure the synthetic ability of the liver. These include measurement of the prothrombin time and serum albumin concentration. These are relatively insensitive indicators of acute liver damage, although they may (in particular the albumin concentration) be good indicators of the severity of chronic liver disease. An exception to this is the measurement of prothrombin time in acute hepatic failure induced by acetaminophen (paracetamol) overdose where hypoprothrombinemia precedes jaundice.
3. Tests that measure levels of substances released into the blood stream. These tests do not measure liver function as such, their serum levels merely representing their release from a damaged hepatocyte. Although many substances are released into the blood stream which can be measured, those which are routinely available include the transaminases, alkaline phosphatase and γ-glutamyl transferase. This reflects the ease by which the activity of these enzymes can be measured using automated procedures. The transaminases include aspartate aminotransferase (AST), which is also known as aspartate transaminase or glutamic oxaloacetic transaminase (GOT), and alanine aminotransferase (ALT), which is also known as 2-oxoglutarate aminotransferase (GPT). Normal serum levels are a result of enzyme release from cells undergoing turnover, while elevation of serum levels is an indication of tissue injury, in the case of the liver reflecting hepatocellular injury (KONTINNEN 1971). Alkaline phosphatase (ALP) is present in kidney, intestine, placenta, and bone in addition to the liver (WHITBY et al. 1984; STOLZ and KAPLOWITZ 1990). A large elevation in serum ALP levels which is of hepatic origin indicates cholestatic liver injury while minor elevations [<3x upper limit of normal (ULN)] occur in both cholestatic and hepatocellular injury (KONTINNEN 1971; WHITBY et al. 1984). γ-Glutamyl transferase (GGT) is more sensitive than ALP in the detection of cholestasis (WHITBY et al. 1984; STOLZ and KAPLOWITZ 1990). However, it can also be elevated in hepatocellular injury and its elevation may be a "normal" finding in patients on enzyme-inducing drugs, reflecting its subcellular location in the smooth endoplasmic reticulum (KEEFFE et al. 1986).

II. Spectrum of Drug-Induced Hepatotoxicity and Hypertransaminemia

The spectrum of drug-induced liver injury is broad, and indeed can mimic any form of naturally occurring liver disease. The situation is further complicated by the fact that the same drug can produce completely different forms of injury in different individuals. Given that the third category of liver function tests is a measure of enzyme release from damaged hepatocytes, it is not surprising that in most forms of hepatic injury there is some elevation of the enzymes, although the pattern of elevation is variable and may depend on the form of the injury (DAVIS and WILLIAMS 1991). Table 1 lists the different

Table 1. Spectrum of drug-induced hepatotoxicity and the pattern of elevation of the hepatic enzymes measurable in the serum. Classification adapted from DAVIS and WILLIAMS (1991)

Hepatic abnormality	Elevation of enzymes[a]		Drug examples
	Transaminases	Alkaline phosphatase	
Acute parenchymal			
Hepatocellular necrosis	+++	+	Acetaminophen, halothane
Microvesicular fat	+++	+	Valproate
Cholestasis	+	+++	Erythromycin, oral contraceptive
Granulomatous	++	++	Allopurinol
Chronic parenchymal			
Chronic active hepatitis	++	+	Methyldopa
Chronic cholestasis	+	++	Chlorpromazine
Fibrosis/cirrhosis	++	+	Methotrexate
Phospholipidosis/alcoholic hepatitis-like lesions	++	+	Amiodarone, perhexilene
Biliary			
Sclerosing cholangitis	+	+++	5-Fluorouracil
Vascular			
Budd-Chiari syndrome	+	+	Oral contraceptives
Veno-occlusive disease	++	++	Cytotoxics
Sinusoidal dilatation and peliosis	++	++	Azathioprine, sex hormones
Liver tumors			
Adenoma	+/–	++	Oral contraceptive
Focal nodular hyperplasia	+/–	++	Oral contraceptive
Hepatocellular carcinoma	+/–	++	Sex hormones
Angiosarcoma	+/–	++	Thorotrast
Cholangiocarcinoma	+/–	++	Thorotrast

+/–, minimal or no elevation of enzymes; +, minimal elevation of enzymes; ++, moderate elevation of enzymes; +++, marked elevation of enzymes.

[a] The pattern of enzyme elevation depicted represents what has been reported in the majority of cases. Clearly, in individual cases, the pattern may be completely different.

forms of hepatic injury together with the pattern of elevation of the hepatic enzymes.

III. Clinical Correlates of Transaminase Measurement

1. Sensitivity and Specificity of Hypertransaminemia

Sensitivity refers to the ability of transaminase measurements to detect small amounts of tissue damage. Since transaminases are present in high concentrations intracellularly, even minor tissue damage will lead to their significant elevation in plasma, and thus measurement of transaminases represents a highly sensitive marker of hepatic damage (STOLZ and KAPLOWITZ 1990). Usually values which are twofold above the ULN are regarded as clinically significant (KONTINNEN 1971; WHITBY et al. 1984; STOLZ and KAPLOWITZ 1990). Both AST and ALT are equally sensitive in the detection of acute hepatic injury, although ALT is less sensitive than AST for chronic hepatic injury (SKREDE et al. 1976; WHITBY et al. 1984).

The specificity of transaminase measurements refers to the ability of the enzymes to identify not only which tissue has been damaged but also the type of hepatic injury. Overall, the specificity of hypertransaminemia is much less than its sensitivity (WHITBY et al. 1984; STOLZ and KAPLOWITZ 1990). With regard to the type of hepatic injury, AST values less than eightfold above the ULN have been seen in both cholestatic and hepatocellular hepatic injury (KONTINNEN 1971; SKREDE et al. 1976). However, the higher the value, the more likely it is that the injury will be hepatocellular (STOLZ and KAPLOWITZ 1990). With regard to tissue specificity, both AST and ALT are widely distributed throughout the body, being found in skeletal muscle, myocardium, kidney, and brain (WHITBY et al. 1984; STOLZ and KAPLOWITZ 1990). Therefore, increased plasma concentrations of these enzymes may also reflect injury to the extrahepatic tissues. However, ALT is more specific than AST for hepatic injury since its concentration in the extrahepatic tissues is much less than that of AST, while in the liver the activities of the two enzymes are the same order of magnitude (WHITBY et al. 1984; STOLZ and KAPLOWITZ 1990).

It is interesting to note that AST is present in both mitochondria and cytosol, the two forms being distinguishable immunochemically (MORINO et al. 1964), while ALT is present only in the cytosol (STOLZ and KAPLOWITZ 1990). In order to improve specificity, a measurement of the ratio of mitochondrial to cytosolic AST has been proposed (STOLZ and KAPLOWITZ 1990). Normally, this ratio is quite low, but massive tissue necrosis leads to outpouring of the mitochondrial isoenzyme and an elevation of the ratio (STOLZ and KAPLOWITZ 1990). However, its usefulness as an indicator of drug-induced damage requires further research particularly with regard to whether it represents an advance on currently available methods.

A low ratio of AST to ALT has also been advocated as an indicator of hepatitis (COHEN and KAPLAN 1979), although its discriminatory value is no greater than a high serum ALT level (>300 IU/l) (De Ritis et al. 1972). A high ratio, usually more than 2, is considered to be highly suggestive of alcoholic liver disease (Cohen and Kaplan 1979). This results from a normal or minimal increase in serum ALT coupled with a modest elevation in AST and reflects a deficiency of pyridoxal 5′-phosphate in alcoholics (Lumeng and Li 1974).

2. Correlation Between Severity of Hepatic Injury and Degree of Hypertransaminemia

Hepatocellular necrosis caused by any hepatic insult (drug or nondrug) usually passes through several phases, culminating in some cases in fulminant hepatic failure and death (Fig. 1). If each etiological factor is considered separately, then the level of hypertransaminemia observed will depend not only on the absolute amount of enzyme released but also on the rate of release of the enzyme. Thus, for example, with acetaminophen poisoning, in the most severe cases, transaminase levels may exceed 20000 U/l (Rumack 1983; Nelson 1990). However, the relationship between the degree of hypertransaminemia and the extent of liver cell necrosis from acetaminophen overdosage is imperfect. Thus, although almost all patients who die from acetaminophen overdosage have transaminase levels higher than 1000 U/l, most patients with transaminases in this range will survive (Ferguson et al. 1977; Thomas 1993).

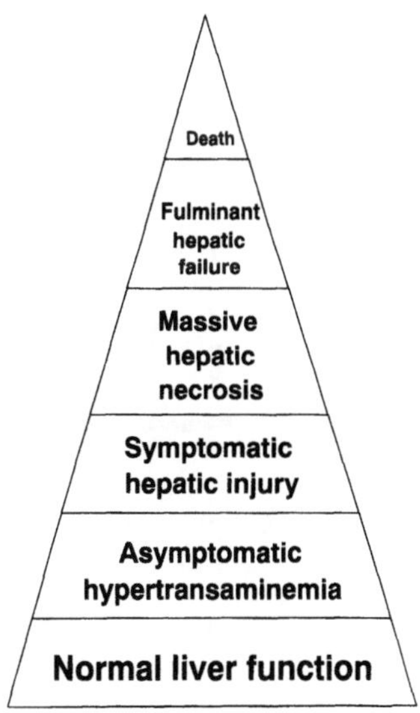

Fig. 1. A schematic representation of the phases of hepatic injury passing from normal liver function to death. The passage from the bottom of the triangle, i.e., normal liver function, which is by far the most common clinical scenario, to the top of the triangle, i.e., death, which fortunately is the rarest, can pass through the different phases as illustrated, although this may not be clinically evident. Additionally, the rate of passage from one phase to another may vary according to the drug as well as the patient

Furthermore, when different etiological factors are considered, there may not be such a clear-cut relationship between degree of hypertransaminemia and the severity of the injury. For example, despite the fact that both viral hepatitis and acetaminophen poisoning lead to fulminant hepatic failure, the degree of hypertransaminemia may be much less in the former than in the latter, suggesting that factors other than hepatocyte cell death may be contributing to severity of the clinical syndrome seen with different etiological factors. Therefore, relating a single time-point measurement of the transaminase level (i.e., the peak level) to the severity of hepatic injury with different agents may produce a misleading picture. Much better would be multiple measurements of the transaminases during the course of the hepatic injury so that an estimate of the overall degree of hypertransaminemia can be obtained. Thus, the overall degree of hypertransaminemia may be similar (or less) when acute short-lasting hepatic injury is compared to more chronic forms of liver damage which can run a prolonged course stretching over many years. However, despite these reservations, it is possible to construct a conceptualized diagram which shows the peak levels of transaminases observed with different hepatotoxins (Fig. 2).

3. Clinical Significance of Minor Degrees of Hypertransaminemia

Much more common than massive drug-induced increases in transaminase levels are the minor increases in enzyme levels which are usually

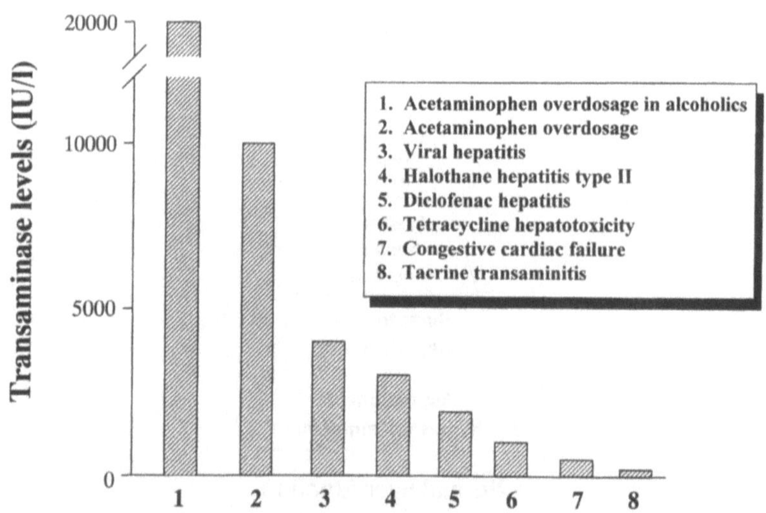

Fig. 2. A conceptualized diagram of the peak levels of serum transaminases attained in different forms of hepatocellular injury. For comparison, non-drug-induced causes of liver injury such as viral hepatitis and congestive cardiac failure are also included. The levels depicted are those which have been reported in the literature. Clearly, in individual cases, the level of serum transaminases may be lower or, on occasions, higher than those depicted

asymptomatic and detected on routine biochemical testing. Their clinical interpretation is more difficult than when there is a massive increase in transaminases.

Fluctuations in serum enzyme levels are often seen in drug-naive, apparently normal individuals (SHERLOCK 1989). In addition, underlying diseases such as AIDS may cause nonspecific liver dysfunction resulting in mild, often transient, elevation of the transaminases (BAYARD et al. 1992). Thus, changes in transaminase levels observed following the initiation of drug therapy which subside despite continuation of the drug are difficult to interpret both in terms of their clinical significance and possible mechanisms. Although such changes may not be drug related, it is equally possible that adaptive phenomena or repair processes as a result of drug exposure may be occurring within the liver, which leads to normalization of enzyme levels. The antioxidant response element which is present in the promoter regions of many of the detoxication enzymes may represent a mechanism by which adaptation occurs in response to drug exposure (JAISWAL 1994), although at present there is little direct evidence to support this with regard to drug-induced hepatic injury. Transient changes in serum transaminase levels have been reported with many drugs including sodium valproate, amiodarone, and isoniazid (Table 2).

If minor changes in serum transaminase levels occur with a particular drug, this may represent the potential of the drug to cause severe toxicity in a small number of patients. Thus, the rare cases of severe hepatotoxicity may then be regarded as the tip of an iceberg while the submerged part represents the frequent minor changes. However, extrapolation of such minor changes to a level of toxicological significance can only be arrived at if the mechanism of the hepatic injury is known, which for most drugs is not possible at present. Drugs such as acetaminophen which cause dose-dependent hepatotoxicity are relatively safe only if the maximum recommended daily dosage (4 g/day) is not exceeded (THOMAS 1993). For drugs causing hepatotoxicity by such a mechanism, it can be speculated that minor degrees of hypertransaminemia at low dose levels will predict the occurrence of more severe toxicity at higher dose levels. In contrast, with drugs which cause idiosyncratic hepatotoxicity, there is no clear dose-response relationship; hypertransaminemia of variable degree occurs at all dose levels. For example, with isoniazid, asymptomatic hypertransaminemia occurs in up to 20% of patients, while clinical hepatitis is up to 20 times less common (PESSAYRE and LARREY 1988). Furthermore, it is important to note that the mild form of hepatic injury has no long-term adverse effect on liver function, morbidity, mortality, or successful completion of the course of chemotherapy, and it does not predict the increased susceptibility to developing the more severe form of liver injury (MITCHELL et al. 1975).

In the assessment of a patient with minor degrees of hypertransaminemia, non-drug-induced causes should obviously be excluded (discussed later). In addition, the self-administration of other hepatotoxic drugs such as tranquilizers, analgesics, and herbal medicines must be excluded by careful clinical evaluation of the patient. A careful and accurate assessment of alcohol intake should also be performed.

When a drug is thought to be responsible for the minor degrees of hypertransaminemia, further management depends on the level of the transaminases. If the transaminase level is clinically insignificant, i.e., <2x ULN, and the patient is clinically asymptomatic, then the drug can be continued as long as the patient is monitored regularly. When the degree of hypertransaminemia is clinically significant, the drug may need to be withdrawn particularly when alternative drugs of equivalent efficacy are available. If the drug was responsible, then the transaminase level should rapidly return back to within normal limits.

Table 2. Frequency of asymptomatic and symptomatic hypertransaminemia reported with different drugs

Drug	Frequency		Reference
	Asymptomatic hypertransaminemia	Symptomatic liver injury	
Amiodarone	25%	1%–3%	LEWIS et al. (1989)
Carbamazepine	22%	<0.1%	PELLOCK (1987), OKUMA et al. (1989)
Clozapine	50%	<0.01%	KELLNER et al. (1993)
Diclofenac	18%–25%	<0.1%	ATRA et al. (1990), SCHIFF (1994)
Imipramine	20%	<1%	BUI and CHANEY (1989)
Iproniazid	20%	1%	DANAN et al. (1983)
Isoniazid	10%–20%	1%–3%	THOMPSON (1982), TIMBRELL (1983)
Isoniazid + rifampicin	44%–82%	7%–10%	PARTHASARATHY et al. (1986), GENDREL et al. (1989)
Halothane	20%	<0.1%	NEUBERGER and KENNA (1987)
Ketoconazole	10%–15%	<0.1%	ROLLMAN et al. (1985)
Methyldopa	6%	<1%	TYSELL and KNAUER (1971), MADDREY and BOITNOTT (1975)
Perhexilene	30%	Unknown	PILCHER et al. (1985)
Propylthiouracil	28%	<1%	LIAW et al. (1993)
Simvastatin	20%	Unknown	MOL et al. (1986)
Tacrine	50%	28%	O'BRIEN et al. (1991)
Valproic acid	44%–67%	<0.1%	SUSSMAN and MCLAIN (1979), VINING et al. (1979), COULTER et al. (1980)

C. Classification of the Causes of Hypertransaminemia

From a mechanistic perspective, the causes of hypertransaminemia can be divided into two categories, chemical and idiosyncratic reactions, each of which can be further subdivided into acute and chronic (Table 3). The mechanisms of acute and chronic hepatic injuries will be dealt with separately.

D. Mechanisms of Acute Hepatic Injury Leading to Hypertransaminemia

I. Role of Drug Metabolism

Drug metabolism can, in most cases, be considered to be a detoxification mechanism, its function being the conversion of lipid-soluble, nonpolar compounds to more water-soluble, polar compounds which can then be excreted from the body via the kidneys or the biliary tract (PARK 1986; PARK and KITTERINGHAM 1987). In certain circumstances, however, the metabolic pathways can also bioactivate the drug, resulting in the formation of chemically

Table 3. A mechanistic classification of the causes of hypertransaminemia

Type	Features	Subtype	Example
Chemical	Toxicity which can be rationalized in terms of either the physicochemical properties or chemical reactivity of the drug or its metabolites. These reactions are dependent on the relative rates of accumulation and clearance of the compound. A dose-response relationship may be discernible, although this is not always the case. Such toxicity may occur either with therapeutic doses of the compound or after overdosage	Acute Chronic	Acetaminophen overdose Amiodarone hepatitis
Idiosyncratic	Aberrant effects that are not predictable from the known pharmacological actions of a drug. There is no simple dose-response relationship and factors within the affected patient may be important in the pathogenesis of the reactions. Reactions are undetectable by preclinical toxicology testing in animals and indeed cannot be reproduced in animal models. Although relatively uncommon, this type accounts for many drug-induced deaths	Acute Chronic	Halothane hepatitis Oxyphenisation chronic active hepatitis

reactive metabolites or free radicals which, if inadequately detoxified, can bind irreversibly to various cellular macromolecules such as nucleic acids and proteins, and lead to carcinogenicity, teratogenicity, cellular necrosis, and hypersensitivity (Fig. 3) (PARK et al. 1992). All drug-metabolizing enzymes including those with a primary detoxication role (such as the glutathione-*S*-transferases) can bioactivate drugs to toxic metabolites, although it is the cytochrome P450 enzymes which catalyze the phase I metabolic pathways that are responsible in most cases (GUENGERICH and LIEBLER 1985; PARK 1986; PARK et al. 1992). The liver is quantitatively the most important site of drug metabolism in the body (WOOLF and JORDAN 1987; PESSAYRE and LARREY 1988), and therefore, in some instances, it is not surprising that this leads to drug-induced hepatic injury.

Many drugs that are metabolized can be bioactivated to chemically reactive metabolites. Fortunately, the formation of such toxic metabolites is counterbalanced by detoxication processes such as glutathione conjugation and epoxide hydrolysis, leading to excretion of the harmless metabolite from the body (PARK et al. 1992). Thus, only individuals who have an imbalance between bioactivation and detoxication will be susceptible to acute hepatic injury (PARK et al. 1992). With chemical injury (Table 3), this only occurs when the burden of the toxic metabolite is so high that the detoxication mechanisms are overwhelmed. Overdose with acetaminophen represents the best example (NELSON 1990). In contrast, for idiosyncratic toxicity, the basis of individual susceptibility to toxicity may be multifactorial and may include a combination of metabolic and immunological factors (PARK et al. 1992; PIRMOHAMED et al. 1992).

The type of toxicity caused by bioactivation of a drug depends on several factors including the site of metabolism, the chemical reactivity and stability of

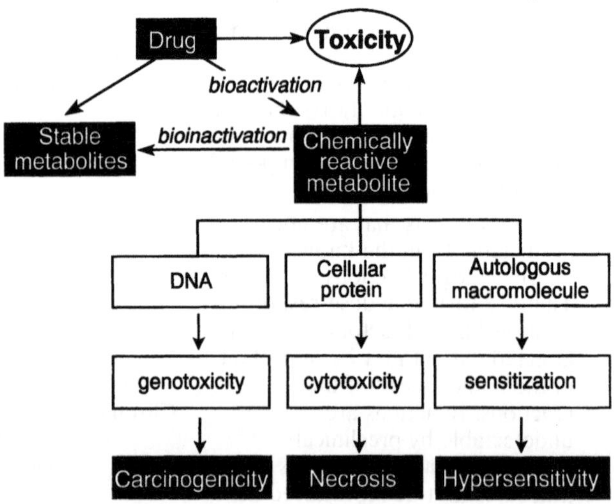

Fig. 3. The relationship between drug metabolism and drug toxicity. The drug can be bioactivated to a chemically reactive metabolite, which by binding to different cellular macromolecules can mediate different forms of toxicity, including necrosis, carcinogenesis, and hypersensitivity

the toxic intermediate, and the nature of the macromolecule to which the intermediate binds (PARK et al. 1987; BOELSTERLI 1993). The liver is the primary site of metabolism, and hence is a major site of formation of chemically reactive metabolites (PESSAYRE and LARREY 1988). Within the liver itself, the combination of a high cytochrome P450 level and a relatively low glutathione level in the centrilobular region makes this part of the liver particularly prone to toxicity mediated by chemically reactive intermediates (PESSAYRE and LARREY 1988).

The reactivity of an intermediate also depends on its chemical "hardness" or "softness" (high or low polarized charge density), which to a large extent determines the selectivity of its binding (PESSAYRE and LARREY 1988; BOELSTERLI 1993). In general, soft electrophiles react with soft nucleophiles such as the thiol groups of cysteine and amino groups of lysine, arginine, or histidine, while hard electrophiles react more readily with DNA. Binding to DNA is particularly important with respect to chemical carcinogenesis (GUENGERICH 1992).

The stability of the chemically reactive metabolite also varies; some are so unstable as to react immediately at their site of generation, while others may be stable enough to leave the organ in which they are formed to cause toxicity in other organs (GILLETTE et al. 1984). Within the cell itself, the reactive metabolite may bind to proteins in the endoplasmic reticulum, plasma membrane, cytosol, or nucleus. The nature of the protein to which the chemically reactive metabolite binds may be an important determinant of the type of toxicity, i.e., either direct toxicity or indirect toxicity caused by an immune-mediated mechanism (BOELSTERLI 1993). For example, binding to a critical cellular protein may result in death of the cell. Thus, alkylation and inactivation of the plasma membrane Ca^{2+}-APTase will result in the disruption of intracellular calcium homeostasis with cellular death. Conversely, where the alkylated protein does not have a critical physiological or catalytic function, direct toxicity may not ensue, but may result in the formation of an immunogenic drug-protein conjugate, thus resulting in immune-mediated toxicity (BOELSTERLI 1993). With respect to the latter, the ability of the chemically reactive metabolite to translocate from the endoplasmic reticulum may allow it to bind covalently to plasma membrane proteins which will facilitate antigen presentation (PARK et al. 1987; POHL et al. 1988). There is also evidence for the presence of functionally active cytochrome P450 enzyme in plasma membrane, which will allow local bioactivation of the drug and subsequent covalent binding (LOEPER et al. 1993).

II. Evidence for the Formation of Chemically Reactive Metabolites

A chemically reactive metabolite is by definition unstable, and therefore it may not be possible to characterize it directly by analytical methods such as high-performance liquid chromatography (HPLC) and mass spectroscopy (KITTERINGHAM et al. 1988). Thus, evidence for the formation of a chemically reactive metabolite is often indirect, usually based on techniques such as covalent binding (KITTERINGHAM et al. 1988; BOELSTERLI 1993), adduct formation with nucleophile (PARK and KITTERINGHAM 1990), immunological methods (BOELSTERLI 1993), and formation of cytotoxic metabolites (SPIELBERG 1984). The most widely used of these methods is covalent binding. Irreversible binding to protein or other macromolecules is the hallmark of covalent binding. It can be determined both in vivo and in vitro. Nucleophiles such as glutathione and *N*-acetylcysteine usually result in a reduction in the covalent binding while, at the same time, they may also result in the reactive metabolite being "trapped" as a stable adduct which can then be isolated and its chemical structure resolved by analytical methods such as mass spectrometry. For drugs such as acetaminophen, it has been shown that the degree of covalent binding reflects the severeity of toxicity (JOLLOW et al. 1973; POTTER et al. 1973). However, the relevance of covalent binding may sometimes be overestimated, particularly when it is determined in vitro in systems which do not contain phase II metabolic pathways (MAGGS et al. 1983; KITTERINGHAM et al. 1988). The role of covalent binding may also be underestimated since a cell may be damaged long before covalent binding reaches its maximum (BOELSTERLI 1993). Furthermore, with covalent binding, overall binding is determined without consideration of the specific protein(s) targeted by the reactive metabolite (BOELSTERLI 1993), a factor which may be of importance in determining the nature of toxicity.

III. Acute Chemical Hepatotoxicity

The mechanisms involved in drug-induced acute chemical hepatotoxicity are complex, and at present still not fully understood. In many of the cases, more than one mechanism may be operating (Fig. 4) (PESSAYRE and LARREY 1988). Bioactivation of a drug to free radicals or electrophiles is the initial event. This results in membranous lipid peroxidation and covalent binding to protein as well as conjugation with and consequent depletion of glutathione. The ultimate consequence of these initial events is the oxidation of protein thiols, which in turn leads to secondary molecular events, finally resulting in cellular death (Fig. 4). An additional factor which may contribute to hepatocellular death is the infiltration of the injured area by activated macrophages (LASKIN and PILARO 1986; LASKIN et al. 1986), which release pro-inflammatory mediators such as leukotrienes and tumor necrosis factor, and active oxygen intermediates. To illustrate the various mechanisms of acute chemical hepatotoxicity, two examples will be considered here: acetaminophen hepatotoxicity and carbon tetrachloride-induced liver necrosis.

1. Acetaminophen Hepatotoxicity

Hepatic failure from acetaminophen overdosage causes 160 deaths/year in England and Wales (BRAY 1993). Serum transaminase levels are elevated 1–3 days after ingestion, and reach levels as high as 10000 IU/l on the 4 day (RUMACK 1983). The role of metabolism in acetaminophen hepatotoxicity has been extensively investigated. In therapeutic doses, acetaminophen undergoes sulfation and glucuronidation in the liver (NELSON 1990), with only a small proportion (5%–10%) undergoing oxidative metabolism by the cytochrome P450 isozymes CYP2E1, CYP1A2 (RAUCY et al. 1989), and CYP3A4 (THUMMEL et al. 1993). The product of oxidative metabolism, *N*-acetyl-*p*-benzoquinoneimine, is normally detoxified by glutathione (PRESCOTT 1983), thus maintaining the balance between activation and detoxication. However, after overdosage, this balance is disturbed because of saturation of sulfation and depletion of the liver glutathione stores, resulting in inadequate detoxification of the reactive metabolite and subsequent hepatic necrosis. The liver

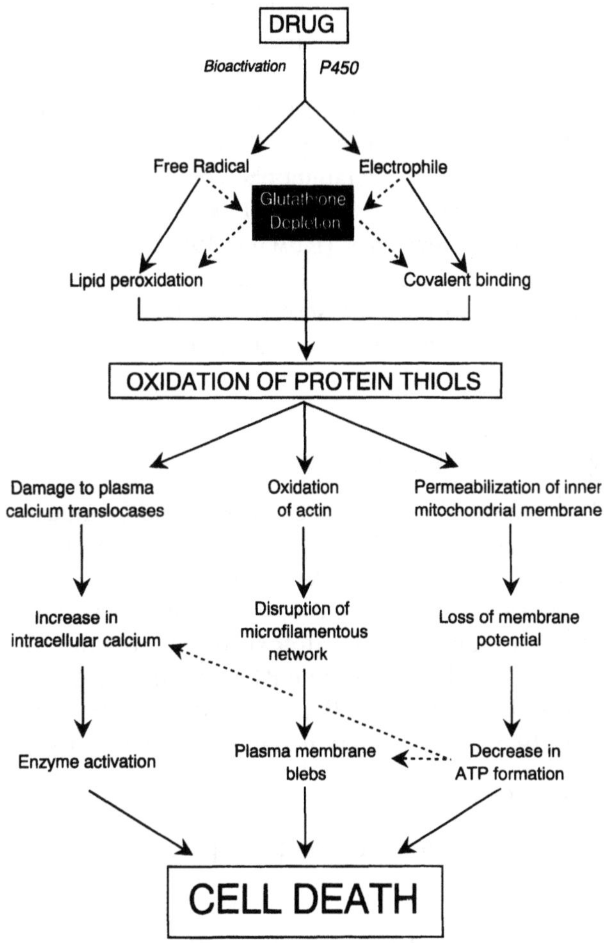

Fig. 4. Mechanism by which bioactivation of a compound to a chemically reactive metabolite results in direct hepatic injury. The initial event, which is enhanced by glutathione depletion, is the oxidation of protein thiols, which in turn leads to several secondary molecular events, ultimately culminating in hepatocyte death. (Adapted from PESSAYRE and LARREY 1988)

injury is predominantly centrilobular (RUMACK 1983), reflecting the high cytochrome P450 content in this region (PESSAYRE and LARREY 1988). The observation that depletion of glutathione was of importance in the pathogenesis of acetaminophen hepatotoxicity has led to the widespread use of *N*-acetylcysteine as an antidote, a treatment which is highly effective, particularly if given in the early stages after overdose (BRAY 1993). There are several possible mechanisms by which the reactive metabolite of acetaminophen may cause the hepatocellular necrosis including modification of free sulfydryl groups, lipid peroxidation, oxidative stress, and arylation of cell macromolecules (PIRMOHAMED et al. 1994).

Although acetaminophen hepatotoxicity is dose dependent, there is interindividual variability in susceptibility, since some individuals who ingest large amounts of acetaminophen do not develop hepatotoxicity, while others can develop liver failure after taking only a few tablets more than the maximum recommended daily dosage (BRAY 1993). Two groups who are more susceptible are chronic alcoholics (SEEFF et al. 1986; LAUTERBURG and VELEZ 1988; LIEBER 1988) and patients on enzyme-inducing anticonvulsants (BRAY et al. 1992). In chronic alcoholics, acetaminophen hepatotoxicity is characterized by extremely high transaminase levels (20000–30000 IU/l), although these rapidly decrease after a few days (RUMACK 1983). Patients with Gilbert's syndrome, an inherited condition characterized by deficient bilirubin glucuronidation, may also be more susceptible (DE MORAIS et al. 1992). In contrast, children seem to be less susceptible, possibly because of enhanced sulfation (LIEH-LAI et al. 1984).

2. Carbon Tetrachloride Hepatotoxicity

Cases of CCl_4 hepatotoxicity have been reported after industrial exposure, indiscrete domestic use, and accidental ingestion (WILLIAMS and BURK 1990). Liver toxicity, which occurs 1–4 days after exposure, is characterized by centrilobular necrosis and massive elevation of transaminases (WILLIAMS and BURK 1990). The mechanism of hepatotoxicity involves the bioactivation of CCl_4 to a free radical by the cytochrome P450 enzymes (RECKNAGEL 1973), in particular by the P450 isoform CYP2E1 (JOHANSSON and INGELMAN-SUNDBERG 1985; BURK et al. 1988). The primary metabolism yields a free radical:

$$CCl_4 \rightarrow Cl- + CCl\cdot_3$$

This radical then reacts with oxygen to give a peroxyl radical:

$$CCl\cdot_3 + O_2 \rightarrow CCl_3O_2\cdot$$

The peroxyl radical leads to lipid peroxidation (HALLIWELL 1994).

Alcoholics are more susceptible to CCl_4 hepatotoxicity (WILLIAMS and BURK 1990). This is probably due to the induction of the P450 isoform CYP2E1 by alcohol (TSUTSUMI et al. 1993), thereby increasing the bioactivation of CCl_4. Hyperbaric oxygen, which has been recommended as a treatment for the hepatic injury, acts by reversibly inhibiting some P450 isoforms and promotes the destruction of CYP2E1, thereby preventing the formation of the $CCl_3\bullet$ radical (BURK et al. 1986).

IV. Acute Idiosyncratic Hepatotoxicity

Acute idiosyncratic hepatotoxicity may be due to direct toxicity of the chemically reactive metabolite ("metabolic" idiosyncrasy) or the toxicity may be indirect, occurring as a result of an immune reaction ("immune-mediated" idiosyncrasy) (PARK et al. 1992, 1994; PIRMOHAMED et al. 1994).

1. Metabolic Idiosyncrasy Causing Hypertransaminemia

The mechanisms of hypertransaminemia secondary to metabolic idiosyncrasy are thought to be similar to those of acute chemical hepatotoxicity described above. However, in most cases, evidence that the hepatic injury is due to direct toxicity of a chemically reactive metabolite is indirect. Features which allow distinction between metabolic idiosyncrasy and direct chemical hepatotoxicity include the absence of a clear dose-response relationship, the occurrence of the liver injury in only a minority of individuals, and the inability to produce the toxicity in animal models (PARK et al. 1992, 1994).

Liver injury associated with the use of the antitubercular drug isoniazid represents a good example of metabolic idiosyncrasy (TIMBRELL 1983). A mild and transient elevation of the transaminases is seen in 10%–20% of individuals (THOMPSON 1982; TIMBRELL 1983). The hypertransaminemia often subsides despite continuation of drug therapy. A more severe form of hepatitis occurs in 0.5%–2% of individuals and is characterized by transaminase levels 10- to 20-fold higher than normal, consistent with the histological picture of hepatic necrosis (BLACK et al. 1975; KOPANOFF et al. 1978; THOMPSON 1982; TIMBRELL 1983). A case fatality rate as high as 10% has been reported with the severe form (BLACK et al. 1975). Isoniazid hepatitis is rare in children, the risk increasing with increasing age, reaching about 3% in patients over 50 years of age (BLACK et al. 1975; MITCHELL et al. 1976; KOPANOFF et al. 1978).

A toxic metabolite produced from isoniazid is thought to be responsible for the severe hepatic injury (TIMBRELL 1983). The mechanism of the mild liver injury is unknown, but again metabolism to directly acting hepatotoxins may be important. Acetylisoniazid, the first product of isoniazid, undergoes hydrolysis to acetylhydrazine, which is either acetylated again to form diacetylhydrazine (a detoxification pathway) or is bioactivated to a reactive acetyl radical which can undergo covalent binding (Fig. 5) (TIMBRELL 1983). The latter pathway is considered to be important in the pathogenesis of hepatic injury, although the relationship between the degree of covalent binding and hepatic damage remains unclear (WOODWARD and TIMBRELL 1984). The relative rates of metabolism of acetylhydrazine to either the diacetyl derivative or the radical may determine individual susceptibility (TIMBRELL et al. 1977; TIMBRELL 1983; LAUTERBURG et al. 1985). The role of acetylator phenotype in predisposing to isoniazid hepatotoxicity is unclear, with associations having been found with both the slow and fast acetylator phenotypes (PARK et al. 1992). It is likely fast acetylators form acetylhydrazine at a faster rate, but also detoxify it to diacetylhydrazine at a faster rate (PARK et al. 1992).

The increased susceptibility of alcoholics may be explained by a higher degree of bioactivation (because of induction of CYP2E1) relative to the acetylation (TIMBRELL 1983). Similarly, concomitant treatment with rifampicin, a potent inducer of the cytochrome P450 enzymes, leads to an increase in transaminases in up to 80% of patients, and to clinical hepatitis in 5%–8% of patients possibly by enhancing the bioactivation of isoniazid (PESSAYRE and LARREY 1988). A recent study has shown that the incidence of clinical isoniazid hepatotoxicity was tenfold higher in slow acetylators than among rapid acetylators receiving combination treatment, which may reflect accumulation of monoacetylhydrazine in slow acetylators (PARTHASARATHY et al. 1986).

An alternative pathway of bioactivation of isoniazid may be the direct hydrolysis of the drug to isonicotinic acid and the direct hepatotoxin, hydrazine (SCALES and TIMBRELL 1982). The formation of the toxic metabolite is increased tenfold in slow acetylators and by concomitant rifampicin treatment (RAGUPATI SARMA et al. 1986).

2. Immune-Mediated Drug-Induced Hypertransaminemia

Bioactivation of a drug by the P450 enzymes may lead to immune-mediated idiosyncratic toxicity, which may be manifest as either asymptomatic

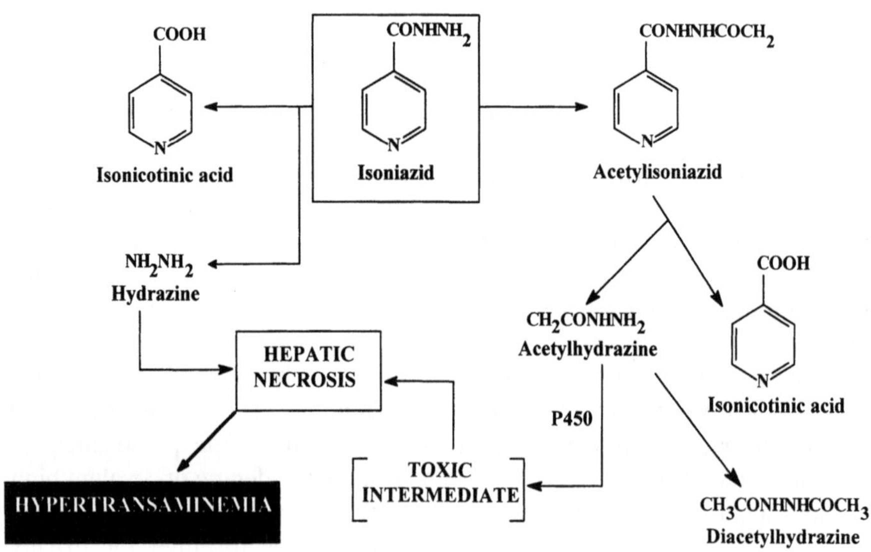

Fig. 5. Role of metabolism in the hepatotoxicity produced by isoniazid, a widely used antitubercular drug. (Adapted from TIMBRELL 1983)

hypertransaminemia or clinical hepatitis. Our understanding of the mechanism by which a drug can induce immune-mediated toxicity is based on the hapten hypothesis (Fig. 6) (PARK et al. 1987). It is well known that the molecular weight of an organic molecule is one of the main factors determining whether it can act as an immunogen (PARK et al. 1987). Most drugs are less than 1000 daltons, and according to classical immunological theory are unlikely to be immunogenic per se (PARK et al. 1987; POHL et al. 1988). Thus, bioactivation of drugs to chemically reactive metabolites which bind covalently to autologous macromolecules leads to the formation of haptenic drug-protein conjugates which are immunogenic, and result in a specific immune response (PARK et al. 1987; POHL et al. 1988). It is important to note that a stable covalent bond is required to carry the hapten through antigen processing and presentation, and thus allow it to function as an immunogen (PARK et al. 1987). The importance of drug bioactivation by the cytochrome P450 en-

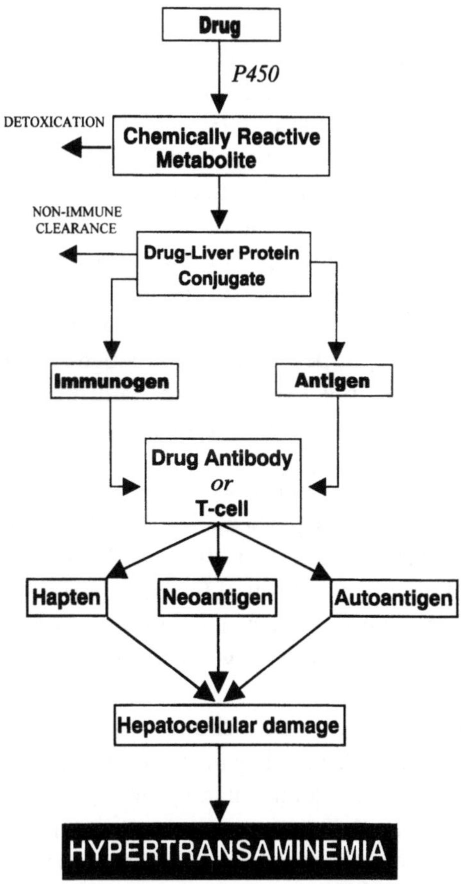

Fig. 6. Hapten hypothesis of drug hypersensitivity. The chemically reactive metabolite can act as a hapten and initiate an immune response (humoral and/or cellular) which is directed against the hapten, neoantigen, or autoantigen, resulting in hepatocellular damage and hypertransaminemia. (Adapted from PARK et al. 1987)

zymes is emphasized by the fact that the liver, which has the highest levels of these enzymes, is often the organ involved in immune-mediated toxicity (BOELSTERLI 1993).

The mechanism of induction of an immune response to a hapten-protein conjugate is not fully understood. The postulated mechanism outlined here is an extrapolation of in vitro studies carried out with model compounds which are intrinsically immunogenic (POHL et al. 1988).

The immune response to a hapten-protein conjugate will involve both B lymphocytes, which mediate humoral immunity, and T lymphocytes, which mediate cellular immunity (POHL et al. 1988). The mechanism of antigen recognition by the T- and B-lymphocyte subsets varies in that B cells are able to bind free antigen (particularly at low antigen concentrations) without any help from antigen-presenting cells (APCs) for their activation, while T cells require antigen processing and presentation by the APCs (KLAUS and HUMPHREY 1993; UNANUE 1993). The immune response elicited by direct interaction of an antigen with a B lymphocyte is usually weak, and, indeed, a stronger B-cell response is known to require stimulation via the secretion of lymphokines by activated T-helper cells (POHL et al. 1988).

The APCs include macrophages, Langerhans cells, and B lymphocytes themselves (KLAUS and HUMPHREY 1993). The B cells are in fact APCs par excellence since they can present antigen to T cells at concentrations 10^3- to 10^4-fold lower than those required by macrophages. Processing refers to the binding, uptake, and intracellular catabolism of the antigen, with the ultimate re-expression of recognizable epitopes on the surface of the APCs. The exact nature of the metabolic events which occur in antigen processing is incompletely understood, although they are likely to vary according to the nature of the antigen and of the epitopes ultimately recognized. For the processed antigen to be recognized by the T lymphocyte, it must be presented in association with class II MHC molecules (UNANUE 1993). An antigen may contain many possible epitopes, although only a few are recognized by the immune system. The predominance of one epitope ("immunodominance") may be dictated by the expression of a particular MHC allele. This phenomenon is known as MHC "restriction" (UNANUE 1993), and in essence what this means is that the high level of polymorphism of the MHC genes results in a subset of individuals in the population who can respond vigorously to drug-related antigens, and thus are more likely to develop drug hypersensitivity (PARK et al. 1992).

Model immunization studies have shown that an immune response, be it cellular or humoral, can be directed against the drug (haptenic epitopes), the carrier protein (autoantigenic determinants), or the novel antigen created by the binding of hapten to the carrier protein (new antigenic determinants) (POHL et al. 1988). More recent evidence, however, suggests that this distinction although useful is to a large extent artificial since an epitope which is part of a carrier moiety under one circumstance may behave like a haptenic determinant in another (KLAUS and HUMPHREY 1993).

Once an immune response against a hapten-protein conjugate has been elicited, the interaction between the antigen and the immune system causes tissue damage through four general mechanisms of hypersensitivity (Table 4) (COOMBES and GELL 1968). Such mechanisms are not exclusive since a particular drug reaction may involve more than one type of hypersensitivity.

Halothane hepatitis can be regarded as a model for immune-mediated hepatotoxicity (NEUBERGER and KENNA 1987). The National Halothane Study (NATIONAL HALOTHANE STUDY 1966) showed that two forms of hepatic injury occur with halothane, the first a mild increase in transaminases in up to 20% of patients, and a second, more severe form ("halothane hepatitis") characterized by liver cell necrosis, occurring in 1 in 35000 patients on first exposure and 1 in 3700 patients on multiple exposure. In both forms of toxicity, metabolism of halothane to reactive species by CYP2E1 is a prerequisite for the development of the liver injury (GUT et al. 1993). The milder form of hepatic injury (type I) is thought to be due to direct toxicity of a reactive intermediate formed by the reductive metabolism of halothane (Fig. 7). The more severe form, halothane hepatitis (type II), is caused by the formation of acyl halide intermediates by the oxidative metabolic pathway (Fig. 7). Consistent with the immune nature of the toxicity, patients frequently exhibit pyrexia, eosinophilia, circulating immune complexes, and liver-kidney microsomal autoantibodies (KENNA et al. 1993). Transaminase levels approaching 5000 IU/l have been reported with halothane hepatitis (type II). More direct evidence of the immune basis of the toxicity has been provided by the finding of specific lymphocytes and antibodies directed against halothane-derived liver neoantigens expressed predominantly in the microsomal fraction of the liver (POHL et al. 1989; GUT et al. 1993; KENNA et al. 1993). Although patients can be sensitized against different neoantigens, each neoantigen has covalently bound to it the same trifluoroacetyl (TFA) hapten, which is formed from the reactive metabolite, trifluoroacetyl chloride (KENNA et al. 1988).

Table 4. Classification of hypersensitivity reactions. (Adapted from COOMBES and GELL 1968)

Type of reaction	Consequence
Type I (immediate)	IgE binds to mast cell surface, leading to degranulation and release of inflammatory mediators
Type II (cytolytic)	Antibody combines with antigen on cell surface and is followed by cellular lysis in the presence of complement
Type III (immune-complex disease)	Formation of antigen-antibody complexes in the extracellular space, followed by deposition in the vascular endothelium and local damage
Type IV (delayed hypersensitivity)	Antigen destruction by activated T lymphocytes, with subsequent inflammatory response

Extensive research over the years into the mechanism of halothane hepatitis has uncovered some important findings, the general principles of which may be applicable to immunotoxicities induced by other drugs:

1. The reactive metabolite binds covalently to abundant luminal proteins of the endoplasmic reticulum such as carboxylesterase which are in the vicinity but are not directly involved in its formation (BOELSTERLI 1993). In addition, those adducts which are relatively long lived (100kDa and 80kDa) are recognized by patient sera more often than those adducts which are short lived (54kDa) (KENNA et al. 1993). The mechanism by which transaminases are released into the blood stream is unknown but presum-

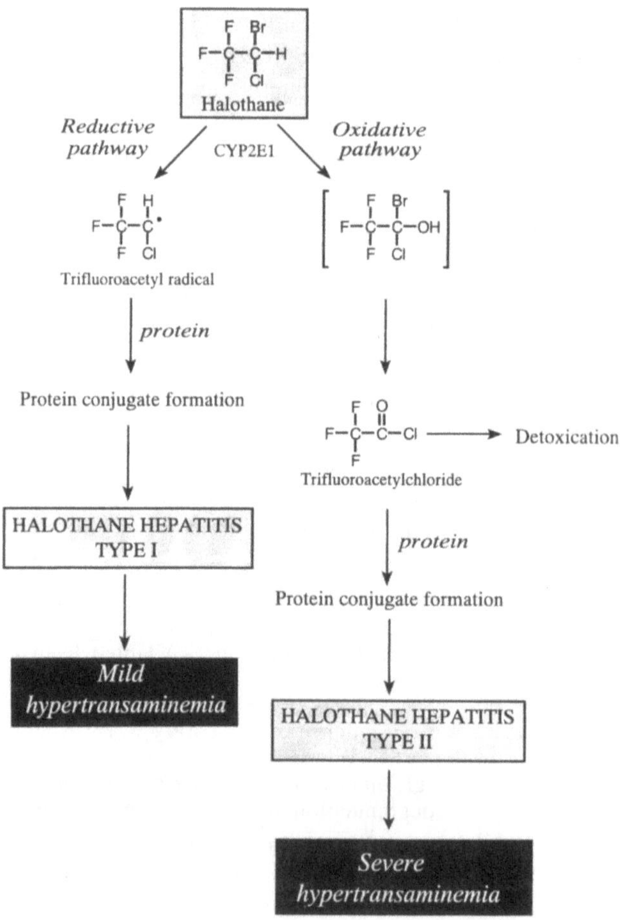

Fig. 7. Role of metabolism in halothane hepatotoxicity. Reductive biotransformation of halothane can lead to a mild form of hypertransaminemia, while the oxidative pathway leads to immune-mediated hepatic damage and a more severe degree of hypertransaminemia. (Adapted from POHL et al. 1989; GUT et al. 1993)

ably reflects a combination of both antibody- and T-cell-mediated cellular lysis.

2. Although formed in the endoplasmic reticulum, TFA-labeled proteins have also been demonstrated on the cell surface, which may be important for antigen presentation (GUT et al. 1993; KENNA et al. 1993). The mechanism by which the antigen is translocated from the endoplasmic reticulum to the cell surface is not known. It is interesting to note that TFA-protein adducts have also been demonstrated in Kupffer cells (CHRISTEN et al. 1991), which are the liver resident macrophages, and thus can act as APCs (RUBINSTEIN et al. 1987).
3. All individuals exposed to halothane produce TFA-protein adducts, although only a minority go on to develop an immune response and, thus, liver injury. It has been suggested that the lack of immune responsiveness might be due to tolerance induced by a presumed repertoire of self-peptides that molecularly mimic TFA-protein adducts. Therefore, individuals who develop the immune response may have a breakdown in tolerance as a result of an irregularity in the expression of the self-peptide (GUT et al. 1993).

E. Mechanisms of Chronic Hepatic Injury Causing Hypertransaminemia

As with acute hepatic injury, the mechanisms of chronic hepatic injury can be subdivided into chemical and idiosyncratic (Table 3). Chronic hepatic injury will lead to hypertransaminemia, although the rise in levels is much lower than that seen with acute hepatic injury. Many of the drugs which cause chronic hepatic injury can also result in acute forms of hepatotoxicity. Drug metabolism also plays an important part in chronic hepatic injury.

I. Chronic Chemical Hypertransaminemia

Selective accumulation and trapping of a drug within the hepatocyte because of its chemical characteristics may lead to a chronic form of hepatic injury. This has been observed with amiodarone and perhexilene, which are cationic, ampiphilic compounds with a lipophilic moiety and an ionizable nitrogen (PESSAYRE and LARREY 1988). In their uncharged state, the drugs enter lysosomes, and become trapped there because of the acidic conditions, which leads to protonation of the nitrogen atom. The drugs inhibit the actions of phospholipases and form stable complexes with the phospholipids, resulting in the accumulation of phospholipids in the lysosomes. By virtue of the fact that amiodarone contains iodine, its accumulation in the liver can visualized by the increased hepatic density on CT scanning (GOLDMAN et al. 1985). In most cases, the result is mild liver dysfunction which is often clinically silent (POUCELL et al. 1984). Approximately 25% of patients on amiodarone (HARRIS et al. 1983; McGOVERN et al. 1983; LEWIS et al. 1989) and 30% of those on perhexilene (PILCHER et al. 1985) developed an elevation of transaminases over two times normal. The incidence of hypertransaminemia with both drugs has been related to their plasma concentrations (HOROWITZ et al. 1982; POUCELL et al. 1984). Severe symptomatic disease clinically and histologically similar to that seen with alcohol can result occasionally (McDONALD 1977; SIMON et al. 1984), although the reasons for this are not known. The time to the development of symptomatic disease with both drugs varies, an insidious onset being more common than an acute onset (McDONALD 1977; HARRIS et al. 1983; McGOVERN et al. 1983). With perhexilene, subjects who have a mutant form of CYP2D6, an enzyme involved in the oxidation of perhexilene, have a higher risk of developing liver disease than subjects who are extensive metabolizers of CYP2D6 (MORGAN et al. 1984). Whether the CYP2D6 status is important in predisposing to amiodarone-induced liver injury in man is not known.

II. Chronic Idiosyncratic Drug-Induced Hypertransaminemia

Several drugs (oxyphenisatin, nitrofurantoin, α-methyldopa, isoniazid, acetaminophen, etretinate, dantrolene) have been reported to cause chronic symptomatic hepatic injury, known as chronic active hepatitis, which is characterized by a mild and insidious elevation of the transaminases occurring after drug intake for at least 6 months, and improving on drug withdrawal (MADDREY 1980; SEEFF 1981). Cirrhosis may develop if the drug is not discontinued. Females are more commonly affected. Features suggestive of immune involvement such as hypergammaglobulinemia, antinuclear antibodies, and smooth muscle antibodies may be present. Some of the drugs which cause chronic hepatic injury have also been reported to cause more acute forms of hepatotoxicity. The mechanism(s) by which the same drug can produce different forms of hepatic injury in different patients is unknown. A similar situation is seen with the hepatitis B and hepatitis C viruses, some patients developing acute hepatitis while others develop chronic liver disease (SHERLOCK 1989). It has been proposed that drug-induced chronic hepatic injury may be the consequence of continued damage to hepatocytes because of prolonged exposure to a drug or (more likely) its chemically reactive metabolite (PESSAYRE and LARREY 1988).

α-Methyldopa, an antihypertensive drug, causes a wide spectrum of hepatic injury, ranging from asymptomatic hypertransaminemia to acute and chronic active hepatitis, to fatal massive hepatic necrosis (TYSELL and KNAUER 1971; MADDREY and BOITNOTT 1975; RODMAN et al. 1976). Methyldopa can be bioactivated by the cytochrome P450 enzymes to a chemically reactive semiquinone or quinone metabolite (DYBING and NELSON 1978). Haptenation of liver cell membrane proteins may initiate an immune reaction directed against the hapten as well as towards unaltered "self" proteins, which may culminate in liver injury (DELPRE et al. 1979). Such an immune response may be enhanced by the fact that methyldopa inhibits suppressor T-cell function (AMMUS and YUNIS 1989), and thus may lead to unregulated antibody production. The factors determining individual predisposition are unknown, although these may be (at least partly) genetic as suggested by the occurrence of hepatotoxicity in four members of a family (SOTANIEMI et al. 1977).

F. Diagnosis of Drug-Induced Hypertransaminemia

I. Distinction Between Drug- and Non-Drug-Induced Etiologies

The diagnosis of drug-induced hypertransaminemia depends on the drug responsible for the injury as well as the nature of the injury. Thus, acetaminophen hepatotoxicity is easy to diagnose from the clinical history of overdosage, plasma acetaminophen levels, and the degree of hypertransaminemia. In contrast, it is much more difficult to diagnose idiosyncratic drug hepatotoxicity since (1) there are no drug-specific diagnostic tests available and (2) many of the drug-induced liver diseases resemble nondrug causes such as viral hepatitis. Even histological examination may be unhelpful because the features of injury are often nonspecific, although the presence of an eosinophilic infiltrate, granulomas, or fatty change is more likely with drug injury than with nondrug causes such as viral hepatitis. Therefore, in such cases, a diagnosis of drug-induced hepatic injury is one of association and exclusion, being dependent on a clear temporal relationship between the onset of drug therapy and the occurrence of toxicity, and elimination of non-drug-induced disorders by the use of specific tests such as viral serology, autoantibody screen, and ultrasonography (NEUBERGER 1990; DAVIS and WILLIAMS 1991).

Problems in diagnosis also arise when the patient is on more than one potentially hepatotoxic agent. The only way to make a diagnosis in such cases may be to rechallenge the patient with the suspect drug, although this decision should not be taken lightly as rechallenge can precipitate a severe reaction.

II. Distinction Between Direct and Immune-Mediated Acute Idiosyncratic Toxicity

As stated above, chemically reactive metabolites formed from drugs can induce injury either directly by binding to essential cellular proteins or indirectly by initiating an immune reaction. Such a distinction is important to make because it may affect treatment of the acute injury, future treatments with alternative related agents, and future drug design. Often the distinction is empirical, being based on the clinical features, although more specific pointers may also be available with certain drugs (Table 5).

G. Conclusions

The measurement of serum transaminases represents a highly sensitive marker of hepatocellular injury. Its specificity, however, is lower than its sensitivity, since hypertransaminemia can occur with damage to extrahepatic tissues and it may not always be possible to determine the type of hepatic injury which has occurred. With respect to the latter, the higher the elevation in transaminases, the more likely it is that the injury is hepatocellular rather than cholestatic. Even when the injury is hepatocellular, it is not always possible to distinguish between acute and chronic forms of hepatic injury solely by measurement of serum transaminases, the distinction usually being afforded by the clinical history and associated features. Additionally, the correlation between the peak level of the rise in transaminases and severity of hepatic injury is imperfect, a relationship which could be strengthened by

Table 5. Criteria which suggest that drug-induced hepatotoxicity is immune-mediated

Criteria	Features	Example
Clinical symptomatology	Fever, rash, arthralgia, lymphadenopathy, eosinophilia	Allopurinol-induced hepatitis
Cellular immunity	a)Infiltration by lymphocytes with specific cell markers indicative of an inflammatory response secondary to recent encounter with antigen	Alcoholic hepatitis
	b) Demonstration by techniques such as lymphocyte transformation of specifically primed lymphocytes reactive against the drug and/or drug-altered antigen	Ticlopidine-induced hepatitis
Humoral immunity	a) Presence of anti-drug antibodies	Amodiaquine-induced hepatotoxicity
	b) Presence of antibodies directed against drug-altered antigens (neoantigens)	Halothane hepatitis type II
	c) Presence of non-organ-specific autoantibodies, for example: i) Antinuclear antibody ii) Antimitochondrial (anti-M_6) autoantibody	i) Methyldopa hepatitis ii) Iproniazid-induced hepatitis
	d) Presence of liver-specific autoantibodies: i) Directed against cytochrome P450 enzymes which metabolize the drugs ii) Directed against other hepatic proteins	i) Hepatotoxicity due to dihydralazine or tienilic acid ii) Carbamazepine-induced hepatotoxicity

multiple transaminase measurements through the course of the toxicity so as to obtain an "area under the curve" for hypertransaminemia. Despite these reservations, there is no doubt that the measurement of serum transaminases represents a useful early marker of hepatocellular injury of various types.

Drug metabolism plays an important part in the pathogenesis of most causes of hypertransaminemia, usually by the formation of a chemically reactive intermediate. The toxicity of the intermediate may be direct in that cellular function may be adversely affected, leading to cellular death, or it may be indirect, in that the toxic metabolite may act as a hapten and initiate an immune cascade, resulting in hepatocellular injury. The distinction between these two forms is usually empirical, being based on clinical criteria, since definitive laboratory tests are not routinely available. For some drugs such as acetaminophen, the hepatic injury is dose dependent and can be predicted from the known pharmacology of the drug, while for the majority of drugs toxicity is usually dose independent and is unpredictable, only a minority of individuals being affected.

References

Ammus S, Yunis AA (1989) Drug-induced red cell dyscrasias. Blood Rev 3:71–82

Atra E, Metz CA, Brown BL, Teoh KW (1990) Flurbiprofen versus diclofenac for the treatment of osteoarthritis of the knee, DICP. Ann Pharmacother 24:920–923

Bayard PJ, Berger TG, Jacobson MA (1992) Drug hypersensitivity reactions and human immunodeficiency virus disease. J Acquir Immune Defic Syndr 5:1237–1257

Black M, Mitchell JR, Zimmerman HJ, Ishak KG, Epler GR (1975) Isoniazid-associated hepatitis in 114 patients. Gastroenterology 69:289–302

Boelsterli UA (1993) Specific targets of covalent drug-protein interactions in hepatocytes and their toxicological significance in drug-induced liver injury. Drug Metab Rev 25:395–451

Bray GP (1993) Liver failure induced by paracetamol. Br Med J 306:157–158

Bray GP, Harrison PM, O'Grady JG, Tredger JM, Williams R (1992) Long-term anticonvulsant therapy worsens outcome in paracetamol-induced fulminant hepatic failure. Hum Exp Toxicol 11:265–270

Bui HD, Chaney RH (1989) Transient hepatitis due to low-dose neuroleptic medication. Am J Gastroenterol 84:578–579

Burk RF, Hill KE, Lane JM (1988) Inhibition of CCl_4 metabolism by oxygen varies between isoenzymes of cytochrome-P450. Biochem Biophys Res Commun 152:1463–1467

Burk RF, Reiter R, Lane JM (1986) Hyperbaric oxygen protection against carbon tetrachloride hepatotoxicity in the rat. Association with altered metabolism. Gastroenterology 90:812–818

Christen U, Burgin M, Gut J (1991) Halothane metabolism: Kupffer cells carry and partially process trifluoroacetylated protein adducts. Biochem Biophys Res Commun 175:256–262

Cohen JA, Kaplan MM (1979) The SGOT/SGPT ratio – an indicator of alcoholic liver disease. Dig Dis Sci 24:835–838

Coombes RRA, Gell PGH (1968) Classification of allergic reactions responsible for clinical hypersensitivity and disease. In: Gell PGH (ed) Clinical aspects of immunology. Oxford University Press, Oxford, pp 575–596

Coulter DL, Wu H, Allen RJ (1980) Valproic acid therapy in childhood epilepsy. J Am Med Assoc 244:785–788

Danan G, Homberg JC, Bernuau J, Rochesicot J, Pessayre D (1983) Iproniazid hepatitis – diagnostic value of a novel anti-mitochondrial antibody, anti-M_6. Gastroenterol Clin Biol 7:529–532
Davis M, Williams R (1991) Hepatic disorders. In: Davies DM (ed) Textbook of adverse drug reactions. Oxford University Press, Oxford, pp 245–304
Delpre G, Grinblat J, Kadish J, Livni E, Shohat B, Lewitus Z, Joshua H (1979) Immunological studies in a case of hepatitis following methyl dopa administration. Am J Med Sci 277:207–213
De Morais SMF, Uetrecht JP, Wells PG (1992) Decreased glucuronidation and increased bioactivation of acetaminophen in Gilbert's syndrome. Gastroenterology 102:577–586
De Ritis F, Coltorti M, Giusti G (1972) Serum transaminase activities in liver disease. Lancet I:685–687
Dybing E, Nelson SD (1978) Metabolic activation of methyldopa and other catechols. Arch Toxicol [Suppl] 1:117–124
Ferguson DR, Snyder SK, Cameron AJ (1977) Hepatotoxicity in acetaminophen poisoning. Mayo Clin Proc 52:246
Gendrel D, Nardou M, Mouba JF, Gahouma D, Moussavou A, Boguikouma JB (1989) Hepatic toxicity following the use of isoniazid-rifampin in African children – role of malnutrition and HBV. Arch Franc Pediatr 46:645–648
Gillette JR, Lau SS, Monks TJ (1984) Intra- and extracellular formation of metabolites from chemically reactive species. Biochem Soc Trans 12:4–7
Goldman IS, Winkler ML, Raper SE, Barker ME, Keung E, Goldberg HI, Boyer TD (1985) Increased hepatic density and phospholipidosis due to amiodarone. Am J Roentgenol 144:541–546
Guengerich FP (1992) Metabolic activation of carcinogens. Pharmacol Ther 54:17–61
Guengerich FP, Liebler DC (1985) Enzymatic activation of chemicals to toxic metabolites. CRC Crit Rev Toxicol 14:259–307
Gut J, Christen U, Huwyler J (1993) Mechanisms of halothane toxicity: novel insights. Pharmacol Ther 58:133–155
Halliwell B (1994) Free radicals, antioxidants, and human disease: curiosity, cause or consequence? Lancet 344:721–724
Harris L, Mckenna WJ, Rowland E, Holt DW, Storey GCA, Krikler DM (1983) Side effects of long-term amiodarone therapy. Circulation 67:45–51
Horowitz JD, White HD, Goble AJ (1982) Liver-disease induced by perhexilene maleate. Med J Aust 2:9–10
Jaiswal AK (1994) Antioxidant response element. Biochem Pharmacol 48:439–444
Johansson I, Ingelman-Sundberg M (1985) Carbon-tetrachloride-induced lipid peroxidation dependent on an ethanol-inducible form of rabbit liver microsomal cytochrome P-450. FEBS Lett 183:265–269
Jollow DJ, Mitchell JR, Potter WZ, Davis DC, Gillette JR, Brodie BB (1973) Acetaminophen-induced hepatic necrosis. II. Role of covalent binding in vivo. J Pharmacol Exp Ther 187:195–202
Keeffe EB, Sunderland MC, Gabourel JD (1986) Serum gamma-glutamyl transpeptidase activity in patients receiving chronic phenytoin therapy. Dig Dis Sci 31:1056–1061
Kellner M, Wiedemann K, Krieg JC, Berg PA (1993) Toxic hepatitis by clozapine treatment. Am J Psychiatry 150:985–986
Kenna JG, Neuberger J, Williams R (1988) Evidence for expression in human liver of halothane-induced neoantigens recognized by antibodies in sera from patients with halothane hepatitis. Hepatology 8:1635–1641
Kenna JG, Knight TL, Van Pelt FNAM (1993) Immunity to halothane metabolite-modified proteins in halothane hepatitis. Ann NY Acad Sci 685:646–661
Kitteringham NR, Lambert C, Maggs JL, Colbert J, Park BK (1988) A comparative study of the formation of chemically reactive drug metabolites by human liver microsomes. Br J Clin Pharmacol 26:13–21

Klaus GGB, Humphrey JH (1993) The fate of antigens. In: Lachmann PJ, Peters DK, Rosen FS, Walport MJ (eds) Clinical aspects of immunology, 5th edn. Blackwell Scientific, Oxford, pp 107–126
Kontinnen A (1971) Serum enzymes as indicators of hepatic disease. Scand J Gastroenterol 6:667–669
Kopanoff DE, Snider DE, Caras GJ (1978) Isoniazid-related hepatitis. A US Public Health Service Cooperative Surveillance Study. Am Rev Respir Dis 117:991–1001
Laskin DL, Pilaro AM (1986) Potential role of activated macrophages in acetaminophen hepatotoxicity. I. Isolation and characterisation of activated macrophages from rat liver. Toxicol Appl Pharmacol 86:204–215
Laskin DL, Pilaro AM, Ji S (1986) Potential role of activated macrophages in acetaminophen hepatotoxicity. II. Mechanism of macrophage accumulation and activation. Toxicol Appl Pharmacol 86:216–226
Lauterburg BH, Velez ME (1988) Glutathione deficiency in alcoholics: risk factor for paracetamol hepatotoxicity. Gut 29:1153–1157
Lauterburg BH, Smith CV, Todd EL, Mitchell JR (1985) Pharmacokinetics of the toxic hydrazino metabolites formed from isoniazid in humans. J Pharmacol Exp Ther 235:566–570
Lewis JH, Ranard RC, Caruso A, Jackson LK, Mullick F, Ishak KG, Seeff LB, Zimmerman HJ (1989) Amiodarone hepatotoxicity – prevalence and clinicopathologic correlations among 104 patients. Hepatology 9:679–685
Liaw YF, Huang MJ, Fan KD, Li KL, Wu SS, Chen TJ (1993) Hepatic injury during propylthiouracil therapy in patients with hyperthyroidism – a cohort study. Ann Intern Med 118:424–428
Lieber CS (1988) Biochemical and molecular basis of alcohol induced injury to liver and other tissues. N Engl J Med 319:1639–1650
Lieh-Lai MW, Sarnaik AP, Newton JF, Miceli JN, Fleischmann LE, Hook JB, Kauffman RE (1984) Metabolism and pharmacokinetics of acetaminophen in a severely poisoned young child. J Pediatr 105:125–128
Loeper J, Descatoire V, Maurice M, Beaune P, Belghiti J, Houssin D, Ballet F, Feldmann G, Guengerich FP, Pessayre D (1993) Cytochromes P-450 in human hepatocyte plasma membrane: recognition by several autoantibodies. Gastroenterology 104:203–216
Lumeng L, Li T-DK (1974) Vitamin B6 metabolism in chronic alcohol abuse. Pyridoxal phosphate levels in plasma and the effects of acetaldehyde on pyridoxal phosphate synthesis and degradation in human erythrocytes. J Clin Invest 53:693–704
Maddrey WC (1980) Drug-related acute and chronic hepatitis. Clin Gastroenterol 9:213–224
Maddrey WC, Boitnott JK (1975) Severe hepatitis from methyl dopa. Gastroenterology 68:351–360
Maggs JL, Grabowski PS, Park BK (1983) Drug protein conjugates V: sex-linked differences in the metabolism and irreversible binding of [^{3}H]ethinyloestradiol in the rat. Biochem Pharmacol 32:2793–2830
McDonald GSA (1977) Liver damage after perhexilene maleate. Lancet I:1056
McGovern B, Garan H, Kelley E (1983) Adverse reactions during treatment with amiodarone hydrochloride. Br Med J 287:175
Mitchell JR, Long MW, Thorgeirsson UP (1975) Acetylation rates and monthly liver function tests during one year of isoniazid preventive therapy. Chest 68:181–190
Mitchell JR, Zimmerman HJ, Ishak KG, Thorgiersson UP, Timbrell JA, Snodgrass WR, Nelson SD (1976) Isoniazid liver injury: clinical spectrum, pathology, and probably pathogenesis. Ann Intern Med 84:181–192
Mol MJTM, Leuven JAG, Erkelens DW, Schouten JA, Stalenhoef AFH (1986) Effects of synvinolin (MK-733) on plasma-lipids in familial hypercholesterolemia. Lancet II:936–939

Morgan MY, Reshef R, Shah RR, Idle JR, Smith RL (1984) Impaired oxidation of debrisoquine in patients with perhexilene liver injury. Gut 10:1057–1064
Morino Y, Kagamiyama H, Wada H (1964) Immunochemical distinction between glutamic-oxaloacetic transaminases from soluble and mitochondrial fractions of mammalian tissues. J Biol Chem 239:943–944
National Halothane Study (1966) Summary of the national halothane study. J Am Med Assoc 197:121–134
Nelson SD (1990) Molecular mechanisms of the hepatotoxicity caused by acetaminophen. Semin Liver Dis 10:267–278
Neuberger JM (1990) Halothane and hepatitis. Incidence, predisposing factors and exposure guidelines. Drug Saf 5:28–38
Neuberger J, Kenna JG (1987) Halothane hepatitis: a model of immune mediated drug hepatotoxicity. Clin Sci 72:263–270
O'Brien JT, Eagger S, Levy R (1991) Effects of tetrahydroaminoacridine on liver function in patients with Alzheimer's disease. Age Ageing 20:129–131
Okuma T, Yamashita I, Takahashi R, Itoh H, Otsuki S, Watanabe S, Sarai K, Hazama H, Inanaga K (1989) A double-blind study of adjunctive carbamazepine versus placebo on excited-states of schizophrenic and schizoaffective disorders. Acta Psychiatr Scand 80:250–259
Park BK (1986) Metabolic basis of adverse drug reactions. J R Coll Phys 20:195–200
Park BK, Kitteringham NR (1987) Adverse drug reactions and drug metabolism. Adv Drug React Bull 122:456–459
Park BK, Kitteringham NR (1990) Drug-protein conjugation and its immunological consequences. Drug Metab Rev 22:87–144
Park BK, Coleman JW, Kitteringham NR (1987) Drug disposition and drug hypersensitivity. Biochem Pharmacol 36:581–590
Park BK, Pirmohamed M, Kitteringham NR (1992) Idiosyncratic drug reactions: a mechanistic evaluation of risk factors. Br J Clin Pharmacol 34:377–395
Park BK, Pirmohamed M, Tingle MD, Madden S, Kitteringham NR (1994) Bioactivation and bioinactivation of drugs and drug metabolites: relevance to adverse drug reactions. Toxicol in vitro 8:613–621
Parthasarathy R, Sarma GR, Janardhanam B, Ramachandran P, Santha T, Sivasubramanian S, Somasundaram PR, Tripathy SP (1986) Hepatic toxicity in south Indian patients during treatment of tuberculosis with short-course regimens containing isoniazid, rifampicin and pyrazinamide. Tubercle 67:99–108
Pellock JM (1987) Carbamazepine side effects in children and adults. Epilepsia 28 [Suppl 3] :S64–S70
Pessayre D, Larrey D (1988) Acute and chronic drug-induced hepatitis. Bailliere's Clin Gastroenterol 2:385–423
Pilcher J, Cooper JDH, Turnell DC, Matenga J, Paul R, Lockhart JDG (1985) Investigations of long-term treatment with perhexiline-maleate using therapeutic monitoring and electromyography. Ther Drug Monit 7:54–60
Pirmohamed M, Kitteringham NR, Park BK (1992) Idiosyncratic reactions to antidepressants: a review of possible mechanisms and predisposing factors. Pharmacol Ther 53:105–125
Pirmohamed M, Kitteringham NR, Park BK (1994) The role of active metabolites in drug toxicity. Drug Saf 11:114–144
Pohl LR, Satoh H, Christ DD, Kenna JG (1988) Immunologic and metabolic basis of drug hypersensitivities. Annu Rev Pharmacol 28:367–387
Pohl LR, Kenna JG, Satoh H, Christ D (1989) Neoantigens associated with halothane hepatitis. Drug Metab Rev 20:203–217
Potter WZ, Davis DC, Mitchell JR, Jollow DJ, Gillette JR, Brodie BB (1973) Acetaminophen-induced hepatic necrosis. III. Cytochrome P-450-mediated covalent binding in vitro. J Pharmacol Exp Ther 187:203–210
Poucell S, Ireton J, Valenciamayoral P, Downar E, Larratt L, Patterson J, Blendis L, Phillips MJ (1984) Amiodarone-associated phospholipidosis and fibrosis of the

liver – light, immunohistochemical and electron-microscopic studies. Gastroenterology 86:926–936
Rescott LF (1983) Paracetamol overdosage. Pharmacological considerations and clinical management. Drugs 25:290–314
Ragupati Sarma G, Immanuel C, Kailasam S, Narayana ASL, Venkatesan P (1986) Rifampicin-induced release of hydrazine from isoniazid. A possible cause of hepatitis during treatment of tuberculosis with regimens containing isoniazid and rifampicin. Am Rev Respir Dis 133: 1072–1075
Raucy JL, Lasker JM, Lieber CS, Black M (1989) Acetaminophen activation by human liver cytochromes P-450IIE1 and P-450IA2. Arch Biochem Biophys 271:270–283
Recknagel RO (1973) Carbon tetrachloride hepatotoxicity: an example of lethal cleavage. CRC Crit Rev Toxicol 2:263–297
Rodman JS, Deutsch DJ, Gutman SI (1976) Methyldopa hepatitis. A report of six cases and review of literature. Am J Med 60:941–948
Rollman O, Jameson S, Lithell H (1985) Effects of long-term ketoconazole therapy on serum-lipid levels. Eur J Clin Pharmacol 29:241–245
Rubinstein D, Roska AK, Lipsky PE (1987) Antigen presentation by liver sinusoidal lining cells after antigen presentation in vivo. J Immunol 138:1377–1382
Rumack BH (1983) Acetaminophen overdose. Am J Med 75 [Suppl]:104–112
Scales MD, Timbrell JA (1982) Studies on hydrazine hepatotoxicity. 1. Pathological findings. J Toxicol Environ Health 10:941–953
Schiff ER (1994) Can we prevent nonsteroidal anti-inflammatory drug-induced hepatic failure? Gastroint Dis Today 3:7–13
Seeff LB (1981) Drug-induced chronic liver disease, with emphasis on chronic active hepatitis. Semin Liver Dis 1:104–115
Seeff LB, Cuccherini BA, Zimmerman HJ, Adler E, Benjamin SB (1986) Acetaminophen hepatotoxicity in alcoholics. A therapeutic misadventure. Ann Intern Med 104:399–404
Sherlock S (1989) Diseases of the liver and biliary system, 8th edn. Blackwell Scientific, Oxford
Simon JB, Manley PN, Brien JF, Armstrong PW (1984) Amiodarone hepatotoxicity simulating alcoholic liver disease. N Engl J Med 311:167–172
Skrede S, Blomhoff JP, Gjone E (1976) Biochemical features of acute and chronic hepatitis. Ann Clin Res 8:182–199
Sotaniemi EA, Hokkanen OT, Ahokas JT, Pelkonen RO, Ahlqvist J (1977) Hepatic injury and drug metabolism in patients with alpha-methyldopa-induced liver damage. Eur J Clin Pharmacol 12:429–435
Spielberg SP (1984) In vitro assessment of pharmacogenetic susceptibility to toxic drug metabolites in humans. Fed Proc 43:2308–2313
Stolz A, Kaplowitz N (1990) Biochemical tests for liver disease. In: Zakim D, Boyer TD (eds) Hepatology. A textbook of liver disease. Saunders, Philadelphia, pp 637–667
Stricker BHC (1992) Drug-induced hepatic injury, 2nd edn, vol 5. Elsevier Science, Amsterdam
Sussman NM, McLain LW (1979) A direct hepatotoxic effect of valproic acid. J Amer Med Assoc 242:1173–1174
Thomas SHL (1993) Paracetamol (acetaminophen) poisoning. Pharmacol Ther 60:91–120
Thompson NJ (1982) Efficacy of various durations of isoniazid preventive therapy for tuberculosis – 5 years of follow-up in the IUAT trial. Bull WHO 60:555–564
Thummel KE, Lee CA, Kunze KL, Nelson SD, Slattery JT (1993) Oxidation of acetaminophen to N-acetyl-p-aminobenzoquinone imine by human CYP3A4. Biochem Pharmacol 45:1563–1569
Timbrell JA (1983) Drug hepatotoxicity. Br J Clin Pharmacol 15:3–14
Timbrell JA, Wright JM, Baillie TA (1977) Monoacetylhydrazine as a metabolite of isoniazid in man. Clin Pharmacol Ther 22:602–608

Tsutsumi M, Lasker JM, Takahashi T, Lieber CS (1993) In vivo induction of hepatic P4502E1 by ethanol – role of increased enzyme synthesis. Arch Biochem Biophys 304:209–218
Tysell JE, Knauer CM (1971) Hepatitis induced by methyl dopa. Report of a case and review of the literature. Dig Dis Sci 16:848–855
Unanue ER (1993) Antigen processing and presentation. In: Lachmann PJ, Peters DK, Rosen FS, Walport MJ (eds) Clinical aspects of immunology, 5th edn. Blackwell Scientific, Oxford, pp 661–672
Vining EP, Botsford E, Freeman JM (1979) Valproate sodium in refractory seizures: a study of efficacy. Am J Dis Child 133:274–276
Whitby LJ, Percy-Robb IW, Smith AF (1984) Lecture notes on clinical chemistry, 3rd edn. Blackwell Scientific, Oxford
Williams AT, Burk RF (1990) Carbon tetrachloride hepatotoxicity: an example of free radical-mediated injury. Semin Liver Dis 10:279–284
Woodward KN, Timbrell JA (1984) Acetylhydrazine hepatotoxicity: the role of covalent binding. Toxicology 30:65–74
Woolf TF, Jordan RA (1987) Basic concepts in drug metabolism: part 1. J Clin Pharmacol 27:15–17

CHAPTER 19

Diagnostic Tools and Clinical Pathology

D.C. Snover

A. General Features and Clinical Evaluation of Drug-Induced Liver Diseases

Hepatic drug reactions occur in a variety of clinical settings. In many cases the association of liver disease with the use of a particular drug is obvious because of a temporal association of developing liver function abnormalities to beginning use of the drug. This scenario generally leads to discontinuation of the drug and resolution of the dysfunction. In this setting biopsy is rarely indicated. With many drugs there is no long-term consequence as long as the drug is not reintroduced.

A more difficult presentation is the patient who develops liver dysfunction with several possible causes. Such a patient often has multiple medical problems and is receiving a variety of medications, several of which may be potentially hepatotoxic. In this patient the detective work required to identify the offending agent may be very difficult and require staged withdrawal and/or substitution of drugs, as well as careful analysis of the pattern of liver enzyme elevation, association of the reaction with use of particular medications in the regimen, and liver biopsy. In these patients assessment should include a listing of medications that the patient is or has been on, analysis of the probability of any of these medications causing liver disease, analysis of the pattern of liver dysfunction in the patient and comparison with known toxicity of the drugs in question (e.g., cholestatic versus hepatitic), analysis of known time to onset of disease with the drugs in question and comparison with known duration of use of these medication in the patient, and analysis of reported histological features of the drugs in question in comparison with the histological findings in the biopsy of the individual patient.

A third presentation is the patient who develops liver disease and is taking no apparent drugs or toxic agents at the time of presentation. Subsequently the patient is discovered to be receiving a toxic agent that the patient and/or physician failed to consider as a drug, or which the patient had been receiving but discontinued prior to development of liver disease. This type of patient stands as a reminder that the history for drug reactions should include not only the question of what medications the patient is currently taking, but also what drugs the patient had been taking in the recent past, and what other food supplements, vitamins, herbal medications, and over-the-counter medications the patient is taking. A dramatic example of failure to recognize that a patient was taking a drug involved the case of a young woman who began developing a series of odd medical ailments including pseudotumor cerebri resulting in the placement of cranial burr holes to relieve increased intracranial pressure, bone pain resulting in placement of a total-body cast for a year, and multiple skin manifestations including pruritus, hyperpigmentation, and alopecia. She had carried diagnoses of brain tumor, serous meningitis, chronic encephalitis, and psychoneurosis. After ten hospitalizations over the course of 8.5 years it was finally realized that the patient had been given high-dose vitamin A as a treatment for "ichthyosis" and had never discontinued its use. The patient had chronic vitamin A toxicity (in 20–20 hindsight) and recovered after discontinuation of the vitamin (i.e., "drug") (Gerber et al. 1954). Other patients with such unsuspected vitamin A toxicity have not been so lucky (Kowalski et al. 1994).

Another common variation on this theme is hepatotoxicity due to the antibiotic Augmentin. With this drug the onset of liver disease often occurs several weeks after discontinuation of the drug, and resolution of the liver dysfunction caused by the drug may not occur for several months (Stricker et al. 1989; Verhamme et al. 1989). This scenario often leads to great confusion and/or mistaken assignment of the etiology of an episode of liver disease.

B. General Mechanisms of Drug Reactions

Traditionally drug reactions are classified by their presumed mechanism and by their clinical/biochemical manifestations (Zimmerman 1978; Stricker 1992). Both of these features influence the histological pattern of disease. Mechanisms of usual drug reactions include the categories of toxic and idiosyncratic reactions. Although we generally try to categorize a drug reaction into one or the other category, it is not always an easy assignment, and it is possible for a drug to manifest both toxic and idiosyncratic effects. The clinical/biochemical pattern of disease includes cholestatic, hepatitic, and mixed patterns. Tumor formation and vascular abnormalities are additional manifestations of drug reactions.

I. Toxic Reactions

Toxic reactions refer to those which are the result of a direct effect of the drug or toxin on the liver and are hence dose dependent and independent of individual variation. Essentially all individuals, if given a large enough dose, suffer the toxic effect of the agent. This is not to say, however, that host factors may not influence the toxicity of a reagent. A common example of host-dependent alteration of a toxic reaction is that of acetaminophen toxicity (Chap. 18). This analgesic is well known for causing characteristic centrilobular (zone 3) hepatocellular necrosis when taken in large doses (Zimmerman 1981). Generally 10g is considered hepatotoxic to a normal individual. However, since the mechanism of toxicity involves the conversion of acetaminophen into toxic intermediate metabolites in the liver, factors that stimulate the production of these metabolites increase the toxicity of a give dose. This may be the mechanism of increased sensitivity associated with chronic alcoholism (LICHT et al. 1980). In addition, since the toxic metabolite is initially bound to glutathione, depletion of glutathione by malnutrition or fasting also increases the toxicity of a given dose (WHITCOMB and BLOCK 1994). Under such circumstances the lethal dose may be considerably less than the average lethal dose.

II. Idiosyncratic Reactions

Idiosyncratic drug reactions are those in which there is individual susceptibility to a drug, based on immunological or other genetic factors (ZIMMERMAN 1978; STRICKER 1992) (Chap. 24). Here relatively few individuals receiving the drug manifest a reaction, and those who do develop a reaction usually do so after a variable length of time and variable dose. Often there is a sensitizing dose, with a more severe reaction to a second exposure to the drug. Idiosyncratic reactions are subdivided on the basis of the presumed pathogenesis of the reaction into allergic, autoimmune, and rare other reactions.

Allergic (hypersensitivity) reactions are often characterized by eosinophilia (peripheral and/or in the tissue) and may be accompanied by other organ involvement such as skin rash. With the allergic reactions the drug effect usually becomes manifest only after a second exposure to the agent, the first exposure being required for sensitization. Allergic reactions are the most common of the idiosyncratic reactions.

Autoimmune reactions are characterized by similarities to other known autoimmune diseases such as primary biliary cirrhosis. In these patients an autoimmune phenomenon seems to be produced, perhaps with the drug acting as a cross-reacting agent which sets off an immune attack in the liver. These diseases usually manifest histologically by lymphocytic destruction of specific epithelial targets in the liver and sometimes other organs as well. An example of this type of reaction is the reaction to thiabendazole, which produces a systemic disease very similar to primary biliary cirrhosis with ductopenia and sicca syndrome (REX et al. 1983; MANIVEL et al. 1987).

Occasional other types of reactions fall into the idiosyncratic group. These include specific enzyme deficiencies that alter the ability of the liver to metabolize a drug. An example of this phenomenon is genetic variation in the acetylation of isoniazid, which may account for observed racial variation in isoniazid toxicity (BLACK et al. 1975) (Chap. 24).

III. Tumor Formation

Tumor induction and vascular reactions are difficult to place into "toxic" or "idiosyncratic" categories, and the distinction is perhaps not too important. In many ways tumor formation is a form of idiosyncratic reaction since in general only a small subset of patients receiving a drug develop tumors. There is variation in the frequency of tumor formation from agent to agent, however, with some producing a rate of occurrence strongly suggesting direct toxicity. A relatively straightforward example of direct toxicity is the radioactive agent thorium dioxide (Thoratrast), which produces its damage by direct irradiation of the liver (ITO et al. 1988; GEUBEL et al. 1988), leading to the development of hepatocellular carcinoma, cholangiocellular carcinoma, and/or angiosarcoma. Since few tumors associated with drugs occur most often as drug-associated phenomenon (i.e., sporadic tumors are more common than drug-induced ones), it is difficult if not impossible to prove that a single case is caused by the drug in question. The burden of demonstrating that a tumor is caused by a drug rests on statistical association unless a direct mechanism for tumor formation can be demonstrated, or the tumor can be shown to regress on discontinuation of the drug, as may occur with contraceptive-associated adenomas. Tumors caused by drugs and their etiological agents are shown in Table 1. Notably, most of the major tumor types seen in the liver have been associated with drugs.

IV. Vascular Reactions

Vascular diseases caused by drugs are listed in Table 2. These cover a wide spectrum and, as opposed to the tumors, are more often than not associated with drug use implying a direct toxic effect. This is especially true for those diseases involving hepatic venous outflow, veno-occlusive disease, and Budd-Chiari syndrome. The association of these reactions with drugs is therefore well established. Many if not most drug-induced vascular disease appear to occur on the basis of tissue toxicity, although the variability in occurrence for

Table 1. Representative tumors associated with drug usage

Drug	Tumor type reported
Androgenic steroids	Hepatocellular adenoma (MULVIHILL et al. 1975; BIRD et al. 1979) Hepatocellular carcinoma (JOHNSON et al. 1972) Cholangiocellular carcinoma (STROMEYER et al. 1979) Angiosarcoma (FALK et al. 1979)
Oral contraceptives	Hepatocellular adenoma (KNOWLES et al. 1978) Hepatocellular carcinoma (LADAGA et al. 1979) Cholangiocellular carcinoma (LITTLEWOOD et al. 1980)
Thorium dioxide (Thoratrast)	Hepatocellular carcinoma (ITO et al. 1988) Cholangiocellular carcinoma (ITO et al. 1988) Angiosarcoma (ITO et al. 1988)
Methyldopa	Cholangiocellular carcinoma (LITTLEWOOD et al. 1980)
Arsenic	Angiosarcoma (LANDER et al. 1975)
Vinyl chloride	Angiosarcoma (THOMAS et al. 1975)

some suggest individual susceptibility and an "idiosyncratic" component of the disease.

V. Interactions

It is important to keep in mind when evaluating possible drug reactions that some liver disease is associated with specific combinations of drugs rather than with single drugs alone. In some cases these drugs are given as part of a compound (example, with Augmentin) or are given as separate agents (GEUBEL et al. 1988).

C. General Biochemical and Histological Types of Drug Reactions

I. Hepatocellular Reactions

Hepatocellular reactions are characterized clinically by elevations of serum transaminase and histologically by hepatocellular necrosis. The necrosis may occur in any of its forms, including zonal necrosis, spotty (or focal) necrosis, and massive necrosis, or it may manifest as chronic hepatitis with piecemeal necrosis. Necrosis associated with fatty change (steatohepatitis) represents a vary characteristic form of hepatitis often associated with drug reactions.

Zonal necrosis is the type of necrosis most often associated with toxic reactions to drugs. The centrilobular zone (zone 3) is the most commonly affected although some drugs affect predominantly the other zones. In addition to being a good marker for toxic reactions, the zone involved may give a clue to the most likely responsible agent.

Table 2. Representative vascular lesions caused by drugs

Drug	Vascular disease reported
Androgenic steroids	Peliosis hepatis (NADELL and KOSEK 1977) Sinusoidal dilatation (PARADINAS et al. 1977)
Azathioprine	Sinusoidal dilatation (ZAFRANI et al. 1983) Peliosis hepatis (ZAFRANI et al. 1983) Venoocclusive disease (ZAFRANI et al. 1983)
Arsenic	Hepatoportal sclerosis (THOMAS et al. 1985)
Busulfan	Venoocclusive disease (SHULMAN et al. 1980)
Contraceptive steroids	Sinusoidal dilatation (ALPERT 1976) Budd-Chiari syndrome (LALONDE et al. 1982)
Organic tea (Comfrey tea)	Venoocclusive disease (WESTON et al. 1987)
Tamoxifen	Peliosis hepatis (LOOMUS et al. 1983)
Vinyl chloride	Hepatoportal sclerosis (THOMAS et al. 1985)

Spotty necrosis giving a histological appearance similar to acute viral hepatitis may be associated with toxic or idiosyncratic reactions. In the case of toxic reactions there is often associated cholestasis leading to a cholestatic hepatitis. The presence of granulomas or significant numbers of eosinophils in the infiltrate is characteristic of an idiosyncratic reaction.

Granulomatous reactions are commonly associated with drug reactions, particularly of the idiosyncratic type. The granulomas of drug reactions are usually associated with a hepatitic picture. They are typically epithelioid, nonnecrotizing, with or without giant cells, and usually located in the lobule. Representative examples of drugs associated with granulomas include:

Allopurinol (Koch et al. 1985)
Clavulanic acid (Stricker et al. 1989)
Halothane (Koch et al. 1985)
Hydralazine (McMaster and Hennigar 1981)
Methyldopa (McMaster and Hennigar 1981)
Nitrofurantoin (Sippel and Agger 1981)
Penicillin and derivatives (McMaster and Hennigar 1981)
Phentoin (McMaster and Hennigar 1981)
Procainamide (McMaster and Hennigar 1981)
Quinidine (Bramlet et al. 1980)
Sulfonamides (McMaster and Hennigar 1981)

Massive necrosis may be associated with toxic or idiosyncratic reactions as well. When due to toxic drugs this reaction is often a response to a massive overdose of the drug, and the association is therefore easily characterized. Idiosyncratic reactions of this type may occur following a known reaction to the drug with inadvertent readministration (Ransohoff and Jacobs 1981).

Chronic hepatitis caused by drugs usually demonstrates piecemeal necrosis and hence is histologically a form of chronic active hepatitis. The pattern of chronic hepatitis without piecemeal necrosis is rarely caused by drugs. When a drug causes a picture of chronic hepatitis, it is usually of the idiosyncratic type. Some representative drugs causing chronic hepatitis are the following (Ishak 1982; Ludwig and Axelsen 1983; Seeff 1981):

Chlorpromazine
Erythromycin
Halothane
Haloperidol
Isoniazid
Methyldopa
Nitrofurantoin
Pentamidine
Procainamide
Prophythiouracil

Sulfonamides
Tolazmide

Fatty change of the liver is common in drug reactions, particularly toxic reactions. It is often of mixed micro- and macrovesicular pattern, although occasionally a purely microvesicular reaction occurs, as with tetracycline toxicity (KUNELIS et al. 1965). When the fatty change is associated with an infiltrate and hepatocellular necrosis or with significant hepatocellular enzyme changes, the diagnosis of steatohepatitis is rendered.

Steatohepatitis may be caused by a variety of drugs in addition to alcohol. It is also commonly identified as a cause of liver dysfunction in obese patients and those with diabetes (POWELL et al. 1990). Therefore it is a nonspecific although characteristic reaction. The finding of steatohepatitis should always lead to a careful review of drug usage.

II. Cholestatic Reactions

Cholestatic reactions may be caused by toxic or idiosyncratic reactions and represent one of the more common types of drug reactions. When the reaction is characterized biochemically by isolated bilirubin elevation with minimal or no elevation of alkaline phosphatase or transaminases, the clinical differential diagnosis includes sepsis, familial cholestasis, and other rare cholestatic reactions such as postoperative cholestasis as well as drug reaction.

The histological pattern of canalicular cholestasis without an inflammatory infiltrate or portal tract changes is characteristic of a number of drugs including the classic example of contraceptive steroids (VALLA and BENHAMOU 1988) (Chap. 23) This pattern is the most characteristic histology of any drug reaction. In addition to the cholestasis one may also find mixed micro- and macrovesicular fatty change.

The second pattern of cholestatic injury is that associated with a portal inflammatory infiltrate and often bile duct damage. This pattern may resemble obstructive liver disease with bile ductular proliferation and a mixed portal infiltrate, leading to the term "cholangiolytic" drug reaction. Although there is a resemblance to obstruction, the degree of cholestasis is often out of proportion to the degree of portal tract change, a useful clue to the drug etiology of the injury. The following drugs are some of those showing this pattern with associated bile duct damage or loss (VERHAMME et al. 1989; MANIVEL et al. 1987; WOOLF and VIERLING 1993; ALTRAIF et al. 1994; DAVIES et al. 1994; ISHII et al. 1993):

Augmentin
Amoxicillin
Flucloxacillin
Chlorpromazine
Barbiturates

Phenytoin
Allopurinol
Carbamazapine
Floxuridine
Paraquat
Clindamycin
Glycyrrhicin
Thiabendazole

III. Mixed Hepatocellular-Cholestatic

Many drugs produce a mixed pattern of hepatocellular injury with cholestasis, with the degree of cholestasis often greater than seen with typical viral infections.

IV. Tumors

The variety of tumors that have been associated with drugs are listed in Table 1. In general there is nothing histopathologically distinctive about tumors associated with drugs compared with those which arise without drugs. One exception to this is the fact that hepatocellular adenomas associated with androgens are often atypical and histologically resemble hepatocellular carcinoma (CRAIG et al. 1989). Despite an ominous histological appearance these tumors generally act in a benign fashion.

Other histological peculiarities include the fact that angiosarcoma associated with vinyl chloride and arsenic may arise in a context of hepatoportal sclerosis a vascular lesion characterized by narrowing of the intrahepatic portal vein branches, and chronic hepatic ischemia (THOMAS et al. 1975; MORRIS et al. 1974). Some drugs may cause multiple types of carcinoma. Perhaps the most classic of these is the association of hepatocellular carcinoma, cholangiocellular carcinoma, and angiosarcoma with thorium dioxide (Thorotrast) (ITO et al. 1988). It is not uncommon to see two of these malignancies in the same liver in this circumstance.

V. Vascular Lesions

The nonneoplastic vascular lesions associated with drug use are listed in Table 2. Some of these, such as peliosis hepatis, nodular regenerative hyperplasia, and hepatoportal sclerosis, may occur with or without an associated drug history. Others, including veno-occlusive disease, are usually associated with drug use. There is considerable overlap in this group in that the many drugs are associated with more than one of these lesions, and there is histological overlap between the diseases as well. For example, most cases of peliosis hepatis are associated with sinusoidal dilatation, although the converse is not true. There is considerable overlap between those agents causing veno-occlusive disease and nodular regenerative hyperplasia (NRH).

There are generally no features that distinguish these entities when associated with drug use from those cases occurring sporadically or in association with other conditions. Therefore, when one of these conditions is diagnosed, the appropriate drug history should be elicited. Although many of these conditions are irreversible, even if the drug is withheld, early discontinuation should always be considered. Note that for veno-occlusive disease certain foodstuffs (in particular herbal teas) should be evaluated in addition to more obvious drug use.

The most serious drug-induced vascular disease is that associated with obstruction to hepatic outflow (veno-occlusive disease and Budd-Chiari syndrome). The distinction between veno-occlusive disease and Budd-Chiari syndrome is mainly one of the size of vessels involved, and hence somewhat arbitrary. Nevertheless, it is of interest that the drugs associated with each of these diseases are somewhat different.

In contrast with the situation in veno-occlusive disease and Budd-Chiari syndrome, the lesions of sinusoidal dilatation, NRH, and hepatoportal sclerosis are somewhat more related. Since the histological features of these three processes show marked overlap, misclassification may occur. This may be particularly true for NRH, which is often undiagnosed on needle biopsy because the findings are subtle and often go unrecognized, especially if the reticulin stain is not used to identify the characteristic regenerative change. It is possible, if not probable, that many cases of drug-induced sinusoidal dilatation (e.g., those due to steroids) would in fact represent NRH if examined carefully.

D. Clinical Evaluation and Diagnosis of Hepatic Drug Reactions

Clinical evaluation of a possible drug reaction starts with a high index of suspicion, remembering that essentially all patterns of liver disease have at one point been linked to a drug reaction, followed by a careful history, laboratory evaluation, possibly a liver biopsy, and withdrawal of the potentially offending agent. These data are then evaluated by looking at the known reported drug reactions of drugs which the patient has been receiving and then comparing the clinical and laboratory features with known aspects of the drug in question. Items to be considered are listed below. The goal is to determine the most likely candidate drug, so that a trial withdrawal of the drug may be attempted. The questions to be asked in this regard are:

1. What agents was the patient receiving?
2. What was the dosage of drug received?
3. What was the duration between beginning use of drug and onset of disease?
4. Was there associated evidence of hypersensitivity (fever, rash, etc)?

5. What was the biochemical nature of the liver disease (hepatitic, cholestatic, or mixed)?
6. What was the histological pattern of the liver disease if biopsied?
7. If the drug was discontinued, what was the duration prior to resolution of disease?

I. History

As implied in the introductory remarks, the importance of an appropriate and complete history vis-à-vis use of drugs or medications cannot be overemphasized. If the physician evaluating a patient dose not know about the presence of a potential drug reaction, it is obvious that an accurate etiological diagnosis cannot be rendered. A complete drug history should involve not only a review of current medications, but also past medications (especially the recent past), use of over-the-counter medications, use of food supplements or "health foods," possible environmental toxic agents (occupational or recreational), and use of illicit drugs. Obtaining this history may not always be easy and is influenced in part by the degree of comfort of the history taker and the patient. Use of the word "medication" instead of "drug" may be preferred since the implication of the word "drug" as possibly meaning "illicit drug" may lead to resistance by the patient. Repeated questioning may be very useful since some persons often do not recall all drug information during the initial interview. Patients should be encouraged to keep thinking about potential toxic agents and report them to the physician as they are recalled.

II. Laboratory Findings

Laboratory abnormalities in liver-associated enzymes are always nonspecific as to the cause of a liver disease, and this is not less true for drug reactions than for liver disease in general. However, this is not to say that careful evaluation of the pattern of enzyme elevations is of no value in identifying the agent responsible for liver disease. Various drugs cause relatively characteristic abnormalities that may allow some discrimination of the most likely agent when encountering a patient with liver dysfunction who is taking several agents. Perhaps the relatively most "typical" abnormality caused by a drug is a more or less pure elevation of bilirubin with minimal elevation of transaminase and/or alkaline phosphatase. Although this pattern can be seen in other liver diseases including Dubin-Johnson syndrome, benign recurrent familial cholestasis, progressive familial intrahepatic cholestasis, cholestasis of sepsis, and cholestasis of pregnancy, the differential diagnosis is more limited than the more generic hepatitis picture of transaminase elevation, and most of the items in the differential diagnosis other than drug reaction can usually be eliminated on clinical grounds. Evaluating the patient with liver dysfunction in whom drug reaction is considered always requires the consideration of other possible etiological agents, and usually the patient undergoes testing for viral hepatitis, autoimmune hepatitis, primary biliary cirrhosis, and perhaps metabolic diseases such as hemochromatosis or Wilson's disease, depending on the clinical situation. Careful clinical and laboratory evaluations theoretically allow a more selective use of diagnostic tests; however, the testing is usually performed as a battery to expedite evaluation.

III. Histopathological Findings

The histopathological findings of drug reactions are described in general above. The need for a biopsy in the case of possible drug reaction depends on the uncertainty of the diagnosis, as with most other liver diseases. Most of the time biopsy is performed because there is little or no suspicion of a drug reaction, and the etiology of the liver disease is unknown. In these circumstances the pathology may provide an initial clue leading to the evaluation of a drug etiology. In a few cases the biopsy is taken specifically to assess the effect of a drug known to cause liver disease. The most common example of this use of biopsy is to assess the degree of liver damage caused by methotrexate in patients with psoriasis. In this case the patient is generally known to be suffering some effect of the drug based on laboratory tests, and the biopsy is performed to assess the degree of fibrosis present as a guide to further use of the drug.

E. Some Specific Illustrative Drug Reactions

I. Unsuspected Acetaminophen Overdose Caused by Consumption of Nyquil

A 28-year-old man with a history of chronic alcohol abuse presented with recent onset of liver failure. He had had a febrile illness the week prior and had stayed home from work, before developing rapidly progressive liver disease characterized by abdominal pain, emesis, and shortness of breath. At presentation to the University of Minnesota Hospital his aspartate aminotransferase level was 32000 units/liter, alanine aminotransferase 12000 units/liter and bilirubin 2.7 μmols/liter. His only reported medication was occasional acetaminophen taken for his fever. He died of his liver disease prior to liver transplantation. Acetaminophen level drawn in the hospital more than 24h after the last known dose of acetaminophen was 5.3. Hepatitis A and B serology was negative. At autopsy the liver showed extensive necrosis with a predilection for the centrilobular region to be necrotic, a pattern highly suggestive of acetaminophen overdose. Careful reevaluation of the clinical history revealed that prior to going to bed several nights before his death he had consumed an 8oz bottle of Nyquil. Nyquil contains 1g/oz acetaminophen; he thus received a one-time dose of 8g, in addition to the tablets he was taking. This fact, together with his chronic alcoholism which predisposed him to the effects of acetaminophen, resulted in his death.

II. Suspected Fatal Isoniazid Toxicity Disproven by Autopsy Examination

Occasionally a drug is suspected to be the cause of a patient's liver disease when in fact another process is leading to the disease. This is illustrated by the case of a 28-year-old pregnant woman who was being treated for prophylaxis of tuberculosis because of a positive PPD result. The patient developed symptoms of fatigue and was hospitalized with mildly elevated serum transaminase levels. She delivered a term baby, but during hospitalization the patient suddenly developed cardiac arrest from which she was successfully resuscitated, followed the next day by marked elevation of transaminases into the 2000 range. Her course was progressively downhill from that point, and she died several days later. Her death was thought to be the result of massive liver necrosis due to isoniazid hepatotoxicity. Review of the histology of the liver at autopsy was not consistent with this diagnosis, however. There was marked centrilobular necrosis and congestion consistent with shock liver and congestive heart failure. Isoniazid typically produces diffuse massive necrosis or chronic hepatitis, not the pattern of necrosis seen in this case. The heart showed features of postpartum cardiomyopathy, which was determined to be the cause of death, not liver disease.

III. Toxicity Due to Health Food ("Hot Stuff")

A 20-year-old man presented with sudden onset of jaundice and elevated transaminase and bilirubin levels. Workup was negative for hepatitis A, B, and C serologies as well as for antimitochondrial, anti-smooth-muscle, and antinuclear antibodies. Liver biopsy was performed, which showed diffuse hepatocellular necrosis with a portal and lobular infiltrate composed mainly of lymphocytes with numerous eosinophils but very few plasma cells. The biopsy was considered most consistent with a drug reaction due to the presence of numerous eosionophils in the face of a diffuse hepatitic process, although autoimmune hepatitis was also considered in the differential diagnosis despite the paucity of plasma cells and the negative serology. Review of the history failed to disclose any medication or drug use, and the patient was placed on steroids with the presumptive diagnosis of possible autoimmune hepatitis. There was a gradual response to these steroids although complete resolution did not occur quickly. Despite the initial failure to identify a drug exposure, the patient eventually confided to a member of the house staff that although he took no medications, he did take a food supplement called "Hot Stuff" as part of a body-building program. The label from a container of "Hot Stuff" was obtained and revealed a bewildering array of organic substances, including multiple exotic tree barks and various desiccated animal organs. Since most of the items listed were, to say the least, not easily identifiable as known causes of liver disease, the patient was instructed to avoid "Hot Stuff" since it may have been the cause of his liver disease. Since withdrawal he has shown continued improvement in his liver function tests. Although it is not possible to prove a relationship between this "health food" and the liver disease, the presumptive diagnosis is that of drug-induced liver disease, of an odd sort.

F. Summary of the Clinical Approach to Drug Toxicity

1. Make sure the drug history is complete and includes past and present medications, over-the-counter drugs, food supplements, and environmental exposures.
2. Correlate the onset of liver disease to the use of each agent.
3. Review the typical biochemical features, time to onset, usual toxic dosage, and typical histological patterns known to be produced by each drug in the patient's drug list.
4. Compare the features determined in step 3 with the patient's known clinical situation to determine the most likely candidate drug(s).
5. Discontinue the drug.

References

Alpert LI (1976) Veno-occlusive disease of the liver associated with oral contraceptives. Case report and review of literature. Hum Pathol 7:709–718

Altraif I, Lilly L, Wanless IR, Heathcote J (1994) Cholestatic liver disease with ductopenia (vanishing bile duct syndrome) after administration of clindamycin and trimethoprim-sulfamethoxazole. Am J Gastroenterol 89:1230–1234

Bird D, Vowles K, Anthony PP (1979) Spontaneous rupture of a liver cell adenoma after long term methyltestosterone. Report of a case treated by emergency right hepatic lobectomy. Br J Surg 66:212–213

Black M, Mitchell JR, Zimmerman HJ et al. (1975) Isoniazid associated hepatitis in 114 patients. Gastroenterology 69:289–302

Bramlet DA, Posalaky Z, Olson R (1980) Granulomatous hepatitis as a manifestation of quinidine hypersensitivity. Arch Intern Med 140:395–397

Craig JR, Peters RL, Edmondson HA (1989) Tumors of the liver and intrahepatic bile ducts. In: Craig JR (ed) Atlas of tumor pathology, 2nd series, fascicle 26. Armed Forces Institute of Pathology, Washington DC

Davies MH, Harrison RF, Elias E, Hubscher SG (1994) Antibiotic-associated acute vanishing bile duct syndrome: a pattern associated with severe, prolonged, intrahepatic cholestasis. J Hepatol 20:112–116

Falk H, Thomas LB, Popper H, Ishak KG (1979) Hepatic angiosarcoma associated with androgenic-anabolic steroids. Lancet 2:1120–1123

Gerber A, Raab AP, Sobel AE (1954) Vitamin A poisoning in adults, with description of a case. Am J Med 16:729

Geubel AP, Nakad A, Rahier J, Dive C (1988) Prolonged cholestasis and disappearance of interlobular bile ducts following chlorpropamide and erythromycin ethylsuccinate. Case of drug interaction? Liver 8:350–353

Ishak KG (1982) The liver. In: Riddell RH (ed) Pathology of drug-induced and toxic diseases. Churchill-Livingstone, New York

Ishii M, Miyazaki Y, Yamamoto T, Miura M, Ueno Y, Takahashi T, Toyota T (1993) A case of drug-induced ductopenia resulting in fatal biliary cirrhosis. Liver 13:227–231

Ito Y, Kojiro M, Nakashima T, Mori T (1988) Pathomorphologic characteristics of 102 cases of Thorotras-related hepatocellular carcinoma, cholangiocarcinoma, and hepatic angiosarcoma. Cancer 62:1153–1162

Johnson FL, Feagler JR, Lerner KG et al. (1972) Association of androgenic-anabolic steroid therapy with development of hepatocellular carcinoma. Lancet 2:1273–1276

Knowles DM, Casarella WJ, Johnson PM, Wolff M (1978) The clinical, radiologic, and pathologic characterization of benign hepatic neoplasms: alleged association with oral contraceptives. Medicine 57:223–237

Koch HK, Gropp A, Oehlert W (1985) Drug-induced liver injury in liver biopsies of the years 1981 and 1983, their prevalence and type of presentation. Pathol Res Pract 179:469–477

Kowalski TE, Falestiny M, Furth E, Malet PF (1994) Vitamin A hepatotoxicity: a caustionary note regarding 25 000 IU supplements. Am J Med 97:523–528

Kunelis CT, Peters JL, Edmondson HA (1965) Fatty liver of pregnancy and its relationship to tetracycline toxicity. Am J Med 38:359–377

Ladaga L, Kay S, Melcher M, King JN (1979) Combined epithelial and sarcomatous elements in a liver cancer associated with oral contraceptive use. Am J Surg Pathol 3:185–190

Lalonde G, Theoret G, Daloze P et al. (1982) Inferior vena cava stenosis and Budd-Chiari syndrome in a woman taking oral contraceptives. Gastroenterology 82:1452–1456

Lander JJ, Stanley RJ, Sumner HW, Boswell DC, Aach RD (1975) Angiosarcoma of the liver associated with Fowler's solution (potassium arsenite). Gastroenterology 68:1582–1586

Licht H, Seiff LB, Zimmerman HJ (1980) Apparent potentiation of acetaminophen hepatotoxicity by alcohol. Ann Intern Med 92:511

Littlewood E, Barrison I, Murray-Lyon IM, Paradinas FJ (1980) Cholangiocarcinoma and oral contraceptives. Lancet 1:310–311

Loomus GN, Aneja P, Bota RA (1983) A case of peliosis hepatis in association with tamoxifen therapy. Am J Clin Pathol 80:881–882

Ludwig J, Axelsen R (1983) Drug effects on the liver: an updated tabular compilation of drugs and drug-related hepatic diseases. Dig Dis Sci 28:651–666

Manivel JC, Bloomer JR, Snover DC (1987) Progressive bile duct injury after thiabendazole administration. Gastroenterology 93:245–249

McMaster KR III, Hennigar GR (1981) Drug-induced granulomatous hepatitis. Lab Invest 44:61–73

Morris JS, Schmid M, Newman S, Scheuer PJ, Sherlock S (1974) Arsenic and noncirrhotic portal hypertension. Gastroenterology 66:86–94

Mulvihill J, Ridolfi R, Schultz F, Borzy MS, Haughton PBT (1975) Hepatic adenoma in fanconi anemia treated with oxymetholone. J Pediatr 87:122–124

Nadell J, Kosek J (1977) Peliosis hepatis. Twelve cases associated with oral androgen therapy. Arch Pathol Lab Med 101:405–410

Paradinas FJ, Bull TB, Westaby D, Murry-Lyon IM (1977) Hyperplasia and prolapse of hepatocytes into hepatic veins during longterm methyltestosterone therapy: possible relationships of these changes to the development of peliosis hepatis and liver tumours. Histopathology 1:225–246

Powell EE, Cooksley WGE, Hanson R, Searle J, Halliday JW, Powell LW (1990) The natural history of nonalcoholic steatohepatitis: a follow-up study of forty-two patients for up to 21 years. Hepatology 11:74–80

Ransohoff DF, Jacobs G (1981) Terminal hepatic failure following a small dose of sulfamethoxazole-trimethoprim. Gastroenterology 80:816–819

Rex D, Lumeng L, Eble J, Rex L (1983) Intrahepatic cholestasis and sicca complex after thiabendazole: report of a case and review of the literature. Gastroenterology 85:718–721
Seeff LB (1981) Drug-induced chronic liver disease, with emphasis on chronic active hepatitis. Semin Liver Dis 1:104–115
Shulman HM, McDonald GB, Mathews D (1980) An analysis of hepatic veno-occlusive disease and centrilobular hepatic degeneration following bone marrow transplantation. Gastroenterology 79:1178–1191
Sippel PJ, Agger WA (1981) Nitrofurantoin-induced granulomatous hepatitis. Urology 18:177–178
Stricker BHC (1992) Drug-induced hepatic injury, 2nd edn. Elsevier Science, Amsterdam
Stricker BH, Van der Broek JW, Keuning J et al. (1989) Cholestatic hepatitis due to antibacterial combination of amoxicillin and clavulanic acid (augmentin). Dig Dis Sci 34:1576–1580
Stromeyer FW, Smith DH, Ishak KG (1979) Anabolic steroid therapy and intrahepatic cholangiocarcinoma. Cancer 43:440–443
Thomas LB, Popper H, Berk PD, Selikoff I, Falk H (1975) Vinyl-chloride-induced liver disease. From idiopathic portal hypertension (Banti's syndrome) to angiosarcomas. N Engl J Med 292:17–22
Thomas LB, Popper H, Berk PD, Selikoff I, Falk H, Koch HK, Gropp A, Oehlert W (1985) Drug-induced liver injury in liver biopsies of the years 1981 and 1983, their prevalence and type of presentation. Pathol Res Pract 179:469–477
Valla D, Benhamou JP (1988) Liver diseases related to oral contraceptives. Dig Dis 6:76–86
Verhamme M, Ramboer C, Van de Bruaene P, Inderadjaja N (1989) Cholestatic hepatitis due to amoxycillin/clavulanic acid preparation. J Hepatol 9:260–264
Weston CF, Cooper BT, Davies JD, Levine DF (1987) Veno-occlusive disease of the liver secondary to ingestion of comfrey. Br Med J 295:183
Whitcomb DC, Block GD (1994) Association of acetaminophen hepatotoxicity with fasting and ethanol use. JAMA 272:1845–1850
Woolf GM, Vierling JM (1993) Disappearing intrahepatic bile ducts: the syndromes and their mechanisms. Semin Liver Dis 13:261–275
Zafrani ES, Pinaudeau Y, Dhumeaux D (1983) Drug-induced vascular lesions of the liver. Arch Intern Med 143:495–502
Zimmerman HJ (1978) Hepatotoxicity. Appleton-Century-Crofts, New York
Zimmerman HJ (1981) Effects of aspirin and acetaminophen on the liver. Arch Intern Med 141:333–342

CHAPTER 20

Antimicrobial Drugs

H.J. ZIMMERMAN and K.G. ISHAK

Among the large number of antimicrobial agents, there are some that lead to little or no injury (e.g., streptomycin, penicillin k), some that lead to idiosyncratic injury (e.g., erythromycin), and some that are intrinsic hepatotoxins (e.g., tetracycline). Some can lead to cytotoxic (hepatocellular) injury with either necrosis (Figs. 1, 2) or steatosis (Fig. 3). Some lead to cholestasis (Fig. 4) or mixed injury (Fig. 5). The necrosis is usually nonzonal (Fig. 1) and uncommonly zonal (Fig. 2). Several drugs can lead to chronic hepatitis (Fig. 6) and some to chronic cholestasis (Fig. 7). In Table 1 are listed the various antimicrobial agents and the hepatic injury associated with their use.

A. Antibiotics

I. Aminoglycosides

Hepatic injury is very rarely attributable to this group. Increased levels of aminotransferase and alkaline phosphatase have been reported in some recipients of gentamicin and of amikacin (STRICKER 1992), and rare instances of cholestatic jaundice have been attributed to tobramycin (VANDERCARR and DRIER 1981). At least one instance of hepatocellular injury has been attributed to Kanamycin (IMOTO and MATSUMOTO 1979). Despite wide usage of streptomycin, hepatic injury has hardly been attributed to this drug.

II. Cephalosporins

These agents rarely provoke significant hepatic injury. Rare instances of mixed cholestatic injury have been attributed to cefazolin, cefotoxime ceftazidime, cepalothin cepachlor, cephalexin and maxolactam. Transient elevation of aminotransferase levels has been seen in recipients of each of these agents (STRICKER 1992).

III. Chloramphenicol

This agent, far more infamous for adverse hematologic reactions than for adverse hepatic effects, has been incriminated in at least 25 instances of hepatic injury. Some appear to have been hepatocellular and others cholestatic. The mechanism is unclear (ZIMMERMAN 1978).

IV. Clindamycin

Elevated levels of aminotransferases develop in 40%–50% of recipients of this drug (FASS and SASLOW 1972). So high an incidence suggests intrinsic, mild hepatotoxicity. Nevertheless, instances of clinically overt hepatocellular injury have been rare (ELMORE et al. 1974). Lincomycin, which is structurally almost identical, only lacking the chlorination at the C-7 position, appears to have no adverse effects on the liver (ZIMMERMAN 1978).

V. Colimycin

Only one individual report of hepatic injury attributable to this drug has been reported, an unimportant event in the career of an unimportant antibiotic.

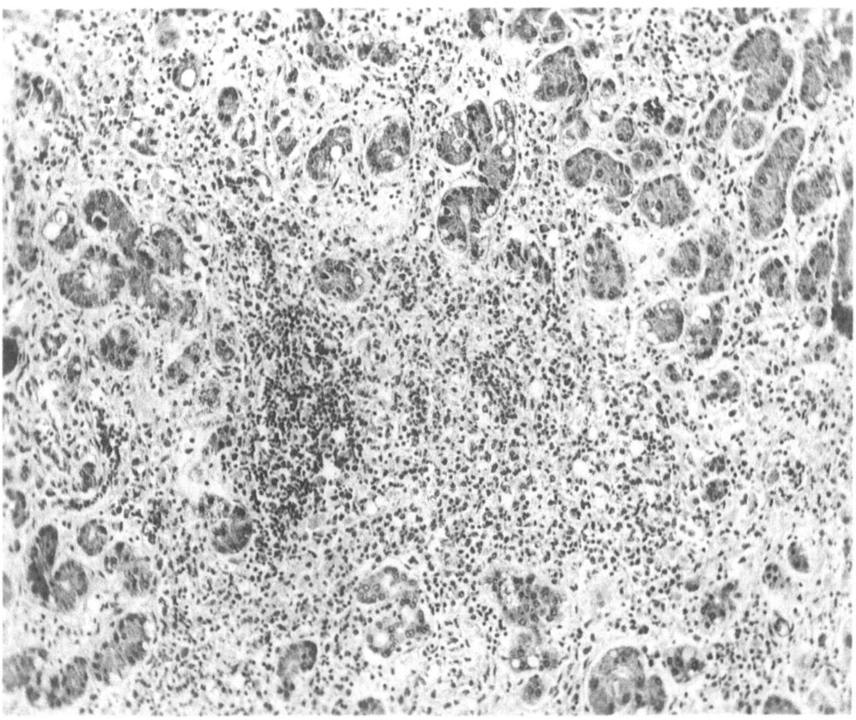

Fig. 1. Massive necrosis secondary to isoniazid therapy. Only a few isolated liver plates have survived. Note the stromal and portal area (*left, center*) inflammation. H&E, ×90

VI. Erythromycin

Although erthythromycin estolate has received the most attention, all preparations except erthromycin base can lead to hepatic injury, and even erythromycin base has been incriminated in one case (ZIMMERMAN and MADDREY 1993). Jaundice occurs in 1%–2% of adult recipients of erythromycin estolate but very rarely in children taking the drug (BRAUN 1973). The jaundice is usually cholestatic. Liver biopsy shows bile casts and a prominent portal inflammatory infiltration, usually rich in eosinophils (Fig. 4). There may be minor parenchymal injury and in some patients hepatic necrosis occurs, yielding a mixed picture (Fig. 5). Ductal injury can occur.

Jaundice, pruritus, abdominal pain, and elevated aminotransferase levels appear 2–21 days after initiation of treatment (ZIMMERMAN 1978). Abdominal pain occurs in approximately 75% of patients and may be so severe that it leads to needless laparotomy (FISCHER and HOAK 1964). The symptoms of liver disease usually subside promptly when the drug is withdrawn. Rarely, jaundice may remain for 6 months or more.

The blood and tissue eosinophilia, fever, and rash that accompany the hepatic injury all suggest the mechanism to be immunologic idiosyncrasy

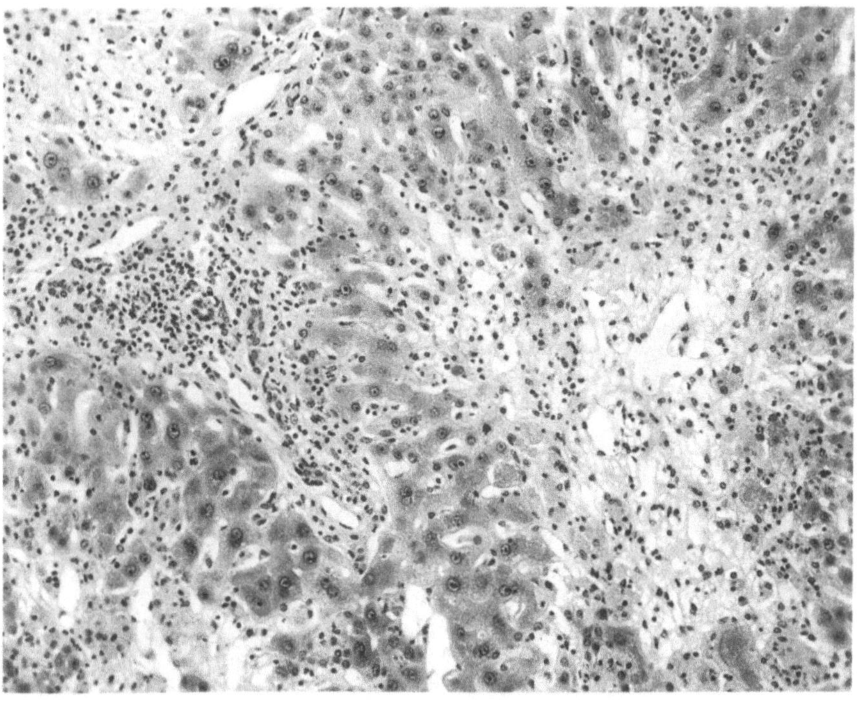

Fig. 2. Zone 3 necrosis associated with ketoconazole therapy. There is dropout of hepatocytes around a terminal hepatic venule (*right*). Portal area (*left*) is infiltrated with a moderate number of inflammatory cells. H&E, ×250

(hypersensitivity). However, the high incidence of hepatic dysfunction in patients taking erythromycin estolate (TICKIN and ROBINSON 1963) and the demonstration that this compound can damage isolated hepatocytes (DUJOVNE et al. 1972) and the ex vivo perfused liver (KENDLER et al. 1972) suggest that intrinsic hepatotoxicity of the agent and its congeners may contribute to the hepatic injury.

VII. Fusidic Acid

This steroid-like antibiotic, used primarily in the treatment of staphylococcal infections, can lead to cholestatic jaundice (HUMBLE et al. 1980).

VIII. Roxithromycin

This semisynthetic derivative of erythromycin has seemed less likely to produce hepatic injury than erythromycin. However, PILLANS and MALING (1993) have recently reported six cases of cholestatic or mixed hepatic injury.

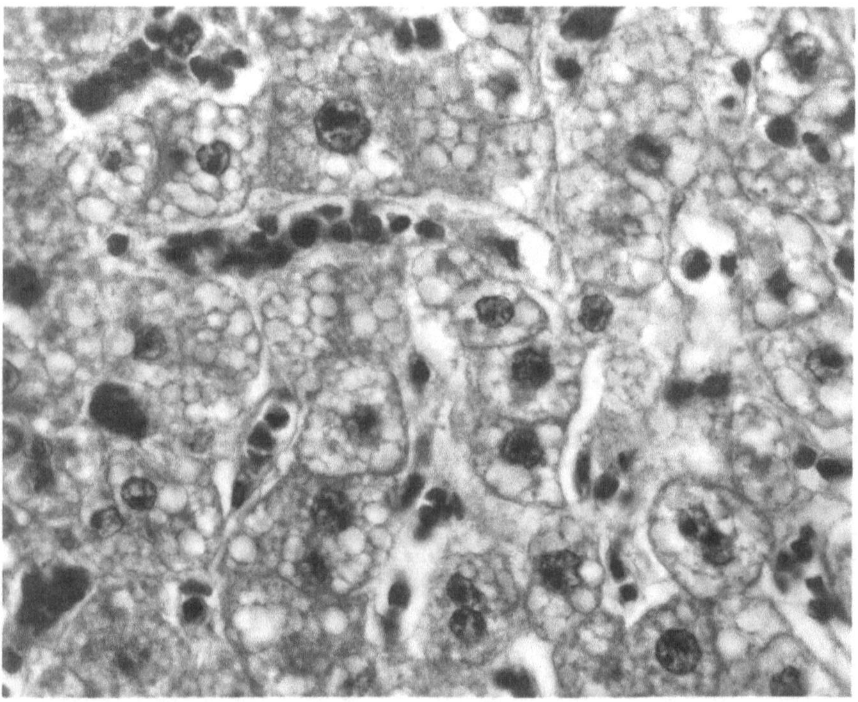

Fig. 3. Microvesicular steatosis associated with tetracycline therapy. Note the multiplicity and small size of the vacuoles in the cytoplasm of the liver cells, and the centrally located nuclei. H&E, ×630

IX. Tetracyclines

This group of drugs has been known since midcentury to produce hepatic injury (LEPPER et al. 1951). Large doses (>1.5 g) of oxytetracycline (Terramycin), chlortetracycline (Aureomycin), or tetracycline (Achromycin) administered intravenously can produce hepatic injury in humans and in experimental animals. The lesion, which is microvesicular steatosis, and the clinical syndrome resemble fatty liver of pregnancy and Reye's syndrome (Fig. 3). While all tetracyclines presumably can lead to the lesion, the potential for the injury differs. However, the lesser incidence with minocycline (Minocin) and doxycycline (Vibramycin) has been attributed (STRICKER 1992) to the lower doses used and the nonparenteral route of administration.

Doxycycline and minocline have also led to a different type of lesion. Doxycycline has led to cholestatic jaundice (SCHRUMPF and NORDGARD 1986) and minocycline has been reported to lead to macrovesicular steatosis in one case (CHATHAM and ROSS 1983).

X. Troleandomycin (Triacetyloleandomycin, TAO)

This drug produced jaundice in 4% and hepatic dysfunction in over 50% of one group of patients who had been taking 2 g/day for 2 or more weeks (TICKIN

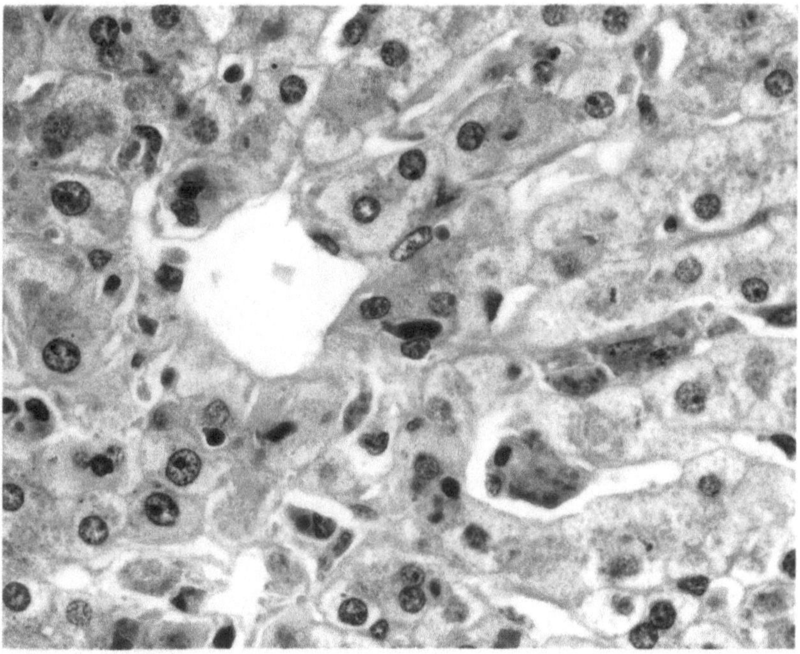

Fig. 4. Intrahepatic cholestasis associated with erythromycin estolate therapy. Bile plugs are present in several canaliculi around the terminal hepatic venule. Bile is also present in the cytoplasm of hypertrophied Kupffer cells (*right*). H&E, ×600

and ZIMMERMAN 1962). The histologic features and the pattern of hepatic dysfunction produced by this drug have been those of mixed injury with hepatocellular and cholestatic features. Mild parenchymal damage and bilirubin casts are seen. TAO appears to be a mild intrinsic hepatotoxin. Individual metabolic differences between different persons presumably determine the extent of hepatic injury. Administration of TAO to patients who are taking oral contraceptives (OCs) can provoke jaundice, a phenomenon attributed to inhibition of OC metabolism by TAO (FEVERY et al. 1983).

XI. Penicillin

Hypersensitivity reactions from penicillin, especially with fever and rashes, are common, but reports of hepatic injury due to penicillin are very rare (DAVIES and HOLMES 1972). Among the huge number of patients who have been given penicillin, very few instances of liver damage have been reported. A few have had reversible cholestatic or hepatocellular injury (ZIMMERMAN 1978). One instance of prolonged cholestasis has been attributed to penicillin (WILLIAMS and MALTJALINE 1981).

Several semisynthetic penicillin derivatives, however, seem to produce jaundice or biochemical evidence of hepatic injury more commonly

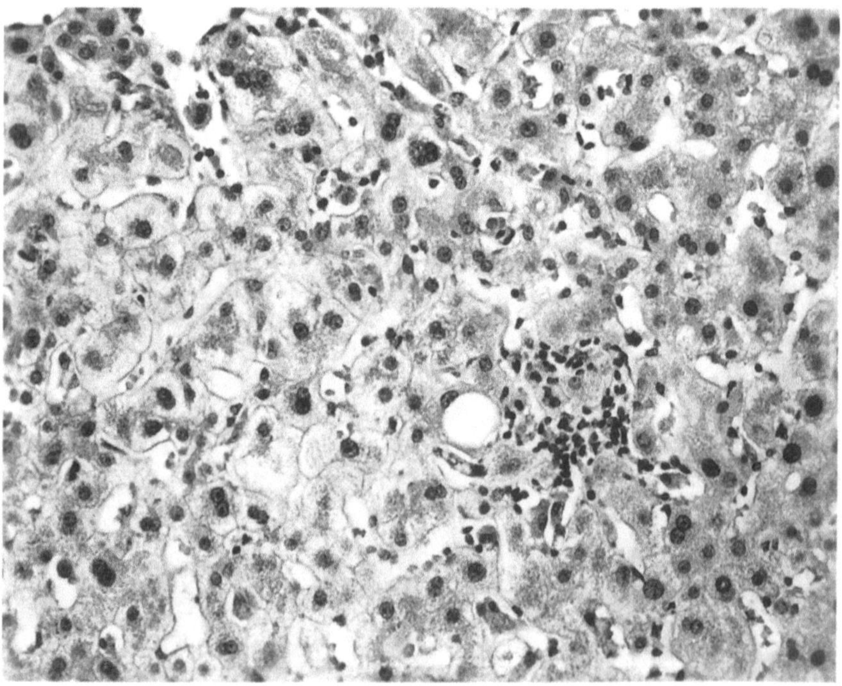

Fig. 5. Acute hepatocellular injury due to erythromycin estolate. Note ballooning degeneration and focal necrosis. H&E, 250

(ZIMMERMAN and MADDREY 1993). Carbenicillin can cause mild hepatic injury (WILSON et al. 1975). Intravenous oxacillin has also been reported to cause cholestasis (TEN-PAS and QUIN 1965) and nonspecific hepatitis that returned on rechallenge (FREEDMAN 1965; DISMUKAS 1973). Cloxacillin (ENAT et al. 1980), dicloxicillin (KLEINMAN and PRESBERG 1984), and flucloxacillin (ECKSTEIN et al. 1993) can each lead to severe cholestasis. Indeed, flucloxacillin has been implicated as the cause of cholestatic liver damage in more than 50 cases. Several have had prolonged cholestasis, even proceeding to a syndrome resembling primary biliary cirrhosis (ECKSTEIN et al. 1993). Amoxacillin-clavulanic acid (Augmentin) has led to a number of instances of cholestatic jaundice (REDDY et al. 1989). One had a prolonged and ultimately fatal course (HEBBARD et al. 1992).

B. Synthetic Antimicrobials

I. Organic Arsenicals

Intrahepatic cholestasis due to a drug reaction was first described in recipients of arsphenamine. The careful description by HANGER and GUTMAN (1940) of

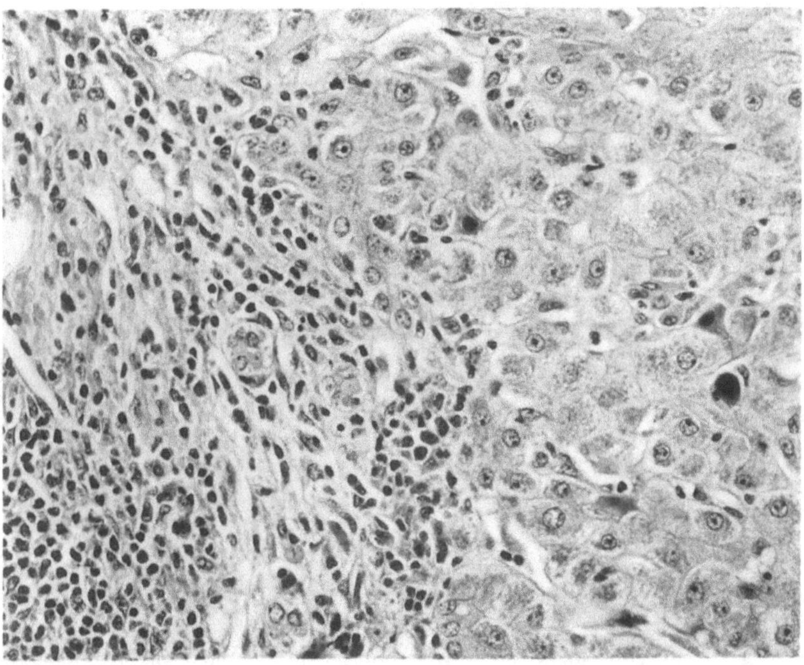

Fig. 6. Chronic hepatitis in patient on nitrofurantoin. There is marked portal inflammation (*left*) and periportal piecemeal necrosis. Note apoptotic (acidophilic) body (*right*). H&E, ×300

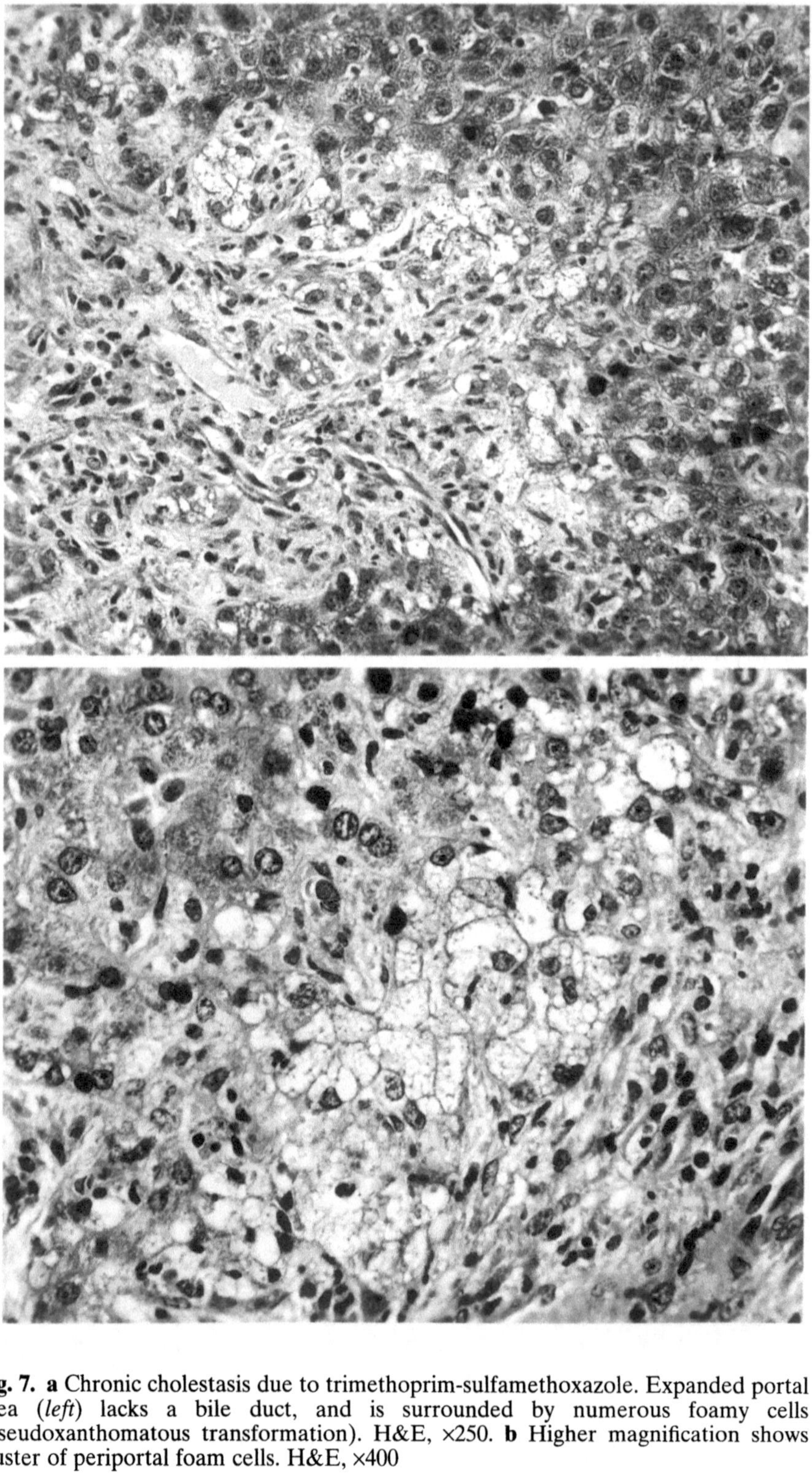

a

b

Fig. 7. **a** Chronic cholestasis due to trimethoprim-sulfamethoxazole. Expanded portal area (*left*) lacks a bile duct, and is surrounded by numerous foamy cells (pseudoxanthomatous transformation). H&E, ×250. **b** Higher magnification shows cluster of periportal foam cells. H&E, ×400

Table 1. Hepatic injury associated with antimicrobial agents

Agent	Injury	Speculated mechanism	Other injury or comments
Antibiotics			
Amikacin	AT	[a]	
Amphotericin	See antifungal agents		
Cephaclor	Ch	I[b]	
Cephalexin	H cell	I[b]	
Cephalothin	Ch	I[b]	
Cephazolin	Ch	I[b]	
Chloramphenicol	h cell, Ch	I	
Clindamycin	H cell	I	
Erythromycin base	Ch (?)	[b]	One case reported
Erythromycin estolate	Ch	HS	
Erythromycin ethylsuccinate	Ch	HS	
Erygthromycin gluceptate	None		
Erythromycin lavtobionate	H cell	I[b]	One case reported
Flucytosine	See antifungal agents		
Fusidic acid	Ch	Intr.	
Gentamicin	AT	[a]	
Griseofulvin	See antifungal agents		
Imipenem-cilastin	AT	[a]	
Josamycin	H cell, Ch	[b]	
Kanamycin	H cell	[b]	One case reported
Ketonconazole	See antifungal agents		
Lincomycin	None		
Moxalactam	AT	[a]	
Novobiocin	H cell	HS	[c]
Rifampin	H cell	HS	[c]
Roxithromycin	CH		
Spectinomycin	AT	[a]	
Tetracycline	Microvesicular	Intr.[d]	
Thiamphenicol	H cell	[b]	One case reported
Troleandomycin	M	MI	
Pencillins			
Pencillin K	H cell, Ch	HS	Extraordinarily rare
Amoxicillin	AT	[a]	
Amoxicillin clavulanate	Ch	HS	
Ampicillin	H cell, Ch	HS	Chronic cholestasis[f]
Carbenicillin	AT	[a]	
Cloxacillin	Ch	HS	
Dicloxacillin	Ch	HS	
Flucloxacillin	Ch	HS	
Methicillin	AT	[a]	
Nafcillin	AT	[a]	
Oxacillin	H cell, Ch	HS	
Piperacillin	AT	[a]	
Ticarcillin	AT	[a]	
Synthetic antimicrobials			
Arsenicals, organic	Ch	HS	Chronic cholestasis
Cinoxacin	J	I[c]	
Ciproflaxacin	H cell	HS[h]	Personal case
Furazolidone	H cell, Ch	HS	
Nalidixic acid	H cell, Ch	HS	
Nitrofurantoin	H cell, Ch	HS	
Norfloxacin	H cell	I[h]	Personal case
Ofloxcin	H cell, Ch	I	
Para-aminosalicylic acid	H cell	HS	

Table 1. (*Contd.*)

Agent	Injury	Speculated mechanism	Other injury or comments
Synthetic antimicrobials			
Sulfonamides[g]	H cell, Ch, M	HS	
Sulfasalazine	H cell	HS	
Sulfamethoxazole-trimethoprim	Ch, H cell, M	HS	Chronic cholestasis
Sulfadoxine-pyrimethamine	h cell, Ch	HS	
Sulfadiazine-trimethoprim	J	HS	In dogs
Sulfones (dapsone)	H cell	HS	
Antifungal agents			
Amphotericin	H cell	I[b]	Very rare
Fluconazole	AT	[a]	
Flucytosine	Ch	MI	
Griseofulvin	Ch	MI	Porphyria relapse
Itraconazole	None		
Ketoconazole	H cell	MI	
Miconazole	AT	[a]	
Saramycetin	Hyperbilirubinemia	Intr.[c]	
Antituberculosis agents			
Cycloserine	AT	[a]	
Ethionamide	H cell	MI	
Isoniazid	H cell	MI	
p-Aminosalicylic acid	H cell	HS	
Prothionamide	H cell	MI	
Pyrazinamide	H cell	MI	
Rifampin	H cell	HS	[c]
Streptomycin	None		
Thiosemicarbazone	H cell	MI	Fat, necrosis
Antiviral agents			
Acyclovir	AT	[a]	
Amantadine	None		
Cytosine arabinoside	H cell	I	
2,3′-Dideoxygrosine	AT	Inh.	65% incidence
2,3′-Dideoxycytidine	None		
Foscarnet	None		
Gancyclovir	AT	[a]	
Idoxyuridine	Ch	I	
Interferons	H cell	?	
Interferon inducers	AT	[a]	
Ribavirin	AT	[a]	
Rimantidine	None		
Xenazoic acid	Ch	HS	
Zidovudine	H cell	I	Steatosis
Antiprotozoal agents			
Amodiaquine	H cell	I	
Carbarsone	Ch	HS	Chronic cholestasis
Chiniofon	H cell	Intr.[e]	
Chloroquine	H cell	I	Phospholipidosis
Diliodoquine	H cell	Intr.[e]	
Emetine	H cell	Intr.[e]	
Hydroxychloroquine	H cell	I	
Mefloquine	AT	[a]	
Mepacrine	H cell	I	
Metronidazole	H cell, Ch	I[b]	Mutagenic
Nifurtimox		?	
Pentamidine	AT	[a]	
Primaquine	H cell	[a]	
Quinine	H Cell	[e]	Granulomas

Table 1. (*Contd.*)

Agent	Injury	Speculated mechanism	Other injury or comments
Pyrimethamine	See sulfodoxine	HS	
Stilbamidine	H cell	I	
Suramin	AAT	[a]	Phospholipidosis
Tryparsamide	H cell, Ch	I	
Vioform	H cell		
Antimetazoan			
Albendazole	H cell	I	
Amoscanate	AT	[a]	
Antimonials	H cell	Intr.	Variable
Dichlorophen	H cell	Intr.	
Diethylcarbarzine	H cell	?	
Flavaspidic acid	Hyperbilirubinemia	Intr.	[c]
Hycanthone	H cell	Intr.	Carcinogenic
Levimasole	AT	[g]	
Mebendazole	H cell	I	
Niclofolan	Ch	I[b]	One case reported
Niridozole	AT	[a]	
Oxaminiquine	AT	[a]	
Praziquantel	AT	[a]	
Pyrantel	AT	[a]	
Thiabendazole	Ch	I	Chronic cholestasis[f]

Ch, cholestatic injury; H cell, hepatocellular injury; M, mixed hepatocellular-cholestatic injury; J, jaundice, not further characterized in reports; HS, hypersensitivity; I, idiosyncratic reaction, type not clear; MI, metabolic idiosyncrasy; Intr., intrinsic toxicity of agent.

[a] Abnormality shows only as elevated aminotransferase levels presumed to reflect minor intrinsic toxicity of agents.

[b] Too few cases for clear picture.

[c] Dose-related dysfunction leads to hyperbilirubinemia.

[d] One derivative, minacycline, has led to a case of apparent hypersensitivity-provoked hepatic injury.

[e] Dose-related hepatic injury in experimental animals. No apparent hepatotoxic effects.

[f] Resembles primary biliary cirrhosis.

[g] Sulfoamides that have been incriminated in hepatic injury include sulfadiazine, sulfadimethoxine, sulfadoxine, sulfanilamide, sulfapyridine, sulfasuccidine, sulfathalidine, sulfathiazole and sulfasoxazole.

the first clearly recognized cases of cholestatic jaundice, apparently resulting from drug allergy, is a milestone in the history of drug-induced hepatic disease. Based on the occurrence of fever and eosinophilia, the syndrome was ascribed to drug hypersensitivity.

The pattern of biochemical abnormality in arsphenamine jaundice closely simulated that of obstructive jaundice. Prolonged cholestasis and a syndrome resembling that of primary biliary cirrhosis was reported to follow arsenical jaundice (Haubrich and Sancetta 1954).

II. Quinolones

There has been little evidence of important hepatic injury attributable to agents of this group. Cinoxacin (Cinobac), norfloxacin (Noroxin), ciprofloxacin (Cipro), nalidixic acid, and ofloxacin (Taravid) have each been incriminated in isolated instances of hepatocellular or cholestatic injury (Stricker 1992).

III. Sulfonamides

Many instances of acute hepatic injury have appeared to be due to sulfonamides during the past half-century (DUJOVNE et al. 1967). Most have shown hepatic necrosis and hepatocellular or mixed jaundice, although cholestatic jaundice has been described (GUTMAN 1957), and an instance of chronic hepatitis has been sttributed to a sulfonamide (TONDER et al. 1974). The rash, fever, eosinophilia, and tissue eosinophil aggregation and granulomas seen in many of the patients, and the relatively fixed latent period of 5–14 days that usually precedes the jaundice, suggest that hypersensitivity is the mechanism for the hepatic damage (DUJOVNE et al. 1967). One published report describes cholestatic jaundice from use of a sulfonamide-containing vaginal cream (MAGEE et al. 1982).

IV. Sulfamethoxazole-Trimethoprim (SMZ-TMP, Bactrim, Septra)

This preparation has led to jaundice in a number of patients. The injury has been reported to be cholestatic or mixed in most instances, but hepatocellular injury can occur. Indeed, severe hepatic necrosis has occurred in some cases. The clinical features are consistent with hypersensitivity as the mechanism (ZIMMERMAN and MADDREY 1993). In at least one instance, injury has been reprovoked by a challenge dose of trimethoprim (TANNER 1986). Patients with AIDS seem particularly likely to develop hepatic injury while taking the preparation (GORDIN et al. 1984). Prolonged cholestasis (Fig. 4) has been reported (MUNOZ et al. 1990).

V. Sulfasalazine (Azulfidine)

This sulfonamide has also been associated with a number of instances of liver injury, usually hepatocellular (ZIMMERMAN and MADDREY 1993). The syndrome resembles other sulfonamide-induced injury in that fever, rash, arthralgias, and hepatitis develop within 1–4 weeks of starting the drug. Low serum complement and circulating immune complexes support the assumption of immunologic idiosyncrasy as the mechanism (MIHAS et al. 1978).

VI. Sulfones

This group of drugs produces hepatic injury similar to that of the sulfonamides. Sulfones appear to produce hepatic injury more often than do the sulfonamides. The incidence has been reported to be about 5% in recipients of the prototypic compound dapsone (BASS 1965). Jaundice appears to be mixed-hepatocellular. The hepatic changes mimic those of infection mononucleosis. The mechanism for the hepatic injury is not clear; hypersensitivity presumably plays a role (ZIMMERMAN 1978).

VII. Nitrofurantoin

Acute hepatic injury from nitrofurantoin may be cholestatic or hepatocellular (ZIMMERMAN and MADDREY 1993). Clinical features suggest that the mechanism is hypersensitivity, although toxic metabolites have been suspected in some cases. Many instances of "chronic active hepatitis" (Fig. 6) have been attributed to this drug (ZIMMERMAN and MADDREY 1993). Females are affected predominantly. The syndrome resembles the autoimmune type of chronic hepatitis (SHARP et al. 1980). Granulomatous hepatitis has also been reported (SIPPEL and AGGER 1981).

VIII. Furazolidone

This furan antimicrobial is related to nitrofurantoin. It has also been reported to lead to both hepatocellular and cholestatic injury (ZIMMERMAN 1978). One report describes cholestatic jaundice provoked by intravaginal administration of furazolidone to a patient who had developed jaundice when taking nitrofurantoin (ENGEL et al. 1975).

C. Antituberculous Drugs

Clarification of the hepatotoxic role of a particular agent in this group has been complicated by the use of drugs in combination. Nevertheless, former use of *P*-aminosalicylic acid (PAS) alone or with streptomycin, and the current use of isoniazid (INH) alone to treat "tuberculin-converters," has permitted deductions regarding the ability of individual agents to produce hepatic injury. Streptomycin, dihydrostreptomycin, and ethambutol appear largely free of hepatotoxic potential, but PAS, INH, and rifampin can cause liver damage (ZIMMERMAN 1978). Rifampin appears to potentiate by enzyme induction the ability of INH to produce hepatic injury (PESSAYRE 1982). The rarity of INH toxicity during its use with PAS suggests that PAS may inhibit INH hepatotoxicity. Injury caused by congeners of INH (pyrazinamide and ethionamide) probably also reflects conversion to a toxic metabolite, and the injury may be regarded as metabolic idiosyncrasy (ZIMMERMAN 1978).

I. *p*-Aminosalicylic Acid (PAS)

Hepatic injury induced by the drug is part of a generalized hypersensitivity reaction characterized by fever, rash, eosinophilia, lymphadenopathy, and "atypical" circulating lymphocytes ("pseudomononucleosis"). The liver shows mixed hepatocellular injury. Necrosis may be massive in fatal cases. In some nonfatal cases, there may be striking periportal necrosis (ZIMMERMAN 1963). While the drug sees little use today, its injury is an important example of immunologic idiosyncrasy.

II. Isoniazid

The huge number of reports of INH-induced liver injury and the great importance of the drug in treatment of tuberculosis demonstrate INH to be one of the most important causes of drug-induced liver injury. The incidence of jaundice among recipients approximates 1%. It is very rare under the age of 20 years and exceeds 2% in patients above 50 years of age (Black et al. 1975). Females and alcoholics appear to be more susceptible than others to injury (Kopanoff et al. 1978).

Clinical features resemble acute viral hepatitis. Anorexia, fatigue, nausea, and vomiting are usual prodromal features, but jaundice and dark urine may be the first evidence of injury. Hepatocellular injury may be severe, with peak values for aminotransferases as high as 4000 IU. Continued administration of isoniazid after prodromal symptoms have appeared may enhance the severity of injury (Black et al. 1975). The liver shows diffuse degeneration and necrosis (Fig. 1). Fatal cases show massive necrosis (Fig. 1). The fatality rate for jaundiced patients is in excess of 10% (Black et al. 1975). In a few patients the liver, on biopsy, has shown changes consistent with chronic hepatitis and cirrhosis (Black et al. 1975). However, ongoing chronic hepatitis after the isoniazid is removed has not been reported.

Minor elevations (less than threefold) of aminotransferases occur in 10%–20% of patients during the first 2 months of isoniazid therapy (Zimmerman 1978). In most of these, the abnormality does not progress and may even subside despite continued administration of the drug. Such patients show minor histologic abnormalities on liver biopsy (Sharer and Smith 1969).

The mechanism for hepatic necrosis appears to be the production of toxic, reactive intermediates that bind covalently to cell macromolecules (Mitchell et al. 1976). Earlier studies suggesting that rapid acetylators of isoniazid are at greater risk of developing hepatic injury have not been confirmed. Indeed, more recent studies suggest the converse to be true (Zimmerman and Maddrey 1993). An important property of rifamipin is the enhancement of hepatotoxic effects of INH, presumably due to its ability to induce the isoform of cytochrome p450 involved in converting INH to its toxic metabolite (Pessayre et al. 1977; Pessayre et al. 1982).

III. Rifampin

Patients can develop jaundice while taking rifampin and INH. Hepatic injury that appears during the 1st month of combined therapy has appeared attributable to rifampin in contrast to INH injury, which usually (85%) appears 2–12 months after starting treatment (Zimmerman and Maddrey 1993). Nevertheless, the recognition that either drug may be responsible is only possible by observing the effects of withdrawal of either or both and readministration. Rifampin-induced injury in this setting is mainly hepatocellular. Degeneration and necrosis are characteristic and tend to be most prominent in zone 3

(SCHEUER et al. 1974). Whether rifampin, by itself without INH, can lead to hepatic injury is not clear.

Presumably unrelated to this hepatic injury is the ability of rifampin to produce unconjugated hyperbilirubinemia. Apparently, the drug competes with other substances cleared by the liver for excretion into bile or uptake from sinusoidal blood by the hepatocyte (ZIMMERMAN 1978).

D. Antifungal Agents

I. Griseofulvin

This agent is a known experimental hepatotoxin. It produces hepatic necrosis, hepatocellular carcinoma, and toxic porphyria (BARICH et al. 1961; HURST and PAGET 1963) as well as lesions similar to "alcoholic hyaline" (Mallory's bodies) in mice (DENK et al. 1975). Humans have developed porphyrinuria, and those with acute intermittent porphyria in remission may experience a relapse while taking the drug (BERMAN and FRANKLIN 1965). We are aware of only two reported cases of jaundice, both cholestatic. Other vague references to liver damage in humans have appeared (ZIMMERMAN 1978).

II. Ketoconazole

Rare hepatocellular necrosis (Fig. 2) and frequent (12%–48%) abnormalities in biochemical tests are found in recipients of this drug (LEWIS et al. 1983). Fatal instances have occurred. Symptomatic hepatic reactions occur mainly within the first few months of treatment. Most instances of injury have occurred in patients over 40 years old, and females outnumber males (ZIMMERMAN and MADDREY 1993). Rash or eosinophilia is rare, and the presumed mechanism of injury is metabolic idiosyncrasy. The incidence of symptomatic hepatic injury has been estimated to be as low as 1 in 10000 cases or as high as 1 in 2000 (JANSEN and SYMOENS 1983; STRICKER et al. 1986).

III. Other Imidazoles

Clotrimazole, econazole, and fluconazole have each led to elevated aminotransferase levels in 5%–15% of patients. However, "econazole" has been reported to lead to "hepatitis" and fluconazole has also led to cases of hepatocellular injury (STRICKER 1992).

IV. Flucytosine

Flucytosine is converted to 5-fluorouracil, a transformation on which its antifungal activity depends. It leads to transient elevations of aminotransferases in 10% of recipients and has been incriminated in the case of hepatic necrosis (RECORD et al. 1971; BENNETT 1977).

E. Antiviral Agents

Information on the hepatotoxicity of these agents is limited. Idoxyuridine has been reported to produce cholestatic jaundice (DAYAN and LEWIS 1969) as well as hepatocellular injury (BREEDEN et al. 1966; SILK and ROOME 1970). Xenelamine (Xenazoic Acid) has led to instances of cholestatic jaundice (HECHT et al. 1965; HERBEUVAL 1966) and cytarabine has led to jaundice of uncertain type (HRYNICK et al. 1972). Acyclovir and gancyclovir can lead to elevated aminotransferase levels (STRICKER 1992). Vidarabine can also lead to elevated levels of bilirubin and aminotransferases (WHITLEY et al. 1981). Zidovudine has led to cholestatic jaundice (DUBIN and BRAFFMAN 1989) and has been associated with instances of massive steatosis (FREIMAN et al. 1993).

2,3-Dideoxinosine (didanosine, ddI) can produce hepatic injury. It was found to lead to elevated aminotransferase levels in 11 of 17 patients with AIDS (LAMBERT et al. 1990) and has been reported to lead to fulminant hepatic failure, with histologic changes resembling those of Reye's syndrome (LAI et al. 1991).

Fialuridine, a nucleoside, when studied for its effects on chronic hepatitis B was found to lead to severe hepatic and pancreatic injury with several fatalities. The hepatic lesion included microvesicular steatosis and in some cases necrosis. Lactic acidosis accompanied the hepatic injury (HOOFNAGLE and KLEINER 1993).

The interferons (IFNs) can lead to minor hepatic injury. These preparations lead to steatosis and necrosis in mice (GRESSER et al. 1981), and to impaired drug metabolism and elevated aminotransferase levels in patients (GOEPFERT et al. 1982; OLDHAM 1982).

F. Antiprotozoal Agents

Most of the agents used to treat malaria, amebiasis, and other protozoan diseases have had little overt hepatotoxic effects. The antimalarial amodiaguine has led to cases of hepatocellular injury, some fatal (LARREY et al. 1986; NEFTEL et al. 1986; RAYMOND et al. 1989). The mechanism has been judged to be immunologic idiosyncrasy. Fatal multisystemic toxicity with hepatic necrosis, oliguria, renal failure, and bullous exfoliative dermatitis has been reported in patients taking pyrimethamine and sulfadoxine for malaria prophylaxis (CURLEY and MACFARLEANE 1988; STRICKER 1992). Pentamidine, stilbamidine, and hydroxystilbamidine have all been reported to lead to minor hepatic injury (STRICKER 1992). Metronidazole has been rarely incriminated in hepatic injury. To our knowledge only three cases have been reported (FAGIN 1965; APPLEBY and VOGTLAND 1983; UCHICHARA et al. 1984).

I. Anthelmintics

Chlorinated hydrocarbons and organic antimonials, long used as anthelmintics, are known to cause hepatic injury. Hycanthone formerly used for the treatment of schistosomiasis, has also been found to produce hepatocellular injury and, in some cases, fatal necrosis (COHEN 1978). Thiabendazole has led to instances of intrahepatic cholestasis, which can progress to a syndrome resembling primary biliary cirrhosis (JALOTA and FRESTON 1974; REX et al. 1983).

Albendazole, a drug used to treat echinoccus disease, can lead to hepatocellular injury (MORRIS and SMITH 1987; WILSON et al. 1987). Mebendazole, an anthelminthic used in human and veterinary medicine, has led to hepatocellular injury in humans (SEITZ et al. 1983; BEKKTI and PIROTTE 1987) and dogs (POLGIN et al. 1981; SWANSON and BREIDER 1982).

References

Appleby DH, Vogtland HD (1983) Suspected metronidazole hepatotoxicity. Clin Pharm 2:373

Barich LL, Schwarz J, Barich DJ, Horowitz MG (1961) Toxic liver damage in mice after prolonged intake of elevated doses of griseofulvin. Antibiot Chemother 11:566

Bass AD (1965) Chemotherapy of bacterial infections. III. Sulfones. In: Di Plama JR, (ed) Drill's pharmacology in medicine, 3rd edn. McGraw-Hill, New York, p 1312

Bekkti A, Pirotte J (1987) Hepatotoxicity of mebendazole. Relationship with serum concentration of the drug. Gastroenterol Clin Biol 11:706

Bennett JE (1977) Flucytosine. Ann Intern Med 86:319

Berman A, Franklin RL (1968) Precipitation of acute intermittent porphyria by griseofulvin therapy. JAMA 192:1005

Black M, Mitchell JR, Zimmerman HJ et al. (1975) Isoniazid associated hepatitis in 114 patients. Gastroenterology 69:289–302

Braun P (1973) Hepatotoxicity of erythromycin. J Infect Dis 119:300

Breeden CJ, Hall TC, Tyler HR (1966) Herpes simplex encephalitides treated with systemic 5-idio-2-deoxyuridine. Ann Intern Med 65:1050

Chatham WW, Ross DW (1983) Leukemoid blood reaction to tetracycline. South Med J 76:1195

Cohen C (1978) Liver pathology in hyacinthine hepatitis. Gastroenterology 75:103

Curley RK, MacFarleane AW (1988) Fatal multisystem toxicity associated with Fansidar. Lancet I:854

Davies GE, Holmes JE (1972) Drug-induced immunological effects on the liver. Br J Anaesth 44:941

Dayan AD, Lewis PD (1969) Idoxyuridine and jaundice. Lancet II:1073

Denk H, Gschnait F, Wolff K (1975) Hepatocellular hyalin (Mallory bodies) in long term griseofulvin treated mice: a new experience made for the study of hyalin formation. Lab Invest 32:773–776

Dismukas WE (1973) Oxacillin-induced hepatic dysfunction. JAMA 226:861

Dujovne CA, Chan CH, Zimmerman HJ (1967) Sulfonamide hepatic injury. N Engl J Med 277:785

Dujovne CA, Shoeman DW, Lasagna L (1972) Experimental basis for the different hepatotoxicity of erythromycin preparation in man. J Lab Clin Med 79:832

Dubin G, Braffman MN (1989) Zidovudine-induced hepatotoxicity. Ann Intern Med 110:85–86

Elmore M, Rissing JP, Rink L, Brooks GF (1974) Clindamycin associated hepatotoxicity. Am J Med 57:627–630

Eckstein RP, Dowsett JF, Lunzer MR (1993) Flucloxacillin induced liver disease. Histopathological findings at biopsy and autopsy. Pathology 25:223

Enat R, Pollack S, Ben-Arieh Y et al. (1980) Cholestatic jaundice caused by cloxacillin: macrophage inhibition factor test in preventing rechallenge with hepatotoxic drugs. Br Med J 1:982
Engel JS, Vogt TR, Wilson DE (1975) Cholestatic hepatitis after administration of furan derivatives. Arch Intern Med 135:733
Fagin ID (1965) Jaundice associated with metronidazole. JAMA 193:1128
Fass RJ, Saslow S (1972) Clindamycin: clinical and laboratory evaluation of parenteral therapy. Am J Med Sci 263:369–376
Fevery J, Van Steenbergen W, Desmet V et al. (1983) Severe intrahepatic cholestasis due to the combined intake of oral contraceptives and triacetyoleandomycin. Acta Clin Belg 28:242–245
Fischer HW, Hoak JC (1964) Mimicry of acute cholecystitis by erythromycin estolate reactions. Reports of two cases. Am J Med 2:47
Freedman MA (1965) Oxacillin: apparent hematologic and hepatic toxicity. Rocky Mt Med J 62:34
Freedman MA, Helfert KE, Hamrell MR, Stein DS (1993) Hepatomegaly with severe steatosis in HIV-seropositive patients. AIDs 7:395
Freiman JP, Hlfort KE, Hamoth MR, Stein DS (1993) Hepatomegaly with severe steatosis in HIV-seropositive patients. AIDS 7:395
Goepfert H, Gutterman JU, Dichtel WJ (1982) leukocyte interferon in patients with juvenile laryngeal papillomatosis. Ann Otol Rhintol Laryngol 91:431
Gordin FM, Simon GL, Wofsy CB, Mills JM (1984) Adverse reactions to trimethoprim-sulfamethoxazole in patients with the acquired immunodeficiency syndrome. Ann Intern Med 100:495
Gresser I, Aguet M, Morel-Maroger L et al. (1981) Electronphoretically pure mouse interferon inhibits growth, induces liver and kindney lesions and kills suckling mice. Am J Pathol 102:396
Gutman AB (1959) Drug reactions characterized by cholestasis associated with intrahepatic biliary tree obstruction. Am J Med 51:1230
Hanger FM Jr, Gutman AB (1940) Post-arsphenamine jaundice. JAMA 115:263
Haubrich WS, Sancetta SM (1954) Spontaneous recovery from hepatobiliary disease with xanthomatosis. Gastroenterology 26:658
Hebbard GS, Smith KG, Gibson PR, Bhathal PS (1992) Augmentin-induced jaundice with a fatal outcome. Med J Aust 156:285
Hecht Y, Levy VG, Agnolucci MT, Caroli J (1965) Hepatitis cholestatique dues a la xenalamine. Arch Mal Appar 54:615
Herbeuval R (1966) Hepatitie cholestatique a la xenalamine. Arch Mal Appar 54:615
Hoofnagle J, Kleiner D (1993) Presentation at meeting (American Association for the Study of Liver Diseases) in hepatotoxicity effects of fialuridine. Chicago, Illinois
Hryniuk W, Foerster J, Shifania M, Charv A (1972) Cytarabine for herpes virus infection. JAMA 219:715
Humble MW, Eykien S, Phillips I (1980) Staphylococcal bacteremia, fusidic acid and jaundice. Br Med J 280:1415
Hurst EW, Paget GE (1963) Proptoporphyria, cirrhosis and hepatomata in livers of mice given griseofulvin. Br J Derm 75:105
Imoto S, Matsumoto H (1979) Drug-related hepatitis. Ann Intern Med 91:129
Jalota R, Freston JW (1974) Severe intrahepatic cholestasis due to thiabendazole. Am J Trop Med Hyg 23:676
Janssen PAJ, Symoens J (1983) Hepatic reactions during ketoconazole treatment. Am J Med 74:80
Kendler J, Anuras S, Laborda O, Zimmerman HJ (1972) Perfusion of the isolated rat liver erythromycin estolate and other derivatives. Proc Soc Exp Biol Med 1939:1271
Kleinman MS, Presberg JE (1984) Cholestatic hepatitis in association with dicloxacillin sodium exposure. Hepatology 4:1007
Kopanoff DE, Snider DE Jr, Caras GJ (1978) Isoniazid related hepatitis. Am Rev Respir Dis 117:991

Lai KK, Gang DL, Zawacki JK, Cosley TP (1991) Fulminant hepatic failure associated with 2,3'dideoxyuridine (ddI). Ann Intern Med 115:253
Lambert JS, Seidlin M, Reichman RC et al. (1990) 2'3'-dideoxyinosine (ddI) in patients with the acquired immunodeficiency syndrome or AIDs related complex. N Engl J Med 322:1333
Larrey D, Castot A, Pessayre D (1986) Amodiaquine-induced hepatitis. A report of seven cases. Ann Intern Med 104:801
Lepper MH, Wolfe CK, Zimmerman HJ et al. (1951) Effect of large doses of Aureomycin on human liver. Arch Intern Med 88:271
Lewis JH, Zimmerman HJ, Benson GD, Ishak KG (1983) Hepatic injury associated with ketoconazole therapy. Analysis of 33 cases. Gastroenterology 86:503–513
Ludwig JR, Axelsen R (1983) Drug effects on the liver. An updated tabular compilation of drugs and drug-related hepatic disease. Dig Dis Sci 28:651
Magee G, Bokhari S, Layden TJ (1982) Cholestatic hepatitis from use of sulfanilamide vaginal cream. Dig Dis Sci 27:1044
Melamed AJ, Muller RJ, Gold JWM et al. (1987) Possible zidovudine-induced hepatotoxicity. JAMA 258:2063
Mihas AA (1978) Sulfasalazine toxic reactions: hepatitis, fever and skin rash associated with hypocomplementemia and immune complexes. JAMA 239:2590
Mitchell JR, Zimmerman HJ, Ishak KG et al. (1976) Isoniazid liver injury: clinical spectrum, pathology and probable pathogenesis. Ann Intern Med 84:181
Morris DL, Smith PG (1987) Albendazole in hydatid disease – hepatocellular toxicity. Trans Soc Trop Med 81:343
Munoz SJ, Martinez-Hernadex K, Maddrey WC (1990) Intrahepatic cholestasis and phospholipidosis associated with the use of trimethoprim-sulfametoxazole. Hepatology 12:342
Neftel KA, Woodtel W, Schmid M et al. (1982) Is amiodarone (Flavoquin) hepatotoxic? Gastroenterol Clin Biol 10:44
Oldham RR (1982) Toxic effects of interferon. Science 219:902
Pessayre D (1982) Present views on isoniazid and isoniazid rifampin hepatitis. Aggressologie 23:123
Pessayre D, Bentata M, DeGott C et al. (1977) Isoniazid rifampicin fulminant hepatitis: a possible consequence of enhancement of isoniazid hepatotoxicity by enzyme induction. Gastroenterology 72:284–289
Pillans P, Maling T (1993) Roxithromycin and hepatitis. Drug Invest 6:296
Polgin DJ, Stoew CM, O'Leary TD et al. (1981) Acute hepatic necrosis associated with the administration of mebendazole to dogs. JAMA 179:1014
Raymond JM, Dumas F, Baldt C et al. (1989) Fatal acute hepatitis due to amodiaquine. J Clin Gastroenterol 11:602
Record CO, Skinner JM, Sleigth P, Speller DCE (1971) Candida endocarditis treated with 5-fluorocytosine. Br Med J 1:262
Reddy KR, Brillant P, Schiff ER (1989) Amoxcillin-clavulanate potassium-associated cholestasis. Gastroenterology 96:1135
Rex D, Lumengl L, Eble J et al. (1983) Intrahepatic cholestasis and sicca complex after thiabendazole. Report of a case and review of the literature. Gastroenterology 85:718–721
Scheuer P, Summerfield JA, Lal S, Sherlock S (1974) Rifampicin hepatitis. A clinical and histological study. Lancet I:421
Schrumpf E, Nordgard K (1986) Unusual cholestastic hepatotoxicity of doxycycline in a young male? Scand J Gastroenterol 21 [Suppl 220]:68
Seitz R, Schwerks W, Arnold R (1983) Hepatocellular Arzineimittelreaktion unter Mebendazol theraful bei Echinococcus. Apticerkus Z Gastroenterol 21: 324
Sharer L, Smith JP (1969) Serum transaminase elevations and other hepatic abnormalities in patients receiving isoniazid. Ann Intern Med 71:1113
Sharp JR, Ishak KG, Zimmerman HJ (1980) Chronic active hepatitis and severe hepatic necrosis associated with nitrofurantoin. Ann Intern Med 92:141

Silk BR, Roome APCH (1970) Herpes simplex encephalitis treated with intravenous idoxyuridine. Lancet I:411
Sippel PJ, Agger WA (1982) Nitrofurantoin-induced granulomatous hepatitis. Urology 18:177
Stricker BH, Blok AP, Bronkhorst FB, van Paryr GE (1986) Ketoconazole-associated hepatic injury. A clinicopathologic study of 55 cases. J Hepatol 3:339
Stricker BHC (1992) Drug-induced liver injury. Elsevier, Amsterdam, pp 98–149
Swanson JF, Breider DVM (1992) Hepatic failure following mebendazole administration to a dog. JAMA 181:72
Tanner AR (1986) Hepatic cholestasis induced by trimethoprim. Br Med J 293:1072
Ten-Pas A, Quinn EL (1965) Cholestatic hepatitis following the administration of sodium oxacillin. JAMA 191:138
Tickin HE, Robinson MM (1963) Effects of some antimicrobial agents on the liver. Ann NY Acad Sci 104:819
Tickin HE, Zimmerman HJ (1962) Hepatic dysfunction and jaundice in patients receiving triacetyloeandomycin. N Engl J Med 267:964–968
Tonder M, Nordoy A, Elgjo D (1974) Sulfonamide-induced chronic liver disease. Scand J Gastroenterol 9:93
Uchichara M, Marda M, Koyamanda W et al. (1984) A case of metronidazole induced liver injury. Acta Hepatol Jpn 25:1612
Vandecarr S, Drier M (1981) Suspected new, rare unexpected or serious reactions reported to the division of drug experiences. FDR Highlights, FDA 17 Febr 1981
Whitley RJ, Soong SJ, Hirsh MS et al. (1981) Herpes simplex encephalitis: vidarabine therapy and diagnostic problems. N Engl J Med 304:313
Williams CN, Maltjaline DA (1981) Severe penicillin-induced cholestasis in a 91 year old woman. Dig Dis Sci 26:470
Wilson FM, Belamaric J, Lauter CB, Lerner AM (1975) Anicteric carbenicillin hepatitis: eight episodes in four patients. JAMA 32:818
Wilson JF, Rausch RL, McMahon BJ et al. (1987) Albendazole therapy in alveolar hydatid disease. A report of favorable results in two patients after short term therapy. Am J Trop Med 37:162
Zimmerman HJ (1963) Clinical and laboratory manifestation of hepatotoxicity. Ann NY Acad Sci 104:954
Zimmerman HJ (1978) Hepatotoxicity. The adverse effects of drugs and other chemicals on the liver. Appleton-Century Croft, New York
Zimmerman HJ (1990) Update of hepatotoxicity due to classes of drugs in common clinical use: non-steroidal drugs, anti-inflammatory drugs, antibiotics, antihypertensives and cardiac and psychotropic agents. Sem Liv Dis 10:322
Zimmerman HJ, Maddrey WC (1993) Toxic and drug-induced hepatitis. In: Schiff L, Schiff ER (eds) Diseases of the liver, 6th edn. Lippincott, Philadelphia, pp 707–783

CHAPTER 21

Hepatotoxicity of Cardiovascular Drugs

R.G. Cameron, F.A. de la Iglesia, and G. Feuer

A. Introduction

Society often pays a price for the progress achieved in the therapeutic benefits offered by new drugs, namely, an increased incidence of toxic side effects. Fortunately, the benefits of advanced therapy outweigh the risks posed by these side effects. The introduction of a new drug can be followed by various types of unexpected reactions, including hepatotoxicity. It is often difficult to establish an association between a drug and reported liver injury, but it becomes certain when the same liver impairment recurs after repeated administration of the same drug (Elkington et al. 1969; Eliastam and Holmes 1971). Infrequently, the response pattern can be so characteristic as to be diagnostic of toxicity of a specific drug, such as phospholipidosis or alcoholic-like hepatitis in response to coralgil or amiodarone (de la Iglesia et al. 1974; Poucell et al. 1984; Guigui et al. 1988). Impairment of hepatic function is associated with the intake of many drugs (Zimmerman 1990), including several cardiovascular drugs that are the main focus of this chapter. In some cases the mechanism of hepatic injury has been recognized; in others, the side effect profile has not been clearly established. These side effects by drugs may complicate patient treatment and, in particular, restrict the use of drugs that are essential to patient management such as antiarrythmics, antihypertensives, or hypolipidemics. If the drug causing the hepatic toxicity is the only effective agent to control a life-threatening situation, hepatic side effects can be acceptable until pharmacologic control is established. An example is the management of intractable cardiac arrhythmias requiring amiodarone. Hepatic reactions have been attributed to many cardiovascular drugs and will be discussed in detail below.

The clinical, morphologic, and biochemical signs of cardiovascular drug-induced liver injury ranges from mild to severe with acute to chronic pathologic reactions including hepatitis (Rodman et al. 1976; Herlong et al. 1978; Bartoli et al. 1979; Itoh et al. 1981; Kalantzis et al. 1991), fatty change (Kremer et al. 1969; Arranto and Sotaniemi 1981a), cholestasis (Hoffbrand et al. 1974; Fisher 1980; Moses et al. 1989), granulomatous hepatitis (Gelb et al. 1979; Chajek et al. 1974; Geltner et al. 1976; Bramlet et al. 1980), and cirrhosis (Arranto and Sotaniemi 1981a,b). Drugs can induce one or more than one side effects simultaneously, as with α-methyldopa or amiodarone.

Disturbances of liver function and drug-induced hepatic lesions have been reported in 5%–35% of patients receiving these drugs. In this chapter we will integrate clinical, pathologic, and biochemical features and mechanisms underlying the hepatic toxicity of cardiovascular drugs.

B. *α*-Methyldopa

Since its introduction in 1960, *α*-methyldopa (L-*α*-methyl-3,4-dihydroxyphenylalanine; Fig. 1) has been one of the most frequently prescribed drugs for the treatment of moderate and severe hypertension (IRVINE et al. 1962; GILLMORE and FREIS 1965; KALANT et al. 1985). This drug is an α_2-adrenergic agonist and the molecular mechanism of adverse actions of this drug has not been clearly established. Considering the extent of *α*-methyldopa use, the drug is generally safe, although several clinical symptoms and biochemical changes have been reported as side effects (CANNON and LARAGH 1963; KALANT et al. 1985). These included sedation, vertigo, lactation from prolactin release, extrapyramidal signs, and depression. Various alimentary symptoms and postural hypotension have also been reported. Retention of salt and water may result in edema. Besides these clinical reactions, *α*-methyldopa may induce allergic reactions including fever, autoimmune hemolytic anemia, granulocytopenia, and thrombocytopenia. Positive tests for lupus erythematosus cells, rheumatoid factors, and Coomb's antiglobulin may develop (MANOHITHARAJAH et al. 1971; BRELAND and HICKS 1982; PAI and PAI 1988).

Knowledge of *α*-methyldopa-induced hepatic side effects is based on case reports (ELKINGTON et al. 1969; TYSELL and KNAUER 1971; GOLDSTEIN et al. 1973; HOYUMPA and CONNELL 1973; SCHWEITZER and PETERS 1974; MADDREY and BOITNOTT 1975; THOMAS et al. 1976) and epidemiological investigations. Most patients developed hepatic symptoms within 6–10 weeks or up to 4–6 months after initiation of *α*-methyldopa therapy. In some cases, signs of hepatic injury became apparent after 2–11 years of exposure to the drug

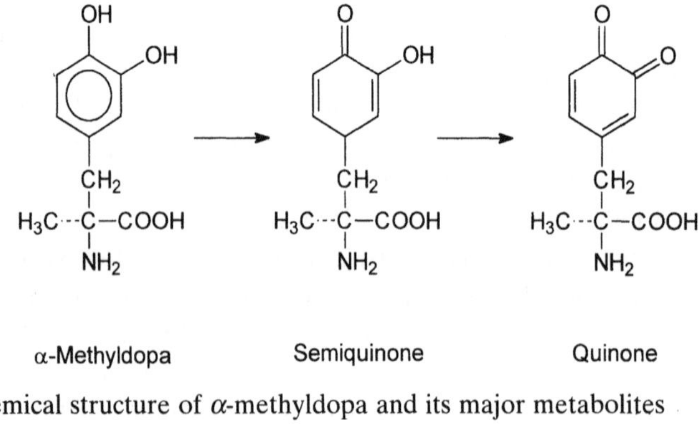

Fig. 1. Chemical structure of *α*-methyldopa and its major metabolites

(HOYUMPA and CONNELL 1973; TOGHILL et al. 1974; SOTANIEMI et al. 1977; SEGGIE et al. 1979; ARRANTO and SOTANIEMI 1981a). This difference suggests that the adverse liver response to α-methyldopa can be divided into two groups based on exposure time, each with a particular subset of biochemical findings, liver histopathology, and clinical symptoms. In the first group the reactions developed short-term; in the second group, the liver lesions manifested after long-term exposures.

Patients exposed for short-term periods became acutely ill, with general malaise, weakness, abdominal pain, nausea, and occasionally jaundice and fever. In many cases the hepatic dysfunction appeared to be mild, and the clinical symptoms and biochemical abnormalities returned to normal upon discontinuation of the drug. Approximately one third of the short-term cases developed persistently high transaminase levels even after being withdrawn from α-methyldopa therapy. Patients in the long-term treatment group developed hepatic injury and had a more chronic progression of the disease. The clinical symptoms indicative of side effects were initially mild and gradually worsened, including severe discomfort, chronic nausea, weakness, epigastric pain, colic, and dyspepsia.

I. Hepatitis

α-Methyldopa hepatitis has been reported in more than 80 cases and the administered dose varied between 250mg to 1g per day. According to a Swedish report, the median age of patients suffering α-methyldopa hepatitis is about 57 years (FURHOFF 1978). Symptoms usually cannot be differentiated from viral hepatitis (THOMAS et al. 1977). The prodromal syndrome includes chills, fever, headaches, fatigue, malaise, anorexia, nausea, diarrhea, and vomiting. Hepatitis is frequently accompanied by fever and other symptoms after 1–4 weeks from the start of drug therapy followed a few days later by frank jaundice. Hepatic dysfunction and jaundice may occur within 8–10 weeks (ELKINGTON et al. 1969) to 6 or 7 months (WILLIAMS and KHAN 1967) after starting α-methyldopa therapy. One patient experienced anorexia, nausea, vomiting, and epigastric pain after 6 weeks of α-methyldopa therapy and then lost weight and became jaundiced 1 week to 10 days later (THOMAS et al. 1977). Upon rechallenge, the hepatic reactions were observed within 4 days (TYSELL and KNAUER 1971). Several deaths were reported due to hepatic coma following prolonged α-methyldopa intake (HOYUMPA and CONNELL 1973; MADDREY and BOITNOTT 1975; RODMAN et al. 1976).

Underlying disease conditions, such as serologic abnormalities, arthritis, and lupus erythematosus cell positivity can contribute to the hepatotoxicity of α-methyldopa (ELIASTAM and HOLMES 1971). The liver is often enlarged and tender, and the clinical symptoms include marked jaundice and cholestasis in about 50% of cases. Liver function tests suggest parenchymal cell damage. Increased bilirubin is a frequent finding and transaminases are elevated, with serum levels frequently exceeding 1000 units. Serum bilirubin levels vary depending on the severity of the hepatic damage. Alkaline phosphatase may be normal or increased. The albumin to globulin ratio is usually within normal limits, but there are reports showing increased globulins, particularly the gamma fraction (ELIASTAM and HOLMES 1971; HOYUMPA and CONNELL 1973).

Histopathologic changes ranged from acute hepatitis to chronic active hepatitis and chronic aggressive hepatitis (ELIASTAM and HOLMES 1971; BALAZS and KOVACH 1981). Morphologic alterations included varying degrees of hepatocytic degeneration, focal, confluent or massive necrosis, and inflammation. In most cases the portal tracts were infiltrated with lymphocytes and mononuclear cells. Occasionally, eosinophils and plasma cells were present, and slight to moderate portal fibrosis may be present (GILLMORE and FREIS 1965; WILLIAMS and KHAN 1967; ELIASTAM and HOLMES 1971). Hepatic endophlebitis associated with central perivenous inflammation is a characteristic change in several cases. Cholestasis, focal necrosis, pleomorphism, ballooning of hepatocytes, and intracytoplasmic eosinophilic bodies are observed in varying degrees and combinations. Massive panlobular necrosis, steatosis, and collapse of the reticulum have been shown in severe hepatic damage.

Electron microscopy revealed definitive, but nonspecific changes in hepatocytes and sinusoidal cells (BALAZS and KOVACH 1981). Destruction of plasma membranes in the vascular and biliary poles and nuclear inclusions in liver cells with increased activity of mesenchymal cells have been found in chronic aggressive hepatitis (SCHMID 1967; GERLACH et al. 1969; POPPER 1971; BALAZS et al. 1973; BALAZS and KOVACH 1981).

α-Methyldopa-induced hepatic damage is attributable to a hypersensitivity reaction rather than to direct toxicity to liver cells (SHERLOCK 1987). In some patients the immune-type reaction is in agreement with positive tests for Coombs' antiglobulin, antinuclear antibodies, and lupus erythematosus cells. The onset and severity of the hepatic injury showed no clear dose relationship or duration dependence in relation to the length of drug exposure. Only relatively small numbers of patients exposed to α-methyldopa are affected, preferentially those with a hypersensitivity or allergic background. A similar lesion has not been reproduced in experimental animals. Thus, immunologically mediated hypersensitivity reactions may be responsible for the hepatic toxicity of α-methyldopa (HOYUMPA and CONNELL 1973; MADDREY and BOITNOTT 1975). Sera from patients with α-methyldopa-induced hepatotoxicity caused significant cytotoxicity to hepatocytes isolated from rabbits pretreated with α-methyldopa after exposure to a cytochrome P-450 inducer (NEUBERGER et al. 1985). Antibody-positive sera caused specific immunofluorescence at the plasma membrane of hepatocytes in liver biopsies from patients taking α-methyldopa. These findings support the hypothesis that immune-mediated mechanisms are involved in hepatic damage and that metabolic activation may be necessary in the generation of α-methyldopa metabolites that can react antigenically. Thus, a combination of immune and metabolic factors is involved in the development of α-methyldopa hepatitis.

α-Methyldopa has been described as the drug most frequently associated with immune drug-induced hemolytic anemia, which may occur simultaneously with hepatitis. Autoimmune-type hemolytic anemia was reported in less than 1% of the patients taking α-methyldopa (MYER and KNELL 1977; BRELAND and HICKS 1982; PAI and PAI 1988). Various mechanisms for the development of hemolytic anemia caused by α-methyldopa were suggested, including an autoimmune mechanism (PAI and PAI 1988; KIRTLAND et al. 1980). The autoimmune hemolytic anemia observed with α-methyldopa is probably caused by an anti-rhesus immunoglobulin G (IgG) antibody directed against intrinsic erythrocyte antigens. This phenomenon can be detected with normal red cells and is not affected by additional administration of α-methyldopa. The mechanism of hemolytic anemia may be caused by α-methyldopa metabolites. These metabolites can affect cyclic adenosine monophosphate (AMP)-mediated inhibition of suppressor lymphocyte function, resulting in uncontrolled production of B lymphocyte autoantibodies (KIRTLAND et al. 1980; BRELAND and HICKS 1982).

II. Fatty Change

After long-term exposure to α-methyldopa, from 1 to 11 years with a mean of 5 years, patients felt mild and gradually increasing discomfort, dyspepsia, nausea, weakness, and epigastric pain. A typical microscopic liver finding was fatty change. Diagnostic leads were present, but less pronounced than in the hepatitis group. Chronic hepatitis-like reaction appeared to be the main finding in liver biopsies of long-term patients (ARRANTO and SOTANIEMI 1981a,b). Liver function tests showed significant increases in serum bilirubin, transaminases, and alkaline phosphatase activities, but these were less pronounced than in patients with acute α-methyldopa hepatitis. Albumin and thrombin were also elevated in long-term patients. Histologic analysis revealed degenerative changes during long-term exposure, although these lesions were more extensive in the short-term group of patients. Mild to moderate focal necrosis, hepatocyte pleomorphism, and variations in nuclear size were seen. Vacuolated nuclei were also present in hepatocytes in long-term patients. In addition, there was infiltration of neutrophils, lymphocytes, eosinophils, plasma cells, and histiocytes. Kupffer cell proliferation with diastase-resistant granules, an indication of necrosis and phagocytic activity, was also present. Fat accumulation was a common finding in the liver cells after chronic exposure to α-methyldopa, and the mechanism of this change is not yet well established (ARRANTO and SOTANIEMI 1981a,b). Hepatic lipid accumulation may involve several factors, such as uncoupling of oxidative phosphorylation or inhibition of triglyceride secretion. Compounds that bind to macromolecules, especially in the endoplasmic reticulum, may inhibit protein synthesis and hence interfere with lipid transport from the cell (KREMER et al. 1969; SOTANIEMI et al. 1977).

Excess α-methyldopa metabolites seemed to affect the hepatic protective mechanism by reducing glutathione content in liver cells. Improvement of antipyrine elimination following withdrawal of α-methyldopa in subjects with normal liver function tests suggested covalent binding or cytochrome P-450 inhibition. The impaired drug metabolism capacity returns to normal levels about 6 months after α-methyldopa withdrawal (YLIKALLIO and SOTANIEMI 1980). In animals, α-methyldopa is oxidized to semiquinone and quinone by way of cytochrome P-450-generated superoxide anions. These reactive metabolites bind covalently with cytoplasmic macromolecules (Fig. 1; MITCHELL and JOLLOW 1975). The liver has a large reserve capacity for drug metabolism, and this functional reserve may account for the delay of symptoms or lesions development over a prolonged period (SHERLOCK 1987). Fatty change, increased collagen deposition, impaired drug metabolism, and decreased cytochrome P-450 and glutathione concentrations contribute to altered hepatic function resulting in chronic liver damage by α-methyldopa.

III. Hepatic Necrosis

Acute submassive necrosis is an unusual complication of α-methyldopa therapy. This serious condition may develop within a short period of treatment, even within 8–10 weeks from initiation of α-methyldopa therapy. Isolated instances of submassive necrosis appear to have repaired after withdrawal from the drug. The most remarkable histologic feature during the acute reaction phase was extensive necrosis in periportal areas. When patients were rechallenged with α-methyldopa, serum transaminases increased within 8 days. The protracted effects of the drug after discontinued therapy have been studied, and liver scans 6–9 months after stopping treatment revealed generalized mottling and hypertrophic left lobe; broad periportal fibrosis and collapsed stroma was noted upon microscopic evaluation (SCHWEITZER and PETERS 1974; PUPPALA and STEINHEBER 1977). Fatal submassive hepatic necrosis occurred after rechallenge (REHMAN et al. 1973).

IV. Cholestasis

Cholestasis is a rare consequence of α-methyldopa hepatotoxicity (TOGHILL et al. 1974; HOFFBRAND et al. 1974; SATALINE and LOWELL 1976; DIENSTAG et al. 1987). A 75-year-old man taking α-methyldopa (250mg daily for 6 years) developed severe cholestatic liver disease (MOSES et al. 1989). There was no evidence of extrahepatic biliary obstruction. The liver biopsy of this patient showed well-preserved liver architecture with marked cholestasis. Edema and inflammation of the portal tract was composed mainly of lymphocytes and neutrophilic polymorphonuclear leukocytes. There was mild ductular proliferation in periportal areas. Withdrawal from the drug resulted in normal transaminase and bilirubin levels within 6 weeks, and alkaline phosphatase activity returned to normal about 22 weeks after α-methyldopa therapy was stopped.

V. Cirrhosis

Cirrhosis or fulminant hepatic failure due to α-methyldopa administration has been reported in patients receiving α-methyldopa for 3 months or 7 weeks (TOGHILL et al. 1974; THOMAS et al. 1976; MYER and KNELL 1977). Increasing malaise, anorexia, nausea, and occasional vomiting occurred after treatment was begun, and jaundice developed after 3 months. Laboratory tests showed increased serum bilirubin, transaminases, and alkaline phosphatase activities, reduced albumin levels, and increased globulin levels. Histologic examination of liver biopsies showed hepatocellular necrosis and collapse bridging adjacent portal tracts. The necrotic areas contained lymphocytes, plasma cells, and macrophages. The remaining parenchymal cells were abnormal, and fine cytoplasmic vacuoles were present. Ballooned cells were scattered throughout the parenchyma (THOMAS et al. 1976). The normal parenchyma was replaced by coarse scars, irregular nodules, and distortion of the lobular architecture, supporting the diagnosis of submassive hepatic collapse with postnecrotic cirrhosis. One case of fulminant hepatic failure after a 7-week period of α-methyldopa treatment has been reported. At autopsy the liver was small, showed massive necrosis, isolated islands of surviving parenchyma, and attempts at regeneration with pseudonodule formation (TOGHILL et al. 1974).

C. Amiodarone

Amiodarone (2-butyl-3-benzofuranyl 4-{2-(diethylamino) ethoxy}-3,5-diiodophenyl ketone; Fig. 2) is an effective antiarrhythmic drug. Its use has been confined to the treatment of refractory ventricular tachyarrhythmias, mainly because of the serious side effects that ensue (MCGOVERN et al. 1983; SHENASA et al. 1984; DE KORWIN et al. 1986; MASON 1987; VROBEL et al. 1989; REASOR and KACEW 1990; WILSON and PODRID 1991; FORNACIERI et al. 1992). The most serious, life-threatening adverse reaction is pulmonary toxicity, characterized by interstitial pneumonitis and fibrosis (MARTIN and ROSENOW 1988a,b). Histologic evidence of amiodarone hepatotoxicity was reported by several investigators (FOGOROS et al. 1983; RAEDER et al. 1985; YAGUPSKY et al. 1985; RIGAS et al. 1986; TJORDMAN et al. 1986; RINDER et al. 1986; BABANY et al. 1986; ANASTASIOU-NANA et al. 1986; PYE et al. 1988; LEWIS et al. 1989, 1990; FLAHARTY et al. 1989). The spectrum of microscopic changes includes features of alcoholic hepatitis, steatosis, Mallory bodies, fibrosis, and cirrhosis (POUCELL et al. 1984; SIMON et al. 1984; VARMA et al. 1985; GOLDMAN et al.

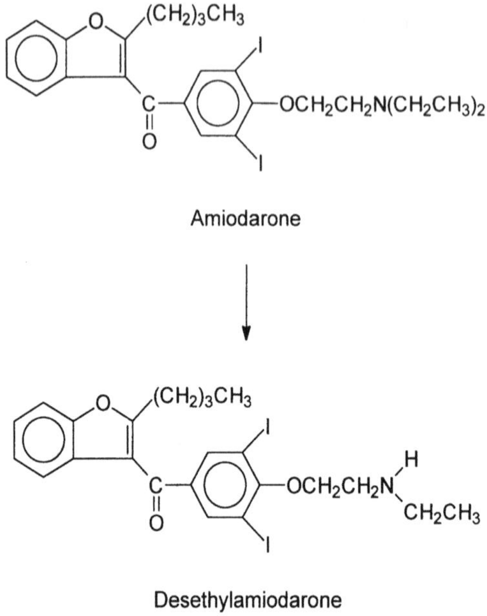

Fig. 2. Chemical structure of amiodarone and major metabolite

1985; LEWIS et al. 1990). The hepatic effects of amiodarone include the accumulation of concentric lamellar bodies indicative of phospholipid fatty liver (Figs. 3, 4). This condition was originally described due to the effects of coralgil, a coronary vasodilator (ODA et al. 1970; IDE 1971; MATSUDA et al. 1971). Phospholipid fatty liver was later identified with amiodarone (POUCELL et al. 1984; DUKE et al. 1985; RIGAS et al. 1986; SHEPHERD et al. 1987; LEWIS et al. 1990). These effects are related to the inability of lysosomes to eliminate the drug and its metabolites, with subsequent massive accumulation of lipid-containing bodies in the hepatocyte cytoplasm (REASOR 1989; REASOR and KACEW 1991; SCHMITZ and MULLER 1991). Symptomatic hepatitis may result from amiodarone treatment (KALANTZIS et al. 1991), and amiodarone modulates polymorphic variants of drug metabolism by interaction with cytochrome P-450 enzymes (SAAL et al. 1984; FUNCK-BRENTANO et al. 1991).

I. Alcoholic-Type Hepatitis

In one study, 17 patients were reported with changes similar to alcoholic liver injury (LEWIS et al. 1990). Histopathologic features included macro- and microvesicular steatosis, hepatocyte ballooning, Mallory bodies, and fibrosis. These pseudoalcoholic hepatitis changes were seen in liver biopsies from asymptomatic, anicteric patients who had taken amiodarone for more than 1 year and had mild elevations of serum transaminases and alkaline phosphatase, although serum bilirubin levels were slightly increased. The incidence

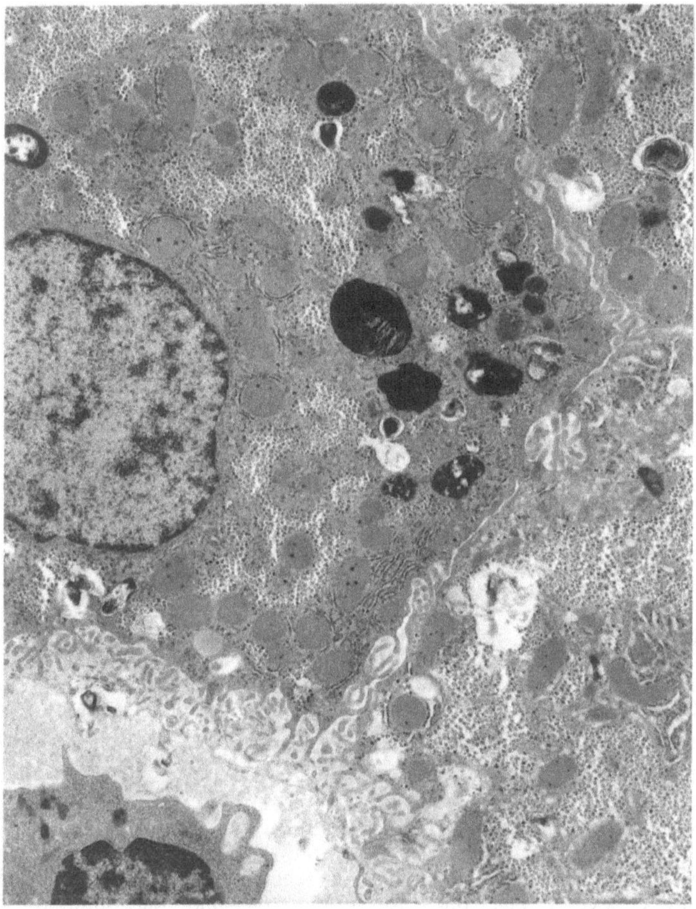

Fig. 3. Electron micrograph of liver biopsy showing phospholipidosis in a 53-year-old man taking amiodarone for treatment of ventricular arrhythmia. (×3000)

of this hepatic reaction is approximately 1% in patients treated with amiodarone (LEWIS et al. 1989). Similar findings were seen in long-term studies (PLONTEUX et al. 1969; HARRIS et al. 1983; RUMESSEN 1986).

Severe amiodarone hepatotoxicity manifested by alcoholic hepatitis symptoms is cytotoxic in character. The liver injury is unpredictable, and it is an expression of an unusual individual susceptibility to the drug rather than to direct toxicity. Despite the resemblance to alcohol-induced liver disease, there were several distinguishing features in amiodarone-induced hepatic lesions. In amiodarone hepatitis, Mallory bodies were located in zone 1 (periportal) of the acinus, whereas in alcoholic liver disease they are found predominantly in zone 2 (midzonal) and zone 3 (pericentral) (ISHAK 1982). Acute foamy changes with massive accumulation of microvesicular cytoplasmic lipid is more

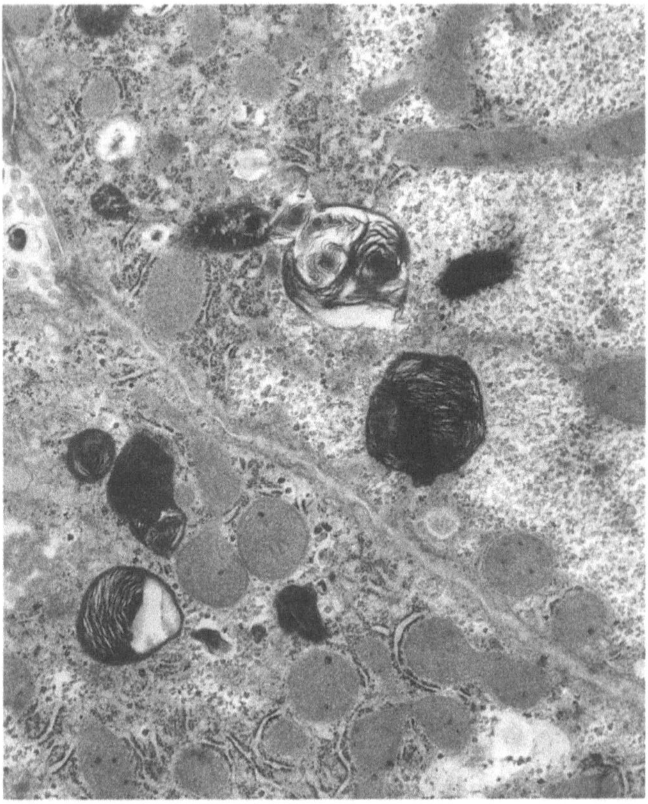

Fig. 4. Electron micrograph of liver biopsy showing phospholipidosis in a 74-year-old man with cardiomyopathy and arrhythmia receiving amiodarone. This photomicrograph shows several electron-dense intracytoplasmic phospholipid inclusions. (×10000)

common in amiodarone hepatitis than in alcoholic injury and is not necessarily accompanied by Mallory bodies or neutrophilic infiltration (Robinson et al. 1989). The presence of phospholipid-laden lysosomal lamellar bodies is characteristic of amiodarone hepatotoxicity and distinguishes this condition from alcoholic liver disease or other causes of hepatic steatosis (Uchida et al. 1983).

Several studies reported clinical hepatitis with steatosis, minimal inflammatory reaction, and mild elevation of serum hepatic enzymes (Waxman et al. 1982). The long-term effects of amiodarone causing mild hepatic lesions or more severe liver dysfunction seem to be unrelated to increases in transaminases, alkaline phosphatase, or bilirubin (Kalantzis et al. 1981; Morelli et al. 1991; Rhodes et al. 1993). Severe hepatitis and fatal outcomes from amiodarone injury have been reported (McGovern et al. 1983; Fogoros et al. 1983; Lim et al. 1984; Yagupsky et al. 1985). Amiodarone causes asymptomatic elevations of serum transaminases between 1.5- and fourfold above the upper limit of normal (WAXMAN et al. 1982; MCGOVERN et al. 1983; FOGOROS et al. 1983; MORADY et al. 1983; ROTMENSCH et al. 1984; SIMON et al. 1984; RAEDER et al. 1985; SMITH et al. 1986; LUPON-ROSES et al. 1986; PYE et al. 1988); a 100-fold increase in serum transaminase levels has also been reported (RHODES et al. 1993; SNIR et al. 1995). In a series of 104 cardiac patients receiving amiodarone, abnormal elevations of transaminases were found (LEWIS et al. 1989). The transaminase elevations were mild in many of the patients and transient in nature, and the levels returned to normal after the dose of amiodarone was lowered or treatment stopped. In contrast to these cases, fibrosis or cirrhosis (POUCELL et al. 1984) and infrequent fatal hepatic injury suggest a wide range of hepatotoxic potential for amiodarone (LIM et al. 1984; POUCELL et al. 1984; RIGAS et al. 1986; BABANY et al. 1986; SHEPHERD et al. 1987; LEWIS et al. 1989; STEVENSON et al. 1989). A number of deaths were reported due to amiodarone-induced hepatic failure (YAGUPSKY et al. 1985; TJORDMAN et al. 1986; RINDER et al. 1986; GILINSKY et al. 1988), and acute confluent, necrotizing hepatitis was described in two cases (KALANTZIS et al. 1991). These patients had received high loading doses of amiodarone and developed jaundice, hypertransaminemia, and prolonged prothrombin time on the second day of treatment. Death followed hepatic coma and acute renal failure on the fourth and 14th day of treatment, respectively. Acute drug-induced hepatitis with confluent and bridging necrosis was diagnosed upon liver biopsy.

II. Phospholipid Fatty Liver

A number of patients taking amiodarone may show clinical phospholipidosis, and liver cells studied by electron microscopy show characteristic concentric, lamellar inclusions (onion-like) with high osmiophilic density within greatly expanded lysosomes (POUCELL et al. 1984; RIGAS et al. 1986; ADAMS et al. 1986; SHEPHERD et al. 1987). Frequently, phospholipid fatty liver may be present without changes representative of pseudoalcoholic hepatitis. Hepatic tissue levels of amiodarone and desethylamiodarone can be detected several months after treatment has been stopped; presence of the drug or its metabolite may account for the persistent hepatic injury (Fig. 2). Phospholipid fatty liver may develop in patients taking the drug for 2 months (CAPRON-CHIVRAC et al. 1985; RIGAS et al. 1986).

The concentric, lamellar inclusion bodies in secondary lysosomes resemble the inclusions seen in primary phospholipidosis from inborn errors of lipid metabolism, such as Tay-Sachs, Niemann-Pick, and Fabry's disease (LÜLLMAN et al. 1975; HRUBAN 1984; POUCELL et al. 1984; DUKE et al. 1985). Similar hepatic inclusion bodies develop with other amphiphilic drugs (MATSUDA et al. 1971; SHENASA et al. 1984; DE LA IGLESIA et al. 1974, 1975; LÜLLMANN et al. 1975; LEWIS et al. 1990). Development of phospholipid fatty liver is related to strong phospholipid binding by the cationic amphiphilic characteristics of the amiodarone molecule, binding to cell membranes and accumulating in lysosomes (Seydel and Wassermann 1976; Ruben et al. 1993). Intralysosomal phospholipid accumulation may inhibit phospholipase A_1 (Shaikh et al. 1987; Reasor et al. 1988; Hostetler et al. 1988). Amiodarone-induced lysosomal inclusions accumulate in the cytoplasm of human hepatocyte cultures within four days in 1%–2% of the cells and in almost all cells by 2 weeks (Yap et al. 1986). Amiodarone-induced phospholipid fatty liver is reversible in experimental animals (Tjordman et al. 1986; Svensson and Chong 1989). In humans, lysosomal phospholipids may persist for several months after the drug administration has been discontinued.

III. Reye's Syndrome-Like Disease

Reye's syndrome-like illness after amiodarone intake has been reported; one patient was an 8-year-old child with acute hepatic injury after 2 months of treatment (Yagupsky et al. 1985; Jones et al. 1988). Characteristic increases of serum transaminases and ammonia levels occurred, and the patient lapsed into coma and died. The clinical symptoms greatly resembled Reye's syndrome, but histologic examination of the liver failed to show the typical microvesicular fatty change. Another patient was given 800mg amiodarone daily for recurrent ventricular fibrillation related to hypertrophic obstructive cardiomyopathy (Jones et al. 1988). After 12 months of treatment the patient contracted an influenza-like illness and shortly afterwards developed clinical, biochemical, and most of the hepatic histologic features of Reye's syndrome. These cases suggest that amiodarone can induce Reye's syndrome in children, similarly to aspirin, including the features of Reye's syndrome hepatic injury (Waldman et al. 1982; Starko and Mullick 1983; Jones et al. 1988). Due to the prolonged half-life of amiodarone, drug levels may remain elevated for several weeks or months following discontinuation of therapy.

D. Aprindine

Aprindine (*N*-(2,3-dihydro-1H-inden-2-yl)-*N*-*N*′-diethyl-*N*-phenyl-1,3-propanediamine); Fig. 5 is an effective agent for the control of arrhythmias because of ischemic heart disease (Fasola and Carmichael 1974; Reid et al. 1977; Stoel and Hagemeijer 1980). Aprindine has been associated with a low incidence of side effects, and liver reactions included lobular hepatitis and cholestasis (Van Leeuwen and Meyboom 1976; Herlong et al. 1978; Elisaf et al. 1992).

I. Hepatitis

Several cases of acute hepatitis caused by aprindine have been reported (Brandes et al. 1976; Elewant et al. 1977; Herlong et al. 1978). In two cases,

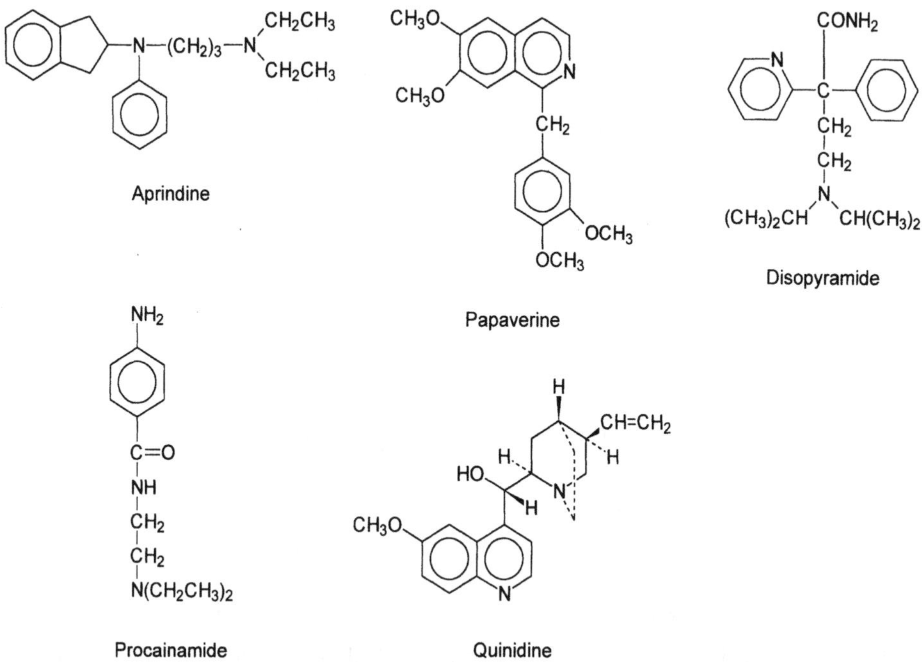

Fig. 5. Chemical structure of aprindine, papaverine, disopyramide, procainamide, and quinidine

the symptoms and pathology were mild, appearing 3 weeks after starting drug therapy and subsiding rapidly after drug withdrawal. Rechallenge in one patient caused mild hepatitis with subsequent recovery, and hypersensitivity signs such as fever, rash, or eosinophilia were not present (HERLONG et al. 1978). Additional case reports of hepatitis due to aprindine indicate that patients developed mild to moderate clinical symptoms within 3 weeks after the initiation of therapy. In all patients aprindine hepatitis resolved after drug withdrawal; rechallenge provoked the reappearance of hepatitis in all patients (ELEWANT et al. 1977). Twenty-two days after the beginning of aprindine therapy, asymptomatic elevations were seen in serum transaminases and alkaline phosphatase levels with slightly increased bilirubin. Clinical, pathologic, and biochemical data suggested aprindine hepatotoxicity. The mechanism of aprindine toxicity is not known, and cholestasis has been reported (STOEL and HAGEMEIJER 1980).

E. Hydralazine and Dihydralazine

Hydralazine (1-hydrazinophthalazine; Fig. 6) is a widely used drug for the treatment of arterial hypertension. It is well tolerated, but some patients develop headache, flushing, palpitations, and electrocardiographic abnormalities (ITOH et al. 1981). Fatal hepatotoxicity attributed to hydralazine has been reported (STUMPF 1991). One major side effect of this drug is the occurrence of

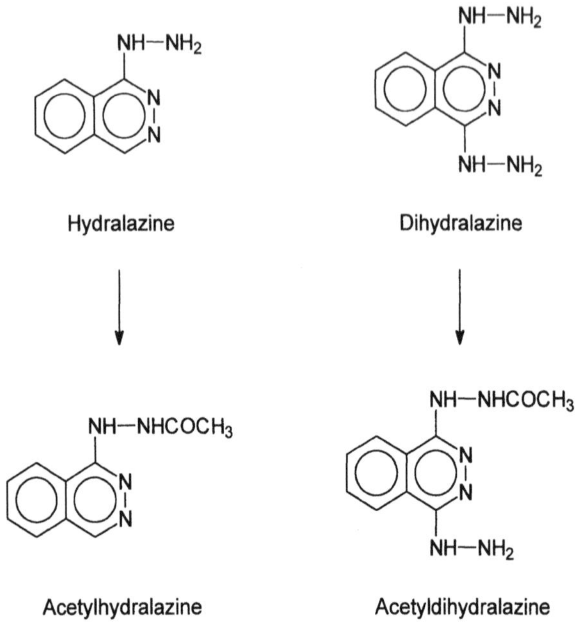

Fig. 6. Chemical structures of hydralazine and dihydralazine and their major metabolites

a systemic lupus erythematosus-like syndrome (ALARCON-SEGOVIA et al. 1967; IRIAS 1975; WECHSLER et al. 1979; BATCHELOR et al. 1980). Review of several clinical cases shows that liver injury induced by hydralazine includes hepatitis, intrahepatic cholestasis, centrilobular necrosis, and granulomata (JORI and PESCHLE 1973; BARTOLI et al. 1979; BARNETT et al. 1980; FORSTER 1980; ITOH et al. 1981; STEWART et al. 1981; PARIENTE et al. 1983; SHAEFER et al. 1989). Dihydralazine administration caused hepatitis in several patients (KNOBLAUCH et al. 1977; WECHSLER et al. 1979; PARIENTE et al. 1983). Hypersensitivity reactions occurred when hydralazine was prescribed for the treatment of hypertension concomitant with epilepsy drugs such as primidone, phenytoin, and phenobarbital. Most clinical manifestations of hydralazine liver reactions returned to normal shortly after drug discontinuation (IRIAS 1975).

I. Hepatitis

Liver injury occurred after 2–6 months in four patients treated with hydralazine (IRIAS 1975; BARTOLI et al. 1979). Other studies show that hepatitis developed within 6–9 months or up to 1 year of treatment (JORI and PESCHLE 1973; KNOBLAUCH et al. 1977; ENAT et al. 1977). Liver function tests showed highly elevated bilirubin and transaminases and slightly increased alkaline phosphatase activities. Histologic examination of liver biopsies revealed submassive to massive focal necrosis, hemorrhage, reticulum collapse, inflammatory cell infiltration, and ductular cell proliferation. Fine fat droplets in hepatocyte cytoplasm were infrequent. Trabecular septa divided the parenchyma into small, dissimilar pseudolobules. Cholestasis was seen in peripheral areas (Itoh et al. 1981). These microscopic findings are compatible with drug-induced toxic hepatitis. In one case the liver showed severe acute hepatitis with bridging necrosis, also called subacute necrosis (Bartoli et al. 1979). Complete remission occurred in all patients approximately 6 months after discontinuation of hydralazine therapy. Thus hydralazine-induced hepatitis was fully reversible in clinical, biochemical, and histologic terms.

The major pathway of hydralazine biotransformation in humans is hepatic acetylation, and the rate of acetylation is controlled by the enzyme *N*-acetyltransferase (Koch-Weser 1976). Non-specific arylamidase is reduced in drug-induced or alcoholic liver injury (Itoh et al. 1980). The liver showed various degrees of centrilobular necrosis together with low arylamidase activity (Itoh et al. 1981). A possible relationship between changes in endoplasmic reticulum function, reduced enzyme activity, and the development of hepatic cell necrosis was proposed, and hydralazine-induced liver injury is related to smooth endoplasmic reticulum dysfunction (Hutterer et al. 1969; Farber 1974).

Dihydralazine (2,3-dihydro-1,4-phthalazine dione dihydrazone; Fig. 6) is a hydralazine analogue and caused hepatitis in four cases (Enat et al. 1977; Knoblauch et al. 1977; Pariente et al. 1983). Hepatitis manifested during dihydralazine administration reversed quickly when drug administration was interrupted and worsened upon rechallenge. The liver reaction due to dihydralazine appears to be similar to hydralazine hepatitis (Barnett et al. 1980; Forster 1980; Itoh et al. 1980, 1981). The onset of dihydralazine hepatitis may vary from a few weeks to several months after drug therapy is initiated. Significant increases of serum transaminase activities were observed clinically. Hepatic encephalopathy and prolonged prothrombin time may accompany the clinical presentation. Histopathologically, the liver shows hepatocytic necrosis, mainly in the centrilobular areas (zone 3), which may expand to bridging necrosis. Most studies reported either centrilobular or bridging severe hepatocytic necrosis as the main lesion, leading occasionally to fibrosis. Dihydralazine induced several cytochrome P-450 enzymes, and anti-liver microsome autoantibodies reacting specifically against some cytochrome P-450 species were found in patients with dihydralazine-induced hepatitis (Nataf et al. 1986; Bourdi et al. 1992).

F. Papaverine

Papaverine (6,7-dimethoxy-1-veratrylisoquinoline; Fig. 5) is a benzylisoquinoline alkaloid with smooth muscle depressant properties, causing relaxation of peripheral arterioles, coronary arteries, and low systemic blood pressure. Papaverine has been widely used in the treatment of cardiac or cerebral circulatory disorders. Other indications for papaverine have been to control smooth muscle spasms in intestinal, urinary, and biliary tracts. Clinical side effects are rare and mild (RONNOV-JESSEN and TJERNLUNG 1969; KIAER et al. 1974; PATHY and REYNOLDS 1980).

I. Hepatitis

Eight patients have been described with a hypersensitivity-type hepatic reaction 1–4 weeks after papaverine treatment. Clinically, there was fever and eosinophilia, and microscopically, eosinophilic infiltration in liver biopsies (KIAER et al. 1974). Eosinophilic infiltration was marked in portal areas and patchy throughout the parenchyma; in addition, diffuse Kupffer cell proliferation was seen.

Biochemical abnormalities included highly elevated transaminases and alkaline phosphatase levels in serum. When papaverine was withdrawn, the transaminases returned to normal levels within a few days. In all cases, liver function tests were within normal limits 2 weeks after papaverine administration was discontinued. A rechallenge test 2 months later resulted in an immediate increase in serum transaminases and alkaline phosphatase, together with moderate eosinophilia. Subsequently, laboratory values returned to normal levels within a few days (KIAER et al. 1974). These data provided clinical, biochemical, and morphologic evidence that the hepatotoxic reaction was clearly caused by papaverine.

G. Procainamide

Procainamide (*p*-amino-*N*-(2-diethylaminoethyl) benzamide; Fig. 5) is an agent for the management of cardiac arrhythmias, and approximately 50% of a single dose is converted into the metabolite *N*-acetylprocainamide (KALANT et al. 1985). Excessive dosage of the drug can impair electrical conduction, and ventricular arrhythmias may occur. Side effects on the central nervous system include depression, psychosis, and hallucinations. Hypersensitivity reactions are associated with occasional fever or chills, agranulocytosis, and the development of a syndrome resembling systemic lupus erythematosus. Only six cases of procainamide-induced liver abnormalities have been reported, and these included intrahepatic cholestasis and granulomatous hepatitis (LEIBOWITZ 1951; HELLMAN 1952; KING and BLOUNT 1963; ROTMENSCH et al. 1978; AHN and TOW 1990; WORMAN et al. 1992; CHUANG et al. 1993).

I. Hepatitis

Hepatitis is an extremely uncommon reaction to procainamide therapy. The features of hepatitis in one of these cases included fever, chills, and granulomatous hepatitis, as determined by biopsy examination. These findings may have developed rapidly, since they were observed within 1 week after the start of procainamide administration (ROTMENSCH et al. 1978). The aggregate of clinical symptoms and liver biopsy findings strongly suggested a hypersensitivity mechanism. When the drug was withdrawn, the fever subsided within 24h and a repeat liver biopsy 12 months later showed normal liver histologic features. Rechallenge with the drug caused the reappearance of fever and mild increases in transaminases and bilirubin, all of which became normal after 24h. An allergic reaction was suspected on account of the results of a positive in vitro mast cell degranulation test detecting mast cell-sensitizing antibodies against procainamide. Other tests of immune cell function in response to procainamide were negative, including lymphocyte stimulation and macrophage migration inhibition tests. A similar type of parenchymal granulomatous reaction has been more commonly seen in response to quinidine.

II. Cholestasis

An unusual case of hypersensitivity reaction associated with acute hepatic dysfunction was reported with procainamide after a large single intravenous dose was administered during cardiac electrophysiology studies (WORMAN et al. 1992). The hypersensitivity reaction was characterized by rash, fever, arthralgia, and myalgia. Several hours after receiving procainamide, serum creatine phosphokinase activity was elevated, indicating rhabdomyolysis. This reaction was accompanied by acute hepatocellular injury manifested by increased serum bilirubin and transaminases. Procainamide-induced intrahepatic cholestatic jaundice associated with serum alkaline phosphatase, γ-glutamyltranspeptidase, transaminases, and bilirubin elevations were reported recently. When procainamide administration was stopped, the hepatic enzymes continued to rise in serum, peaked at 11 days after discontinuation of therapy, and slowly receded over several weeks, while γ-glutamyltranspeptidase showed no improvement (AHN and TOW 1980; CHUANG et al. 1993).

H. Quinidine

Quinidine (6-methoxy-α-(5-vinyl-2-quinuclidinyl)-4-quinolinemethanol; Fig. 5) is an essential drug for the treatment of cardiac arrhythmias. Clinical features of quinidine-induced hepatotoxicity included weakness, nausea or vomiting, chilling, anorexia, vague myalgia, and abdominal pains. The most frequently observed clinical signs were fever and hepatomegaly, occasionally splenomegaly, and rarely jaundice (DEISSEROTH et al. 1982; MURPHY and RYMER 1973; HANDLER et al. 1975; KOCH et al. 1976). No deaths have been reported following hepatotoxic reactions, and normal hepatic function returned after discontinuation of the drug in all cases.

I. Hepatitis

Relevant features of quinidine hepatic reactions are fever within 6–12 days of treatment as the first manifestation of toxicity, followed by clinical laboratory and morphologic liver changes. This sequence was confirmed after rechallenge with small doses of the drug leading to prompt recurrence of fever and hepatic dysfunction. Seven cases of hepatitis have been reported due to quinidine, as confirmed by hepatic morphologic abnormalities. By light microscopy, changes included distinct centrizonal or spotty hepatocellular necrosis and degeneration, pericentral subacute inflammatory reaction, and sinusoid dilatation (HANDLER et al. 1975; KOCH et al. 1976). Electron microscopic sections showed the centrilobular zone with completely destroyed hepatocytes and neighboring intact or viable hepatocytes containing many lysosomes and fat vacuoles. Mitochondria showed variations in size and shape and an increase in the number and size of the granules within the matrix. Endoplasmic reticulum membranes were increased with stacking and dilatation. Kupffer cells in necrotic areas were hyperplastic with marked proliferation of microvilli and variations in nuclear size and shape. The cytoplasm of Kupffer cells contained clumps of darkly stained lysosome-like material (KOCH et al. 1976). Approximately 1 month from the beginning of quinidine therapy, transaminases and alkaline phosphatase activities were increased and then fell rapidly to baseline levels. Biochemical function tests were altered, but returned to normal approximately 4 days after rechallenge (DEISSEROTH et al. 1972; MURPHY and RYMER 1973; KOCH et al. 1976).

These data suggest a hypersensitivity mechanism for quinidine hepatotoxic reactions. In all cases there was a relatively uniform 1- to 2-week sensitization period followed by fever and hepatic dysfunction with eosinophilic infiltration of the liver parenchyma. The centrilobular location of the lesion may represent hepatocellular damage by reactive metabolites upon interaction with a specific cytochrome P-450 (McLEAN et al. 1965; MITCHELL and JOLLOW 1975).

II. Granulomatous Hepatitis

Reversible granulomatous hepatitis was reported in six cases of quinidine sulfate-induced hepatotoxicity (GELB et al. 1979; CHAJEK et al. 1974; GELTNER et al. 1976; BRAMLET et al. 1980). Clinical signs of toxicity were weakness, dizziness, diaphoresis, fever, urticaria, and increased serum hepatic enzymes. The formation of granulomata in liver tissue was detected as early as 3 days after readministration of quinidine. These effects were considered to be the results of hypersensitivity to the drug. Light microscopic examination of liver biopsies showed noncaseating granulomatous hepatitis (BRAMLET et al. 1980). Small, round granulomata were clearly seen randomly scattered throughout the parenchyma. Portal areas contained sparse mononuclear infiltrates, and there were no necrotic changes. Electron microscopic studies revealed that the granulomata contained histiocytes, lymphocytes, and engulfed hepatocytes. Focal necrosis was also observed in surrounding hepatocytes, and significant alterations of cytoplasmic organelles were found, especially dilated smooth endoplasmic reticulum and lysosomes. Immunofluorescence staining was slightly positive for polyvalent antihuman γ-globulin and monovalent antihuman IgG in the granulomata (BRAMLET et al. 1980).

I. Lipid-Regulating Agents

Upon establishment of the relationship of altered lipid metabolism and cardiovascular degenerative disease, regulation or control of lipid profiles has characterized the thrust of pharmacotherapy in this area. Atherosclerosis causes 50% of all mortality in the United States (ROSS 1993). In terms of risk reduction, a 1% decrease in cholesterol levels results in a 2% reduction in coronary artery disease morbidity (FURBERG et al. 1994; TODD and WARD 1988). Traditionally, dietary control, physical exercise, and significant life-style modification were recognized as fundamental paradigms in the control of dyslipidemias. Emerging knowledge on lipoprotein metabolism suggested strong genetic control, and receptor-mediated interactions that determine the phenotype most likely to respond to therapy. Thus, lipid regulation by agents affecting specific cell surface receptors or specific enzyme inhibitors are contemporary pharmacotherapy, encompassing homozygous or heterozygous, familial combined or polygenic dyslipoproteinemias. Therapeutic approaches aimed at modifying basic lipid metabolism might eventually elicit unexpected toxicity, considering the significant role of the liver in lipid and lipoprotein metabolism. Paradoxically, there are not many reports characterizing liver structure in patients receiving hypolipidemics, considering the large population undergoing lipid-regulating therapy.

Modulation of hepatic lipid metabolism and the prolonged exposure of patients to these therapeutic modalities prompted the review of lipid-regulating agents on liver function with three main questions in mind:

1. What is the liver structure and function in hyperlipoproteinemias?
2. Can liver effects be differentiated between treated and naive hyperlipoproteinemias?
3. How well do experimental findings correlate with data?

I. Classes of Lipid-Regulating Agents

Early approaches to the treatment of serum dyslipidemias employed resins, probucol, and nicotinic acid either alone or in combination with fibrates (GOTTO 1993). These agents preferentially influenced triglyceride levels with minor effects on cholesterol metabolism. Inhibition of 3-hydroxy-3-methylglutaryl coenzyme A reductase (HMG-CoA), the rate-limiting enzyme of cholesterol biosynthesis, was possible by compactin or mevinolin; the latter was recognized as lovastatin. Cholesterol control, mainly decreasing the low-

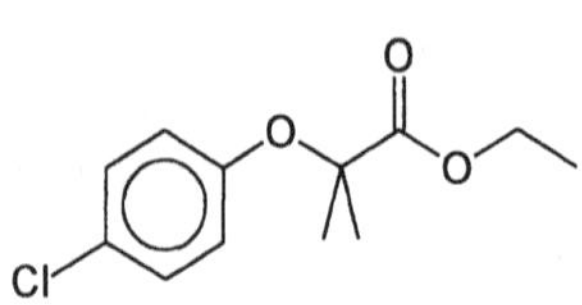

Clofibrate

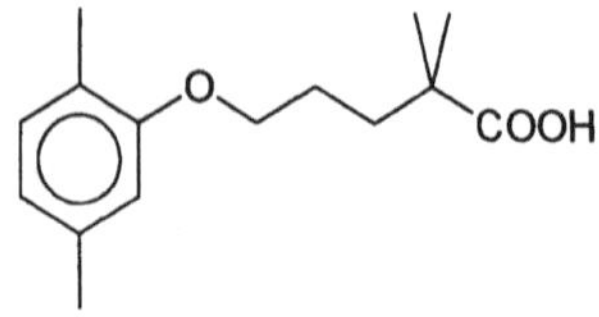

Gemfibrozil

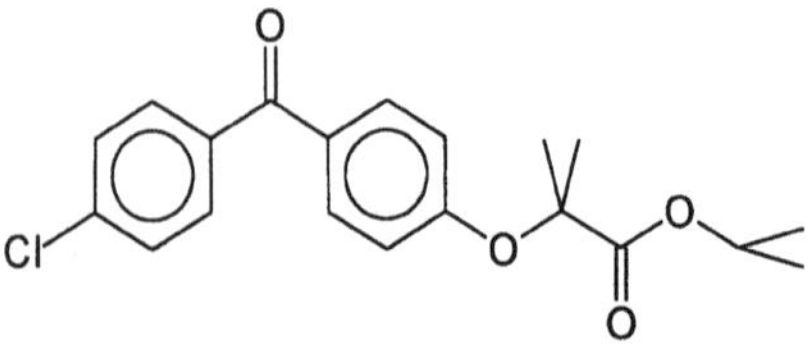

Fenofibrate

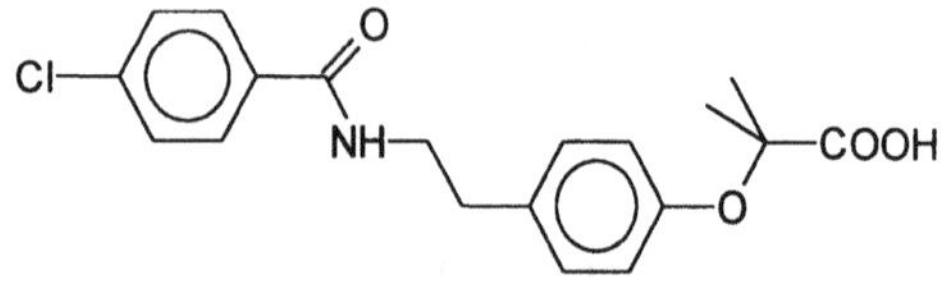

Bezafibrate

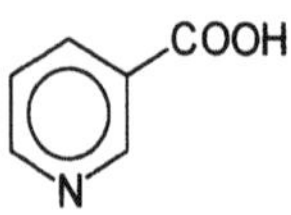

Nicotinic acid

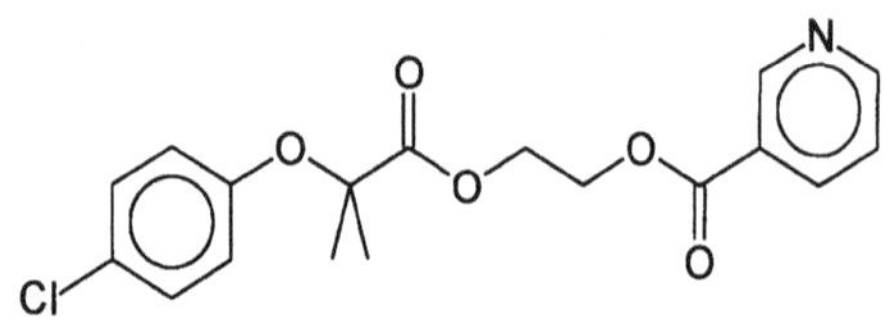

Etofibrate

Fig. 7. Chemical structure of lipid-regulating agents

density lipoprotein (LDL)-cholesterol fraction, became a significant therapeutic approach, and therapeutic regimens for dyslipidemias now include fibrates, statins, or both in association. Most commonly used fibrates include clofibrate, etofibrate, fenofibrate, bezafibrate, and gemfibrozil (Fig. 7); the statins are lovastatin, simvastatin, fluvastatin, mevastatin, pravastatin, and atorvastatin (Fig. 8).

II. Hyperlipoproteinemia and Liver Structure

Changes in serum proteins from hypercholesterolemic patients consist of elevated LDL (NATIONAL CENTER FOR HEALTH STATISTICS 1986). Dyslipidemias occur in later stages of life when several drugs are administered concurrently (i.e., antihypertensives, antirrheumatics, and sedatives being the most frequent association). An early study described the ultrastructure of hepatocytes in two different hyperlipidemias (ANCLA and BEAUMONT 1966), recognizing fatty change as a principal landmark (KOVACS et al. 1972). Some degree of underlying hepatic pathology may be present in response to exogenous factors

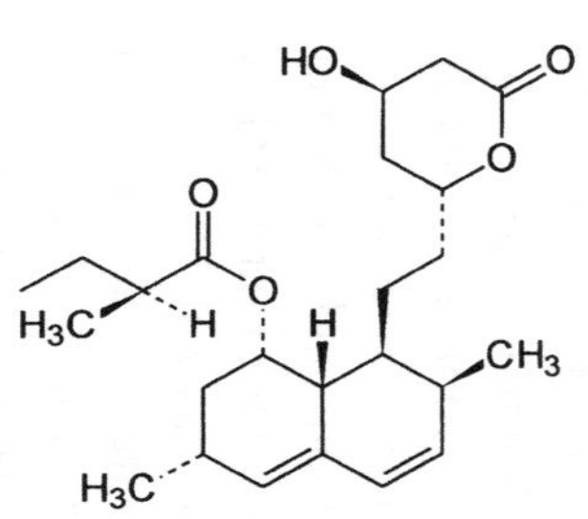

Lovastatin
(MK-803, Mevinolin, MEVACOR)

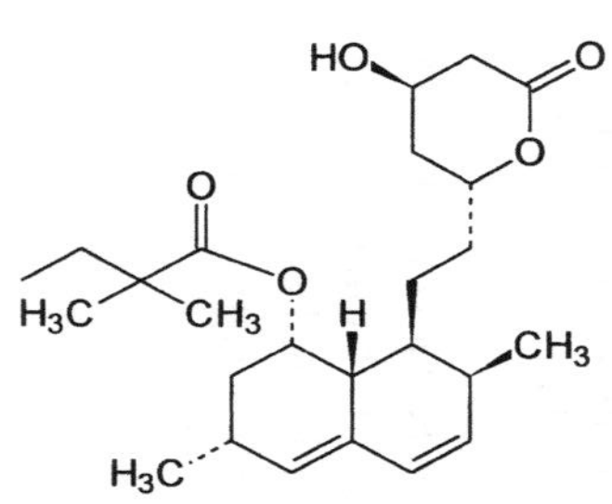

Simvastatin
(MK-733, Synvinolin, ZOCOR)

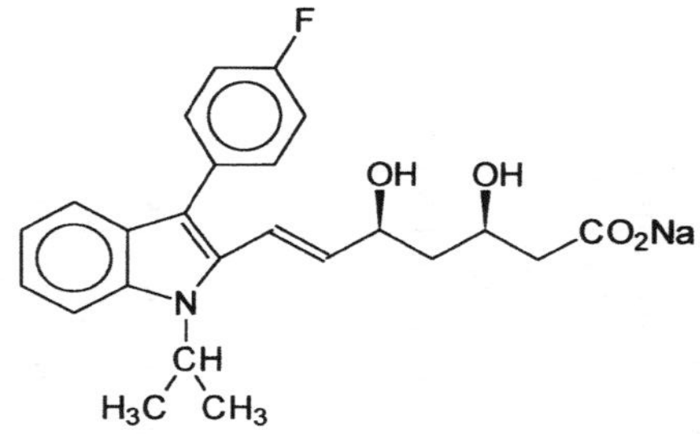

Fluvastatin Sodium
(XU 62-320)

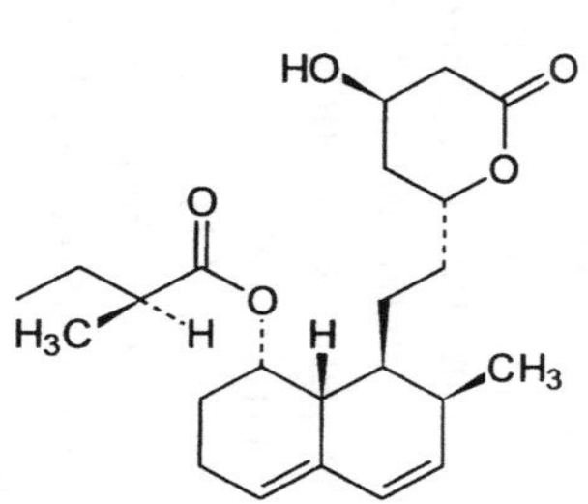

Mevastatin
(ML-236B, CS-500, Compactin)

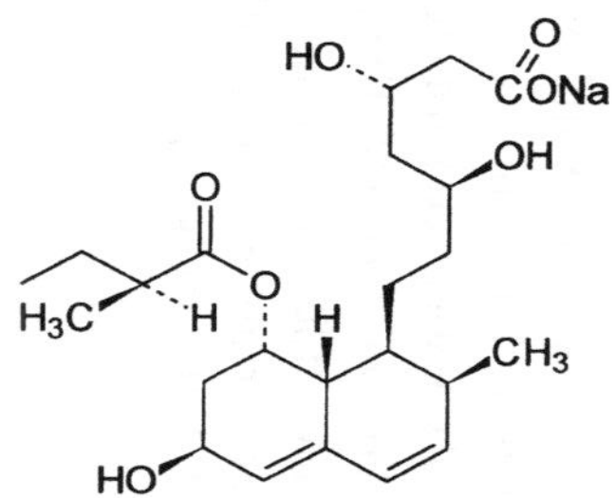

Pravastatin Sodium
(CS-514, SQ-31000)

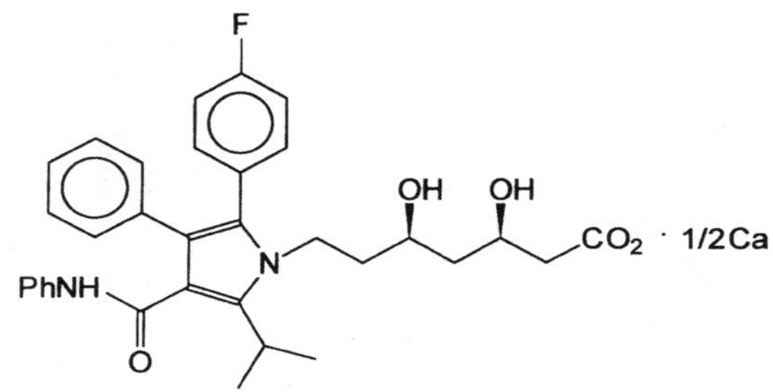

Atorvastatin Calcium
(CI-981)

Fig. 8. Chemical structure of hydroxy-methylglutaryl-coenzyme A reductase inhibitors

such as diet, alcohol intake, or even superimposed drug-related effects by other distinct agents (MA et al. 1972; LIEBER 1991). Nicotinic acid induced ultrastructural changes in the liver within a background of preexisting changes (BAGGENSTOSS et al. 1967; KOHN and MONTES 1969). Several reports have described the liver structure after the administration of other lipid regulators, including clofibrate (KEMMER and HANEFELD 1977; VOSS and KEMMER 1978; HANEFELD et al. 1980), fenofibrate (BLÜMCKE et al. 1983), and gemfibrozil (DE LA IGLESIA et al. 1982).

III. Nicotinic Acid

Nicotinic acid or niacin (pyridine 3-carboxylic acid; Fig. 7) and close derivatives have proved useful lipid-lowering agents; however, nicotinic acid can cause marked peripheral vasodilatation, flushing, gastrointestinal irritation, and hepatotoxicity (WINTER and BOYER 1973; CHRISTENSEN et al. 1962; ISHAK 1982; ETCHASON et al. 1991). The mechanism of this hepatic reaction has not been defined. There are, however, major limiting clinical effects such as flushing, fainting, nausea, and vomiting, and hyperpigmentation of the skin may occur frequently. Large or medium doses of nicotinic acid sometimes cause hepatotoxicity associated with jaundice (RIVIN 1959; KALANT et al. 1985; HENKIN et al. 1990; DALTON and BERRY 1992). Intrahepatic cholestasis was reported during nicotinic acid therapy, characterized with marked pruritus, jaundice, increased serum bilirubin, and alkaline phosphatase (EINSTEIN et al. 1975; RADER et al. 1992; PATEL and TAYLOR 1994).

IV. Fibrates

Clofibrate (2-(4-chlorophenoxy)-2-methyl propanoic acid ethyl ester; Fig. 7) was approved for treatment of hyperlipidemia over 25 years ago. Administration of clofibrate to experimental animals caused significant hepatomegaly, induced hepatic drug metabolizing enzymes (BITEAUX-ANTOINE et al. 1989), and increased peroxisomes and liver tumors. The unknown mechanism for hepatomegaly, the peroxisome proliferation phenomenon, and the tumor formation formed a quizzical triad with apparent relevance for human safety (DE LA IGLESIA and FARBER 1982; REDDY et al. 1980). Fibrates available for use in the last decade were clofibrate, gemfibrozil, fenofibrate, bezafibrate, and others. The prominence of the preclinical findings, together with some of the clinical effects observed, led to an adverse perception as to the long-term safety of fibrates. Like other agents in this group, asymptomatic transaminase elevations over a range of multiples of the upper limit of normal have been recognized (ZIMMERMAN 1990; BLUM 1994). The majority of fibrate-related reactions are related to the gastrointestinal, central nervous, and tegumentary systems (MONK and TODD 1987). No deaths and recovery from these effects other than in liver and muscle was reported in an extensive surveillance study after administration of fenofibrate, ciprofibrate, gemfibrozil, and bezafibrate

(SGRO and ESCOUSSE 1991). One report included a case of fatal hepatitis during treatment with perhexiline maleate and bezafibrate (VALMALLE et al. 1989).

Biopsy data from fibrate-exposed liver and from naive hyperlipidemics show that fatty change is a predominant phenomenon, although qualitatively it may be considered to be different from the steatosis seen in obesity (BACON et al. 1994). A series of reports have described the long-term effects of clofibrate in liver biopsies from dyslipoproteinemic patients (KEMMER and HANEFELD 1977; VOSS and KEMMER 1987; SCHWANDT et al. 1978; HANEFELD et al. 1980, 1983). This series of reports established that no significant changes occurred in subcelluar organelles, including the peroxisomes of human hepatocytes. The number and volume density of peroxisomes increased by 50% and 23% respectively, during the first few months of treatment, and subsequently the values returned to normal limits. Although the morphometric data pointed to volume and numerical density increases, recent criteria indicated that more than twofold increases in the number of peroxisomes are necessary for the expansion of this compartment to be considered biologically relevant (GRAY and DE LA IGLESIA 1984).

Long-term administration of gemfibrozil (5-(2,5-dimethylphenoxy)-2,2-dimethyl pentanoic acid; Fig. 7) was studied in liver biopsies from hyperlipoproteinemic patients (DE LA IGLESIA et al. 1982). Hepatic fatty change appeared as a histopathologic entity irrespective of the pattern of dyslipidemia, and no remarkable effects were reported in the hepatocyte fine structure. No increase in peroxisomes was reported, and a morphometric study confirmed the subjective observations (DE LA IGLESIA et al. 1981).

Fenofibrate (2-[4-(4-chlorobenzoyl) phenoxy]-2-methylpropanoic acid-1-methyl ethyl ester; Fig. 7) has also been studied for liver reactions consistent (BLÜMCKE et al. 1983). Although there have been isolated reports of hepatitis, the incidence is extremely low (SCHWANDT et al. 1978; VACHON 1980; CHATRENET et al. 1993). Organelle antibodies were found against smooth muscle, nucleus, and mitochondria in about 70% of drug-induced hepatitis attributed to a heterogeneous group of drugs which included clometacin, fenpofibrate, oxyphenusatin, and papaverine (HOMBERG et al. 1985). Most frequently recognizable events are moderate, asymptomatic transaminase elevations (ROBERTS 1989). A series of liver biopsies from 28 hyperlipidemic patients on fenofibrate showed no significant hepatic alterations compared to a cohort group of ten naive individuals (BLÜMCKE et al. 1983). Fatty change was also reported. A morphometric study included the evaluation of peroxisomes in liver biopsies from ten patients on fenofibrate and from 15 patients on diet only; no significant differences were found (GARIOT et al. 1983, 1987). Taking all the liver biopsy data together, the proliferation seen in rodents was not reflected in human liver. It is plausible that effects would be seen if humans were to receive higher doses, but species differences in peroxisome ontogenesis are remarkable (DE LA IGLESIA et al. 1992).

V. Statins

Lovastatin and pravastatin (Fig. 8) lower cholesterol and triglycerides in very low density lipoproteins (VLDL), LDL and apoprotein B (ApoB), with minor increases in high-density lipoproteins (HDL) and no changes in ApoA-1 (VEGA and GRUNDY 1990; GRUNDY et al. 1990; JONES et al. 1991). Several studies included coadministration with fibrates, resulting in more pronounced decrease in VLDL and increased HDL. These beneficial effects have been contrasted with a higher risk of myopathy (PIERCE et al. 1990).

Liver transaminase elevations are frequently observed with HMG-CoA inhibitors and these increases usually resolve after withdrawal from therapy. No record of permanent liver damage has been documented (BLUM 1994). Lovastatin increased transaminases in up to 2% of patients receiving the drug for 1 year (FRISMAN et al. 1989). Pravastatin, fluvastatin, simvastatin, or atorvastatin (Fig. 8) caused transaminase elevations above three times the upper limit of normal in a few patients, usually 1%–4% in clinical trials (WALKER 1989; PRAVASTATIN MULTINATIONAL STUDY GROUP FOR CARDIAC RISK PATIENTS 1993; ROBISON et al. 1994; ARKY 1995; NAWROCKI et al. 1995). The low rate of hepatic adverse events with pravastatin may have been the result of the single daily dose mode of administration (JONES et al. 1991).

In experimental studies, lovastatin caused marked hepatocellular atypia and foci of cellular alteration in rats, and bile duct hyperplasia and centrilobular hepatocyte necrosis in rabbits. Transaminase elevation in dogs abated while treatment was continued, and there were no changes in primates (ALBERTS et al. 1989; MACDONALD et al. 1988; GERSON et al. 1989). Fluvastatin caused hepatocellular necrosis in rodents from a carcinogenicity study (ROBISON et al. 1994). An experimental HGM-CoA inhibitor, GR 95030X, increased transaminases and creatine phosphokinase, but no histologic changes in the liver of marmosets (OWEN et al. 1994). Nonhuman primates also did not show liver morphologic changes with simvastatin (MANABE et al. 1989). Similarly, dogs with transaminase increases greater than ten times the control values which resolved spontaneously showed no hepatocellular changes either by light or electron microscopy upon biopsy at the crest of the transaminase elevation (GERSON et al. 1991).

Most of these experimental studies used very high, systemic toxic doses that could have resulted in blood levels intolerable in humans. The pathogenesis of elevated transaminases upon HMG-CoA inhibition is not known. Proposed, but not definitely established mechanisms have been attributed to the extent of inhibitor exposure and to cellular toxicity because of persistent mevalonate synthesis inhibition. The elevated transaminases in humans appear to resolve regardless of whether or not therapy is discontinued. The average increases are not exaggerated and not accompanied by elevated bilirubin or alkaline phosphatase. To our knowledge, there are no literature case reports of liver damage confirmed by biopsy accompanying these transaminase elevations. Considering the experimental evidence reflected in the intense enzyme induction and the metabolic enzyme inhibition, the transaminase elevation may not represent direct liver cell toxicity. Changes in the clearance or metabolism of transaminases might contribute to the high levels observed. Marmosets may represent a good model for studying transaminase elevations, as seen with some experimental compounds. Overall, this class of lipid-regulating agents does not appear to pose a significant hepatotoxicity risk, based on the extent of universal use and the low frequency of reported, documented reactions over the past decade.

J. Miscellaneous Cardiovascular Drugs

Hepatocellular and cholestatic injury has been reported consistently with other drugs in cardiovascular disease (Figs. 5, 9). These included captopril (*S*-[1-(3-mercapto-2-methyl-1-oxypropyl)-L-proline]; Vandenburg et al. 1981; Rychelynck et al. 1982; Hurault de Ligny et al. 1982; Rahmat et al. 1985; Lunel et al. 1987; Bellary et al. 1989; Bailer and Isaac 1989; Hagley et al. 1993), phenindione (2-phenyl-1,3-indanedione; Zimmerman 1963; Ishak 1982), and practolol (*N*-[4-[2-hydroxy-3[(1-methylethyl)-amino]propoxy]-acetamide; Brown et al. 1978). Hepatotoxicity including chronic cholangitis and fatal hepatic injury have been reported in the application of the β-adrenergic blocker labetalol hydrochloride (2-hydroxy-5-[1-hydroxy-2-[9(1-methyl-3-phenylpropyl) aminoethyl] benzamide monohydrochloride; Douglas et al. 1989; Clark et al. 1990; Stumpf 1991). Disopyramide (α-[2-diisopropylamino)ethly]-α-phenyl-2-pyridine-acetamide) has antiarrhythmic effects similar to those of quinidine, and therefore the toxicity is probably

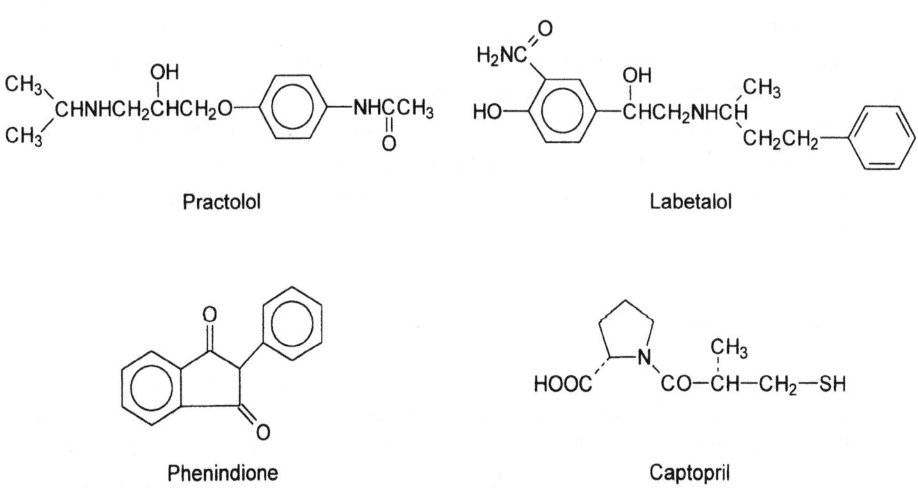

Fig. 9. Chemical structure of phenindione, captopril, labetalol, and practolol

related to a mechanism similar to that described for quinidine (MEINERTZ et al. 1977; MULLEN et al. 1989).

K. Modulation of Hepatotoxicity

Observations from the recent literature suggest that certain cardiovascular drugs can modify or lessen the hepatotoxicity of another drug. Such alternatives may pose interesting opportunities and challenges for future therapeutic applications. Verapamil or chlorpromazine provided protection against carbon tetrachloride- or dimethylnitrosamine-induced liver damage in rats. The mechanism was a reduction of intracellular calcium levels, and these findings were paralleled with the positive effects of calcium channel antagonists on cardiac ischemia (LANDON et al. 1986). When oxidipine was given chronically to rats, transaminase levels decreased even in the presence of microscopic hepatic changes presumed to correlate well with transaminase elevations (WANER et al. 1990). In vitro studies with isolated rat hepatocytes incubated with diltiazem, verapamil, or gallopamil protected the cells from injury by preventing calcium influx into the cytoplasm (THIBAULT et al. 1991). Calcium channel antagonists also inhibited DNA damage and toxic cell death by acetaminophen. Either verapamil or chlorpromazine acting as a calcium calmodulin antagonist had a role in the regulation of intracellular calcium stores and prevented further calcium influx (RAY et al. 1993). These cell-protective effects were also shown after carbon tetrachloride toxicosis, by decreasing transaminase levels and reducing intracellular calcium load (ROMERO et al. 1994). These effects may reflect interactions between the toxicant and the calcium antagonist agent on the cell membrane. After verapamil was infused continuously, sufficient to block P glycoprotein effects, the toxicity of doxorubicin was increased. Elevated transaminases and liver damage ensued, since the verapamil interaction led to increased inflow of the drug into the cell (FUHRMAN et al. 1994). Thus cellular damage can become exaggerated if the calcium channel blocker interacts with nonmetabolic elements of cell defense mechanisms. It is obvious that the protection against cell injury resides in the modulation of calcium channel activity on the cell membrane. This leads to a convergence of thoughts that may bring new opportunities in the approaches to hepatotoxicity management.

L. Conclusions

Many cardiovascular drugs have hepatotoxic potential, and the causative agent has been identified in most studies. In several instances, however, the conclusions derived from the studies have been criticized for the lack of adequate controls, and that the majority of reports describe hospitalized patients with acute disease. This review attempts to evaluate critically hepatic side effects of cardiovascular drugs. The evidence for hepatotoxicity of a particular drug was assessed by reports based on clinical, biochemical, and morphologic liver changes that returned to within normal limits after withdrawal from drug. Rechallenge quickly resulted in overt manifestations of hepatotoxicity with similar symptomatology as in the original reaction.

It is important to consider the significance of side effects in the pathogenesis of drug reactions affecting the liver, since in a high percentage of cases fulminant hepatic failure may be drug related (Trey et al. 1968; Ishak 1982; Clements and Holmes 1987). Cardiovascular drugs in a wide sense include antiarrhythmic, antihypertensive, and lipid-lowering agents and their wide use relates to the high morbidity and prevalence of these diseases. The integral assessment of clinical, biochemical, and morphologic findings showed known types of liver reactions, such as cholestasis, fatty change, hepatitis, granulomatous reactions, necrosis, and cirrhosis. The mechanism of the adverse effect of the drug depends on whether or not it results in microvesicular steatosis, acute hepatocellular injury, cholestasis, or idiosyncratic reaction. Toxic metabolite-dependent or hypersensitivity-related liver injury is frequently associated with immunologic changes. Liver biopsy in patients on cardiovascular drugs with clinical and biochemical changes suggested liver dysfunction and pointed directly to drugs causing autoimmune hepatitis. Unexplained, asymptomatic elevated transaminase levels in the absence of bilirubin or other liver function tests in patients on cardiovascular drugs ranged from spontaneous resolution to significant hepatic injury. The degree of enzyme elevation is not usually synchronized with the cellular damage. Thus hepatonecrogenic potential cannot be ascribed prima facie to elevated transaminases in the absence of confirmatory liver biopsy data.

The diagnosis of fulminant hepatic failure due to drug toxicity is very important. Severe hepatitis during therapy with cardiovascular drugs is rare and has only been reported after exposure to α-methyldopa, amiodarone, hydralazine, or labetalol. In these life-threatening situations, liver biopsy is also an important component in the patient management and treatment, and it can extend to liver transplantation. Major conclusions derived from reports on the hepatoxicity of cardiovascular drugs emphasize the importance of the liver biopsy for understanding the nature and extent of liver injury, for identifying the pattern of liver disease associated to a specific drug, and for predicting the outcome or patient prognosis.

Finally, each of the drugs considered caused a low frequency of hepatic reactions, although in some instances a multifactorial origin may play a role. There are no significant data pointing to synergies that can precipitate serious liver reactions, and perhaps some have been avoided by present trends that reduce the number of concurrent medications a patient may be receiving. Nevertheless, the possibility of hepatic injury needs to be carefully considered when one or more of these drugs are used in the treatment of cardiovascular disease.

References

Adams PC, Bennett MK, Holt DW (1986) Hepatic effects of amiodarone. Br J Clin Pract [Symp Suppl] 44:81–95
Ahn CS, Tow DE (1990) Intrahepatic cholestasis due to hypersensitivity reaction to procainamide. Arch Intern Med 150:2589–2590
Alarcon-Segovia D, Wakim KG, Worthington JW, Ward LE (1967) Clinical and experimental studies on the hydralazine syndrome and its relationship to systemic lupus erythematosus. Medicine (Baltimore) 46:1–33
Alberts AW, MacDonald JS, Till AF, Tobert JA (1989) Lovastatin. Cardiovasc Drug Rev 7:89–109
Anastasiou-Nana MI, Anderson JL, Nanas JN et al. (1986) High incidence of clinical and subclinical toxicity associated with amiodarone treatment of refractory tachyarrhythmia. Can J Cardiol 2:138–145
Ancla M, Beaumont V (1966) Etude du foie au microscope electronique dans deux variétés d'hyperlipidemies majeures. Pathol Biol 14:1167–1177
Arky R (1995) Physicians' desk reference. Montvale, NJ. Medical Economics Data, Division of Medical Economics Company
Arranto AJ, Sotaniemi EA (1981a) Morphological alterations in patients with alpha-methyldopa-induced liver damage after short- and long-term exposure. Scand J Gastroenterol 16:853–863
Arranto AJ, Sotaniemi EA (1981b) Histologic follow up of alpha-methyldopa-induced liver injury. Scand J Gastroenterol 16:865–872
Babany G, Mallat A, Zafrani ES, Saint-Marc Girardin MF, Carcone B, Dhumeaux D (1986) Chronic liver disease after low daily doses of amiodarone. J Hepatol 3:228–232
Bacon BR, Farakvash MJ, Janney CG, Neuschwander-Tetri BA (1994) Nonalcoholic steatohepatitis: an expanded clinical entity. Gastroenterology 107:1103–1109
Baggenstoss AH, Christensen NA, Berge KG, Baldus WP, Spiekerman RE, Ellefson RD (1967) Fine structural changes in the liver in hypercholesterolemic patients receiving long-term nicotinic acid therapy. Proc Mayo Clin 42:385–399
Bailer SO, Isaac DE (1989) Captopril and the liver. Lancet 2:154–156
Balazs MS, Kovach G (1981) Chronic aggressive hepatitis after methyldopa treatment. Hepatogastroenterology 28:199–202
Balazs MS, Varkonyi S, Juhasz J (1973) Elektronmikroskopische Untersuchungen in Fällen von chronisch-aggressiver Hepatitis. Acta Hepatogastroenterol 20:399–409
Barnett DB, Hudson SA, Golightly PW (1980) Hydralazine-induced hepatitis. Br Med J 280:1165–1166
Bartoli E, Massarelli G, Solinas A, Faedda R, Chiandussi L (1979) Acute hepatitis with bridging necrosis due to hydralazine intake. Arch Intern Med 139:698–699
Batchelor JR, Welsh KI, Mansila-Tinoco R, Dollery CT, Hughes GR, Bernstein R, Ryan P, Naish PF, Aber GM, Bing RF, Russell GI (1980) Hydralazine-induced systemic lupus erythematosus. Influence of HLA-DR and sex on susceptibility. Lancet 1:1107–1109
Bellary SV, Isaacs PET, Scott AW (1989) Captopril and liver. Lancet 2:514
Blum CB (1994) Comparison of properties of four inhibitors of 3-hydroxy-3-metylglutaryl-coenzyme-reductase. Am J Cardiol 73:3D–11D
Blümcke S, Schwartzkopff W, Lobeck H, Edmonson NA, Prentice DE, Blane GF (1983) Influence of fenofibrate on cellular and subcellular live structure in hyperlipidemic patients. Atherosclerosis 46:105–116
Boiteaux-Antoine AF, Magdalou J, Fournel-Gigleux S, Siest G (1989) Comparative induction of drug-metabolizing enzymes by hypolipidemic compounds. Gen Pharmacol 20:407–412
Bourdi M, Gautier J-C, Mircheva J, Larry D, Guillouzo A, Andre C, Belloc C, Beaune PH (1992) Anti-liver microsomes autoantibodies and dihydralazine-induced hepatitis: specificity of autoantibodies and inductive capacity of the drug. Mol Pharmacol 42:280–285

Bramlet DA, Posalaky Z, Olson R (1980) Granulomatous hepatitis as a manifestation of quinidine hypersensitivity. Arch Intern Med 40:395–397

Brandes JW, Smitz-Moormann P, Lehmann FG, Martini GA (1976) Gelbsucht nach Aprindin. Eine hepatitis-ähnliche Arzneimittelschädigung. Dtsch Med Wochenschr 101:111–113

Breland BD, Hicks GS (1982) Hepatitis and hemolytic anemia associated with methyldopa therapy. Drug Intel Clin Pharm 16:489–492

Brown PJ, Lesna M, Hamlyn AN, Record CO (1978) Primary biliary cirrhosis after long-term practolol administration. Br Med J 1:1591

Cannon PJ, Laragh JH (1963) Treatment of hypertension with alpha-methyl-dopa. Pharmacotherapie 1:171–184

Capron-Chivrac D, Reis N, Quenum C et al. (1985) Hepatopathie aigue due à l'amiodarone. Etude d'un cas et revue de la literature. Gastroenterol Clin Biol 9:535–539

Chajek T, Lehrer B, Geltner D, Levij IS (1974) Quinidine-induced granulomatous hepatitis. Ann Intern Med 81:774–776

Chatrenet P, Regimbeau C, Ramain JP, Penot J, Bruandet P (1993) Hepatite chronique active cirrhogène au fenofibrate. Gastroenterol Clin Biol 17:612–613

Christensen NA, Anchor RW, Berge KG et al. (1961) Nicotinic acid treatment of hypercholesterolemia. JAMA 177:546

Chuang LC, Tunier AP, Akhtar N, Levine SM (1993) Possible case of procainamide-induced intrahepatic cholestatic jaundice. Ann Pharmacother 27:434–437

Clark JA, Zimmerman HJ, Tanner LA (1990) Labetalol hepatotoxicity. Ann Intern Med 113:485

Clements GL, Holmes AW (1987) Nicotinic acid induced fulminant hepatic failure. J Clin Gastroenterol 9:582–584

Dalton TA, Berry RS (1992) Hepatotoxicity associated with sustained-release niacin. Am J Med 93:102–104

Deisseroth A, Morganroth J, Winokur S (1972) Quinidine-induced liver disease. Ann Intern Med 77:595–597

De Korwin JD, Gagey S, Paille F et al. (1986) Hepatite aigue imputée à l'amiodarone. Gastroenterol Clin Biol 10:688–689

de la Iglesia FA, Farber E (1982) Hypolipidemics carcinogenicity and extrapolation of experimental results for human safety assessments. Toxicol Pathol 10:152–174

de la Iglesia FA, Feuer G, Takada A, Matsuda Y (1974) Morphologic studies on secondary phospholipidosis in human liver. Lab Invest 30:539–549

de la Iglesia FA, Feuer G, McGuire EJ, Takada A (1975) Morphological and biochemical changes in the liver of various species in experimental phospholipidosis after diethylaminoethoxy-hexestrol treatment. Toxicol Appl Pharmacol 34:28–44

de la Iglesia FA, Pinn SM, Lucas J, McGuire EJ (1981) Quantitative stereology of peroxisomes in hepatocytes from hyperlipoproteinemic patients receiving gemfibrozil. Micron 12:97–107

de la Iglesia FA, Lewis JE, Buchanan RA, Marcus EL, MacMahon G (1982) Light and electron microscopy of the liver in hyperlipoproteinemic patients under long-term gemfibrozil treatment. Atherosclerosis 43:19–37

de la Iglesia FA, Gray RH, McGuire EJ (1992) Subcellular organelle biogenesis and dynamics in peroxisome proliferation. J Am Coll Toxicol 11:343–348

Dienstag JL, Wands JR, Koff RS (1987) Acute hepatitis. In: Braunwald E, Isselbacher KJ, Petersdorf RG et al. (eds) Harrison's principles of internal medicine. 11th edn. McGraw-Hill, New York, pp 1325–1338

Douglas DD, Yang RD, Jensen P, Thiele DL (1989) Fatal labetalol-induced hepatic injury. Am J Med 87:235–236

Duke MD, Madison JM, Montgomery CK et al. (1985) Electron microscopic demonstration of lysosomal inclusion bodies in lung, liver, lymph nodes and blood leukocytes of patients with amiodarone pulmonary toxicity. Am J Med 78:506–512

Einstein N, Baker A, Galper J, Wolf H (1975) [illegible] Am J Dig Dis 20:282–286

Elewant A, Van Durme JF, Goethals L, Kauffman JM, Mussche M, Elinck W, Roels H, Bogaert M, Barbier F (1977) Aprindine-induced liver injury. Acta Gastroenterol Belg 40:236–243

Eliastam M, Holmes AW (1971) Hepatitis, arthritis and lupus cell phenomena caused by methyldopa. Dig Dis 16:1014–1018

Elisaf M, Stefanaki-Nikou S, Voulgarelis M, Masalas C, Tsianos EV (1992) Aprindine-induced granulomata. J Hepatol 14:276–279

Elkington SG, Schreiber WM, Conn HO (1969) Hepatic injury caused by L-alpha methyldopa. Circulation 40:589–595

Enat R, Rader G, Barzilai J (1977) Leberschaden durch Adelphan. Schweiz Med Wochenschr 107:657

Etchason JA, Miller TD, Squires RW et al. (1991) Niacin-induced hepatitis: a potential side effect of low-dose time-release niacin. Mayo Clin Proc 66:23–28

Farber HI (1974) Fever, vomiting and liver dysfunction with procainamide therapy. Postgrad Med 56:155–156

Fasola AF, Carmichael R (1974) The pharmacology and clinical evaluation of aprindine – a new antiarrhythmic drug. Acta Cardiol 29 [Suppl 8]:317–333

Fisher MM (1980) Mechanisms of drug-induced cholestasis. Semin Liver Dis 1:151–156

Flaharty KK, Chase SL, Yaghsezian HM, Rubin R (1989) Hepatotoxicity associated with amiodarone therapy. Pharmacotherapy 9:39–44

Fogoros RN, Anderson KP, Winkle RA et al. (1983) Amiodarone: clinical efficacy and toxicity of 96 patients with recurrent drug-refractory arrhythmias. Circulation 68:88–94

Fornacieri G, Monducci I, Barone A, Bassi C, Beltrani M, Tomasi C (1992) Amiodarone-induced acute hepatitis: case report. J Clin Gastroenterol 15:271–273

Forster HS (1980) Hepatitis from hydralazine. N Engl J Med 302:1362

Fuhrman GM, Cromeens DM, Newman RA, Clear KR, Carrasco CH, Wright KC, Guercio S, Guercio A, Curley SA (1994) Hepatic arterial infusion of verapamil and doxorubicin with complete hepatic venous isolation and extracorporeal chemofiltration: pharmacological evaluation of reduction in systemic drug exposure and assessment of hepatic toxicity. Surg Oncol 3:17–25

Funck-Brentano C, Jacqz-Aigrain E, Leenhardt A, Roux A, Poirier J-M, Jaillon P (1991) Influence of amiodarone on genetically determined drug metabolism in humans. Clin Pharmacol Ther 50:259–266

Furberg CD, Byington RP, Crouse JR, Espeland MA (1994) Pravastatin, lipids and major coronary events. Am J Cardiol 73:1133–1134

Furhoff AK (1978) Adverse reactions with methyldopa – a decade's reports. Acta Med Scand 203:425–428

Gariot P, Barrat E, Mejean L, Pointel JP, Drouin P, Debry G (1983) Fenofibrate and human liver. Lack of proliferation of peroxisomes. Arch Toxicol 53:151–163

Gelb A, Grazenas N, Sussman H (1979) Acute granulomatous disease of the liver. Dig Dis 15:842–847

Geltner D, Chajek T, Rubinger D et al. (1976) Quinidine hypersensitivity and liver involvement: a survey of 32 patients. Gastroenterology 70:650–652

Gerlach V, Manitz G, Themann H (1969) Feinstrukturuntersuchungen bei activer chronischer Hepatitis unter besondere Berücksichtigung des Mesenchyms. Acta Hepatospenol 16:90–105

Gerson RJ, MacDonald JS, Alberts AW, Kornbrust DJ, Majka JA, Stubbs RJ, Bokelman DL (1989) Animal safety and toxicology of simvastatin and related hydroxy-methylglutaryl-coenzyme A reductase inhibitors. Am J Med 87 [Suppl 4A]:285–389

Gerson RJ, Allen HL, Lankas GR, MacDonald JS, Alberts AW, Bokelman DL (1991) The toxicity of a fluorinated-biphenyl HMG-CoA reductase inhibitor in Beagle dogs. Fund Appl Toxicol 16:320–329

Gilinsky NH, Briscoe GW, Kuo CS (1988) Fatal amiodarone hepatotoxicity. Am J Gastroenterol 83:161–163

Gillmore BL, Freis ED (1965) Methyldopa in the treatment of hypertension. Med Ann DC 34:13–18

Goldman IS, Winkler ML, Raper SE, Barker ME, Keung E, Goldberg HI, Boyer TD (1985) Increased hepatic density and phospholipidosis due to amiodarone. Am J Roentgenol 144:541–546

Goldstein GB, Lam KC, Mistilis SP (1973) Drug induced active chronic hepatitis. Dig Dis 18:177–184

Gotto AM Jr (1993) Dyslipidemia and atherosclerosis. A forecast of phramaceutical approaches. Circulation 87 [Suppl]:III54–III59

Gray RH, de la Iglesia FA (1984) Quantitative microscopy comparison of peroxisome proliferation by the lipid regulating agent gemfibrozil in several species. Hepatology 4:520–530

Grundy SM, Vega GL, Garg A (1990) Use of 3-hydroxy-3-methyl glutaryl coenzyme A reductase inhibitors in various forms of dyslipidemia. Am J Cardiol 66:31B–38B

Guigui B, Perrot S, Berry JP, Fleury-Feith J, Martin N, Metreau JM, Dhumeaux D, Zafrani ES (1988) Amiodarone-induced hepatic phospholipidosis: a morphological alteration independent of pseudoalcoholic liver disease. Hepatology 8:1063–1068

Hagley MT, Hulisz DT, Burns CM (1993) Hepatotoxicity associated with angiotensin-converting enzyme inhibitors. Ann Pharmacother 27:228–231

Handler SD, Hirsch NR, Haas K et al. (1975) Quinidine hepatitis. Arch Intern Med 135:871–872

Hanefeld M, Kemmer C, Leonhardt W, Kunze KD, Jaross W, Haller H (1980) Effects of p-chlorophenoxyisobutyric acid (CPIB) on the human liver. Atherosclerosis 36:159–172

Hanefeld M, Kemmer C, Kadner E (1983) Relationship between morphological changes and lipid-lowering action of p-chlorophenoxyisobutyric acid (CPIB) on hepatic mitochondria and peroxisomes in man. Atherosclerosis 46P:239–246

Harris L, McKenna W, Rowland E, Storey G, Krikler D (1983) Side effects of long term amiodarone therapy. Circulation 67:45–51

Hellman E (1952) Allergy to procainamide. J Am Med Assoc 149:1393–1394

Henkin Y, Johnson KC, Segrest JP (1990) Rechallenge with crystalline niacin after drug-induced hepatitis from sustained-release niacin. JAMA 264:241–243

Herlong HF, Reid PR, Boitnott JK, Maddrey WC (1978) Aprindine hepatitis. Ann Intern Med 89:359–361

Hoffbrand BI, Fry W, Bunton GL (1974) Cholestatic jaundice due to methyldopa. Br Med J 3:559–561

Homberg JC, Abuaf N, Helmy-Khalil S, Biour M, Poupon R, Islam S, Darnis F (1985) Drug-induced hepatitis associated with anticytoplasmic organelle autoantibodies. Hepatology 5:722–727

Hostetler KY, Giordano JR, Jellison EJ (1988) In vitro inhibition of lysosomal phospholipase Al, of rat lung by amiodarone and desethylamiodarone. Biochem Biophys Acta 959:316–321

Hoyumpa AM, Connell AM (1973) Methyldopa hepatitis: report of three cases. Am J Dig Dis 18:213–222

Hruban Z (1984) Pulmonary and generalized lysosomal storage induced by amphiphilic drugs. Environ Health Perspect 55:53–76

Hurault de Ligny B, Mariot A, Kessler M, Caraman PL, Netter P (1982) Hepatite au cours d'une polythérapie associant de captopril. Therapie 37:698–700

Hutterer F, Klion FM, Wengraf A, Schaffner F, Popper H (1969) Hepatocellular adaptation and injury. Structural and biochemical changes following dieldrin and methyl-butter yellow. Lab Invest 20:455–464

Ide T (1971) A case of phospholipid fatty liver. Hepatosplenol Jpn 12:474–483

Irias JJ (1975) Hydralazine-induced lupus erythematosus-like syndrome. Am J Dis Child 129:862–864

Irvine RO, O'Brien KP, North JDK (1962) Alpha methyldopa in treatment of hypertension. Lancet 1:300–303

Ishak KG (1982) The liver. In: Riddell RH (ed) Pathology of drug-induced and toxic diseases. Churchill Livingstone, London, pp 457–513
Itoh S, Yamada Y, Ichinoe A, Tsukada Y (1980) Hydralazine-induced liver injury. Dig Dis Sci 25:884–887
Itoh S, Ichinoe A, Tsukada Y, Itoh Y (1981) Hydralazine-induced hepatitis. Hepatogastroenterology 28:13–16
Jones DB, Mullick FG, Hoofnagle JH, Baranski B (1988) Reye's syndrome-like illness in a patient receiving amiodarone. Am J Gastroenterol 83:967–969
Jones PH, Farmer JA, Cressman MD et al. (1991) Once-daily pravastatin in patients with primary hypercholesterolemia: a dose-response study. Clin Cardiol 14:146–151
Jori GP, Peschle C (1973) Hydralazine disease associated with transient granulomas in the liver. Gastroenterology 64:1163–1167
Kalant H, Roschlau WH, Sellers EM (eds) (1985) Principles of medical pharmacology, 4th edn. University of Toronto, Toronto, pp 207–208
Kalantzis N, Gabriel P, Mouzas J, Tiniakos D, Tsigas D, Tiniakos G (1991) Acute amiodarone-induced hepatitis. Hepatogastroenterology 38:71–74
Kemmer C, Hanefeld M (1977) Ultrastructural results in liver biopsies from patients with hyperlipoproteinemia. Zentralbl Allg Pathol Pathol Anat 121:243–253
Kiaer HW, Olson S, Ronnov-Jessen V (1974) Hepatotoxicity of papaverine. Arch Pathol 98:292–296
King JA, Blount RE Jr (1963) An unexpected reaction to procainamide. J Am Med Assoc 186:603–604
Kirtland HH, Mohler DN, Horwitz DA (1980) Methyldopa inhibition of suppressor-lymphocyte function – a proposed cause of autoimmune hemolytic anemia. N Engl J Med 302:825–832
Knoblauch M, Cueni B, Spycher M, Schmid M (1977) Dihydralazin-induzierte akute Hepatitis bei IgM-Mangel. Schweiz Med Wolhenschr 107:651–656
Koch MJ, Seeff LB, Crumbley CE, Rabin L, Burns WA (1976) Quinidine hepatotoxicity. A report of a case and review of the literature. Gastroenterology 70:1136–1140
Koch-Weser J (1976) Medical intelligence. Drug therapy hydralazine. N Engl J Med 295:320–323
Kohn RM, Montes M (1969) Hepatic fibrosis following long term nicotinic acid therapy. A case report. Am J Med Sci 258:94–99
Kovacs K, Lee R, Little JA (1972) Ultrastructural changes of hepatocytes in hyperlipoproteinemia. Lancet 1:752–753
Kremer GJ, Kössling FK, Lange HJ, Victor N (1969) Bestimmung des Fettgehalts in der Leber. Dtsch Med Wochenschr 94:163–166
Landon EJ, Naukam RJ, Rama-Sastry BV (1986) Effects of calcium channel blocking agents on calcium and centrilobular necrosis in the liver of rats treated with hepatotoxic agents. Biochem Pharmacol 35:697–705
Leibowitz S (1951) Chills and fever following oral use of procainamide. N Engl J Med 245:1006
Lewis JH, Ranard RC, Caruso A, Jackson LK, Mullick F, Ishak KG, Seeff LB, Zimmerman HJ (1989) Amiodarone hepatotoxicity: prevalence and clinicopathologic correlations among 104 patients. Hepatology 5:679–685
Lewis JH, Mullick F, Ishak KG, Ranard RC, Ragsdale B, Perse RM, Rusnock EJ, Wolke A, Benjamin SB, Seeff LB, Zimmerman HJ (1990) Histopathologic analysis of suspected amiodarone hepatotoxicity. Hum Pathol 21:59–67
Lim PK, Trewby PN, Storey GCA et al. (1984) Neuropathy and fatal hepatitis in a patient receiving amiodarone. Br Med J 288:1638–1639
Lüllmann H, Lüllmann-Rauch R, Wassermann O (1975) Drug-induced phospholipidoses. Crit Rev Toxicol 4:185–218
Lunel F, Griffen P, Cadrenec JF, Victor N, Opolon P (1987) Hepatitie aigue après la prise du maleate d'enalapril. Gastroenterol Clin Biol 11:174–175

Lupon-Roses J, Simo-Canonge R, Lu-Cortez L et al. (1986) Probably early acute hepatitis with parenteral amiodarone. Clin Cardiol 9:223–225
Ma MH, Goldfisher S, Biempica L (1972) Morphology of the normal liver cell. Prog Liver Dis 4:1–17
MacDonald JS, Gerson RJ, Kornbrust DJ, Kloss MW, Prahalada S, Berry PH, Alberts AW, Bokelman DL (1988) Preclinical evaluation of lovastatin. Am J Cardiol 62:16J–27J
Maddrey WC, Boitnott JK (1975) Severe hepatitis from methyldopa. Gastroenterology 68:351–360
Manabe S, Sudo S, Yamashita K et al. (1989) Subacute toxicological study in monkeys treated orally with pravastatin sodium for 5 weeks. J Toxicol Sci 14 [Suppl]:57–83
Manohitharajah SM, Jenkins WJ, Roberts PD, Clarke RC (1971) Methyldopa and associated thrombocytopenia. Br Med J 1(747):494
Martin WJ II, Rosenow EC III (1988a) Amiodarone pulmonary toxicity. Recognition and pathogenesis, part 1. Chest 93:1067–1075
Martin WJ II, Rosenow EC III (1988b) Amiodarone pulmonary toxicity. Recognition and pathogenesis, part 2. Chest 93:1242–1248
Mason JW (1987) Amiodarone. N Engl J Med 316:455–466
Matsuda Y, Ikegami F, Kobayashi K, Hasumura Y, Takada A, Takeuchi J (1971) Phospholipidosis caused by DH. Saishin Igaku 26:2263–2267
McGovern B, Garan H, Kelly E et al. (1983) Adverse reactions during treatment with amiodarone hydrochloride. Br Med J 287:175–180
McLean AEM, McLean EK, Judah JD (1965) Cellular necrosis in the liver induced and modified by drugs. Int Rev Exp Pathol 4:127–137
Meinertz T, Langer KH, Kasper W, Just H (1977) Disopyramide-induced intrahepatic cholestasis. Lancet 2:828–829
Mitchell JR, Jollow DJ (1975) Metabolic activation of drugs to toxic substances. Gastroenterology 68:392–410
Monk JP, Todd PA (1987) Bezafibrate. A review of its pharmacodynamic and pharmacokinetic properties and therapeutic use in hyperlipidemia. Drugs 33:539–576
Morady F, Sauvé MJ, Malone P et al. (1983) Long-term efficacy and toxicity of high-dose amiodarone therapy for ventricular tachycardia or ventricular fibrillation. Am J Cardiol 52:975–979
Morelli S, Guido V, De Marzio P, Aguglia F, Balsano F (1991) Early hepatitis during intravenous amiodarone administration. Cardiology 78:291–294
Moses A, Zahger D, Amir G (1989) Cholestatic liver injury after prolonged exposure to methyldopa. Digestion 42:57–60
Mullen GE, Greenson JK, Mitchell MC (1989) Fulminant hepatic failure after ingestion of sustained release nicotinic acid. Ann Intern Med 111:253–255
Murphy PJ, Rymer W (1973) Quinidine-induced liver disease? Ann Intern Med 78:785–786
Myer S, Knell AJ (1977) Cirrhosis and hemolysis complicating methyldopa treatment. Br Med J 1:879–882
Nataf J, Bernau J, Larry D, Guillin MC, Ruff B, Benhamou JP (1986) A new anti-liver microsome antibody: a specific marker of dihydralazine-induced hepatitis. Gastroenterology 90:1751
National Center for Health Statistics (1986) Total serum cholesterol levels of adults 20 to 74 years of age: United States, 1976–1980. Department of Health and Human Services, Washington DC, publication (DHS) 86–1686, vital and health statistics, series 11, no 236
Nawrocki JW, Weiss SR, Davidson MH, Sprecher DL, Schwartz SL, Lupien PJ, Jones PH, Haber HE, Black DM (1995) Reduction of LDL cholesterol by 25% to 60% in patients with primary hypercholesterolemia by atorvastatin, a new HMG-CoA reductase inhibitor. Arterioscler Thromb Vasc Biol 15:678–682
Neuberger J, Kenna JG, Nouri Aria K, Williams R (1985) Antibody mediated hepatocyte injury in methyl dopa induced hepatotoxicity. Gut 26:1233–1239

Oda T, Shikata T, Naito C, Suzuki H, Kanetaka I, Iino S, Miyake K, Sakai T, Onda H, Fujiwara K, Yamanaka M, Shimizu N, Yoshitoshi Y (1970) Phospholipid fatty liver: a report of three cases with a new type of fatty liver. Jpn Exp Med 40:127–135

Owen K, Pick CR, Libretto SE, Adams MJ (1994) Toxicity of a novel HMG-CoA reductase inhibitor in the common marmoset (callithrix jacchus). Hum Exp Toxicol 13:357–368

Pai RG, Pai SM (1988) Methyldopa-induced revcersible immune thrombocytopenia. Am J Med 85:123

Pariente EA, Pessayre D, Bernuau J, Degott C, Benhamon JP (1983) Dihydralazine hepatitis: report of a case and review of the literature. Digestion 27:47–52

Patel SD, Taylor HC (1994) Intrahepatic cholestasis during nicotinic acid therapy. Cleve Clin J Med 61:70–75

Pathy MS, Reynolds AJ (1980) Papaverine and hepatotoxicity. Postgrad Med J 56:488–490

Pierce LR, Wysowski DK, Gross TP (1990) Myopathy and rhabdomyolysis associated with lovastatin-gemfibrozil combination therapy. JAMA 264:2991–2992

Plonteux G, Heagham C, Ernowald H, Vondeghen N (1969) Long-term hepatic tolerance of amiodarone in the clinic. Eur J Pharmacol 8:369–376

Poucell S, Ireton J, Valencia-Mayoral P, Downar E, Larratt L, Patterson J, Blendis L, Phillips MJ (1984) Amiodarone-associated phospholipidosis and fibrosis of the liver, light, immunohistochemical and electron microscopic studies. Gastroenterol 86:926–936

Pravastatin Multinational Study Group for Cardiac Risk Patients (1993) Effects of pravastatin in patients with serum total cholesterol levels from 5.2 to 7.8 mmol/liter (200–300 mg/dl) plus two additional atherosclerotic risk factors. Am J Cardiol 72:1031–1037

Puppala AR, Steinheber FU (1977) Fulminant hepatic failure associated with methyldopa. Am J Gastroenterol 68:578–581

Pye M, Northcote RJ, Cobbe SM (1988) Acute hepatitis after parenteral amiodarone administration. Br Heart J 59:690–691

Rader JI, Calvert RJ, Hathcock JN (1992) Hepatic toxicity of unmodified and time-release preparations of niacin. Am J Med 92:77–81

Raeder EA, Podrid PJ, Lown B (1985) Side effects and complications of amiodarone therapy. Am Heart J 109:975–983

Rahmat J, Gelfand RL, Gelfand MC, Winchester JF, Schreiner GE, Zimmerman HJ (1985) Captopril associated cholestatic jaundice. Ann Intern Med 102:56–58

Ray SD, Kamendulis LM, Gurule MW, Yorkin RD, Corcoran GB (1993) Ca^{2+} antagonists inhibit DNA fragmentation and toxic cell death induced by acetaminophen. FASEB J 7:453–463

Reasor MJ (1989) A review of the biology and toxicologic implications of the induction of lysosomal lamellar bodies by drugs. Toxicol Appl Pharmacol 97:47–56

Reasor MJ, Kacew S (1990) Amiodarone pulmonary toxicity: morphologic and biochemical features. Proc Soc Exp Biol Med 196:1–7

Reddy J, Azarnoff DL, Hignite CE (1980) Hypolipidaemic hepatic peroxisome proliferators form a novel class of chemical carcinogens. Nature 283: 397–398

Rehman OM, Keith TA, Gall EA (1973) Methyl-dopa induced submassive hepatic necrosis. JAMA 224:1390–1392

Reid PR, Greene HL, Varghese PJ (1977) Suppression of refractory arrhythmias by aprindine in patients with the Wolff-Parkinson-White syndrome. Br Heart J 39:1353–1360

Rhodes A, Eastwood JB, Smith SA (1993) Early acute hepatitis with parenteral amiodarone: a toxic effect of the vehicle? Gut 34:565–566

Rigas B, Rosenfeld LE, Barwick KW, Enriquez R, Helsberg J, Batsford WP, Josephson ME, Riely CA (1986) Amiodarone hepatotoxicity. A clinicopathologic study of five patients. Ann Intern Med 104:348–351

Rinder HM, Love JC, Wexler R (1986) Amiodarone hepatoxicity. N Engl J Med 314:318–319
Rivin AV (1959) Jaundice occurring during nicotinic acid therapy for hypercholesterolemia. JAMA 170:2088–2089
Roberts WC (1989) Safety of fenofibrate – US and worldwide experience. Cardiology 76:169–179
Robinson K, Mulrow JP, Rowland E, McKenna WJ (1989) Long-term effects of amiodarone on hepatic function. Am J Cardiol 64:95–96
Robison RL, Suter W, Cox RH (1994) Carcinogenicity and mutagenicity studies with fluvastatin, a new, entirely synthetic HMG-CoA reductase inhibitor. Fund Appl Toxicol 23:9–20
Rodman JS, Deutsch DJ, Gutman SI (1976) Methyldopa hepatitis: a report of six cases and review of the literature. Am J Med 60:941–948
Romero G, Las Heras B, Sainz-Suberviola L, Cenarruzabeitia E (1994) Protective effects of calcium channel blockers in carbon tetrachloride-induced liver toxicity. Life Sci 55:981–990
Ronnov-Jessen V, Tjernlund A (1969) Hepatotoxicity due to treatment with papaverine: report of four cases. N Engl J Med 281:1333–1337
Ross R (1993) The pathogenesis of atherosclerosis: a perspective for the 1990s. Nature 362:810–809
Rotmensch HH, Yust I, Siegman-Igra Y, Liron M, Ilie B, Vardinon N (1978) Granulomatous hepatitis: a hypersensitivity response to procainamide. Ann Intern Med 89:646–647
Rotmensch HH, Belhassen B, Swanson BN et al. (1984) Steady state serum amiodarone concentrations: relationship with antiarrhythmic efficacy and toxicity. Ann Intern Med 101:462–469
Ruben Z, Rorig KJ, Kacew S (1993) Perspectives on intracellular storage and transport of cationic-lipophilic drugs. Proc Soc Exp Biol Med 203:140–149
Rumessen JJ (1986) Hepatotoxicity of amiodarone. Acta Med Scand 219:235–239
Rychelynck JP, Batho JM, Peny J, Beuve-Mery P (1982) Hepatite au captopril. Nouv Presse Med 11:1950–1951
Saal AK, Werner JA, Greene HL, Sears GK, Graham EL (1984) Effect of amiodarone on serum quinidine and procainamide levels. Am J Cardiol 53:1264–1267
Sataline L, Lowell D (1976) Methyldopa toxicity. Gastroenterology 70:148–149
Schmid M (1967) Zur Frage der chronischen Hepatitis. Dtsch Med Wochenschr 92:257–258
Schmitz G, Muller G (1991) Structure and function of lamellar bodies, lipid-protein complexes involved in storage and secretion of cellular lipids. J Lipids Res 32:1539–1570
Schwandt P, Klinge O, Immich H (1978) Clofibrate and the liver. Lancet 2:325
Schweitzer IL, Peters RL (1974) Acute submassive hepatic necrosis due to methyldopa. Gastroenterology 66:1203–1211
Seggie J, Saunders SJ, Kirsch RE (1979) Alpha-methyldopa-induced hepatotoxicity. S Afr Med J 55:77–83
Seydel JR, Wassermann O (1976) NMR studies on the molecular basis of drug-induced phospholipidosis. II. Interaction between several amphophilic drugs and phospholipids. Biochem Pharmacol 25:2357–2364
Sgro C, Escousse A (1991) Effets indésirables des fibrates (hors de foie et muscle). Therapie 46:351–354
Shaefer MS, Markin RS, Wood RP, Shaw BW (1989) Hydralazine-induced cholestatic jaundice following liver transplantation. Transplantation 47:203–204
Shaikh NA, Downar E, Butany J (1987) Amiodarone – an inhibitor of 5-phospholipase activity. A comparative study of the inhibitory effects of amiodarone, chloroquine and chlorpromazine. Mol Cell Biochem 76:163–172
Shenasa M, Vaisman U, Wojciechowski M, Denker S, Murthy V, Akatar M (1984) Abnormal abdominal computerized tomography with amiodarone therapy and clinical significance. Am Heart J 107:929–933

Shepherd NA, Dawson AM, Crocker PR, Levison DA (1987) Granular cells as a marker of early amiodarone hepatoxicity: a pathological and analytical study. J Clin Pathol 40:418–423
Sherlock S (1987) Diseases of the liver and biliary system, 9th edn. Blackwell Scientific, Oxford, pp 390–424
Simon JB, Manley PN, Brien JF et al. (1984) Amiodarone hepatotoxicity simulating alcoholic liver disease. N Engl J Med 311:167–172
Smith WM, Lubbe WF, Whitlock RM et al. (1986) Long-term tolerance of amiodarone treatment for cardiac arrhythmias. Am J Cardiol 57:1288–1293
Snir Y, Pick N, Riesenberg K, Yanai-Inbar I, Zirkin H et al. (1995) Fatal hepatic failure due to prolonged amiodarone treatment. J Clin Gastroenterol 20:265–266
Sotaniemi EA, Hokkanen OT, Ahokas JT, Pelkonen RO, Ahlquist J (1977) Hepatic injury and drug metabolism in patients with alpha-methyldopa-induced liver damage. Eur J Clin Pharmacol 12:429–435
Starko KM, Mullick FG (1983) Hepatic and cerebral pathology findings in children with fatal salicylate intoxication: further evidence for a causal relation between salicylate and Reye's syndrome. Lancet 1:326–329
Stevenson RN, Nayani TH, Davies JR (1989) Acute hepatic dysfunction following parenteral amiodarone administration. Postgrad Med J 65:707–708
Stewart GW, Peart WS, Boylston AW (1981) Obstructive jaundice pancytopenia and hydralazine. Lancet 1:1207
Stoel I, Hagemeijer F (1980) Aprindine: a review. Eur Heart J 1:147–156
Stumpf JL (1991) Fatal hepatotoxicity induced by hydralazine or labetalol. Pharmacotherapy 11:415–418
Svensson CK, Chong MT (1989) Effect of amiodarone on the disposition of acetaminophen in the rat. J Pharm Sci 78:900–902
Thibault N, Peytavin G, Claude JR (1991) Calcium channel blocking agents protect against acetaminophen-induced cytotoxicity in rat hepatocytes. J Biochem Toxicol 6:237–238
Thomas E, Bhuta S, Rosenthal WS (1976) Methyldopa-induced liver injury. Rapid progression to fatal postnecrotic cirrhosis. Arch Pathol Lab Med 100:132–135
Thomas E, Rosenthal WS, Zapiach L, Micci D (1977) Spectrum of methyldopa liver injury. Am J Gastroenterol 68:125–133
Tjordman K, Katz I, Bursztyn M (1986) Amiodarone and the liver. Ann Intern Med 102:411–412
Todd PA, Ward A (1988) Gemfibrozil. A review of its pharmacodynamic and pharmacokinetic properties and therapeutic use in dyslipidemia. Drugs 36:314–339
Toghill PJ, Smith PG, Benton P, Brown RC, Matthews HL (1974) Methyldopa liver damage. Br Med J 3:545–548
Trey C, Lipworth L, Chalmers T et al. (1968) Fulminant hepatic failure: presumable contribution of halothane. N Engl J Med 279:798–801
Tysell JE, Knauer M (1971) Hepatitis induced by methyldopa (Aldomet). Report of a case and a review of the literature. Dig Dis 16:849–855
Uchida T, Kao H, Quispe-Sjogren M et al. (1983) Alcoholic foamy degeneration – a pattern of acute alcoholic injury of the liver. Gastroenterology 84:683–692
Vachon JM (1980) Hepatite due au procetofene. Nouv Presse Med 9(37):2740
Valmalle R, Bacq Y, Furet Y, Dorval E, Barbieux JP, Metman EH (1989) Hepatite aiguë mortelle lors d'un traitment par maleate de perhexiline et bezafibrate. Gastroenterol Clin Biol 13:530–531
Vandenburg M, Parfrey P, Wright P, Lazda E (1981) Hepatitis associated with captopril treatment. Br J Clin Pharmacol 11:105–106
Van Leeuwen R, Meyboom RH (1976) Agranulocytosis and aprindine. Lancet 2:1137–1139
Varma RR, Troup PJ, Komorowski RA et al. (1985) Clinical and morphological effects of amiodarone on the liver. Gastroenterology 88:1091–1093
Vega GL, Grundy SM (1990) Management of primary mixed hyperlipidemic with lovastatin. Arch Intern Med 150:1313–1319

Voss K, Kemmer C (1987) Image processing in pathology part 8: internal structure of mitochondria during treatment of HLP-patients with regadrin. Exp Pathol 15:311–318

Vrobel TR, Miller PE, Mostow ND, Rakita L (1989) A general overview of amiodarone toxicity: its prevention, detection and management. Prog Cardiovasc Dis 31:393–426

Waldman RJ, Hall WN, McGee H et al. (1982) Aspirin as a risk factor in Reye's syndrome. JAMA 247:3089–3094

Walker JF (1989) Simvastatin: the clinical profile. Am J Med 87 [Suppl 4A]:44S–46S

Waner T, Nyska A, Bogin E, Levy R, Galiano A (1990) Drug-induced decrease of serum alanine and aspartate aminotransferase activity in the rat as a result of treatment with oxidipine, a new calcium channel blocker. J Clin Chem Clin Biochem 28:25–30

Waxman HL, Groh WC, Marchlinski FE et al. (1982) Amiodarone for control of sustained ventricular tachyarrhythmia: clinical and electrophysiologic effects in 51 patients. Am J Cardiol 50:1066–1074

Wechsler B, Brion NO, Colau C, Ximenes H, Godeau P (1979) Lupus erythemateux induit par la dihydralazine. Nouv Press Med 8:3754–3755

Williams ER, Khan MA (1967) Liver damage in patients on methyldopa. J Ther Clin Res 1:5–7

Wilson JS, Podrid PJ (1991) Side effects from amiodarone. Am Heart J 121:158–171

Winter SL, Boyer JL (1973) Hepatic toxicity from large doses of vitamin B3 (nicotinamide). N Engl J Med 289:1180–1182

Worman HJ, Ip JH, Winters SL, Tepper DC, Gomes AJ (1992) Hypersensitivity reaction associated with acute hepatic dysfunction following a single intravenous dose of procainamide. J Intern Med 232:361–363

Yagupsky P, Gazala E, Sofer S, Maor E, Abarbanel J (1985) Fatal hepatic failure and encephalopathy associated with amiodarone therapy. J Pediatr 107:967–970

Yap SH, Rijntjes PJ, Mashage HJ (1987) Amiodarone-induced lyposomal inclusions in primary cultures of human hepatocytes. Gastroenterology 92:272–273

Ylikallio A, Sotaniemi EA (1980) Drug metabolism and liver function after methyldopa withdrawal. Br J Clin Pharmacol 10:115–119

Zimmerman HJ (1963) Clinical and laboratory manifestation of hepatotoxicity. Ann NY Acad Sci 104:954

Zimmerman HJ (1990) Update of hepatotoxicity due to classes of drugs in common clinical use: non-steroidal drugs, anti-inflammatory drugs, antibiotics, antihypertensives, and cardiac and psychotropic agents. Semin Liver Dis 10:322–338

CHAPTER 22

Analgesic Hepatopathy

M.J. ZUCKERMAN and S. ANURAS

A. Introduction

Analgesic hepatopathy refers to a spectrum of drug-induced hepatic injury that may be caused by a large number and variety of both prescription and nonprescription drugs. Data on the epidemiology, pathogenesis, clinical manifestations and outcome, treatment, and prevention of hepatic injury due to acetaminophen, the nonsteroidal antiinflammatory drugs (NSAIDs), and narcotic analgesics are reviewed.

Data on the incidence of analgesic hepatopathy are variable, but the extent of the problem and the number of fatalities is greater for acetaminophen than the NSAIDs. The clinical settings in which analgesic hepatopathy occurs include that of acute overdose, short-term therapeutic use, long-term therapeutic use, intermittent use, and the use of multiple analgesics or other potentially hepatotoxic medications. Mechanisms of hepatotoxicity may be either predictable (intrinsic hepatotoxicity) or unpredictable (metabolic or immunologic idiosyncratic hepatotoxicity). Acetaminophen is a dose-dependent hepatotoxin associated with a particular pattern of liver injury and which has a specific and effective therapy, so treatment is discussed in detail. NSAIDs cause a spectrum of hepatic injury by different mechanisms, and specific antidotes are not available. The importance of recognizing NSAID-induced hepatotoxicity is stressed.

B. Acetaminophen

I. Epidemiology

1. Incidence of Hepatotoxicity

Acetaminophen (paracetamol; *N*-acetyl-para-amino-phenol) is a popular analgesic and antipyretic available over-the-counter as a single medication or in combination with other agents. The standard dosage formulations of acetaminophen in the United States are 325 mg, 500 mg, and 650 mg (BLACK and RAUCY 1986; SEEF et al. 1986). Acetaminophen is generally considered a safe and effective drug with a recommended maximum daily intake of 4 g (BRAY 1993) and a wide margin of safety. However, since the first cases of severe liver injury due to self-poisoning were described in Great Britain (Davidson and Eastham 1966; Proudfoot and Wright 1970; Thomson and Prescott 1966), acetaminophen has become the most common cause of drug-induced acute liver injury and hepatic failure in many countries (George and Farrell 1993; Smilkstein et al. 1991; Zimmerman and Maddrey 1993).

Detailed information on the incidence of acetaminophen-induced hepatotoxicity and associated morbidity and mortality is not available (Mitchell 1988; Prescott 1983). The most common setting for acetaminophen-induced liver injury is that of suicidal overdose, but injury may also occur unintentionally or accidentally in alcoholics and with therapeutic use (Barker et al. 1977; Prescott 1986; Seef et al. 1986). In the acute overdosage setting, liver injury is usually associated with the ingestion of greater than 10–15 g acetaminophen (Stricker 1992). It is a popular means of attempting suicide in many Western countries, but there are differences between countries (Lee 1993a). The incidence rose dramatically in Great Britain in the 1970s (Prescott 1983) and acetaminophen is the most common suicidal agent there (Lee 1993b). It is estimated that acetaminophen overdose is still responsible for at least 100 deaths annually in Great Britain (O'Grady et al. 1991) and is the cause of over half the cases admitted to the liver failure unit at King's College Hospital in London. Acetaminophen is the most common pharmacologic agent involved in drug overdoses in the United States, with more than 97 000 cases reported to poison control centers in 1989 (Litovitz et al. 1990; Smilkstein et al. 1991). Recent reports from other countries show that acetaminophen poisoning is a significant reason for hospitalization in Australia (Brotodihardjo et al. 1992), and has been an increasing problem in Israel over the past decade (Oren and Levy 1992; Winkler and Halkin 1992) with a recent estimated annual incidence of acetaminophen overdoses of 57/100 000. However, hepatic injury due to acetaminophen was not found to be a frequent event (18 of 1100 cases) in an analysis of cases of drug-induced hepatic injury report to the Danish Committee on Adverse Drug Reactions (1978–1987), despite being available over the counter since 1984 (Friis and Andreasen 1992).

2. Hepatotoxicity in Alcoholics

In addition to suicide attempts, the other clinical setting in which the recognition of acetaminophen-induced hepatotoxicity has been emphasized is in chronic alcoholics (Barker et al. 1977; Erickson et al. 1992; Edwards and Oliphant 1992; Floren et al. 1987; Goldfinger et al. 1978; Kumar and Rex 1991; Licht et al. 1980; Maddrey 1987; McClain et al. 1980; Seef et al. 1986; Wooton and Lee 1990). Most of the clinical reports have been in patients taking doses usually considered safe, either in the therapeutic range or slightly above this range (less than 10 g/day) (Schenker and Maddrey 1991). In a review of 47 cases of alcohol-induced hepatotoxicity (Seifert et al. 1993), the average dose of acetaminophen was found to be 7 g/day, with doses as low as

2.5 g/day reported. From a survey of 64 alcoholics at Oklahoma Memorial Hospital (SEIFERT et al. 1993), it was found that 31% were regular acetaminophen users and 3 were chronic daily drinkers who ingested more than 2.5 g daily, suggesting the widespread potential for hepatotoxicity. It has been reported that this alcohol acetaminophen syndrome accounted for 65% of patients admitted for acute liver failure at Parkland Memorial Hospital in Dallas, Texas (LEE 1993a), and suggested that this may be the most common form of acute liver failure in the United States. Although it is recognized that it is difficult to obtain accurate information on drug ingestion from alcoholics (MADDREY 1987), the problem of hepatotoxicity at relatively low doses of acetaminophen in chronic alcoholics is well recognized (SCHENKER and MADDREY 1991).

3. Hepatotoxicity in Therapeutic Settings

There have been several reports of hepatotoxicity from apparently therapeutic doses of acetaminophen in patients who were not chronic alcoholics (BARKER et al. 1977; JOHNSON and TOLMAN 1977; MADDREY 1987; MCCLAIN et al. 1988). Hepatotoxicity from acute or chronic ingestion in this setting may be more common than previously recognized and serum acetaminophen levels are usually not obtained either due to lack of appreciation of the role of the drug or because it has already been discontinued. Factors suggested to increase susceptibility to hepatotoxicity in nonalcoholics at these lower doses, in the range of 5–6 g/day, are starvation and malnutrition, as well as other drug ingestion (BARKER et al. 1977; ERICKSSON et al. 1992; LEE 1993a; SCHENKER and MADDREY 1991). These patients usually recover after discontinuation of the drug. Acute liver injury has also been reported (BONKOVSKY et al. 1994) after short-term ingestion of therapeutic doses (1–3 g/day) of acetaminophen in a patient with chronic cardiopulmonary disease. Studies suggested that hepatic toxicity was due to reduced hepatic and renal clearance, as well as reduced hepatic glutathione concentration possibly related to hepatic hypoxia.

Drug interactions may be responsible for some cases of unintentional acetaminophen-induced toxicity at therapeutic or near-therapeutic doses. There may be enhanced susceptibility due to anticonvulsant drugs (BRAY 1993). There have been several recent reports of liver injury in patients taking both isoniazid and acetaminophen at modest doses, suggesting a possible interaction (CRIPPIN 1993; MOULDING et al. 1991; MURPHY et al. 1990; NOLAN et al. 1994). Acetaminophen-induced hepatotoxicity has been reported with a therapeutic dose in a nonalcoholic patient being treated for human immunodeficiency virus infection (SHRINER and GOETZ 1992). Although increased hepatotoxicity of acetaminophen due to zidovudine may have been responsible, multiple explanations could be considered in the setting, including malnutrition, in addition to other drug interactions and human immunodeficiency virus or other related infections.

II. Pathogenesis

1. Hepatotoxic Dose and Blood Level

The threshold dose for liver toxicity after a single ingestion in humans is generally considered to be above 10–15 g and most cases of poisoning from a single overdose have been over 15 g in adults and 150 mg/kg in children (MITCHELL et al. 1974; PRESCOTT 1983; SMILKSTEIN et al. 1988; ZIMMERMAN and MADDREY 1993). However, there is not a good correlation between dose and severity of liver injury. Additionally, the patient's estimate of the dose ingested may not be reliable and vomiting and gastric lavage may reduce the amount of drug actually absorbed.

The plasma concentration of acetaminophen is more closely related to the risk of liver damage than is the dose (BLACK 1980; PRESCOTT et al. 1971, 1974; PRESCOTT 1983). After a hepatotoxic dose of acetaminophen, metabolism is impaired and there is a prolongation of the half-life which is related to the extent of liver damage. Nomograms estimating the risk of hepatotoxicity, and used for treatment decisions, have been developed based upon these observations. Using a semilogarithmic plot of plasma acetaminophen concentration versus time after ingestion, severe liver damage can be predicted to usually occur if the acetaminophen level exceeds 300 µg/ml at 4 h after ingestion or 50 μg/ml at 12 h, or if the serum half-life exceeds 4 h. Liver damage can be expected above 200 μg/ml at 4 h and is unlikely at values below 150 μg/ml at 4 h.

2. Mechanism

Acetaminophen causes predictable hepatotoxicity related to the production of a toxic metabolite (BLACK 1980; MITCHELL et al. 1973a,b, 1974; PRESCOTT 1983). In therapeutic doses, the major metabolic pathway of acetaminophen is through glucuronide and sulfate conjugation, which is dose dependent. A small fraction (approximately 5%) of the dose is metabolized by the cytochrome P-450 system to a reactive metabolite which is normally inactivated by conjugation with glutathione and eventually excreted as cysteine and conjugates of mercapturic acid. The reactive metabolite, thought to be *N*-acetyl-*p*-benzoquinoneimine, is normally detoxified by conjugation with glutathione. The reactive metabolite causes hepatocellular necrosis when hepatocellular glutathione becomes depleted. With large doses of acetaminophen, the normal metabolic pathway becomes saturated and the toxic metabolite accumulates due to increased production and depletion of glutathione stores due to consumption. The mechanism of cell injury by the reactive metabolite of acetaminophen is probably by covalent binding of the toxic metabolite to hepatocellular constituents or by peroxidative injury (NELSON 1990). The mechanism of liver damage in alcoholics and in the therapeutic setting of patients who present with evidence of acute hepatic necrosis is the same as that in the overdosage setting (PRESCOTT 1986). There may be individual differences in the metabolism of acetaminophen. It has been suggested that some individuals with hepatic injury at low doses of acetaminophen may have an idiosyncratic mechanism of hepatotoxicity (MITCHELL 1988; PRESCOTT 1986; STRICKER 1992).

3. Factors Influencing Hepatotoxicity

Factors which may influence the hepatotoxicity of acetaminophen include alcohol use, drug metabolism, age, diet, and nutrition. Acetaminophen-induced hepatotoxicity due to injury caused by the toxic metabolite is influenced by both the activity of the cytochrome P-450 system and the concentration of intrahepatic glutathione. Individual variation in susceptibility can occur because the rate of metabolite formation is related to dose, rate of absorption, glucuronide and sulfate conjugation capacity, and cytochrome P-450 enzyme activity (MITCHELL 1988). Genetic factors may play a role (BRAY 1993; NELSON 1990). There appears to be a lower incidence of hepatotoxicity in children (RUMACK 1984), even at acetaminophen blood levels toxic in adults. There may be age-related differences in metabolic pathways (RUMORE and BLAIKLOCK 1992).

The clinical association of acetaminophen hepatotoxicity with alcoholism and possible drug interactions may be explained on the basis of acetaminophen metabolism. Although not all animal studies agree, chronic alcohol use is thought to predispose to hepatotoxicity due to increased production of the toxic metabolite by induction of cytochrome P-450 activity (P-450 IIE1) and decreased detoxification of the metabolite due to depletion of glutathione (KUMAR and REX 1991; LAUTERBURG and VELEZ 1988; MADDREY 1987). Decreased glutathione stores may also explain the possible predisposition of malnutrition to hepatotoxicity (BARKER et al. 1977; ERICKSSON et al. 1992; LAUTERBURG and VELEZ 1988). A number of drugs have been shown in models to either inhibit or enhance hepatic injury, some (e.g., caffeine) having different effects at different doses (NELSON 1990; STRICKER 1992). In particular, cysteine precursors, as discussed under treatment, and cimetidine inhibit and phenobarbital and isoniazid enhance hepatotoxicity.

III. Clinical Manifestations and Laboratory Findings

1. Clinical Course

The clinical course after an acetaminophen overdose has a predictable pattern (LINDEN and RUMACK 1992; PRESCOTT 1983; RUMACK and MATTHEW 1975; ZIMMERMAN 1978). Early signs and symptoms are nonspecific. Consciousness is not impaired unless there is an effect from the ingestion of other drugs. The first phase occurs in the first few hours after ingestion of a hepatotoxic dose. There is anorexia, nausea, and vomiting, although some patients are asymptomatic. These symptoms may resolve and the patient appears to have recovered. The second phase occurs 1–3 days after ingestion with evidence of liver injury. There is abdominal pain, right upper quadrant tenderness, and elevated transaminase levels, possibly with associated jaundice. Liver enzymes [both alanine aminotransferase (ALT) and aspartate aminotransferase (AST) are high (>1000 to several thousand IU/l) and at times extremely high (>10000 IU/l). There are lesser increases in alkaline phosphatase and only modest hyperbilirubinemia (usually less than four times normal in the early stages). Coagulation disturbances with prolonged prothrombin time may appear. The patient may become oliguric. The third phase occurs 3–5 days following ingestion, when some patients go on to develop clinically apparent liver disease and possibly fulminant hepatic failure. Additionally, hematologic, renal, and cardiac abnormalities may occur. Severe thrombocytopenia, not associated with disseminated intravascular coagulation, has been described in a few cases of overdose (FISCHEREDER and JAFFE 1994; THORNTON and LOSOWSKY 1990). Acute renal failure may occur in association with hepatotoxicity, usually with severe poisoning, and also can occur as the liver injury is improving (BOYER and ROUFFE 1971; MCCLAIN 1988; PRESCOTT 1983). Patients go on to either death from fulminant hepatic failure and its complications or to recovery. In patients who recover, liver function returns to normal, usually within 7–20 days (PRESCOTT 1983).

The clinical manifestations in patients with acetaminophen-induced hepatotoxicity with therapeutic use may include a short history of malaise, nausea, vomiting, abdominal pain, and jaundice along with typical biochemical abnormalities of high aminotransferases, mild to moderate increase in bilirubin, and normal or mild increase in alkaline phosphatase (PRESCOTT 1986). Patients may not volunteer information on acetaminophen ingestion and confirmation of the exact does of acetaminophen ingested is usually not possible. A characteristic clinical presentation of acetaminophen toxicity in chronic alcoholics has been emphasized (KUMAR and REX 1991; MADDREY 1987; SEEF et al. 1986). Patients may have complaints on presentation similar to those of overdose patients, but laboratory abnormalities may include extremely high serum aminotransferase levels and prolonged prothrombin time, with AST more elevated than ALT. Compared to the usual suicide ingestion patients, acetaminophen hepatotoxicity in alcoholics is associated with elevated aminotransferases on presentation, there is the usual elevated AST/ALT ratio seen in alcoholics, and acetaminophen levels if checked are usually normal or low since the drug has often been discontinued. Aminotransferase levels are generally higher than those seen in alcoholic hepatitis.

2. Pathology

The characteristic histopathologic appearance at biopsy or autopsy is centrizonal hemorrhagic necrosis (BLACK 1980; ZIMMERMAN 1978). Kidneys may also be affected and show proximal and distal tubular necrosis. Typical cases of liver damage occurring in the therapeutic setting associated with marked aminotransferase elevation also show acute centrilobular hepatic necrosis with little or no inflammatory reaction or involvement of the portal tracts (PRESCOTT 1986). Several atypical cases have been described. Acute necrosis associated with overdosage may be superimposed upon chronic lesions (PRESCOTT 1986). Chronic liver injury has rarely been reported (BONKOVSKY et al. 1978; JOHNSON and TOLMAN 1977), either exacerbated by or caused by long-term ingestion of therapeutic doses of acetaminophen.

3. Prognosis

The morbidity and mortality from acetaminophen overdose depends on the source and selection of patients (PRESCOTT 1983). End points may be either clinically significant hepatotoxicity, usually defined as aminotransferase levels greater than 1000 IU/l, or death, and prognosis is clearly affected by the timing and administration of specific therapy. Early reports of mortality from acetaminophen overdose in Great Britain and the United States prior to the use of specific therapy were in the range of 6%–25%, but it is probably now in the 1%–2% range (PRESCOTT 1983). Prognosis on admission can be assessed by measuring plasma acetaminophen concentration in relation to time after ingestion (see Sect. II.1) (PRESCOTT et al. 1971, 1979). Using these nomograms, hepatotoxicity occurs in about 60% of patients with acetaminophen concentrations above the line joining semilogarithmic plots of 200 μg/ml at 4 h and 30 μg/ml at 15 h, and 90% above the line joining 300 μg/ml and 45 μg/ml. According to these investigators, about 15% of overdose patients fall above the treatment line, hepatotoxicity develops in 8%, and fatal hepatic failure in 1%–2%. In an early British treatment trial (PRESCOTT et al. 1979), 58% of patients studied retrospectively who received supportive treatment alone developed hepatotoxicity and 5% died. Using the similar Rumack-Matthew nomogram (LINDEN and RUMACK 1992; RUMACK and MATTHEW 1975), patients treated with suppportive care only who had acetaminophen levels above the probable hepatic toxicity line had a 14%–89% incidence of hepatotoxicity and a mortality of 5%–24%.

In the era of specific treatment for acetaminophen overdose, prognosis is improved (see Sect. IV.2). In the American oral *N*-acetylcysteine trial (SMILKSTEIN et al. 1988), there was a mortality of 0.43% (11 of 2540) and, among those treated in the intravenous *N*-acetylcysteine trial (SMILKSTEIN et al. 1991), mortality attributable to acetaminophen was 1.1% (2 of 179). In a study of 306 overdose patients from Westmead Hospital in Sydney, hepatotoxicity developed in 6.9%, fulminant hepatic failure in 1%, and there were no deaths. In a study of 291 subjects presenting to Jerusalem hospital emergency rooms, toxic range levels were found in only 6, and all patients recovered without evidence of hepatotoxicity.

Prognostic factors have also been studied in patients who develop fulminant hepatic failure. Death due to acetaminophen-induced fulminant hepatic failure usually occurs 4–18 days after drug ingestion (BLACK 1980), and at Kings College Hospital only 12% of patients with fatal outcomes died within 3 days following the overdose (Harrison et al. 1990b). Based upon studies from Kings College Hospital, survival rates were 34.4%. Age was an important variable, with higher mortality in the age group >50 years (O'Grady et al. 1989). The following adverse prognostic factors were identified: an acidosis (arterial pH < 7.30 on admission) or the subsequent development of grade III encephalopathy, a prothrombin time >100s, and a serum creatinine concentration of >300 μmol/l. Another poor prognostic sign identified may be a plasma factor V concentration ≤10% of normal and this has been suggested as being potentially useful for selecting candidates for transplant when present in conjunction with an increase in factor VIII or severe hepatic coma within 2 or 3 days of overdose (Pereira et al. 1992).

The prognosis for patients with acetaminophen-induced hepatotoxicity with therapeutic use is not well defined. Many alcoholics and patients with unintentional liver injury and typical clinical symptoms and biochemical abnormalities resolve without sequelae (Linden and Rumack 1992; Prescott 1986). Acetaminophen levels or half-lives in these settings are usually not known, but it is assumed that patients with potentially toxic levels on the nomogram are at risk of hepatotoxicity. From the literature on acetaminophen hepatotoxicity in alcoholics presenting with high aminotransferase levels (Lee 1993b), mortality is at least 20%.

IV. Treatment

1. General Management

Clinical information should be obtained regarding the amount and formulation of acetaminophen ingested, other drugs ingested or medications being taken, acute or chronic alcohol abuse, and history of liver disease (Smilkstein et al. 1991). Routine laboratory evaluation includes measurements of AST, ALT, bilirubin, alkaline phosphatase, prothrombin time, blood usea nitrogen (BUN), creatinine, electrolytes, amylase, complete blood count, and urinalysis. The plasma acetaminophen level should be measured as soon as possible from 4 to 24h following ingestion (Linden and Rumack 1992; Prescott 1983; Smilkstein et al. 1991). Acetaminophen levels measured less than 4h after ingestion cannot be interpreted since continued absorption may occur. A second acetaminophen level should be determined 4h after the first and some would repeat levels at 16, 24, and 32h after ingestion or until no longer detectable (Smilkstein et al. 1991). Decisions to institute specific therapy are based on acetaminophen levels, acetaminophen half-life determinations, or on the basis of a history of potentially toxic ingestion.

General management includes gastric aspiration and lavage performed within 4h of ingestion, intravenous fluid replacement, and antiemetics in patients with persistent nausea and vomiting. Further management involves the decision whether or not to administer specific therapy with an antidote.

2. Specific Therapy

a) N-*Acetylcysteine Protocols*

Acetaminophen hepatotoxicity can be prevented by the early administration of specific therapy. Specific therapy for acetaminophen overdose is based upon giving a glutathione precursor to prevent glutathione depletion (PRESCOTT et al. 1974, 1976, 1979), although it may also protect against acetaminophen hepatotoxicity by other mechanisms. Exogenously administered glutathione does not penetrate hepatocytes, so early studies used cysteamine and methionine. Current therapy is with *N*-acetylcysteine.

Therapy with *N*-acetylcysteine is initiated if the acetaminophen level is above the lower line of the treatment nomogram (LINDEN and RUMACK 1992; PRESCOTT 1983; RUMACK et al. 1981; RUMACK and MATTHEW 1975) for possible or probable toxicity (150 μg/ml at 4 h). A second level may not be necessary. Therapy should also be initiated if the initial acetaminophen level is above the treatment line but the time of ingestion is not known and a full course administered if the second level 4 h later shows a prolonged half-life (>4 h). Therapy may also be initiated on the basis of an ingestion of more than 7.5–10 g if an acetaminophen level cannot be obtained. Treatment is discontinued if the acetaminophen level at 4 h or longer after ingestion is below the treatment line. Although exact thresholds have not been determined, the threshold for giving *N*-acetylcysteine to patients at possibly increased risk of hepatotoxicity due to alcohol or concomitant medications such as anticonvulsants is often considered to be lower (BRAY 1993). Patients being treated with *N*-acetylcysteine should have daily routine laboratory tests for 3–4 days until returning toward normal. Liver biopsy is not part of routine management.

There are several *N*-acetylcysteine protocols for acetaminophen overdose in use which differ in route of administration, total dose, and duration of treatment (PRESCOTT et al. 1979; SMILKSTEIN et al. 1988, 1991). The protocol used in the United States and approved by the United States Food and Drug Administration is an oral *N*-acetylcysteine protocol with an initial dose of 140 mg/kg followed by 17 doses of 70 mg/kg over 72 h (total dose of 1330 mg/kg) (SMILKSTEIN et al. 1988). The standard treatment protocol in Europe and Canada is a 20-h intravenous *N*-acetylcysteine protocol with an initial dose of 150 mg/kg in 200 ml 5% dextrose over 15 min followed by 50 mg/kg in 500 ml 5% dextrose over 4 h and 100 mg/kg in 11 5% dextrose over the next 16 h (total dose of 300 mg/kg) (PRESCOTT et al. 1979). A 48-h intravenous *N*-acetylcysteine protocol has recently been studied in the United States using an initial dose of 140 mg/kg inflused over 1 h, followed 4 h afterwards by 12 maintenance doses of 70 mg/kg (total dose 980 mg/kg) (SMILKSTEIN et al. 1991). There are no prospective controlled studies comparing the safety and efficacy of these protocols, but they appear to be comparable. Higher than standard doses of *N*-acetylcysteine may be useful in cases of large acetaminophen doses.

Cimetidine has been shown experimentally to have some efficacy in decreasing acetaminophen-induced hepatotoxicity in animals, but it is not recommended for clinical use (ZIMMERMAN and MADDREY 1993).

The advantages of oral *N*-acetylcysteine therapy are potentially higher hepatic concentrations and lack of potentially life-threatening adverse effects; however, it is unpalatable and may cause vomiting and diarrhea. The advantage of intravenous *N*-acetylcysteine therapy is that it can be used more easily in vomiting patients, is more convenient, and results in higher plasma concentrations (SMILKSTEIN et al. 1991). Adverse effects of intravenously administered *N*-acetylcysteine include anaphylactoid reactions, more likely to occur with the initial dose (JANES and ROUTLEDGE 1992) and treatable with intravenous antihistamine and temporary cessation of the *N*-acetylcysteine infusion. In the United States intravenous study (SMILKSTEIN et al. 1991), adverse effects occurred in 14.3% of 223 cases, mostly consisting of skin rashes that did require stopping therapy, and there were no serious side effects.

b) *Efficacy and Timing of* N-*Acetylcysteine Administration*

Both oral and intravenous *N*-acetylcysteine administration are effective in preventing hepatotoxicity (aminotransferase levels >1000 Iu/l) and mortality (PRESCOTT et al. 1979; RUMACK et al. 1981; SMILKSTEIN et al. 1988, 1991). Among patients with acetaminophen levels indicating probable risk of hepatotoxicity, mortality has been reported at 2% with the 20-h intravenous protocol, 0.7% with the oral protocol, and 1.1% with the 48-h intravenous protocol. Efficacy is related to the timing of administration and is greatest when *N*-acetylcysteine is given soon after ingestion of acetaminophen. Controversy exists as to the value of late administration, especially after 24 h.

Early studies (PRESCOTT et al. 1979) found the greatest efficacy of *N*-acetylcysteine administration to be within 8 h following acetaminophen ingestion and with little efficacy in preventing hepatotoxicity after 15 h. More recent studies (BRAY 1993; SMILKSTEIN et al. 1988) suggest that late administration of oral and intravenous *N*-acetylcysteine may be beneficial up to 24 h. Hepatotoxicity using the oral regimen developed in 6.1% of patients at probable risk when *N*-acetylcysteine was started within 10 h of acetaminophen ingestion and in 26.4% when begun 10–24 h after ingestion.

3. Fulminant Hepatic Failure

Fulminant hepatic failure develops in a small percentage of severely poisoned patients. Standard treatment is given for hepatic failure. Both retrospective (HARRISON et al. 1990a) and prospective (KEAYS et al. 1991) studies from Kings College Hospital in London showed benefit from late administration of intravenous *N*-acetylcysteine in improving survival in patients with acetaminophen-induced fulminant hepatic failure. In the retrospective study, treatment after 10–36 h was associated with a mortality of 37% compared to

58% in patients given supportive treatment, and in the prospective study of 50 patients with established liver failure mortality was 20% in the treated group compared to 48% ($P < 0.05$) in the controls. An improvement by *N*-acetylcysteine of hemodynamics and oxygen transport in patients with fulminant hepatic failure (HARRISON et al. 1991) may account for improved survival, but the usefulness and mechanism of *N*-acetylcysteine in the setting is not yet established (SHEINER et al. 1992).

Liver transplantation may be another therapeutic option for patients with acetaminophen-induced fulminant hepatic failure. Poor prognostic factors have been determined from studies at Kings College Hospital (see Sect. III.3) (HARRISON et al. 1990a; O'GRADY et al. 1989; PEREIRA et al. 1992). Early recognition of a poor prognosis may be useful in determining need for transplant and providing time to obtain a donor. However, due to medical, psychiatric, and logistic problems, only 6 of 29 potential candidates referred to Kings College Hospital for a liver transplant actually underwent surgery, with 4 of 6 being survivors (O'GRADY et al. 1991). It has been argued that an advantage of liver transplantation over optimal medical management has not yet been clearly demonstrated (FLORKOWSKI et al. 1991).

V. Prevention

Since acetaminophen causes predictable hepatotoxicity in a dose-dependent manner, prevention consists of either not using the drug or keeping exposure below the toxic level (SCHENKER and MADDREY 1991). Recommendations have been made for increased awareness of both physicians and the general public of the potential for hepatotoxicity by both acute and chronic abuse, including possible injury with modest doses with therapeutic use and in alcoholics (BARKER et al. 1977; BRAY 1993; ERICKSSON et al. 1992; KUMAR and REX 1991; MADDREY 1987; SEEFF et al. 1980; WOOTON and LEE 1990). Specifically, there has been a call for more warnings and dissemination of data. Chronic alcoholics should be cautioned regarding acetaminophen use and warned to limit future use if they develop acetaminophen-induced hepatotoxicity. Acetaminophen should be individually prescribed with doses taking into account conditions of starvation or malnutrition, alcoholism, and concurrent medications that have been associated with possible increased risk of hepatotoxicity. It has been suggested (BONKOVSKY et al. 1994) that physicians should be alert to the possibility of inadvertent or inapparent acetaminophen toxicity in patients with underlying cardiopulmonary disease who develop acute liver injury. For patients who take an intentional overdose of acetaminophen, prevention of hepatotoxicity involves bringing the patient for immediate medical attention so that the antidote may be administered in a timely fashion. Increased public awareness of the danger of taking an excessive dose of acetaminophen might encourage more suicide attempts, but would decrease the likelihood of accidental overdose and help family and friends to recognize the importance of prompt attention in case of an overdose (BRAY 1993). Another approach which has been considered toward preventing acetaminophen-hepatotoxicity is to develop a nonhepatotoxic acetaminophen derivative or a combination pill with methionine (NELSON 1990; BRAY 1993).

C. Nonsteroidal Antiinflammatory Drugs

I. Epidemiology

Nonsteroidal antiinflammatory drugs (NSAIDs) are a popular and commonly prescribed group of drugs which have analgesic, antiinflammatory, antipyretic, and platelet inhibitory properties. There are approximately 74–100 million NSAID prescriptions annually in the United States, accounting for 4.5% of all prescriptions (BROOKS and DAY 1991; KATZ and LOVE 1992), and 20 million annually in Great Britain (BATEMAN 1994). In the United States, only aspirin and ibuprofen are available without prescription. The main mechanism of action is cyclooxygenase inhibition and interference with prostaglandin synthesis, although NSAIDS also have properties of therapeutic importance that are not dependent on prostaglandin metabolism (BROOKS and DAY 1991; FURST 1994). Differences between NSAIDs exist in their chemical class, pharmacokinetics, clinical efficacy in individual patients, and adverse effects. NSAIDs are shown grouped by chemical class in Table 1 (BROOKS and DAY 1991). The most frequent and well-known adverse effects of NSAIDS are gastrointestinal, renal, dermatologic, and central nervous system effects. In addition, probably all NSAIDs can cause hepatic injury.

Historically, hepatotoxicity due to NSAIDS was initially recognized with phenylbutazone and aspirin (GAY 1990; ZIMMERMAN 1986, 1990). Increased recognition and concern about NSAID-induced hepatotoxicity occurred after multiple reports of severe and fatal injury due to benoxaprofen in 1982. The Arthritis Advisory Committee of the United States Food and Drug Administration concluded that hepatic toxicity should be considered a class characteristic of NSAIDs (PAULUS 1982). Drug-related abnormalities of liver enzymes are not unusual, but irreversible and fatal liver injury is rare. Some drugs have been withdrawn from the market because of hepatotoxicity (e.g., benoxaprofen, ibufenac). All NSAIDs have been associated with some type of liver injury and there have been several major reviews of clinically significant liver injury (LEWIS 1984; PRESCOTT 1986; RABINOVITZ and VAN THIEL 1992; STRICKER 1992; ZIMMERMAN 1990). It has been emphasized that individual NSAIDs differ in the frequency with which they are associated with significant liver injury, in their mechanism of hepatotoxicity, and in their clinical manifestations.

It is difficult to determine the actual incidence of NSAID-induced hepatic injury and the relative risks of individual NSAIDs for several reasons. The causal relationship between the drug and liver disease may be difficult to

Table 1. Clinical manifestations and outcome of nonsteroidal antiinflammatory drug-induced hepatotoxicity

Drug	Clinical manifestations	Outcome
A. Salicylic acids		
Benorilate	Hepatocellular injury, similar to acetaminophen	Fatality reported
Diflunisol[a]	Cholestasis, to mainly hepatocellular	Recovery
Salicylates[a]	Hepatocellular injury[b]	Usually mild, reversible, may be severe or fatal
B. Acetic acids		
Clometacine[c]	Hepatocellular injury[b], features of hypersensitivity	Can be fatal
Diclofenac[a]	Hepatocellular injury[b]	Can be fatal
Etodolac[a]	Biochemical abnormality	Not clinically significant
Floctafenine	Biochemical abnormality	Not clinically significant
Indomethacin[a]	Hepatocellular injury, cholestasis	Can be fatal
Sulindac[a]	Cholestasis, hepatocellular injury, mixed features of hypersensitivity	Can be fatal
Tolmetin[a]	Hepatocellular injury, features of hypersensitivity, multisystem toxicity reported	Possible fatalities reported
Zomepirac[c]	Biochemical abnormality	Not clinically significant
C. Propionic acids		
Benoxaprofen[c]	Cholestatic syndrome	High case-fatality
Carprofen	Biochemical abnormality	Insufficient data
Fenbufen	Hepatocellular injury	Recovery
Fenoprofen[a]	Hepatocellular injury	Insufficient data
Flurbiprofen[a]	Biochemical abnormality	Not clinically significant
Ibufenac[c]	Hepatocellular injury	Can be fatal
Ibuprofen[a]	Hepatocellular injury	Fatality reported
Ketoprofen[a]	Biochemical abnormality, possible cholestasis report	Not clinically significant
Naproxen[a]	Cholestasis or mixed	Can be fatal
Oxaprozin[a]	Hepatocellular	Not clinically significant
Pirprofen[c]	Hepatocellular injury[b]	Can be fatal
D. Fenamic acids		
Meclofenamic acid[a]	Biochemical abnormality	Insufficient data
Mefenamic acid[a]	Hepatocellular injury	Insufficient data
Niflumic acid	Hepatocellular injury	Fatality reported
E. Enolic acids		
Oxyphenbutazone	Similar to phenylbutazone	Fatality reported
Phenylbutazone[a]	Hepatocellular injury, cholestatic syndrome, granulomatous hepatitis, hypersensitivity features may occur	Can be fatal
Piroxicam[a]	Hepatocellular injury, cholestasis or mixed	Can be fatal
Tenoxicam	Biochemical abnormality	Insufficient data
F. Nonacidic compounds		
Nabumetone[a]	Biochemical abnormality	Not clinically significant

[a] Available in the United States.
[b] Cases reported which resemble chronic active hepatitis.
[c] Withdrawn from the market.

ascertain since the underlying rheumatologic disorder may have hepatic involvement or there may be underlying liver disease, patients are often taking multiple medications, rechallenge with the potentially offending agent is usually not attempted, and there usually is not a single clear pattern of injury with which to associate the drug. Inferences regarding incidence based on reports of NSAID-induced hepatotoxicity in the literature have several sources of bias since they are related to the frequency of drug use, publicity, particular and unusual side-effects, and the timing of drug release (DOUBE 1990; FURST 1994; KATZ and LOVE 1992). In addition to case reports and series of variable quality and detail, however, there have been several recent epidemiologic studies, as well as data reported to various national agencies. As with studies showing that some NSAIDs are more frequently associated with the gastrointestinal complications of bleeding and perforation (BATEMAN 1994), there is also some information on the relative risks of hepatotoxicity.

There is a distinction between the incidence of laboratory abnormalities (elevated aminotransferases) and clinically significant liver disease. Mild biochemical abnormalities are frequent, while overt liver injury is rare and is the basis for case reports. The relationship between the propensity of an NSAID to produce aminotransferase elevations and mild hepatic injury to the development of significant hepatic injury is not clear (ZIMMERMAN 1986).

There have been four epidemiologic studies demonstrating a low incidence of significant NSAID-associated liver injury. Studies vary in the methods of data collection and analysis, NSAIDs included, clinical end points, years the study was conducted, and the country studied. A British population-based study (JICK et al. 1992) derived from computers used by general practitioners between 1988 and 1991 estimated the frequency of clinically important liver disease associated with diclofenac, naproxen, and piroxicam to be 1/100000 users. A British retrospective study (GARCIA RODRIGUEZ et al. 1994) found 23 cases of acute liver injury in outpatients and hospitalized patients between 1987 and 1991 among 600000 NSAID users for an incidence of 3.7/100000 NSAID users. Among the 12 non-aspirin NSAIDs, sulindac had the greater risk, although no cases were severe. A Canadian retrospective population-based study (GARCIA RODRIGUEZ et al. 1992) of patients hospitalized for acute liver injury between 1982 and 1986 found an incidence of 9/100000 person years. The age- and sex-adjusted risk ratio for NSAID use was 1.7. An American case-control study (CARSON et al. 1993) of hepatitis between 1980 and 1987, however, did not find an association of NSAID use with acute hepatitis requiring hospitalization.

Data collected from reports to the United States Food and Drug Administration of adverse hepatic effects provide an estimate of the incidence of NSAID-induced hepatotoxicity and the relative risks of the non-aspirin NSAIDs on the market between 1984 and 1989 (KATZ and LOVE 1992). There were 1182 reports of NSAID-associated hepatic toxicity, most frequently with ibuprofen (18%), sulindac (17%), diclofenac (16%), naproxen (13%), and piroxicam (12%), reflecting reporting incidences, not occurrence incidences. There was a disproportionately greater occurrence of adverse drug reports for diclofenac, sulindac, and phenylbutazone based upon spontaneous reports and estimates of tablets sold, and the lowest occurrences were with ibuprofen, ketoprofen, indomethacin, and naproxen. Fatalities were reported in 8% of cases. According to other statistics, there were a disproportionate number of reports of hepatic injury due to sulindac, accounting for about 10% of NSAID prescriptions, but 25% of reported cases (TARAZI et al. 1993). Of 338 reports on sulindac hepatotoxicity between 1978 and 1986, 91 were thought to represent a causal relationship. The Adverse Drug Reactions Advisory Committee of Australia received more reports between 1981 and 1989 of hepatic reactions to diclofenac than to any other drug (PURCELL et al. 1991). The incidence of severe hepatic injury due to diclofenac in Australia has been roughly estimated to be on the order of 1 case/50000–100000 prescriptions (SALLIE et al. 1991) and by others to be 1.8 validated cases/million prescriptions based on adverse drug reaction reports of 26 nonfatal cases between 1981 and 1989 (PURCELL et al. 1991). Data from the Danish Committee on Adverse Drug Reactions based on anecdotal reports found 97 cases of NSAID-induced hepatic injury from 1978 to 1987, of which 18 were related to sulindac and 17 to ibuprofen, indicating a disproportionate incidence, based on consumption data, due to sulindac (FRIIS and ANDREASEN 1992).

There are many case reports of the association of NSAIDs with clinical liver injury. Based upon the clinical evidence, causality for NSAIDs causing symptomatic liver injury is most established for salicylates, diclofenac, sulindac, pirprofen, phenylbutazone, and clometacin (STRICKER 1992). The more frequent reports of significant liver injury of those on the market are with diclofenac, sulindac, phenylbutazone, pirprofen, and the least with mefenamic acid, meclofenamic acid, and ketoprofen (LEWIS 1984; PRESCOTT 1986), despite the introduction of newer NSAIDS (e.g., etodolac, oxaprozin, nabumetone). Each NSAID must be assessed individually, since the frequency of NSAID-induced hepatotoxicity is not related to the structural class (TARAZI et al. 1993; ZIMMERMAN 1986).

Elevations of aminotransferases are common in patients taking salicylates, ranging from 5% to 50% (FREELAND et al. 1988; PRESCOTT 1986; SEAMAN and PLOTZ 1976; ZIMMERMAN 1974, 1981), usually associated with high doses (e.g., 3–5 g/24 h) in patients being treated for connective tissue disorders (e.g., systemic lupus erythematosus, juvenile rheumatoid arthritis, acute rheumatic fever), but are also seen in healthy volunteers. Underlying illness appears to play a role, although these disease often were treated with high doses of salicylates, now a less commonly used drug. An estimated 3% of all reported early cases of aspirin-associated liver injury were severe (ZIMMERMAN 1981).

II. Pathogenesis

The mechanisms of NSAID-induced liver injury, in contrast to that of acetaminophen, are poorly understood. Hepatotoxicity does not appear to be related to the inhibition of prostaglandin synthesis, unlike gastrointestinal toxicity. Mechanisms of NSAID injury to the liver include both intrinsic toxicity and idiosyncrasy, although in many cases the mechanism is not established. The apparent mechanism of injury of non-salicylate NSAIDS is idiosyncrasy, either metabolic or immunologic (LEWIS 1984; STRICKER 1992; ZIMMERMAN 1990). Idiosyncratic hepatotoxicity is unpredictable injury which occurs in a small percentage of people taking the drug (ZIMMERMAN and MADDREY 1993). Metabolic idiosyncrasy is assumed to be related to the accumulation of toxic metabolities, and is associated with a more variable duration of exposure (weeks to months) and a delayed response to challenge. Metabolic idiosyncrasy is the more common mechanism of injury. It has been suggested that drugs with this mechanism cause mild hepatic injury to which tolerance develops, but can also rarely cause cases of overt hepatic injury. Immunologic idiosyncrasy is associated with clinical features of hypersensitivity (e.g., fever, rash, eosinophilia), a short duration of exposure (days to weeks), and a prompt response to rechallenge. Features of hypersensitivity suggest immunologic idiosyncrasy in at least some cases, for phenylbutazone, sulindac, tolmetin, clometacin, and diclofenac.

The mechanism of hepatotoxicity is not characteristic of NSAID chemical class. An adverse effect to one NSAID does not necessarily predict that another NSAID will cause the same reaction in that person (PAULUS 1982). Repeat exposure to a drug of the same class does not predictably lead to a reaction, but there has been a case report (ANDREJAK et al. 1987) of cross-reactivity between naproxen and fenoprofen, two propionic acid derivatives. Isolated cases have suggested that hepatotoxicity does not recur if an NSAID of a different class is used (HELFGOTT et al. 1990; SCULLY et al. 1993).

Salicylates have intrinsic toxicity and injury is dose-related (ZIMMERMAN 1981). Determinants of injury are salicylate dosage, serum levels, and duration of exposure (PRESCOTT 1986; SEAMAN and PLOTZ 1976; ZIMMERMAN 1981). Hepatic injury is associated with high serum levels more than dosage. Two-thirds of injury occurs with levels >25 mg/dl and only 10% with <15 mg/dl. Duration of exposure is usually 6 days to weeks or more, while single large overdoses usually are not associated with significant hepatic injury. Hypoalbuminemia appears to be a risk factor for salicylate hepatotoxicity, presumably by increasing the ratio of free to bound salicylate (GITLIN 1980). Injury from aspirin (acetylsalicylic acid) and other salicylates (e.g., choline salicylate, sodium salicylate, choline magnesium trisalicylate) is probably due to the accumulation of a toxic metabolic (STRICKER 1992). Toxicity may be related to uncoupling of oxidative phosphorylation. Salicylates have been implicated in Reyes' syndrome, which is characterized by liver dysfunction, hypoglycemia, acidosis, and encephalopathy in children and young adults usually associated with a viral-type illness (DOUBE 1990) (see Chap. 14, this volume).

In some instances, there appears to be more than one mechanism for an individual NSAID, often based upon the clinical pattern or setting, and there may be a contribution of intrinsic toxicity. Drugs which may have more than one mechanism of hepatotoxicity are phenylbutazone, sulindac, and diclofenac. The major mechanism for phenylbutazone appears to be immunologic idiosyncrasy, based on the clinical association with occurrence after a short duration of exposure, fever, and rash, while there is also evidence for intrinsic hepatotoxicity from patients with hepatocellular injury without hallmarks of hypersensitivity, toxicity from overdoses, and experimental hepatotoxic effects (BENJAMIN et al. 1981; PRESCOTT 1986; ZIMMERMAN 1990). Based on the frequent association with clinical hallmarks of hypersensitivity, brief periods of exposure, and response to challenge, the usual mechanism of injury of sulindac is thought to be immunologic idiosyncrasy, but some cases without the hallmarks and associated with longer exposure may be mediated by metabolic idiosyncrasy (TARAZI et al. 1993). The mechanism of injury of diclofenac is idiosyncrasy, probably metabolic idiosyncrasy in most cases (ZIMMERMAN and MADDREY 1993), but immunologic idiosyncrasy has been suggested in the few cases with features of hypersensitivity (HELFGOTT et al. 1990; IVESON et al. 1990).

Benoxaprofen was withdrawn from the market due to reports of fatalities. It was suggested that benoxaprofen toxicity may be due to progressive accumulation of this NSAID with a long serum half-life due to a vicious cycle of injury and impaired biliary and renal excretion (PRESCOTT 1986; PRESCOTT and LESLIE 1982).

III. Clinical Manifestations and Laboratory Findings

1. General Observations

Analgesic hepatopathy due to NSAIDs is associated with a spectrum of clinical manifestations, biochemical abnormalities, and histopathology. Few NSAIDs have a distinct pattern of toxicity. The clinical patterns and outcomes of NSAID-associated hepatic injury are summarized in Table 1. NSAIDs are organized by chemical class, but within each class there are a variety of chemical manifestations and NSAIDs vary in frequency of reports of severe injury. There may be a prodrome of fatigue, malaise, nausea, pruritus, abdominal pain, jaundice, or flu-like symptoms. Hepatocellular injury is more likely to be associated with anorexia, fatigue, nausea, and jaundice and cholestatic injury associated with pruritus and jaundice (KATZ and LOVE 1992). Features of hypersensitivity (fever, rash, eosinophilia) have been associated more with certain NSAID: phenylbutazone (BENJAMIN et al. 1981), sulindac (TARAZI et al. 1993), diclofenac (HELFGOTT et al. 1990; IVESON et al. 1990), tolmetin, and clometacin (see Sect. C.II). There have also been reports of liver injury associated with multisystem toxicity with some NSAIDs, e.g., tolmetin (SHAW and ANDERSON 1991) and mefenamic acid (CHAN et al. 1991).

Clinical patterns of injury may be categorized as those with evidence of biochemical injury (elevated aminotransferases) or those with clinically significant liver injury, hepatocellular, cholestatic, or mixed (Table 1), with some NSAIDs producing multiple patterns. The hepatocellular injury pattern is more common than the cholestatic pattern. Cholestatic patterns have been associated most often with benoxaprofen, sulindac, naproxen, diflunisal, and phenylbutazone. NSAIDs associated with histologic evidence of chronic active hepatitis include aspirin, diclofenac, clometacin, and pirprofen. Granulomatous hepatitis, present in occasional case reports, has been associated most often with phenylbutazone (BENJAMIN et al. 1981). Microvesicular steatosis has been associated with injury due to piroxicam (HEPPS et al. 1991), tolmetin (SHAW and ANDERSON 1991), indomethacin (KELSEY and SCHARYJ 1967), and pirprofen (DANAN et al. 1985).

The duration of drug use prior to the onset of clinically significant liver injury is extremely variable and generalizations can only be made for the NSAIDs for which a number of cases have been reported.

The outcome of patients with clinically significant NSAID-induced liver injury is also variable. Most NSAID liver injury is reversible after the drug is discontinued. Cases of severe and fatal hepatic injury have been described for many of the NSAIDs and have led to the withdrawal from the market of some (e.g., benoxaprofen, ibufenac). Fatal hepatic injury has been described most often with diclofenac, sulindac, pirprofen, phenylbutazone, naproxen, piroxicam, indomethacin, clometacin, and salicylates. Some NSAIDs have been associated with a prolonged course despite withdrawal of the medications, e.g., diclofenac with autoimmune hepatitis (IVESON et al. 1990; SALLIE et al. 1991), responding to courses of steroids, but the long-term prognosis is uncertain.

2. Specific NSAIDs

There are enough cases reported to generalize about the clinical features of only some of the NSAIDs. Hepatic injury due to salicylates is usually mild and reversible (PRESCOTT 1986; ZIMMERMAN 1981, 1990). Patients are usually asymptomatic, although in more severe cases may have malaise, nausea, anorexia, and upper abdominal discomfort. Onset is usually within 4 weeks of initiation of therapy. Biochemical features are mild to moderate aminotransferase elevations (one-third less than 100 IU/ml and 90% below 1000 IU/ml), with AST often greater than ALT, mild to modest elevations of alkaline phosphatase, and bilirubin usually normal or only mildly elevated. Liver biopsies show evidence of focal hepatic necrosis and inflammation. A few cases of chronic hepatitis have been reported and a single case of reversible cholestatic hepatitis (LOPEZ-MORANTE et al. 1993). Injury is usually reversible after salicylates are discontinued, but fatalities have been described. Other salicylates are thought to have a pattern of injury similar to aspirin. Benorilate is an ester of acetylsalicylic acid and acetaminophen with clinical toxicity more related to that of acetaminophen. Diflunisal may cause reversible cholestatic jaundice or a hepatocellular pattern (WARREN 1978).

Diclofenac is a phenylacetic acid derivative. Aminotransferase elevations less than three times normal are seen in about 15% of patients and are typically reversible (ZIMMERMAN 1990). There have been many cases and series in the last decade of significant liver injury (BREEN et al. 1986; DUNK et al. 1982; HELFGOTT et al. 1990; IVESON et al. 1990; OUELLETTE et al. 1991; SALLIE et al. 1991; SCHAPIRA et al. 1986; SCHIFF and MADDREY 1994; SCULLY et al. 1993). Two clinical patterns have been described, the more common hepatocellular injury pattern resembling acute hepatitis, as well as several cases with the picture of chronic active hepatitis. A review of 29 cases reported in the literature (SCULLY et al. 1993) found that about half the patients were jaundiced, 6 had features of hypersensitivity, and 4 had autoimmune markers with features suggestive of autoimmune hepatitis. Onset of injury was variable, but often within the first 3 months, and liver biopsies usually showed some degree of periportal inflammation. Several cases had a histologic picture of chronic active hepatitis (IVESON et al. 1990; SALLIE et al. 1991; SCULLY et al. 1993). Most patients improved when the drug was discontinued, but there were four fatalities and two received steroid treatment. Of 26 patients of diclofenac-induced liver injury reported to the Adverse Drug Reaction Advisory Committee in Australia, one-fourth were asymptomatic, while the others often had anorexia or nausea, and half were jaundiced. Features of hypersensitivity were not seen. Onset was typically within 6 months. Laboratory data showed a hepatocellular injury predominantly with mild to moderate aminotransferase elevations. Most cases were reversible, while there was one fatality.

Clinical features of sulindac-induced liver injury include systemic manifestations with a predominantly cholestatic clinical pattern, but also hepatocellular or mixed (DHAND et al. 1981; TARAZI et al. 1993; WHITTAKER et al. 1982). Many patients have a short duration of exposure (less than 4 weeks), often correlated with the presence of fever, rash, and eosinophilia. Injury occurs after more than 8 weeks in 20%. Pancreatitis has also been associated and may contribute to cholestasis (ZIMMERMAN 1990). Fatalities have been reported, but of the 91 reports to the United States. Food and Drug Administration, only 1 death was due to fulminant liver failure, with 3 others due to hypersensitivity (TARAZI et al. 1993). Another acetic acid derivative, indomethacin, has a clinical pattern of injury which is mainly hepatocellular, but may be cholestatic (KELSEY and SCHARYJ 1967; ZIMMERMAN 1990). Histology in the most commonly cited case was centrilobular necrosis with microvesicular steatosis. Few fatalities have been described.

The propionic acid derivatives include benoxaprofen, which was withdrawn from the market soon after its introduction in the United States after a number of reports of severe liver injury and fatalities (GOUDIE et al. 1982; PRESCOTT 1986; PRESCOTT and LESLIE 1982; TAGGART and ALDERDICE 1982). This injury was not apparent in the clinical trials. Most deaths were in elderly women. Few cases of liver injury with ibuprofen have been reported, suggesting a lower incidence than related drugs. Aminotransferase elevations were reported in up to 16% of patients in some clinical trials, but in a study of clinical trials looking at drug-related incidence, as opposed to total incidence, there were no cases associated with ibuprofen, compared to 5.2% for aspirin and 3.2% for oxaprozin (Freeland et al. 1988). Only a few cases of hepatic injury have been reported with naproxen (Bass 1974; Victorino et al. 1980). Information on oxaprozin from clinical trials (Miller 1992; Zimmerman 1986) found aminotrasferase elevations in up to 15% of patients, but probably drug related in only 3.2% (Freeland et al. 1988), and only 1.1% > three times normal, with most returning toward normal despite continuing therapy, and only one case of anicteric hepatitis. For pirprofen, asymptomatic aminotransferase elevations > three times normal have been reported in 2.8% of pooled clinical trials (Danan et al. 1985), and there have been over 14 cases of overt hepatic injury (Danan et al. 1985; Lohse et al. 1993; Prescott 1986; Zimmerman 1990). Clinically significant liver injury has been suggested in a patient taking ketoprofen (Nores et al. 1991), and with fenoprofen in a patient previously with naproxen-induced hepatotoxicity (Andrejak et al. 1987), but these NSAIDs and flurbiprofen are poorly documented causes of liver injury (Stricker 1992).

Mefenamic acid and meclofenamic acid have little reported hepatoxicity other than mild aminotransferase elevations (Stricker 1992).

Phenylbutazone is an NSAID of established hepatoxicity which is no longer in frequent clinical use. Multiple cases of hepatic injury have been reported, occurring with both therapeutic use and in the overdose setting (Benjamin et al. 1981; Prescott 1986). Several different syndromes have been described. Overdose can lead to acute hepatic necrosis. Hypersensitivity features are common, with fever and rash, eosinophilia, and onset of illness in less than 6 weeks. Other patients present with anorexia, nausea and vomiting, fever, and abdominal pain. Histopathology varies; hepatocellular injury is more common than cholestatic injury, and there may be granulomatous hepatitis, usually associated with clinical features of hypersensitivity and mild hepatocellular injury. Fatalities have occurred in about one-fourth of cases in reviews.

Several cases of liver injury associated with piroxicam have been reported (Bismuth et al. 1987; Hepps et al. 1991; Lee et al. 1986; Paterson et al. 1992; Planas et al. 1990; Sherman and Jones 1992). Symptomatic hepatic injury has been described as hepatocellular, cholestatic, and mixed. Duration of exposure has varied from days to months. Fatal hepatic failure may occur despite withdrawal of the drug.

Nabumetone is a non-acidic NSAID. It has not been associated with significant liver injury. In a series of 1677 patients, significant elevations of aminotransferases occurred in 0.4% of patients (Friedel et al. 1993) and in a comparative 12-week study (Eversmeyer et al. 1993) elevated aminotransferases were reported in 0.5% of patients.

IV. Treatment

Treatment of analgesic hepatopathy due to NSAIDs is encountered in two settings, that of finding abnormal liver function tests in a patient taking

NSAIDs and that of over liver injury. Elevated aminotransferases may be found in patients taking NSAIDs (see Sect. C.V). In the absence of symptoms, guidelines vary as to the necessity for stopping NSAIDs in the presence of mild elevations. The treatment of NSAID-induced hepatic injury is to discontinue the drug following recognition of injury and to follow the patient and laboratory values. Clinical follow-up should continue with attention to possible progression of liver injury despite withdrawal. Specific therapy is not available, so treatment is otherwise supportive. A trial of corticosteroid therapy has been suggested to be of possible benefit in rare cases of patients with NSAID-associated (e.g., diclofenac) liver disease with features of chronic active hepatitis (SALLIE et al. 1991). In the case of development of fulminant hepatic failure, liver transplant is an option in appropriate candidates and successful outcomes have been reported for hepatic failure due to piroxicam (BISMUTH et al. 1987; PATERSON et al. 1992) and pirprofen (LOHSE et al. 1993).

V. Prevention

Recommendations for NSAID use in general include restricting their use to situations where they are clearly indicated and using the lowest effective dose, the latter recommendation being more relevant to the prevention of gastrointestinal rather than hepatic toxicity. Hepatotoxicity due to NSAIDs is generally unpredictable and not dose dependent, with the major exception being salicylates. Both patients and physicians should be aware of the small but definite risk of clinically significant hepatic injury occurring with NSAID use.

Monitoring of liver function tests, especially aminotransferases, is recommended during NSAID use (GAY 1990; RABINOVITZ and VAN THIEL; SCHIFF and MADDREY 1994; ZIMMERMAN 1986). The optimal method for monitoring patients on NSAIDs in general, or for individual NSAIDs, as well as efficacy and cost-effectiveness have not been established. In general, baseline liver chemistries should be obtained and repeated at preplanned intervals, e.g., monthly for 6–12 months. The NSAID may be continued if aminotransferases are less than three times the upper limit of normal and the patient is asymptomatic. The use of the NSAID should be reassessed and possibly discontinued if greater than three times normal or discontinued if aminotransferases continue to rise. The drug should be withdrawn if the patient has signs and symptoms of hepatitis (e.g., fatigue, malaise, anorexia, nausea, vomiting, fever) or features of hypersensitivity (fever, rash). Monitoring may also be indicated when altering the dose of an NSAID or changing concomitant medications, in addition to when starting an NSAID (KATZ and LOVE 1992). Despite monitoring at monthly or more frequent intervals, there may be rapid onset of overt liver injury and prevention may not be successful. It has been suggested that monitoring is likely to be more effective with NSAIDs whose mechanism of hepatotoxicity is metabolic idiosyncrasy rather than hypersensitivity (ZIMMERMAN 1986). For NSAIDs such as sulindac, known to be associated with hypersensitivity, routine monitoring of asymptomatic patients may add little to monitoring for signs and symptoms of hepatic injury and manifestations of hypersensitivity especially during the first 4–8 weeks (TARAZI et al. 1993).

Abnormal liver function tests unrelated to drug-induced hepatotoxicity may occur in patients taking NSAIDs and baseline clinical and laboratory assessments of patients prior to starting on NSAIDs may reveal evidence of underlying liver disease, possibly identifying the patient as being at increased risk for NSAID-induced hepatotoxicity and making interpretation of further laboratory tests more difficult. NSAIDs may be carefully used in patients with mild hepatic dysfunction (RABINOVITZ and VAN THIEL 1992) and an option would be to use an NSAID with a lower reported incidence of hepatic injury.

Another special clinical setting is the use of NSAIDs in patients with a previous history of NSAID-associated hepatic injury. Patients should not be rechallenged with the same NSAID (GAY 1990), but if hepatic enzyme abnormalities have resolved, another NSAID, preferably of a different class (see Sect. C.II) may be instituted with careful monitoring.

D. Narcotic Analgesics

Narcotic analgesics rarely cause hepatic injury, although they may cause biliary spasm (STRICKER 1992). Propoxyphene, a formerly popular analgesic, is the only one with established hepatotoxicity (BASSENDINE et al. 1986; DAIKOS and KOSMIDIS 1975; KLEIN and MAGIDA 1971; LEE and REES 1977; ROSENBERG et al. 1993). There have been approximately 24 reported cases, including a recent series of 9 cases from one British institution (ROSENBERG et al. 1993). The mechanism of hepatotoxicity appears to be immunologic idiosyncrasy. Symptoms are often malaise, nausea, abdominal discomfort, jaundice, and sometimes fever. Duration of exposure is usually less than 3 months. The liver chemistries usually have a cholestatic pattern and the clinical picture is suggestive of biliary tract disease. Histology shows predominantly cholestasis and portal tract inflammatory changes, at times with mild periportal fibrosis. There have been several reports of rechallenge (BASSENDINE et al. 1986; DAIKOS and KOMIDIS 1975; KLEIN and MAGIDA 1971) with the onset of recurrent symptoms usually within a few days. Post-challenge biopsies have shown portal tract infiltrates of eosinophils and lymphocytes (BASSENDINE et al. 1986). Injury is reversible and no fatalities have been reported. Treatment consists of withdrawal of the drug in cases of suspected propoxyphene-induced hepatic injury and evaluation for possible biliary tract disease. It has been suggested that propoxyphene-induced liver injury may be more common than previously realized due to confusion with biliary disease (ROSENBERG et al. 1993).

References

Andrejak M, Davion T, Gineston JL, Capron JP (1987) Cross-hepatotoxicity between non-steroidal anti-inflammatory drugs. BMJ 295:180–181

Barker JD, de Carle DJ, Anuras S (1977) Chronic excessive acetaminophen use and liver damage. Ann Intern Med 87:299–301

Bass BH (1974) Jaundice associated with naproxen. Lancet I:998

Bassendine MT, Woodhouse KW, Bennet M, James OFW (1986) Dextropropoxyphene induced hepatotoxicity mimicking biliary tract disease. Gut 27:444–449

Bateman DN (1994) NSAIDs: time to re-evaluate gut toxicity. Lancet 343:1051–1052

Benjamin SB, Ishak KG, Zimmerman HJ, Grushka A (1981) Phenylbutazone liver injury: a clinical-pathologic survey of 23 cases and review of the literature. Hepatology 1:255–263

Bismuth H, Samuel D, Gugenheim J, Castaing D, Bernuau J, Rueff B, Behamou J-P (1987) Emergency liver transplantation for fulminant hepatitis. Ann Intern Med 107:337–341

Black M (1980) Acetaminophen hepatotoxicity. Gastroenterology 78:382–392

Black M, Raucy J (1986) Acetaminophen, alcohol, and cytochrome p-450. Ann Intern Med 104:427–429

Bonkovsky HL, Mudge GH, McMurty RJ (1978) Chronic hepatic inflammation and fibrosis due to low doses of parcetamol. Lancet I:1016–1018

Bonkovsky HL, Kane RE, Jones DP, Galinsky RE, Banner B (1994) Acute hepatic and renal toxicity from low doses of acetaminophen in the absence of alcohol abuse or malnutrition: evidence for increased susceptibility to drug toxicity due to cardiopulmonary and renal insufficiency. Hepatology 19:1141–1148

Boyer TD, Rouff SL (1971) Acetaminophen-induced hepatic necrosis and renal failure. JAMA 218:440–441

Bray GP (1993) Liver failure induced by paracetamol. Avoidable deaths still occur. BMJ 306:157–158

Breen EG, McNicholl J, Cosgrove E, McCabe J, Stevens FM (1986) Fatal hepatitis associated with diclofenac. Gut: 27:1390–1393

Brooks PM, Day RO (1991) Nonsteroidal antiinflammatory drugs – differences and similarities. N Engl J Med 324:1716–1725

Brotodihardjo AE, Batey RG, Farrell GC, Byth K (1992) Hepatotoxicity from paracetamol self-poisoning in Western Sydney: a continuing challenge. Med J Aust 157:382–385

Carson JL, Strom BL, Duff A, Gupta A, Das K (1993) Safety of nonsteroidal anti-inflammatory drugs with respect to acute liver disease. Arch Intern Med 153:1331–1336

Chan JCN, Lai FM, Critchley JAJH (1991) A case of Stevens-Johnson syndrome, cholestatic hepatitis and haemolytic anaemia associated with use of mefenamic acid. Drug Saf 6:230–234

Crippin JS (1993) Acetaminophen hepatotoxicity: potentiation by isoniazid. Am J Gastroenterol 88:590–592

Daikos GK, Kosmidis JC (1975) Propoxyphene jaundice. JAMA 323:835

Danan G, Trunet P, Bernuau J, Degott C, Babany G, Pessayre D, Rueff B, Benhamou JP (1985) Pirprofen-induced fulminant hepatitis. Gastroenterology 89:210–213

Davidson DGD, Eastham WN (1966) Acute liver necrosis following overdose of paracetamol. BMJ 2:497–499

Dhand AK, LaBrecque DR, Metzger J (1981) Sulindac (Clinoril) hepatitis. Gastroenterology 80:585–586

Doube A (1990) Hepatitis and non-steroidal anti-inflammatory drugs. Ann Rheum Dis 49:489–490

Dunk A, Walt R, Jenkins W, Sherlock S (1982) Diclofenac hepatitis. BMJ 284:1605–1606

Edwards R, Oliphant J (1992) Paracetamol toxicity in chronic alcohol abusers – a plea for greater consumer awareness. NZ Med J 105:174–175
Ericksson LS, Broome U, Kalin M, Lindholm M (1992) Hepatotoxicity due to repeated intake of low doses of paracetamol. J Intern Med 231:567–570
Eversmeyer W, Poland M, DeLapp RE, Jensen CP (1993) Safety experience with nabumetone versus diclofenanc, naproxen, ibuprofen, and piroxicam in osteoarthritis and rheumatoid arthritis. Am J Med 95 [Suppl 2A]:10S–18S
Fischereder M, Jaffe JP (1994) Thrombocytopenia following acute acetaminophen overdose. Am J Hematol 45:258–259
Floren CH, Thesleff P, Nilsson A (1987) Severe liver damage caused by therapeutic doses of acetaminophen. Acta Med Scand 222:285–288
Florkowski CM, Ferner RE, Jones AF (1991) Liver transplantation after acetaminophen overdose. BMJ 303:420
Freeland GR, Northington RS, Hedrich DA, Walker BR (1988) Hepatic safety of two analgesics used over the counter: ibuprofen and aspirin. Clin Pharmacol Ther 43:473–479
Friedel HA, Langtry HD, Buckley MM (1993) Nabumetone. A reappraisal of its pharmacology and therapeutic use in rheumatic diseases. Drugs 45:131–156
Friss H, Andreasen PB (1992) Drug-induced hepatic injury: an analysis of 1100 cases reported to The Danish Committee on Adverse Drug Reactions between 1978 and 1987. J Intern Med 232:133–138
Furst DE (1994) Are there differences among nonsteroidal antiinflammatory drugs? Arthritis Rheum 37:1–9
Garcia Rodriguez LA, Pere Z, Gutthann S, Walker AM, Leuck L (1992) The role of nonsteroidal anti-inflammatory drugs in acute liver injury. BMJ 305:865–868
Garcia Rodriguez LA, Williams R, Derby LE, Dean AD, Jick H (1994) Acute liver injury associated with nonsteroidal anti-inflammatory drugs and the role of risk factors. Arch Intern Med 154:311–316
Gay GR (1990) Another side effect of NSAID. JAMA 264:2677–2678
George J, Farrell GC (1993) Drug-induced liver disease. In: Gitnick G (ed) Current hepatology, vol 13. Mosby, St Louis, pp 105–157
Gitlin N (1980) Salicylate hepatotoxicity: the potential role of hypoalbuminemia. J Clin Gastroenterol 2:281–285
Goldfinger R, Ahmed KS, Pitchumoni CS, Weseley SA (1978) Concomitant alcohol and drug abuse enhancing acetaminophen toxicity. Am J Gastroentero 170:385–388
Goudie BM, Birnie GF, Watkinson G, MacSween RNM, Kissen LH, Cunningham NE (1982) Jaundice associated with the use of benoxaprofen. Lancet I:1799
Harrison PM, Keays R, Bray GP, Alexander GJM, Williams R (1990a) Improved outcome of paracetamol-induced fulminant hepatic failure by late administration of acetylcysteine. Lancet 335:1572–1573
Harrison PM, O'Grady JG, Keays RT, Alexander GJM, Williams R (1990b) Serial prothrombin time as prognostic indicator in paracetamol induced fulminant hepatic failure. BMJ 301:964–966
Harrison PM, Wendon JA, Gimson AES, Alexander GJM, Williams R (1991) Improvement by acetylcysteine of hemodynamics and oxygen transport in fulminant hepatic failure. N Engl J Med 324:1852–1857
Helfgott SM, Sandberg-Cook J, Zakim D, Nestler J (1990) Diclofenac-associated hepatotoxicity. JAMA 264:2660–2662
Hepps KS, Maliha GM, Estrada R, Goodgame RW (1991) Severe cholestatic jaundice associated with piroxicam. Gastroenterology 101:1737–1740
Iveson TJ, Ryley NG, Kelly PMA, Trowell JM, McGee JOD, Chapman RWG (1990) Diclofenac associated hepatitis. J Hepatol 10:85–89
Janes J, Routledge PA (1992) Recent developments in the management of paracetamol (acetaminophen) poisoning. Drug Saf 7:170–177

Jick H, Derby LE, Garcia Rodriguez LA, Jick SS, Dean AD (1992) Liver disease associated with diclofenac, naproxen, and piroxicam. Pharmacotherapy 12:207–212
Johnson GK, Tolman KG (1977) Chronic liver disease and acetaminophen. Ann Intern Med 87:302–304
Katz LM, Love PY (1992) NSAIDs and the liver. In: Famaey JP, Paulus HE (eds) Therapeutic applications of NSAIDs: subpopulations and new formulations. Dekker, New York
Keays R, Harrison PM, Wendon JA, Forbes A, Gove C, Alexander GJM, Williams R (1991) Intravenous acetylcysteine in paracetamol induced fulminant hepatic failure: a prospective controlled trial. BMJ 303:1026–1029
Kelsey WM, Scharyj M (1967) Fatal hepatitis probably due to indomethacin. JAMA 199:586–587
Klein NC, Magida MG (1971) Propoxyphene (Darvon) hepatotoxicity. Am J Dig Dis 16:467–469
Kumar S, Rex DK (1991) Failure of physicians to recognize acetaminophen hepatotoxicity in chronic alcoholics. Arch Intern Med 151:1189–1191
Lauterburg BH, Velez ME (1988) Glutathione deficiency in alcoholics: risk factor for paracetamol hepatotoxicity. Gut 29:1153–1157
Lee SM, O'Brien CJ, Williams R, Whitaker S, Gould SR (1986) Subacute hepatic necrosis induced by piroxicam. BMJ 293:540–541
Lee TH, Rees PJ (1977) Hepatotoxicity of dextropropoxyphene BMJ 2:296–297
Lee WM (1993a) Drug-induced hepatotoxicity. Aliment Pharmacol Ther 7:477–485
Lee WM (1993b) Acute liver failure. N Engl J Med 329:1862–1872
Lewis JH (1984) Hepatic toxicity of nonsteroidal anti-inflammatory drugs. Clin Pharm 3:128–138
Licht H, Seeff LB, Zimmerman HJ (1980) Apparent potentiation of acetaminophen hepatotoxicity by alcohol. Ann Intern Med 92:511–512
Linden CH, Rumack BH (1992) Acetaminophen poisoning. In: Tintinalli JE, Krome RL, Ruiz E (eds) Emergency medicine: a comprehensive study guide, 3rd edn. McGraw-Hill, New York, pp 593–597
Litovitz TL, Schmitz BF, Bailey KM (1990) 1989 annual report of the American Association of Poison Control Centers National Data Collection System. Am J Emerg Med 8:394–442
Lohse AW, Otto G, Hermann E, Poralla T, Meyer zum Buschenfelde KH (1993) Remission of severe rheumatoid arthritis following liver transplantation. Br J Rheumatol 32:827–828
Lopez-Morante AJ, Saez-Royvela F, Diez-Sanchez V, Martin-Lorente JL, Yoguero L, Ojeda C (1993) Aspirin-induced cholestatic hepatitis. J Clin Gastroenterol 16:270–272
Maddrey WC (1987) Hepatic effects of acetaminophen. Enhanced toxicity in alcoholics. J Clin Gastroenterol 9:180–185
McClain CJ, Kromhout JP, Peterson FJ, Holtzman JL (1980) Potentiation of acetaminophen toxicity by alcohol. JAMA 244:251–253
McClain CJ, Holtzman J, Allen J, Kromhout J, Shedlofsky S (1988) Clinical features of acetaminophen toxicity. J Clin Gastroenterol 10:76–80
Miller LG (1992) Oxaprozin: once-daily nonsteroidal anti-inflammatory drug. Clin Pharm 11:591–603
Mitchell JR (1988) Acetaminophen toxicity. N Engl J Med 319:1601–1602
Mitchell JR, Jollow DJ, Potter WZ, Davis DC, Gillette JR, Brodie BB (1973a) Acetaminophen-induced hepatic necrosis. I. Role of drug metabolism. J Pharmacol Exp Ther 187:185–194
Mitchell JR, Jollow DJ, Potter WZ, Gillette JR, Brodie BB (1973b) Acetaminophen-induced hepatic necrosis. IV. Protective role of glutathione. J Pharmacol Exp Ther 187:211–217

Mitchell JR, Thorgeirsson SS, Potter WZ, Jollow DJ, Keiser H (1974) Acetaminophen-induced hepatic injury. Protective role of glutathione in man and rationale for therapy. Clin Pharmacol Ther 16:676–684

Moulding TS, Redeker AG, Kanel GC (1991) Acetaminophen, isoniazid, and hepatic toxicity. Ann Intern Med 114:431

Murphy R, Swartz R, Watkins PB (1990) Severe acetaminophen toxicity in a patient receiving isoniazid. Ann Intern Med 113:799–800

Nelson SD (1990) Molecular mechanisms of the hepatotoxicity caused by acetaminophen. Semin Liver Dis 10:267–278

Nolan CM, Sandblom RE, Thummel KE, Slattery JT, Nelson SD (1994) Hepatotoxicity associated with acetaminophen usage in patients receiving multiple drug therapy for tuberculosis. Chest 105:408–411

Nores JM, Rambaud S, Remy JM (1991) Acute hepatitis due to ketoprofen. Clin Rheumatol 10:215–216

O'Grady JG, Alexander GJM, Hayllar KM, Williams R (1989) Early indicators of prognosis in fulminant hepatic failure. Gastroenterology 97:439–445

O'Grady JG, Wendon J, Tan KC, Potter D, Cottam S, Cohen AT, Gimson AES, Williams R (1991) Liver transplantation after paracetamol overdose. BMJ 303:221–223

Oren R, Levy M (1992) Paracetamol overdose in Jerusalem, 1984–1989. Isr J Med Sci 28:795–796

Ouellette GS, Slitzky BE, Gates JA, Lagarde S, West AB (1991) Reversible hepatitis associated with diclofenac. J Clin Gastroenterol 13:205–210

Paterson D, Kerlin P, Walker N, Lynch S, Strong R (1992) Piroxicam induced submassive necrosis of the liver. Gut 33:1436–1438

Paulus HE (1982) FDA Arthritis Advisory Committee meeting. Arthritis Rheum 25:595–596

Pereira LMMB, Langley PG, Hayllar KM, Tredger JM, Williams R (1992) Coagulation factor V and VIII/V ratio as predictors of outcome in paracetamol induced fulminant hepatic failure: relation to other prognostic indicators. Gut 33:98–102

Planas R, de Leon R, Quer JC, Barranco C, Broguera M, Gassull MA (1990) Fatal submassive necrosis of the liver associated with piroxicam. Am J Gastroenterol 85:468–470

Prescott LF (1983) Paracetamol overdosage. Pharmacological considerations and clinical management. Drugs 25:290–314

Prescott LF (1986) Effects of non-narcotic analgesics on the liver. Drugs 32 [Suppl 4]:129–147

Prescott LF, Leslie PJ (1982) Side effects of benoxaprofen. BMJ 284:1783

Prescott LF, Wright N, Roscoe P, Brown SS (1971) Plasma-paracetamol half-life and hepatic necrosis in patients with paracetamol overdosage. Lancet I:519–522

Prescott LF, Newton RW, Swainson CP, Wright N, Forrest ARW, Matthew H (1974) Successful treatment of severe paracetamol overdosage with cysteamine. Lancet I:588–592

Prescott LF, Park J, Sutherland GR, Smith IJ, Proudfast AT (1976) Cysteamine, methionine, and penicillamine in the treatment of paracetamol poisoning. Lancet I:109–113

Prescott LF, Illingworth RW, Critchley JAJH, Stewart MJ, Adam RD, Proudfast AT (1979) Intravenous *N*-acetylcysteine: the treatment of choice for paracetamol poisoning. BMJ 2:1097–1100

Proudfoot AT, Wright N (1970) Acute paracetamol poisoning. BMJ 3:557–558

Purcell P, Henry D, Melville G (1991) Diclofenac hepatitis. Gut 32:1381–1385

Rabinovitz M, Van Thiel DH (1992) Hepatotoxicity of nonsteroidal anti-inflammatory drugs. Am J Gastroenterol 87:1696–1704

Rosenberg WMC, Ryley NG, Trowell JM, McGree JOD, Chapman RW (1993) Dextropropoxyphene induced hepatotoxicity: a report of nine cases. J Hepatol 19:470–474

Rumack BH (1984) Acetaminophen overdose in young children. Treatment and effects of alcohol and other additional ingestants in 417 cases. Am J Dis Child 138:428–433

Rumack BH, Matthew H (1975) Acetaminophen poisoning and toxicity. Pediatrics 55:871–876

Rumack BH, Peterson RC, Koch GG, Amara IA (1981) Acetaminophen overdose. 662 cases with evaluation of oral acetylcysteine treatment. Arch Intern Med 141:380–385

Rumore MM, Blaiklock RG (1992) Influence of age-dependent pharmacokinetics and metabolism on acetaminophen hepatotoxicity. J Pharm Sci 81:203–207

Sallie RW, Quinlan MF, McKenzie T, Shilkin KB, Reed WD (1991) Diclofenac hepatitis. Aust NZ J Med 21:251–255

Schapira D, Bassan L, Nahir AM, Scharf Y (1986) Diclofenac-induced hepatotoxicity. Postgrad Med J 62:63–65

Schenker S, Maddrey WC (1991) Subliminal drug-drug interactions: users and their physicians take notice. Hepatology 13:995–998

Schiff ER, Maddrey WC (1994) Can we prevent nonsteroidal anti-inflammatory drug-induced hepatic failure? Gastrointest Dis Today 3:7–13

Scully LJ, Clarke D, Barr RJ (1993) Diclofenac induced hepatitis. 3 cases with features of autoimmune chronic active hepatitis. Dig Dis Sci 38:744–751

Seaman WE, Plotz PH (1976) Effect of aspirin on liver tests in patients with RA or SLE and in normal volunteers. Arthritis Rheum 19:155–160

Seeff LB, Cuccherini BA, Zimmerman HJ, Adler E, Benjamin SB (1986) Acetaminophen hepatotoxicity in alcoholics. A therapeutic misadventure. Ann Intern Med 104:399–404

Seifert CF, Lucas DS, Vondracek TG, Kastens DJ, McCarty DL, Bui B (1993) Patterns of acetaminophen use in alcoholic patients. Pharmacotherapy 13:391–395

Shaw GR, Anderson R (1991) Multisystem failure and hepatic microvesicular fatty metamorphosis associated with tolmetin ingestion. Arch Pathol Lab Med 115:818–821

Sheiner P, de Majo W, Levy GA (1992) Acetylcysteine and fulminant hepatic failure. Hepatology 15:552–554

Sherman KE, Jones C (1992) Hepatotoxicity associated with piroxicam use. Gastroenterology 103:354–355

Shriner K, Goetz MB (1992) Severe hepatotoxicity in a patient receiving both acetaminophen and zidovudine. Am J Med 93:94–96

Smilkstein MJ, Knapp GL, Kulig KW, Rumack BH (1988) Efficacy of oral *N*-acetylcysteine in the treatment of acetaminophen overdose. Analysis of the national multicenter study (1976 to 1988). N Engl J Med 319:1557–1562

Smilkstein MJ, Bronstein AC, Linden C, Augenstein WL, Kulig KW, Rumack BH (1991) Acetaminophen overdose: a 48-hour intravenous N-acetylcysteine treatment protocol. Ann Emerg Med 20:1058–1063

Stricker BHC (1992) Drug-induced hepatic injury, 2nd edn. Elsevier, Amsterdam

Taggart HM, Alderdice JM (1982) Fatal cholestatic jaundice in elderly patients taking benoxaprofen. BMJ 284:1372

Tarazi EM, Harter JG, Zimmerman HJ, Ishak KG, Eaton RA (1993) Sulindac-associated hepatic injury: analysis of 91 cases reported to the Food and Drug Administration. Gastroenterology 104:569–574

Thomson JS, Prescott LF (1966) Liver damage and impaired glucose tolerance after paracetamol overdosage. BMJ 2:506–507

Thornton JR, Losowsky MS (1990) Severe thrombocytopenia after paracetamol overdose. Gut 31:1159–1160

Victorino RMM, Silveira JCB, Baptista A, de Moura MC (1980) Jaundice associated with naproxen. Postgrad Med J 56:368–470

Warren JS (1978) Diflunisal-induced cholestatic jaundice. BMJ 2:736–737

Whittaker SJ, Amar JN, Wanless IR, Heathcote J (1982) Sulindac hepatotoxicity. Gut 23:875–877

Winkler E, Halkin H (1992) Paracetamol overdose in Israel – 1992. Isr J Med Sci 28:811–812

Wooton FT, Lee WM (1990) Acetaminophen hepatotoxicity in the alcoholic. South Med J 83:1047–1049

Zimmerman HJ (1974) Aspirin-induced hepatic injury. Ann Intern Med 80:103–105

Zimmerman HJ (1978) Hepatotoxicity: the adverse effects of drugs and other chemicals on the liver. Appleton-Century-Crofts, New York

Zimmerman HJ (1981) Effects of aspirin and acetaminophen on the liver. Arch Intern Med 141:333–342

Zimmerman HJ (1986) Hepatic effects of oxaprozin. Semin Arthritis Rheum 15 [Suppl 2]:35–39

Zimmerman HJ (1990) Update of hepatotoxicity due to classes of drugs in common clinical use: non-steroidal drugs, anti-inflammatory drugs, antibiotics, antihypertensives, and cardiac and psychotropic agents. Semin Liver Dis 10:322–338

Zimmerman HJ, Maddrey WC (1993) Toxic and drug-induced hepatitis. In: Schiff L, Schiff ER (eds) Diseases of the liver, 7th edn. Lippincott, Philadelphia, pp 707–783

CHAPTER 23

Steroids and Other Hormones

H.J. ZIMMERMAN and K.G. ISHAK

This chapter deals with the effects of gonadal steroids and their synthetic equivalents, glucocorticoids, and several anterior hypophysical hormones. It also describes the effects of oral hyglycemic and antithyroid drugs.

A. Gonadal Steroids and Their Derivatives

Hepatic injury that appears to be attributable to derivatives of male and female sex steroids (Table 1) includes hepatic dysfunction, cholestatic jaundice, and benign hepatic tumors. While these effects appear to be shared by the C-17-alkylated anabolic steroids and by the C-17-ethinylated female sex steroids, production of the Budd-Chiari syndrome seems attributable only to the estrogenic component of the contraceptive steroids (ZIMMERMAN and MADDREY 1987), and exacerbation of hepatic porphyria is relatable mostly to derivatives of progesterone (SONG and KAPPAS 1975). Both anabolic and contraceptive steroids have been implicated in the production of peliosis hepatis and associated changes (ZIMMERMAN and MADDREY 1987); and oral contraceptive steroids can also provoke a unique form of sinusoidal dilatation (POULSON and WINKLER 1973).

B. Anabolic Steroids

Several forms of hepatic injury are attributable to the anabolic steroids (ISHAK and ZIMMERMAN 1987). For the most part, these have involved the synthetic or semisynthetic agents, although natural androgens may play a role in the development of vascular and neoplastic lesions.

The hepatic lesions have been associated with use of the steroids for a variety of conditions, including aplastic anemia, transsexualism of females, and impotence, and use by athletes for body-building and muscle enhancement (ISHAK and ZIMMERMAN 1987). The lesions seen consist of two main groups: those that occur after a relatively short period (1–6 months) of taking the drug, namely cholestasis and associated hepatic dysfunction; and those that develop after prolonged use of the anabolic agent, namely neoplasms (ISHAK and ZIMMERMAN 1987) and vascular lesions (ZAFRANI et al. 1983).

Table 1. Comparison of hepatic lesions produced by oral contraceptives and anabolic steroids

Lesion	Oral contraceptives	C-17-alklated anabolic-androgen steroids
Cholestasis and hepatic dysfunction	+	+
Nodular regenerative hyperplasia	+	+
Peliosis hepatis	+	++
Hepatic adenoma	++	+
Hepatocellular carcinoma	+	+
Hepatic vein thrombosis	+	–
Sinusoidal dilatation (zone 1)	+	–
Porphyria exacerbation	+	–

I. Cholestasis

Cholestatic jaundice induced by methyltestosterone was first described over 40 years ago (WERNER et al. 1950). Instances of jaundice caused by other structurally related steroids have now been identified (ZIMMERMAN 1978). First labeled an idiosyncratic reaction, even attributed to hypersensitivity (WERNER et al. 1950), the adverse effect of methyltestosterone on the liver is now recognized to be an expression of an intrinsic hepatotoxic effect of the steroids, albeit a mild one (ZIMMERMAN 1978).

1. Structural Characteristics of Icterogenic Steroids

The anabolic steroids that can cause jaundice and hepatic dysfunction all have an alkyl group in the C-17 position (Fig. 1). Testosterone, 19-nontestosterone, and their esters do not cause jaundice or hepatic dysfunction. An anecdotal reference over 40 years ago (WERNER 1947) to jaundice while the patient was taking testosterone may have been coincidence. Another instance of jaundice attributed to a nonalkylated anabolic steroid occurred in a recipient during the third trimester of her pregnancy (GARRIGUES-GIL et al. 1986). This may have reflected either cholestatic jaundice of pregnancy or the combined effect of the drug and pregnancy.

2. Incidence

Only a small minority of recipients of ordinary therapeutic doses of the anabolic steroids develop jaundice, although the majority develop hepatic dysfunction (FOSS and SIMPSON 1959; KORY et al. 1959). High therapeutic doses, employed to treat aplastic anemia, have led to a 17% incidence of jaundice (PECKING et al. 1980). Jaundice in the usual case has not developed until the drug had been taken for at least 1 month; and in most patients for 2–5 months or even longer (ZIMMERMAN 1963).

The rate of development and the severity of hepatic dysfunction are dose dependent (KORY et al. 1959; TICKTIN and ZIMMERMAN 1966). Furthermore, the

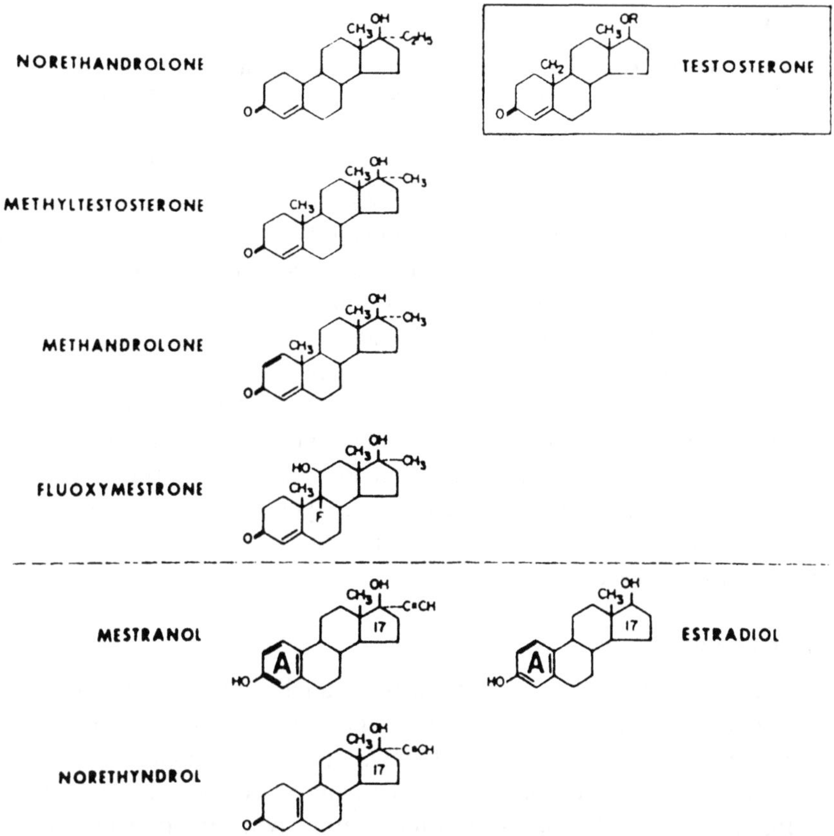

Fig. 1. Structure of anabolic and contraceptive steroids that can lead to cholestasis compared to testosterone and estradiol. Note C-17 alkylation of anabolic steroids and C-17 ethinylation of mestranol and norethyndrol critical to the cholestasis-producing effect. Also note unsaturation of ring A, also a feature enhancing cholestatic effects of mestranol

larger the daily dose, the more likely is jaundice to develop; and it is probable that jaundice would develop in all individuals given large enough doses of one of these agents (SCHAFFNER and RAISFIELD 1969). However, the development of jaundice from the usual therapeutic doses appears to depend on individual susceptibility.

3. Clinical Features

The syndrome of hepatic disease produced by the alkylated anabolic steroids includes few clinical manifestations other than jaundice. Malaise, mild anorexia, and nausea may precede the jaundice by several days to several weeks, although jaundice may appear in an otherwise asymptomatic patient. Pruritus occurs in some cases and may be severe. Jaundice may be intense with values for bilirubin above 20 mg/dl, or it may be slight.

4. Biochemical Features

Laboratory studies reveal a cholestatic pattern of hepatic injury (ZIMMERMAN 1963). Values for aminotransferases [AST (SGOT) and ALT (SGPT)] are usually less than fivefold elevated, even when bilirubin levels are very high. Alkaline phosphatase (ALP) values differ from those seen in the intrahepatic cholestasis caused by chlorpromazine (CPZ). They are normal or only modestly elevated in most patients with steroid jaundice. Less than 5% of patients have values more than three times the normal upper limit (ZIMMERMAN 1963). The relatively slight elevation of the aminotransferase values is similar to the pattern of the cholestatic jaundice produced by CPZ or even lower. The lack of striking elevations of ALP, however, is a feature that distinguishes the cholestatic jaundice of anabolic steroids from that of CPZ (ZIMMERMAN 1978). These biochemical features and the histologic ones that are discussed in the next section warrant a terminologic distinction between forms of cholestatic jaundice – canalicular jaundice to refer to the type of cholestasis due to the anabolic steroids and hepatocellular jaundice to describe the type caused by CPZ (ZIMMERMAN 1978).

5. Histopathology

Liver biopsy usually shows only bile casts in canaliculi and bilirubin-staining of hepatocytes, mainly in zone 3 (ISHAK and ZIMMERMAN 1987) (Fig. 2). A few hepatocytes may show the foamy, reticulated appearance called "pseudoxanthomatous degeneration" (ISHAK and ZIMMERMAN 1987; SHAFFNER et al. 1959). Occasional patients show mild parenchymal injury manifested by sinusoidal ("free") acidophilic bodies (apoptosis) and by foci of necrosis; portal areas usually appear normal. The lack of inflammation in the portal area ("bland" cholestasis) associated with the canalicular jaundice of anabolic steroids thus provides a histologic difference from the portal inflammation associated with the hepatocanalicular jaundice of CPZ.

Electron microscopic studies of the liver show changes in the canaliculi, Golgi apparatus, and lysosomes (SCHAFFNER et al. 1960; ORLANDI and JEZEQUEL 1966; PHILLIPS et al. 1978). The canaliculi show blunting and loss of microvilli, a nonspecific manifestation of cholestasis of any etiology. The Golgi apparatus contains dark granules; lysosomes show degenerative changes. Administration of an anabolic steroid (norethandrolone) to rats also leads to injury of the pericanalicular microfilaments with loss of filament structure and replacement by a granular zone (PHILLIPS et al. 1978, 1986). These abnormalities apparently lead to impaired canalicular contraction, a physiologic defect that presumably contributes to cholestasis.

6. Prognosis

The outlook for complete recovery from steroid-induced injury is excellent. In the anicteric patient with dysfunction, return to normal begins almost as soon as the drug is stopped. In the jaundiced patient, however, subsidence of icterus

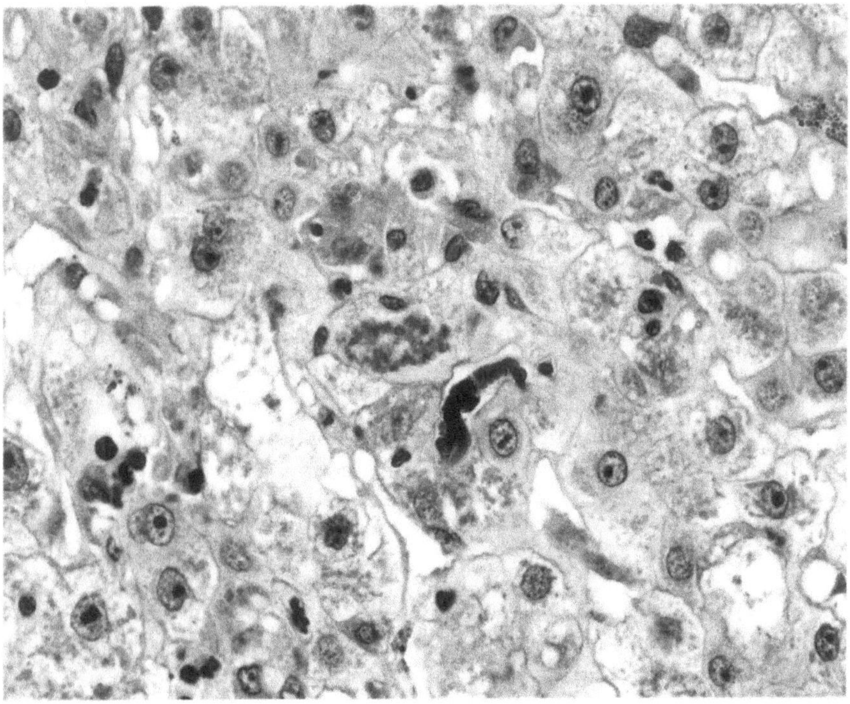

Fig. 2. Chronic cholestasis due to methyltestosterone therapy. A canalicular bile plug overlies an hepatocyte harboring a Mallory's body. H&E, ×630

may require weeks to months (ZIMMERMAN 1963). An instance of chronic cholestasis and cirrhosis accompanied by a syndrome resembling "primary biliary cirrhosis" has been ascribed to methyltestosterone (GLOBER and WILKINSON 1968).

Death, as the outcome of jaundice caused by an anabolic steroid, has been extremely rare. Several reported fatalities have involved debilitated patients (KOSZALKA 1957; WILDER 1962; GILBERT et al. 1963) or patients with necrosis associated with peliosis hepatis (BOYER 1978).

7. Mechanism

The physiologic defects imposed by the anabolic steroid are mainly excretory (HEANEY and WHELDON 1958; LEEVY et al. 1961). Clearance of bilirubin from the blood is impaired less than is canalicular excretion, which is strikingly depressed (ARIAS 1963; PLAA and PRIESTLEY 1977).

The cholestatic effects appear attributable to interference with both the bile salt dependent fraction (BSDF) (DESPOPOULUS 1971) and the bile salt independent fraction (BSIF) (PAUMGARTNER et al. 1976) of bile flow. Presumed sites of injury leading to cholestasis involve the canaliculus and its pericanalicular microfibrillar network as well as the basolateral (sinusoidal) plasma membrane and perhaps the tight junction (PLAA and PRIESTLY 1977; ZIMMERMAN and LEWIS 1987; PHILLIPS et al. 1986). Injury to the basolateral plasma membrane (TUCHWEBER et al. 1986; KREEK 1987) involves inhibition of the $Na^+K^+ATPase$ of the hepatocyte plasma membrane, presumably by decreasing its viscosity.

Susceptibility to the adverse hepatic effects of anabolic steroids appears to be modified by host factors. Differences between species in susceptibility indicate that genetic factors govern vulnerability (ZIMMERMAN 1978). Furthermore, the cholestatic effect of the chemically similar contraceptive steroids, which resembles that of the anabolic steroids, is clearly subject to genetic influences (ADLERCREUTZ and TENHUNEN 1970; KREEK 1987).

Preexisting liver disease enhances the adverse effect of anabolic steroids on liver function. The impairment of hepatic function induced by the steroids is additive to pretreatment abnormality of function (LEEVY et al. 1961).

II. Peliosis Hepatis

Peliosis hepatis is a vascular lesion that has been reported in more than 50 recipients of anabolic steroids. It consists of blood-filled lakes (Fig. 3). The

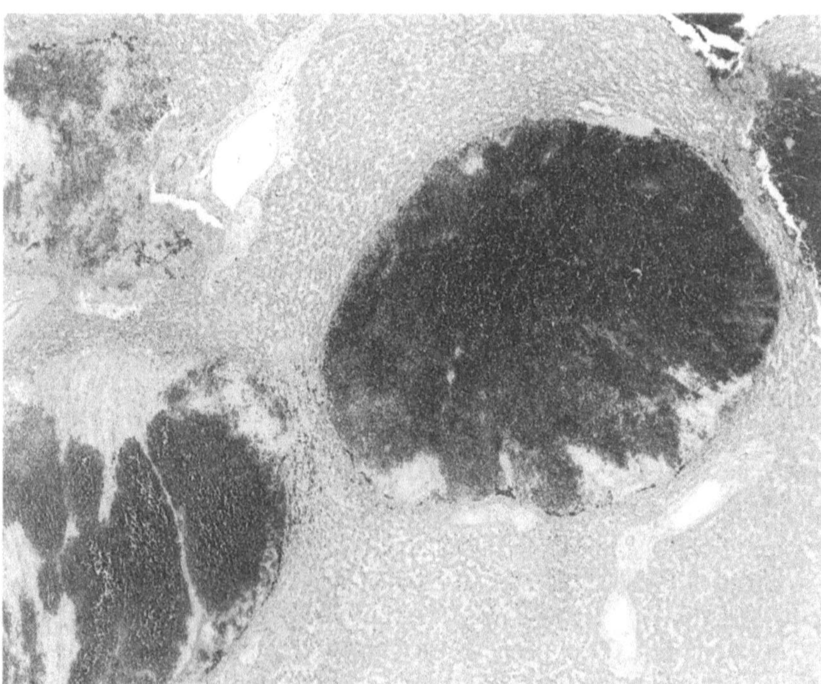

Fig. 3. Peliosis hepatis associated with oxymetholone therapy for aplastic anemia. Several blood-filled cavities are scattered in the section. H&E ×630

pathogenesis of the lesion is unknown, but it may be quite separate from that of the hepatic dysfunction induced by the C-17-alkylated steroids. Testosterone, which has no C-17 alkylation and no adverse effect on liver function, has been incriminated as the cause of Peliosis (BURGER and MARCUSO 1952). All of the C-17-alkylated steroids have been incriminated (ISHAK and ZIMMERMAN 1987). Danazol has also led to the lesion (NESHER et al. 1985).

The reported cases of peliosis have occurred in both sexes and have shown no age predilection. The only clinical manifestation is hepatomegaly, except for the infrequent instances of rupture and hemoperitoneum or of jaundice and liver failure due to compression and necrosis of the remaining parenchyma (NADEL and KOSEK; BOYER 1978).

III. Neoplasms

Both benign and malignant tumors have been reported in recipients of the anabolic steroids. Also diffuse hyperplasia, nodular regenerative hyperplasia (NRH), and even focal nodular hyperplasia (FNH) have been attributed to these agents (ISHAK and ZIMMERMAN 1987). Acceptance of the association between the administration of the steroids and these hyperplastic and neoplastic lesions is based on reports of regression of some of these lesions on cessation of steroid administration (LOWDELL and MURRAY-LYON 1985), the demonstration of androgen receptors in normal hepatocytes and cells of hepatocellular carcinoma (BANNISTER et al. 1985; NAGASUE et al. 1985), and the reproduction of hyperplastic and neoplastic lesions in mice by prolonged treatment with methyltestosterone (TAYLOR and SNOWBALL 1984).

1. Nodular Regenerative Hyperplasia

Nodular regenerative hyperplasia (NRH) and diffuse hyperplasia have been described in recipients of anabolic steroids. Nodular regenerative hyperplasia, sometimes referred to as hepatic adenomatosis, is a somewhat nonspecific lesion which is seen in association with a number of systemic and hepatic diseases (ISHAK and ZIMMERMAN 1987).

2. Hepatocellular Adenoma

Hepatocellular adenomas have been reported in a number of recipients of C-17-alkylated steroids (ISHAK and ZIMMERMAN 1987) and in at least one instance of a C-17-nonsubstituted steroid, testosterone enanthate (CARRASCO et al. 1985). However, the adenoma has been attributed to anabolic steroid (AS) administration far less frequently than to oral contraceptive (OC) use. Furthermore, in at least half of the reported instances of AS-associated hepatic adenoma there were multiple tumors; most were asymptomatic and rupture was infrequent, occurring in only 10% of a group of 30 cases collected from the literature (PELLETIER et al. 1984). In contrast, OC-associated adenomas are most often solitary, often present with abdominal pain, and may rupture in up to 40% of reported cases (KLATSKIN 1977). Indeed, one gains the impression that the multiple adenomas seen in AS recipients are part of nodular regenerative hyperplasia; and only about half of the reported instances appear to be solitary adenomas that are similar clinically and histologically to the OC-associated ones (ISHAK and ZIMMERMAN 1987).

3. Hepatic Carcinoma

At least 40 recipients of anabolic steroids have developed hepatocellular carcinoma (ISHAK and ZIMMERMAN 1987). Usually the drug had been administered for 2–4 years, with the longest recorded period 11 years. Age at the time of recognition of the carcinoma has averaged 18 years; and about 70% of reported cases have been males. The average interval between initiation of steroid therapy and appearance of the carcinoma has been 72 months, but it has been distinctly shorter in patients with Fanconi's aplastic anemia than in others (WESTABY and WILLIAMS 1981). These and other features of the cases led WESTABY and WILLIAMS (1981) to speculate that the oncogenic potential of Fanconi's chromosomal abnormality combined with that of the steroid to lead to the neoplasm. That the steroids can provoke carcinoma in other types of patients, however, is clear from the total number now reported.

Acceptance of the reported cases as carcinoma, however, has by no means been unanimous. ANTHONY (1975), in a critical analysis of the first 12 reported cases, accepted only two as valid examples of carcinoma. He emphasized that the absence of α-fetoprotein from the blood, in 11 of 12 cases, the extraordinarily benign course in many of them, and the rarity of metastases led him to question the validity of the diagnosis of hepatocellular carcinoma. Nevertheless, instances of deaths and of metastases from these carcinomas have been recorded (ISHAK and ZIMMERMAN 1987). While the steroid-associated carcinomas are less rapidly progressive, less inevitably death-dealing, and less compellingly malignant than the usual hepatocellular carcinoma, they are carcinomas, albeit distinctive ones. The microscopic appearance of steroid-associated carcinomas does not differ from that of other hepatic carcinomas. In any event, the reports (MCGAUGHAN et al. 1985) of apparent regression of putative carcinoma after withdrawal of the steroid have practical implications. Indeed, two patients have been reported to be alive and well 10 and 14 years after androgen withdrawal.

4. Other Neoplasms

Several reports have drawn attention to the association of angiosarcoma with anabolic steroid therapy (FALK et al. 1979; NORDSTEN 1985). Two cases of cholangocarcinoma (CHC) and one of mixed CHC-HCC have also been reported in recipients of the steroids (TURANI et al. 1983).

C. Female Sex Hormones and the Contraceptive Steroids

I. Estrogenic Hormones and Related Drugs

A large number of studies have established the ability of natural and synthetic estrogenic steroids to impair hepatic function, especially that associated with bile flow (KREEK 1987; MUELLER and KAPPAS 1964; KLAASSAN and WATKINS 1984; SCHREIBER and SIMON 1983). The adverse hepatic effects on the liver of the estrogenic hormones (estradiol, estriol, estrone) and their derivatives (ethinyl estradiol, mestranol) appear to be qualitatively different from those of the nonhormone (stilbestrol, diethylstilbestrol). The hormonal estrogens and their derivatives produce cholestatic injury; they interfere with bile flow. They can also play a role in tumorigenesis. Diethylstilbestrol (DES) is more likely to produce hepatocellular injury (ELIAS and SCHWINNER 1945; ZIMMERMAN and MADDREY 1987).

The cholestatic effects of estrogenic hormones and their derivatives became apparent as cholestatic jaundice of pregnancy came under scrutiny (KREEK 1987) and the icterogenic effects of oral contraceptive preparations (OCs) began to be studied (EISALO et al. 1964; ROMAN and HECKER 1968). These estrogens interfere selectively with excretion of BSP and bilirubin by the liver of rats (GALLAGHER et al. 1966) and humans (KREEK 1987; SCHREIBER and SIMON 1983). They interfere with canalicular excretion far more than with removal of the dye from blood. Alteration of the phenolic character of ring A of the estrogen by hydroxylation and methoxylation at the C-1 or C-2 position inhibits or destroys the adverse effect on liver function (GALLAGHER et al. 1966). Interestingly, the addition of an ethinyl substituent at the C-17 position restores or enhances the ability to impair hepatic function, an effect analogous to the effect of C-17 alkylation in anabolic steroids.

The demonstration of adverse effects of estrogens on hepatic function has led to the deduction that the estrogenic component of the OC preparations is mainly responsible for the hepatic dysfunction produced by the preparations (PLAA and PRIESTLY 1977; EISALO et al. 1964; ROMAN and HECKER 1968; METREAU et al. 1972; KREEK 1987). A contributory role for the progestin, however, remains tenable (KREEK 1987). The available evidence suggests that the cholestatic jaundice of pregnancy may be a manifestation of exaggerated responsiveness to the cholestatic effects of high estrogen levels (ADLERCREUTZ and TENHUNIN 1970; HAEMMARI and WYSS 1967; REYES et al. 1976; REYES 1982).

The interference with bile secretion appears to involve decreased formation of canalicular bile and debatably increased regurgitation of bile at "leaky" tight junctions (PLAA and PRIESTLEY 1977; ZIMMERMAN and LEWIS 1987; ELIAS et al. 1983). Decreased formation of canalicular bile seems attributable to decreased uptake of bile acids, leading to decreased bile-salt-dependent flow (BSDF), as well as decreased electrolyte secretion and decreased bile-salt-independent flow (BSIF) (KLAASSEN and WATKINS 1984; REICHEN and SIMON 1984).

The impaired uptake of bile acids is attributable to a decrease in fluidity and $Na^{+}K^{+}$ATPase activity of the basolateral plasma membrane of the hepatocyte (KEEFFE et al. 1980). That estrogenic hormones may also have an effect at the canalicular level similar to that of the anabolic steroids would be a reasonable supposition, in view of the similarity in structure, but remains to be demonstrated.

Most of the attention to estrogen-produced hepatic dysfunction has related to the effects of contraceptive steroids, and of hormonal derivatives. Reports of impaired liver function, hyperbilirubinemia, and overt liver disease in patients with prostatic carcinoma who were treated with stilbestrol [diethylstilbestrol (DES)] have also appeared (KONTURRI et al. 1972; DAHL and SCHMID 1969). Indeed, DES has been found to lead to the "alcoholic hyaline" (Mallory's bodies) type of hepatocyte degeneration in several strains of hamsters (COE et al. 1983) and in a patient being treated for prostatic carcinoma (SEKI et al. 1983).

II. Progestational Steroids

Progesterone has no demonstrable adverse effect on hepatic function. There appears to be little evidence that progesterone or a derivative is the endogenous steroid responsible for cholestatic jaundice of pregnancy, despite the 20- to 40-fold increase in production of progesterone during the last trimester of pregnancy. Indeed, studies of the related syndrome of jaundice caused by the contraceptive steroids and other data have led to a consensus that estrogens, blood levels of which are increased up to 1000-fold in late pregnancy (KREEK 1987), play the key role in producing jaundice of pregnancy. ADLERCREUTZ and TENHUNEN (1970) concluded that the cholestatic jaundice of pregnancy is the result of enhanced sensitivity to the cholestatic effects of "normal amounts of estrogens," and is an exaggerated manifestation of the slight cholestatic effect observed in normal late pregnancy.

Synthetic progestins include two main groups of compounds. In one group, characterized by a methyl group in the C-19 position, are derivatives of progesterone. Members of the other group lack the C-19 methyl group (C-19 nor-compounds). They are derivatives of 19-nortestosterone (ADLERCREUTZ and TENHUNEN 1970). The nortestosterone derivatives used as oral contraceptives also have a C-17 ethinyl group, while the progesterone derivatives have an acyl group in the C-17 position. Only the derivatives of nortestosterone (e.g., norethynodrel, lynestrenal, and norethisterone) can cause impaired liver function and jaundice (ADLERCREUTZ and TENHUNAN 1970; METREAU et al. 1972). They have led to cholestatic jaundice, especially in larger than contraceptive doses (ADLERCREUTZ and TENHANAN 1970; LANGLANDS and MARTIN 1975). While these ethinylated norprogestins have some adverse effect on hepatic function, they clearly produce less impairment than do the C-17 ethinyl estrogens. However, the progestins, when given with the C-17 ethanol estrogens, seem to enhance the hepatic injury produced by the estrogens, and seem to add a component of hepatocellular injury to the cholestatic effect of the estrogens (KREEK 1987; METREAU et al. 1972). Instances of hepatocellular injury attributed to norethindrone (ROUTIER et al. 1967) and cyproterone acetate (MEIJERS et al. 1986) are consistent with this view.

III. Adverse Effects of Contraceptive Steroids on the Liver

Cholestatic jaundice and impaired hepatic function were the first to command special interest (KREEK 1987; PEREZ-MERA and SHIELDS 1962; ROMAN and HECKER 1968; METREAU et al. 1972). Other effects include the development of benign and malignant tumors (ISHAK 1979; KLATSKIN 1977; PORTER et al. 1987; STURVETANT 1979; NEUBURGER et al. 1980), aggravation of hemangioma or of lesions of familial hemorrhagic telangiectasia (KOSITICHEK and CULLEN 1970; ROWLEY et al. 1970), production of Budd-Chiari syndrome (LEWIS et al. 1983; VALLA et al. 1986), sinusoidal changes (POULSEN and WINCKLER 1973), peliosis hepatis (KARASAWA et al. 1979; SCHONBERG 1982), hepatic rupture (FREDERICK et al. 1974; BOTTGER et al. 1981), and provocation of bouts of porphyria (SONG and KAPP 1975; KAPPAS and GRANNICK 1968).

Jaundice had been reported, by 1972, in at least 300 recipients of these steroids (METREAU et al. 1972), and it has been estimated (SCHAFFNER 1966) that the actual number may be tenfold the number described in the literature. Estimates of 1 in 10000 recipients in most parts of the world and of 1 in 4000 recipients in Sweden have been offered (METREAU et al. 1972).

Hepatic dysfunction is much more frequent. As many as 40%–50% of recipients of these agents have been reported to develop impaired excretion of BSP and a lesser proportion elevated serum aminotransferase levels (METREAU et al. 1972). However, some reports have stressed the rarity of hepatic dysfunction in recipients of these steroids. The disparity between the various reports may be the result of several factors. Monitoring during the course of taking the steroids may fail to detect abnormal function unless it is performed early. Moderate impairment may develop and then subside as compensatory adjustments take place (METREAU et al. 1972). Differential susceptibility of different groups of patients may also contribute to disparate results. Postmenopausal women appear to be more sensitive than younger women to adverse effects of steroids on hepatic function (METREAU et al. 1972). Some ethnic groups (Swedes, Chileans) are particularly sensitive to the icterogenic effects of the oral contraceptives (METREAU et al. 1972; ORELLANA-ALCADE and DEMINGUEZ 1966), and accordingly also more likely to develop dysfunction. Nevertheless, with sensitive measures of liver function such as fractional BSP clearance, almost all recipients of contraceptive steroids show impaired function.

IV. Syndrome of Contraceptive Steroid Jaundice

1. Clinical Features

Onset of the jaundice is usually during the first six cycles of treatment, and often during the first cycle (Metreau et al. 1972). Malaise, anorexia, nausea, and especially pruritus may precede the onset of jaundice by several days to 2 weeks. Vomiting is rare. Pruritus may be the first symptom.

2. Biochemical Features

Bilirubin levels are usually moderately elevated, uncommonly above 10mg/dl (Metreau et al. 1972), and rarely as high as 20mg/dl (Lieberman et al. 1984). Other biochemical features also resemble the jaundice produced by the alkylated, anabolic steroids. Alkaline phosphatase levels are only modestly elevated. Cholesterol levels are rarely increased. Values for AST and ALT are elevated in about two-thirds of cases, usually to less than threefold the ULN (Metreau et al. 1972). In 15% of patients, the cholestasis is less pure and there is some evidence of parenchymal injury (Schaffner 1966; Orellana-Alcade and Deminguez 1966).

3. Histologic Characteristics

These features also resemble those of anabolic steroid jaundice. Bile casts in canaliculi and normal parenchyma are characteristic. The lesion is that of "bland cholestasis," i.e., there is little or no portal inflammatory response (Schaffner 1966; Metreau et al. 1972). In some patients, parenchymal hepatic injury is shown by the presence of sinusoidal acidophilic bodies (Hartley et al. 1969).

Ultrastructural changes are similar to those of other forms of cholestasis (Metreau et al. 1972; Phillips et al. 1986). The abnormalities include dilatation of canaliculi, and blunting and fragmentation of microvilli. The smooth endoplasmic reticulum shows dilatation and vesiculation and the mitochondria assume bizarre shapes and acquire paracrystalline figures (Metreau et al. 1972; Perez et al. 1969; Martinez-Mandaton et al. 1970).

4. Prognosis

In most patients jaundice is gone within 1 month, although the icteric period may exceed 3 months (Metreau et al. 1972; Lieberman et al. 1984). There are no residua. Biliary cirrhosis reported in one patient was assumed by the authors to have been preexistent (Hartley et al. 1969).

5. Susceptibility

Vulnerability to the OC-induced jaundice appears genetically affected. The importance of genetic factors is shown by: the demonstrations that women with a personal or family history of cholestatic jaundice of pregnancy are particularly susceptible to icterogenic effects of an oral contraceptive or of ethinyl estradiol (REYES 1982; KREECK et al. 1987); and by the much higher incidence of OC-induced jaundice among Scandinavian women (DALEN and WESTERHOLM 1974) and Chilean women of Araucanian extraction (REYES 1982) than among other groups.

V. Tumors Associated with Oral Contraceptives

1. Hepatocellular Adenoma

The striking increase in the incidence of hepatic adenomas is the result of widespread use of contraceptive steroids (KLATSKIN 1977; EDMUNDSON et al. 1976; ROOKS et al. 1979; CHRISTOFFERSON and MAYS 1979; STURVETANT 1979). An extraordinarily rare lesion prior to 1960, adenoma has now been recorded in hundreds of patients. While it is difficult to estimate the total number of cases recorded, an estimate of 300 cases diagnosed per year in the United States was offered in 1979 (ROOKS et al. 1979). The number of published case reports has declined as the association between adenoma and OC use has become an accepted phenomenon. Also, there may have been a decrease in incidence, secondary to reduced dose of the estrogenic component of the OC preparation.

The strong circumstantial evidence for an etiologic relationship between adenoma and OC use is reinforced by the demonstration of a direct relationship between the duration of use of OCs and the development of adenoma (EDMONDSON et al. 1976; LIPSTATE et al. 1981; KERLIN et al. 1983), the regression of the tumors after withdrawal of the OC (EDMONDSON et al. 1977), and the description of multiple adenomas in a patient with an ovarian carcinoma (MOSONYI 1956). Furthermore, the etiologic role of OCs has been established conclusively by the case control studies of EDMONDSON et al. (1976) and of ROOKS and his associates (1979).

While the tumor has been found as early as 6 months after starting the intake of an OC, taking the agent for more than 5 years seems to pose a much greater risk than taking the preparation for less than 3 years (EDMONDSON et al. 1976). Women who had taken OCs for more than 5 years had 100 times the risk of developing an adenoma than those who had taken the pill for less than 1 year. Seven years of OC use raised the relative risk to 500 (ROOKS et al. 1979). However, even the hundreds of reported cases of adenoma are but a tiny fraction of the millions of women who have taken these agents.

Patients with hepatocellular adenoma have been, of course, mainly women in the childbearing years. The few older patients have been mainly those receiving estrogen therapy (ROOKS et al. 1979; STURVETANT 1979). Over 90% of patients with adenoma had been taking an OC.

a) Clinical Features

The clinical manifestations of hepatic adenoma fall into four categories (KLATSKIN 1977; EDMONDSON et al. 1976; KEIFER and SCOTT 1977; TERBLANCHE et al. 1978). These are: (a) an asymptomatic lesion encountered as an incidental finding at laparotomy; (b) a mass found on physical examination or during an imaging procedure; (c) identification of the tumor as the cause of a painful, tender enlarged liver or a specific, tender mass; (d) a sudden, life-threatening intraabdominal hemorrhage secondary to rupture of the tumor and characterized by severe pain and, usually, vascular collapse.

Presentation with pain and tenderness appears to be the result of hemorrhage into the tumor (AMERIKS et al. 1975; TERBLANCHE et al. 1978). Symptoms had generally been present for several days, rarely for weeks or even months. Occasional patients in this group develop jaundice, presumably due to compression of the intrahepatic biliary tree by expanding tumor (STURVETANT 1979). The presence of fever with right upper quadrant pain may yield a syndrome that simulates cholecystitis; and, when accompanied by jaundice, could be mistaken for choledocholithiasis (WILSON 1982).

Hemoperitoneum is the serious sequel to hemorrhage into the adenoma with consequent rupture of the tumor. Symptoms have usually been present for several hours, rarely for 1 or 2 days prior to the recognition of the intraabdominal hemorrhage (EDMONDSON et al. 1976; TERBLANCHE et al. 1978). EDMONDSON et al. (1976) have drawn attention to the temporal relationship between menstruation and rupture of adenoma, "suggesting that constriction of the large arteries supplying the adenoma may occur at the same time as the spasm of the spiral arteries of the endometrium that results in sloughing and bleeding."

Specific diagnosis of adenoma is usually made only after resection, although history, physical examination, and "imaging" procedures should lead to a presumptive diagnosis. Arteriography is a useful means of demonstrating the tumor prior to rupture (KERLIN et al. 1983).

b) Histologic Features

The adenoma is composed of large hepatocytes, often pale, sometimes vacuolated, at times fatty. They form sheets of cells and occasionally prominent cords, without lobular structure, or portal areas. Sinusoids are usually compressed, leading to the sheet-like appearance. Some adenomas have a fibrous capsule (Fig. 4). Others merge with the uninvolved parenchyma (ISHAK 1988).

c) Treatment

Resection of the adenoma is generally readily accomplished and the outlook is good when the lesion has been recognized prior to rupture. Even patients with hemoperitoneum may fare well if the diagnosis is made promptly and the tumor resected. However, there have been fatalities in instances of delayed recognition and late laparotomy, with death the result of hemorrhagic shock,

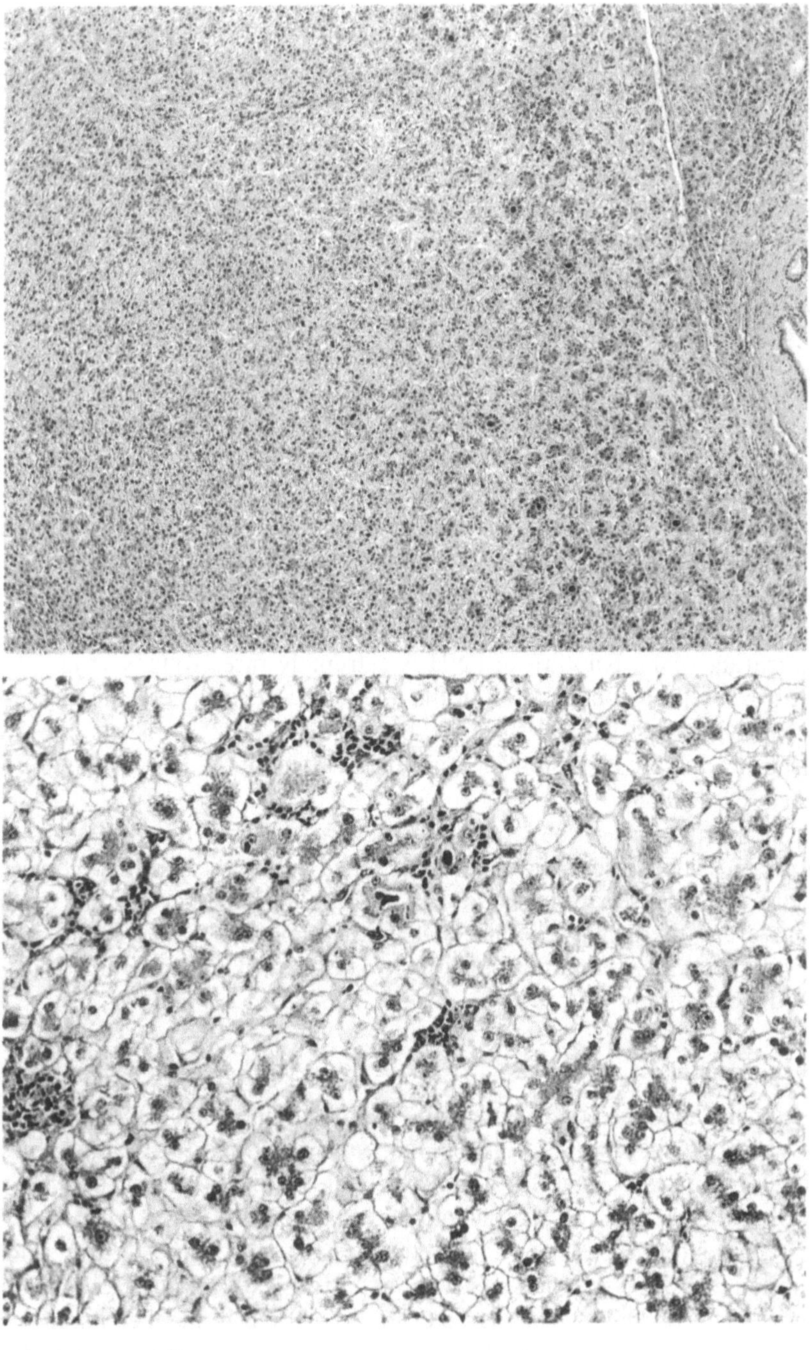

a

b

Fig. 4. a Hepatocellular adenoma induced by long-term oral contraceptive use. The growth is "sheet-like" with some pseudogland formation *to the right*. Part of a portal area is present *at the extreme right* of the photographic field. H&E ×35. **b** Hepatocellular adenoma. Higher magnification of case illustrated in **a**, showing large pale cells with a low nuclear/cytoplasmic ratio. Occasional bile plugs are seen. Note lack of a trabecular pattern. H&E, ×195

coagulation abnormalities, and related complications (AMERIKS et al. 1975; ISHAK and RABIN 1975; EDMUNDSON et al. 1976). These cases account for the case fatality rate of 8%–10% among patients who present with pain and hemorrhage (STURVETANT 1979).

Removal of the tumor is the treatment of choice. Pregancy may lead to recurrence and even rupture in the patient whose tumor has not been removed and carcinoma may develop in an adenoma long after the OCs have been stopped (CHRISTENSON et al. 1981); accordingly, resection of the adenoma seems more appropriate than monitoring the patient for regression.

2. Focal Nodular Hyperplasia

The relationship of this tumor to OCs is much less clear than that of adenoma. The striking sex predilection for adenoma of females is not seen, although females with the lesion appear to be at least twice as frequent as males (ISHAK and RABIN 1975; KERLIN et al. 1983). While over 90% of patients with adenoma had been taking OCs, less than 60% of those with FNH had taken one of the preparations (ISHAK and RABIN 1975). Furthermore, the FNH is seen in all age groups, while adenoma is almost confined to women in the childbearing years. Rupture of FNH is extremely rare (KERLIN et al. 1983), while it is a feared complication of the adenoma. Nevertheless, the increased number of reports of FNH since the introduction of OCs reflects either increased attention to all tumors or, perhaps, an effect of OCs on growth of FNH (KERLIN et al. 1983).

The morphology of the lesion is characteristic (Fig. 5). Grossly, the tumor is nodular, usually lacks a capsule, and has a central scar. Microscopically, there is fibrosis separating nodules of normal hepatocytes, and within fibrous areas there may be bile duct epithelium (ISHAK and RABIN 1975). Many specimens resemble cirrhosis. (This lesion is sometimes called "pseudocirrhosis".)

3. Hepatocellular Carcinoma

There is also evidence that OCs can be hepatocarcinogenic (O'SULLIVAN and ROSSWICK 1976; AMTRUP et al. 1980; HELLING and WOODS 1982; NEUBERGER et al. 1986; HENDERSON et al. 1983; FORMAN et al. 1986; STUBBLEFIELD 1984). By now over 100 users of the contraceptive steroids have developed hepatocellular carcinoma (HCC), a lesion expectedly rare in young women. Furthermore, the lesion has involved patients without cirrhosis, a relatively uncommon circumstance for HCC. The character of the neoplasm has been somewhat atypical, appearing histologically fairly benign, yet leading to metastases (AMERIKS et al. 1975). Furthermore, the tumor is rarely accompanied by high blood levels of α-fetoglobulin, and many of the patients have experienced survival surprisingly long for HCC (STRICKER 1992). Despite the unusual character of the tumor, an hepatocarcinogenic role for the OCs seems confirmed by the case-control studies of HENDERSON et al. (1983) and

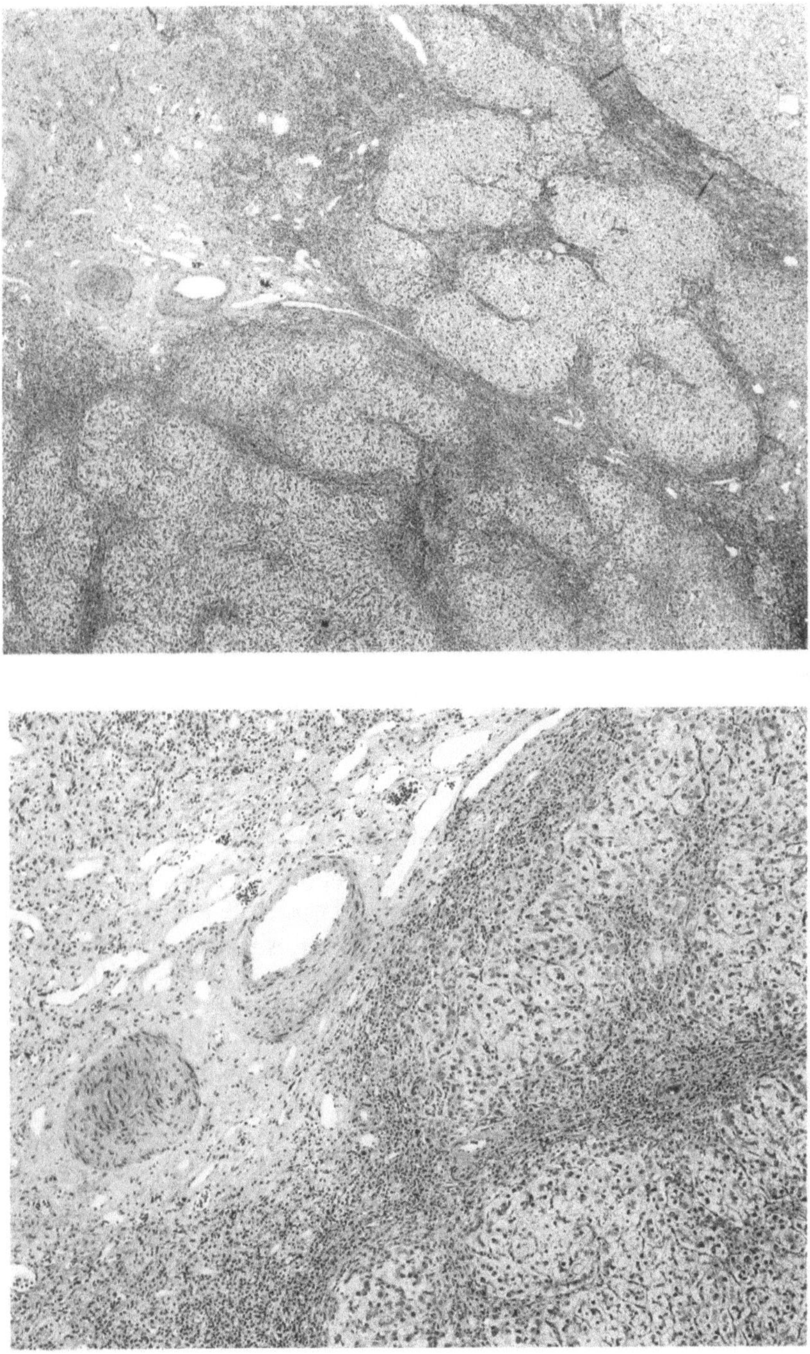

a

b

Fig. 5. **a** Focal nodular hyperplasia. Incidental finding in a woman taking oral contraceptives. Note the cirrhosis-like architecture. Part of the central scar is present *in the left upper corner of the* field. H&E, ×75. **b** Focal nodular hyperplasia. Higher magnification of case illustrated in **a**. Two thick-walled arteries are present (*upper left corner*). A septum is connected to the central scar. H&E, ×75

NEUBERGER et al. (1986). These groups have found significantly greater use of OCs among women with HCC than among matched controls. Indeed, NEUBERGER et al. (1986) found that use of the OCs for 8 years or more is associated with a 4.4-fold increased risk of HCC; and, on exclusion from analysis of patients with serologic markers of hepatitis B infection, the relative risk for OC users rises to 7.2. Several recipients of DES have also been reported to develop HCC (SONTANIEMI et al. 1975; ROSINUS and MAUER 1981; DE PAGTER et al. 1979; BROOKS 1982). Nevertheless the issue remains controversial, with the carcinogenic role dismissed (BROSENS et al. 1986) or considered of little moment (IVERSON and THORESEN 1986).

Several cases of cholangiocarcinoma have been reported in users of OCs (PORTER et al. 1981; LITTLEWOOD et al. 1980; ELLIS 1978). Epidemiologic analysis, however, has provided no evidence for an etiologic role for the agents (FORMAN et al. 1986).

Angiosarcoma has been reported in several recipients of DES (HAM et al. 1980; HOCH-LIGATI 1978) and in a patient who had been taking OCs (MONROE et al. 1981). Also of interest is the report of five cases of epithelioid hemangioendothelioma involving young women taking OCs (DEAN et al. 1985) and of a mesenchymoma in a recipient of OCs (MACHIN and CROSBIE 1986).

VI. Vascular Lesions

1. Effect on Hemangiomas and Related Lesions

Large hepatic hemangiomas have been reported in several women who had been taking an OC (KOSITCHEK and CULLEN 1970; FREEDMAN 1982). The rarity of the association with OCs, however, suggests a preexisting hemangioma, perhaps provoked to a striking increase in size by the steroids. In support of this likelihood is the report of the apparent aggravation of familial hemorrhagic telangiectasia by oral contraceptives and of the apparent production or enhancement of "port-wine angiomas" (ZAFRANI et al. 1983).

2. Sinusoidal Dilatation

Sinusoidal dilatation is a characteristic lesion of OC use (POULSON and WINKLER 1973; MOLLEKEN 1979). The dilatation associated with OC use involves selectively zone 1 (or zone 1 and 2) of the hepatic acinus (Fig. 6). This sharply localized dilatation has been described only with OC use.

3. Peliosis Hepatis

Peliosis hepatis (Fig. 3), a lesion observed in some recipients of anabolic steroids (ZAFRANI et al. 1983; ISHAK and ZIMMERMAN 1987), has also been attributed, but less prominently, to contraceptive steroids (SCHONBERG 1982).

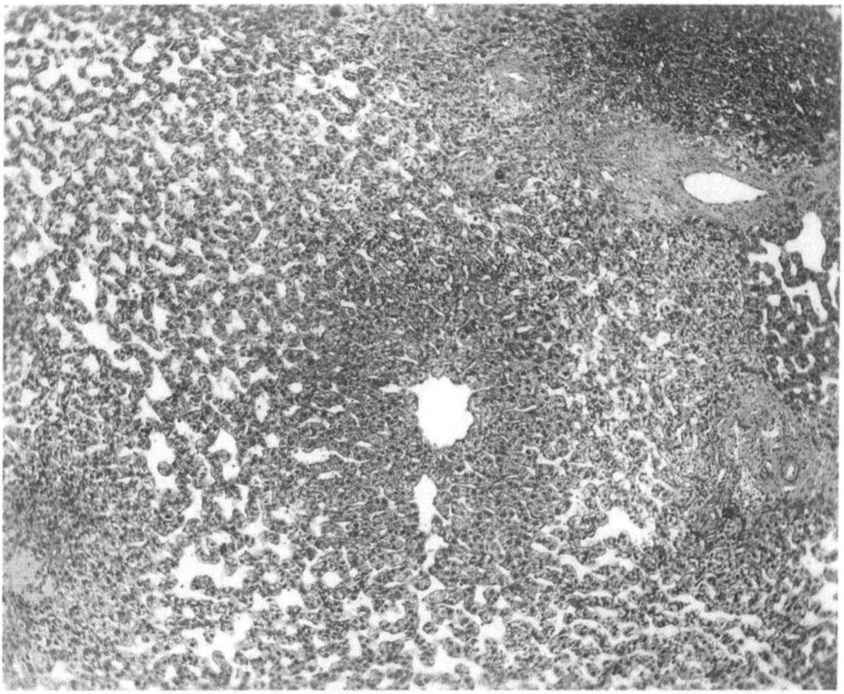

Fig. 6. Striking sinusoidal dilatation (more prominent mid-zonally) is present in the liver biopsy specimen from a patient who was on a long-term oral contraceptive preparation. Masson, ×55

When associated with adenomas the lesion may contribute to the hazard of the adenoma, since the peliotic lesion may itself rupture and lead to hemoperitoneum.

4. Hepatic Vein Thrombosis (Fig. 7)

The Budd-Chiari syndrome has been observed in at least 100 recipients of contraceptive steroids (Lewis et al. 1983; Valla et al. 1986). Indeed, in all but one of these instances the lesion has appeared to be hepatic vein thrombosis. The one exception was described as veno-occlusive disease (Alpert 1976). The hepatic vein thrombosis has been attributed to the thrombogenic effects of the estrogenic components of the OCs (Zafrani et al. 1983). The assumption that steroids have been responsible for the vascular lesion, however, has been doubted (Maddrey 1987; Reynolds 1987); and the association has been attributed to coincidence. However, Valla et al. (1986), in a multicenter case-control study, demonstrated that the risk of hepatic vein thrombosis in women using OCs was more than twice that of the control group.

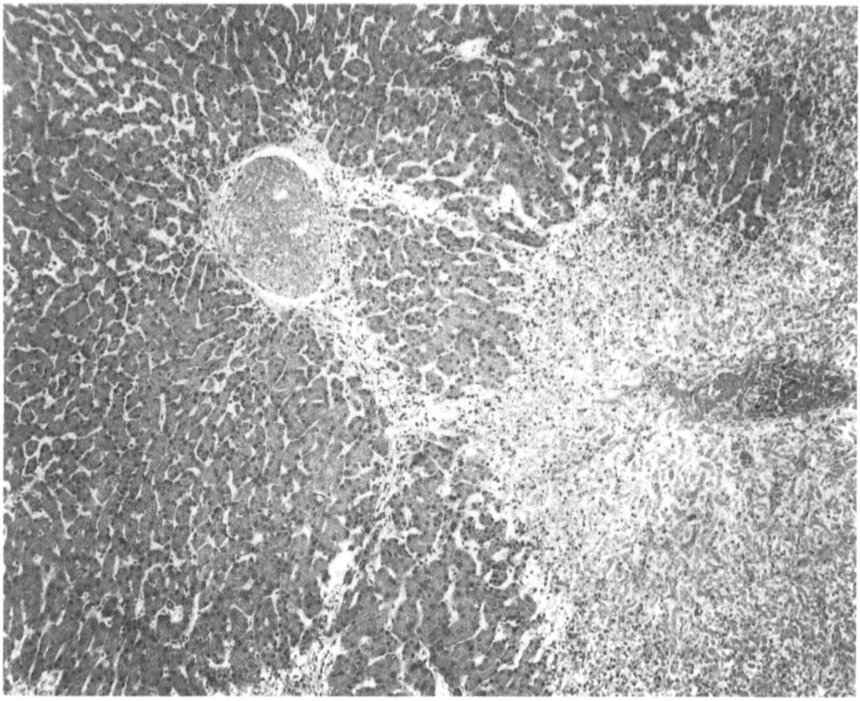

Fig. 7. Hepatic vein thrombosis in patient on long-term oral contraceptives. A terminal hepatic venule (*left*) contains an organized thrombus. Another vein (*right*) is centered in an area of necrosis involving zones 3 and 2, H&E, ×60

Indeed, the enhancement by OC use of the risk of hepatic vein thrombosis appears comparable to that of cerebrovascular accident, myocardial infarction, and venous thromboembolism (VALLA et al. 1986). VALLA et al. (1985) also demonstrated that many of the patients who develop hepatic vein thrombosis have an underlying myeloproliferative state. VALLA et al. (1985) deduced that the thrombosis reflects enhancement by estrogens of the thrombogenic effect of the myeloproliferative state.

Hepatic vein thrombosis is a rare complication of OC use, having been reported in all but a tiny fraction of the millions of women who have used OCs. Nevertheless, the lesion has importance as a frequently fatal entity. Among the causes of this rare syndrome, use of contraceptive steroids appears to be an important precipitant.

5. Rupture of the Liver

One of the modes of presentation f hepatic adenoma and carcinoma, rupture of the liver, has also been reported to occur during pregnancy (HIBBARD 1976; BIS and WAXMAN 1976). The rupture has usually been attributed to preeclampsia and the associated hemorrhages in zone 1. However, the vascular lesions seen in recipients of OCs, the observation that rupture of the liver has been reported in patients who had been taking OCs (FREDERICK et al. 1974; BOTTGER et al. 1981) and in a woman who developed peliosis and rupture after having taken DES for 3 years, suggests that hepatic rupture during pregnancy may be the result of hormonal vascular changes.

6. Other Vascular Changes

Other hepatic vascular abnormalities attributed to OCs include thrombosis of the portal vein and its branches (ZAFRANI et al. 1983), thrombosis of the hepatic artery and its branches (ZAFRANI et al. 1983), and hepatic infarction (JACOBS 1984; PETERSON and NEUMAN 1984). Thrombosis of the portal vein usually occurs in association with hepatic vein thrombosis (ZAFRANI et al. 1983).

VII. Disturbed Porphyrin Metabolism

Female sex hormones appear to play a role in provoking attacks of hepatic porphyria (SONG and KAPPAS 1975; BISSELL and SCHMIDT 1987). Features are a predominance of females among patients with acute intermittent porphyria (AIP), the almost exclusive development of the disease after the age of puberty, the apparent relationship of attacks to pregnancy or to the menstrual cycle, and the apparent clinical exacerbation or enhancement of biochemical abnormalities in patients taking contraceptive steroids.

The consequent hypothesis that endogenous steroids might lead to enhanced synthesis of porphyrins in susceptible individuals has found support in the ability of the derivatives of progesterone to induce the rate-limiting enzyme of porphyrin synthesis, δ-aminolevulinic acid synthetase (ALAS) (RIFKIND et al. 1970; EDWARDS and ELIOT 1975). A role in the porphyrin metabolism, however, is not restricted to steroids of the progesterone family. Patients with alcoholic porphyria cutanea tarda may develop exacerbations of the syndrome while receiving estrogen therapy for prostatic carcinoma (MONCKATON-CAPEMAN et al. 1966), and attacks of acute intermittent porphyria or of porphyria cutanea tarda can be provoked by contraceptive or other sex steroids (BISSELL and SCHMIDT 1987).

VIII. Mechanisms of Injury by Contraceptive Steroids

The pathogenesis of hepatic dysfunction and jaundice by the contraceptive steroids is presumably similar to that of the C-17-alkylated anabolic steroids. Just as the icterogenic anabolic agents all bear a C-17 alkyl group on C-17, so do the derivatives of female sex steroids that can cause jaundice to bear an ethinyl group in that position (Fig. 1). Indeed, the C-17 β-glucuronide is even more cholestasis producing than the ethanol-bearing steroids. The effects of these steroids appear to be mainly on the plasma membrane, especially the basolateral portions. However, injury to the canaliculus, its pericanalicular fibrils and its contracting power and to the tight junction may contribute to the cholestatic effects of the steroids.

The estrogenic component of OCs seems to play a greater role than the progestational one in leading to impaired hepatic function (METREAU et al. 1972). It is clearly more likely to be responsible for the Budd-Chiari syndrome. The component responsible for the peliosis is unclear.

The effects of OCs, and indeed of estrogens, may depend on attachment to specific estrogen receptors (PORTER et al. 1987). Indeed, receptors identified in rat liver appear to bind bilirubin and foreign dye (e.g., BSP), and part of the cholestatic effect imposed by ethinyl estradiol or anabolic steroids may be competition with bilirubin or the dye by blocking at the receptor (PORTER et al. 1987).

Estrogenic components of contraceptive preparations have seemed to be more incriminable than the progestational ones in the genesis of tumors. They can produce adenomas in experimental animals (GOLDFARB 1976) and enhance other tumorigenesis (KOHIGASHI et al. 1986). It seems likely the synthetic estrogens and the anabolic steroids are acting as promoters (PITOT 1985).

Clearly important in the pathogenesis of adenoma is the duration of intake of the OC and the dose of estrogen. Although the early observations led to the inference that the character of the estrogen was also relevant, mestranol being considered more tumorigenic than ehtinyl estradiol, subsequent observations have led to a dismissal of that view (FITZ 1984). The cholestatic effects also appear to depend on dose of steroid. Mestranol and ethinyl estradiol appear to be equivalently cholestasis producing. The use in recent years of OCs containing a lowered dose of the estrogenic component of the OCs has been accompanied apparently by fewer reported instances of cholestasis and of adenoma. The development of hepatic carcinoma is related to duration exposure to OCs (NEUBERGER et al. 1986).

IX. Cholelithiasis

Long-term users of OCs have appeared to have twice the expected prevalence of cholelithiasis, and among patients with gallstones the number of users of OCs has seemed significantly greater than among those without the stones (LEISSNER et al. 1977). The lithogenic effect is consistent with the observation that OCs lead to an increased cholesterol saturation of bile and to a decrease in the rate of bile acid synthesis, and concentration of bile acids in the bile and bile acid pool (BENNION et al. 1976). These effects seem attributable to the estrogen component of the OC. Estrogens alone apparently enhance gallstone formation in postmenopausal women. Nevertheless, the apparent enhancement of lithogenesis by OCs seems to be acceleration of the rate of formation of stones rather than an increase in ultimate incidence.

D. Drugs Related to Sex Hormones

I. Antiestrogens

There are three drugs that have seen use as antiestrogens, acting by attachment to estrogen receptors. In the process, they may have weak estrogenic activity.

1. Clomiphene

This ovulation-inducing agent has been implicated in two instances of tumorigenesis. One involved the hepatoblastoma in a 15-month-old infant whose mother had been treated with clomiphene before conception (MELAMED et al. 1982). The other involved a 25-year-old woman who was found to have an adenoma after 2 years of receiving the drug (CARRASCO et al. 1984). There is also vague reference to "hepatic function" abnormalities in patients receiving clomiphene (STRICKER 1992).

2. Cyclofenil

This antiestrogen has been implicated in an appreciable incidence of hepatic injury (OLSSON et al. 1983; ROSSI et al. 1992). Biochemical evidence has been noted in 35% (OLSSON et al. 1983) or more (GIBSON and GRAHAM 1983) of recipients; and overt hepatitis has been estimated to occur in about 1% of Swedish patients taking the drug (OLSSON et al. 1983). The injury appears to be hepatocellular or mixed, and in one patient the disease included granulomas.

3. Tamoxifen

This antiestrogen is used to treat estrogen-dependent breast carcinoma. It has also been implicated in a number of instances of hepatic injury. Cholestatic (AGRAWAL and ZELKOWITZ 1981) and mixed (BLACKBURN et al. 1984) jaundice, a "benign cyst" (NAND et al. 1982), and peliosis hepatis with rupture (LOOMUS et al. 1983) have been reported. In addition, an instance of hyperlipemia with giant, steatotic hepatomegaly that evolved during treatment with tamoxifen has been described (TANIYA et al. 1987); and cholestatic jaundice has been reported in a patient receiving both tamoxifen and medroxyprogesterone (RIIPA et al. 1984).

II. Antihypophysial Drugs

1. Danazol

This agent, described as an impeded androgen with anabolic effects, is used as an antigonadotropin and for other purposes. It is ethinylated in the C-17 position, as are the oral contraceptive steroids, and there is a five-membered (isoxazol) ring attached to the A ring. Both changes alter the metabolic effects of the steroid molecule strikingly. Danazol, however, shares C-17-alkylated steroid properties in the dose-related impairment of function (dye excretion), and it has led to apparent hepatic injury in man. Elevated aminotransferase levels have been recorded in 17% to over 50% of recipients (Ohsawa and Iwaskito 1986; Vincens et al. 1984), and instances of cholestatic (Boue et al. 1986; Silva et al. 1989) and hepatocellular (Najakima et al. 1986) jaundice have been reported. Also of note are the reports of hepatocellular carcinoma (Buamah 1985; Weill et al. 1988), of hepatocellular adenomas (Middleton et al. 1989; Fermand et al. 1990), and of peliosis involving the liver and spleen (Nesher et al. 1985) in women taking the drug.

2. Octreotide

This analogue of somatostatin can inhibit growth hormone secretion. Several reports have appeared of acute hepatocellular injury that developed during treatment with the drug and subsided after drug withdrawal (Arosio et al. 1988; Minocha and Dean 1991).

E. Glucocorticoids

Large doses can produce fatty changes in the liver of man and experimental animals, apparently mainly as the result of enhanced mobilization of lipids from the depots (Alpers and Isselbacher 1975). Even smaller doses (15–20mg prednisolone/day) can lead to varying degrees of hepatic steatosis.

Hepatic steatosis secondary to glucocorticoid administration is usually of little clinical moment. Occasionally, the fatty liver may have more important clinical implications. At least five instances of proved or suspected embolism of fat, from a glucocorticoid-induced fatty liver, to the vascular bed of the lungs, kidney, and other organs, have been described (Hill 1961; Jones et al. 1965).

Other adverse effects of glucocorticoids on the liver, observed in experimental animals, have not been described in man, Large doses have led to focal necrosis and steatosis in rabbits, rats, and mice (Tanyol and Rehfuss 1955; Antopol 1950).

F. Oral Hypoglycemic Agents

I. Sulfonylureas

Carbutamide and metahexamide produced serious, at times fatal, hepatic injury with sufficient frequency (0.5%–1.5%) to lead to their removal from clinical use in this country (CREUTZFELDT 1975). Chlorpropamide was also associated with an apparently high incidence of overt liver damage, in the early years of its use. However, the mainly cholestatic injury of chlorpropamide (SCHNEIDER et al. 1984) carries less of a threat than the mainly cytotoxic injury that was produced by metahexamide (MACH et al. 1959) and carbutamide (KIRTLEY 1957). Furthermore, employment of lower doses of chlorpropamide since the 1970s appears to have resulted in a reduced incidence of liver damage.

Other sulfonylurea derivatives have been described to have a lower incidence. Acetohexamide had been implicated by 1968, in 21 cases of hepatic injury, of which only 7 are clearly attributable to the drug (ZIMMERMAN 1978). Both hepatocellular (GOLDSTEIN and ROTHENBERG 1966) and cholestatic (RANK and OLSON 1989) jaundice have been recorded. An extremely low incidence of overt liver damage has been associated with administration of tolbutamide (STRICKER 1992), with only a half-dozen instances of jaundice, all cholestatic, having been reported.

Tolazemide has been implicated in at least four instances of cholestatic jaundice (ZIMMERMAN and MADDREY 1993). One was chronic, resembling primary biliary cirrhosis (VAN THIEL et al. 1974), reminiscent of the PBC-like syndrome attributed to tolbutamide (GREGORY et al. 1967). Azapinamide was reported to lead to an instance of cholestatic jaundice (WEINSTEIN et al. 1963).

Glibenclamide (gliburide, Micronase) has led to several instances of cholestatic jaundice accompanied by generalized hypersensitivity (CLARKE et al. 1974); one was fatal (WONGPACTOON et al. 1981). Three instances of hepatocellular injury have also been reported (GOODMAN et al. 1987), and injury accompanied by hepatic granulomas has been described (INGELMO et al. 1980).

The mechanism for injury is unclear. Rash, fever, and eosinophilia, and onset of illness during the first several weeks of taking the respective drug, in some patients with sulfonylurea-induced jaundice, suggest that in these cases hypersensitivity may be responsible for the hepatic injury. In other patients, however, these collateral features of hypersensitivity are not seen.

II. Clinical Syndrome

Onset of hepatic injury is usually during the 1st month of taking the implicated sulfonylurea, although liver damage may not appear until after many months of therapy. Rash and fever are discribed in some patients prior to or concomitant with the appearance of jaundice. These systemic features, however, may occur in patients who are without liver damage, and liver damage may develop in patients who are without rash or fever. Gastrointestinal complaints may also accompany overt hepatic injury.

The clinical manifestations of hepatic disease vary with the sulfonylurea. Elements of both cytotoxic and cholestatic injury are combined in the jaundice

Table 2. Adverse hepatic effects of sul fonylurea hypoglycemic agents

Drug		Hepatic injury
Acetohexamide	(Dimelor)	Rare hepatocellular, very rare cholestatic
Azepinamide		Very rare hepatocellular
Carbutamide	(BZ-55)	Hepatocellular with cholestatic features, incidence 0.5%–1.5%, use abandoned
Chlorpropamide	(Diabinese)	Cholestatic, granulomas seen
Glibuthiazole	(Glypasol)	Incidence of jaundice (hepatocellular) was 20%, use abandoned
Glymidine	(Gonadafon)	Elevated aminotransferase levels, 16% incidence in one study
Glipizide	(Glucotrol)	Elevated aminotransferase levels, very rare cholestatic injury
Glisoxepide	(Prodioban)	Elevated aminotransferase levels, very rare jaundice
Glyburide	(Glibenclamide, Micronase)	Hepatocellular and cholestatic jaundice reported, also granulomas
Glyparamide	(P-1306)	Hepatic injury very rare
Metahexamide	(Euglycin)	Hepatocellular incidence 0.5%–1.0%, abandoned because of toxicity
Tolazamide	(Tolinase)	Rare cholestatic, also chronic cholestasis resembling primary biliary cirrhosis
Tolbutamide	(Orinase)	Rare cholestatic, chronic cholestasis resembling primary biliary cirrhosis

produced by these agents (Table 2). The injury that resulted from carbutamide and metahexamide was predominantly cytotoxic. Levels of the aminotransferases were high, the liver showed necrosis, the clinical pattern resembled viral hepatitis, and there were deaths in hepatic failure. The high alkaline phosphatase levels and prominent cholestasis on biopsy that accompany the overt cytotoxic injury, however, warrant designation of the injury as mixed-hepatocellular. The jaundice provoked by chlorpropamide, on the other hand, appears to have been mainly cholestatic, although it may be accompanied by some evidence of parenchymal injury. Accordingly, it may be categorized as hepatocanalicular jaundice (ZIMMERMAN 1978).

III. Prognosis

As is to be expected of hepatocellular injury, the liver damage induced by carbutamide and metahexamide has led to some fatalities. While no fatal hepatic necrosis has been recorded among patients with acetohexamide-induced liver damage, one patient was described as developing macronodular cirrhosis (GOLDSTEIN and ROTHENBERG 1966). Also, at least one instnce of a fatal biliary cirrhosis-like syndrome that developed while the patient was taking tolbutamide has been described (GREGORY et al. 1967), and an instance of chronic cholestasis has been ascribed to tolazemide (NAKAO et al. 1985).

Recovery has appeared to be complete in most patients who sustained cholestatic jaundice while taking chlorpropamide.

The presence of granulomas in the livers of patients taking sulfonylurea (BLOODWORTH 1963) seems to be quite independent of other histologic, clinical, or biochemical features of hepatic injury, since the granulomas have been found in patients without hepatic injury. There has been little emphasis on sulfonylurea-related granulomas, however, since the report of BLOODWORTH (1963), other than the occasional case of jaundice accompanied by granulomatous inflammation.

IV. Biguanide

We are aware of only two reports (SMETANA 1963; NAMAHISA et al. 1975) of jaundice attributed to a biguanide. The interference by the biguanides with hepatic metabolism that leads to lactic acidosis appears to have no other adverse effect on the liver.

V. Other Oral Hypoglycemic Agents

The hypoglycins are natural hepatotoxins found in the seed and meat of the unripe fruit of the tree *Blighia sapida* (TANAKA et al. 1976). Best known as the cause of "Jamaican vomiting sickness," the unripe fruit (called "akee" in Jamaica), which contains hypoglycins, leads to acute vomiting, convulsions, and death. Convulsions are the result of profound hypoglycemia, which presumably is also responsible for the fatal outcome. The liver in these patients shows microvesicular steatosis similar to that of Reyes syndrome.

G. Antithyroid Drugs (Table 3)

Derivatives of thiourea were among the early drugs recognized to cause hepatic injury as the result of an idiosyncratic reaction. Nevertheless, the number of instances reported in the intervening 4 decades is relatively small (ZIMMERMAN and MADDREY 1993). Jaundice has been a complication of

Table 3. Adverse hepatic effects of antithyroid compounds[a]

Drug	Hepatic injury
Carbimazole	Cholestatic
Methimazole	Cholestatic, often prolonged
Methylthiouracil	Cholestatic
Propylthiouracil	Hepatocellular, rarely cholestatic, chronic active hepatitis reported
Thiouracil	Cholestatic

[a] All are derivatives of thiouracil.

treatment with thiouracil, propylthiouracil, methimazole, carbimazole, and methylthiouracil (ZIMMERMAN 1978). The mechanism of overt hepatic injury with each of these agents is very low, although the incidence of elevated aminotransferase levels approaches 30% in recipients of propylthiouracil.

I. Form of Injury

Jaundice produced by the members of this group, with the exception of propylthiouracil, has been mainly cholestatic (Table 3). In all but one of the 16 described cases of methimazole-induced injury, transaminase levels have been only modestly increased (<eight fold normal), alkaline phosphatase values have been appreciably elevated, and liver biopsies have shown mainly cholestasis. The one instance of fulminant failure involved a hepatitis B carrier in whom the acute injury was attributed to methimazole (KANG et al. 1990). Carbimazole and methylthiouracil-induced jaundice has also been cholestatic. Also all but one of the instances of hepatic injury caused by thiouracil appeared to be cholestatic (ZIMMERMAN 1963).

Propylthiouracil-induced hepatic injury has been hepatocellular in almost all of the reported cases (ZIMMERMAN and MADDREY 1993). While most cases have been acute, hepatocellular injury showing histologic and biochemical features consistent with the chronic active hepatitis has also been reported, and several cases have showed "bridging necrosis" (FEDOTIN and LEFER 1975; MAGGIOR et al. 1989).

II. Clinical Features

Onset of the syndrome may be abrupt or gradual, and in most of the reported cases may be as early as 2–4 weeks after starting the respective drug; or as long as 2 and even 3 months (ZIMMERMAN 1978). Rash, fever, lymphadenopathy, and agranulocytosis in various combinations have preceded or accompanied the jaundice in only some of the patients. All ages are apparently susceptible, and an instance of cholestatic jaundice has even been recorded in a neonatal infant whose mother had been taking propylthiouracil (HAYASHIDA et al. 1991).

III. Prognosis

Subsidence of the cholestatic jaundice associated with methimazole has been extraordinarily slow. In about half of the reported cases, 3–5 months elapsed before the evidence of hepatic injury disappeared. There have been no deaths clearly ascribable to the hepatic injury induced by thiouracil or carbimazole, and only two attributed to methimazole (KOBAYASHI et al. 1981; KANG et al. 1990). Fatal cases of propylthiouracil-induced jaundice have been due to agranulocytosis or to hepatic necrosis (ZIMMERMAN 1978).

IV. Mechanism

The mechanism for injury appears to be at least in part a hypersensitivity reaction to the respective agent. The fairly brief latent period of exposure to the respective drug prior to the development of jaundice in some cases, and the fever and rash that herald the hepatic injury in others, have led to the interpretation of the reaction as being due to hypersensitivity. Demonstration of transformation of lymphocytes from patients with PTU-related jaundice, on exposure in vitro to the respective drug, is consistent with this view (Fedotin and Lefer 1975). However, in many of the reported cases onset of injury is not early, not accompanied by hallmarks of hypersensitivity; and only a minority of cases have shown a positive response to the lymphocyte test in vitro. The role of metabolic idiosyncrasy remains plausible (Stricker 1992).

That intrinsic toxicity of these agents may also play a role is suggested by the high incidence of minor hepatic injury in recipients of PTU. Liaw et al. (1993) have reported that almost 30% of a group of patients receiving PTU developed abnormal aminotransferase levels. Presumably, immunologic idiosyncrasy converts the mild injury to severe hepatocellular disease.

V. Comment

The hepatologic hazard of antithyroid drugs seems to be relatively minor. The low incidence and the benign cholestatic nature of methimazole and carbimazole jaundice indicate the problem to be of little moment and secondary in importance to the generalized hypersensitivity reactions and the hematologic injury. While the incidence of PTU injury is also low, the hepatic injury when it strikes is serious.

References

Adlercreutz H, Tenhunen R (1970) Some aspects of the interaction between natural and synthetic female sex hormones and the liver. Am J Med 49:630

Agrawal BL, Zelkowitz L (1981) Bone "flare", hypercalcemia and jaundice after tamoxifen therapy. Arch Intern Med 141:1240

Alpers DH, Isselbacher KJ (1975) Fatty liver: biochemical and clinical aspects. In: Schiff L (ed) Diseases of the liver, 4th edn. Lippincott, Philadelphia, pp 815–832

Alpert LI (1976) Veno-occlusive disease of the liver associated with oral contraceptives: case report and review of the literature. Hum Pathol 7:709

Ameriks JA, Thompson NW, Frey CF, Appelman HD, Walter JF (1975) Hepatic cell adenomas, spontaneous liver rupture, and oral contraceptives. Arch Surg 110:548

Amtrup F, Slottved J, Svanholm H (1980) Liver cell carcinoma in young women possibly induced by oral contraceptives. Acta Obstet Gynecol Scand 59:567

Anthony AP (1975) Hepatoma associated with androgenic steroids. Lancet I:685

Antopol W (1950) Anatomic changes in mice treated with excessive doses of cortisone. Proc Soc Exp Biol Med 73:262

Arias IM (1963) Effects of a plant acid (icterogenin) and certain anabolic steroids on the hepatic metabolism of bilirubin and sulfobromophthalein (BSP). Ann NY Acad Sci 104:1014

Arosio M, Bazzoni N, Ambrosi B, Faglia G (1988) Acute hepatitis after treatment of acromegaly with octreotide. Lancet II:1498

Bannister P, Sheridan P, Losowsky MS (1985) Identification and characterization of the human hepatic androgen receptor. Clin Endocrinol (Oxf) 23:495
Bennion LJ, Ginsberg RL, Garnick MH, Bennett PH (1976) Effects of oral contraceptives on the gallbladder bile of normal women. N Engl J Med 244:189
Bis KA, Waxman N (1976) Rupture of the liver associated with pregnancy: a review of the literature and report of two cases. Surg Gynecol Obstet 31:763
Bissell DM, Schmidt R (1987) Hepatic porphyrias. In: Schiff L, Schiff ER (eds) Diseases of the liver, 6th edn. Lippincott, Philadelphia
Blackburn AM, Amiel SA, Millis RR et al. (1984) Tamoxifen and liver damage. Br Med J 289:288
Bloodworth JMB Jr (1963) Morphologic changes associated with sulfonylurea therapy. Metabolism 12:287
Bottger G, Schiebold KO, Ulmann B, Rockel A (1981) Liver rupture after several years of hormone contraception. Z Gesamte Inn Med 36:226
Boue F, Caffin B, Oelfraisay J-F (1986) Danazol and cholestatic hepatitis (letter). Ann Intern Med 105:139
Boyer JL (1978) Androgenic-anabolic steroid associated peliosis hepatis in man – a review of 38 reported cases. Adv Pharmacol Ther 8:175
Brooks JJ (1982) Hepatoma associated with diethylstilbestrol therapy for prostatic carcinoma. J Urol 128:1044
Brosens I, Johannisson E, Baulieu E-E et al. (1986) Oral contraceptives and hepatocellular carcinoma. Br Med J 292:1667
Buamah PK (1985) An apparent danazol-induced primary hepatocellular carcinoma. J Surg Oncol 28:114
Burger RA, Marcuse PM (1952) Peliosis hepatis. Report of a case. Am J Clin Pathol 22:569
Carrasco D, Barrachina M, Prieto M, Berenguer J (1984) Clomiphene citrate and liver-cell adenoma. N Engl J Med 310:1120
Carrasco D, Prieto M, Pallardo L et al. (1985) Multiple hepatic adenomas after long-term therapy with testosterone enanetrate. J Hepatol 1:573
Christensen SE, Andersen VR, Vilstrup H (1981) A case of hepatoma in pregnancy associated with earlier oral contraception. A case report. Acta Obstet Gynecol Scand 60:519
Christopherson WM, Mays ET (1979) Relation of steroids to liver oncogenesis. J Toxicol Environ Health 5:207
Clarke BF, Campbell IW, Ewing DJ et al. (1974) Generalized hypersensitivity reaction and visceral arteritis with fatal outcome during glibenclamide therapy. Diabetes 23:739
Coe JE, Ishak KG, Ross MJ (1983) Diethylstilbestrol-induced jaundice in the Chinese and Armenian Hamster. Hepatology 3:489
Creuzfeldt W (1975) Oral antibiabetika. In: Gerok W, Sickinger K (eds) Drugs and the liver Schattauer, Stuttgart, pp 366–373
Dahl P, Schmid E (1969) Arzneimittelikterus durch Ostrogene beim Mann. Z Gastroenterol 7:183
Dalen E, Westerholm B (1974) Occurrence of hepatic impairment in women jaundiced by oral contraceptives and their mothers and sisters. Acta Med Scand 195:459
Dean PJ, Haggitt RC, O'Hara CJ (1985) Malignant epithelioid hemangioepithelioma of the liver in young women. Relationship to oral contraceptive use. Am J Surg Pathol 9:695
De Pagter AG, van Berge Henegouwen GP, Brandt KH, Bronkhorst FB (1979) Orale anticonceptiva en de lever. Ned Tydochr Geneeskd 123:881
Despopoulus AA (1971) Hepatic and renal excretory metabolism of bile salts: a backgroud for understanding steroid-induced cholestasis. J Pharmacol Exp Ther 176:273
Edmondson HA, Henderson B, Benton B (1976) Liver-cell adenomas associated with use of oral contraceptives. N Engl J Med 294:470

Edmondson HA, Reynolds TB, Henderson B, Benten B (1977) Regression of liver cell adenomas associated with oral contraceptives. Ann Intern Med 86:180

Edwards AM, Eliott WH (1975) Induction of δ-aminolevulinic acid synthetase in isolated rat liver cells by steroids. J Biol Chem 250:2750

Eisalo A, Jarvinen PA, Luukkainen T (1964) Hepatic impairment during the intake of contraceptive pills. Clinical trial with postmenopaual women. Br Med J 2:426

Elias E, Igbal S, Knutton S et al. (1983) Increased tight junction permeability: a possible mechanism of estrogen cholestasis. Eur J Clin Invest 13:383

Elias E, Igbal S, Knutton S et al. (1983) Increased tight junction permeability: a possible mechanism of estrogen cholestasis. Eur J Clin Invest 13:383

Elias H, Schwinner D (1945) The hepatotoxic action of diethylstilbesterol with report of a case. Am J Med Sci 209:602

Ellis EF (1978) Oral contraceptives: cholangiocarcinoma-death. Clin Alert 54

Falk H, Thomas LB, Popper H (1979) Hepatic angiosarcoma associated with androgenic-anabolic steroids. Lancet II:1120

Fedotin MS, Lefer LG (1975) Liver disease caused by propylthiouracil. Arch Intern Med 135:319

Fermand JP, Levy Y, Bauscary D et al. (1990) Danazol-induced hepatocellular adenoma. Am J Med 88:5291

Fitz JG (1984) Oral contraceptives and benign tumors of the liver. West J Med 140: 260

Forman D, Vincent TJ, Doll R (1986) Cancer of the liver and the use of oral contraceptives. Br Med J 292:1357

Foss GL, Simpson SL (1959) Oral methyltestosterone and jaundice. Br Med J 1:259

Frederick WC, Howard RG, Spatola S (1974) Spontaneous rupture of the liver in patients using contraceptive pills. Arch Surg 108:93

Freedman AN (1982) Liver lesions and oral contraceptives. Can Med Assoc J 126: 1149

Gallagher TF Jr, Mueller MN, Kappas A (1966) Estrogen pharmacology. IV. Studies on the structural basis for estrogen-induced impairment of liver function. Medicine 45:471

Garrigues-Gil V, Berenguer-Lapuerta JB, Ponce-Garcia J et al. (1986) A non-C17 alkylated steroid and long-term cholestasis. Ann Intern Med 104:135

Gibson T, Graham R (1983) Cyclofenil treatments of scleroderma. A controlled study. Br J Rheum 22:218

Gilbert EF, DaSilvia A-Q, Queen DM (1963) Intrahepatic cholestasis with fatal termination following norethandrolone therapy. JAMA 185:538

Glober GA, Wilkerson JA (1968) Biliary cirrhosis following the administration of methyltestosterone. JAMA 204:170

Goldfarb S (1976) Sex hormones and hepatic neoplasia. Cancer Res 36:2584

Goldstein MJ, Rothenberg AJ (1966) Jaundice in a patient receiving acetohexamide. N Engl J Med 275:97

Goodman R, Dean PJ, Radparvar A et al. (1987) Glyburide-induced hepatitis. Ann Intern Med 106:837

Gregory DH, Zaki GF, Sarosi GA, Carey JB Jr (1967) Chronic cholestasis following prolonged tolbutamide administration. Arch Pathol 84:194

Haemmarli UP, Wyss HI (1967) Recurrent intrahepatic cholestasis of pregnancy. Medicine 46:299

Ham JM, Fracs F, Pirola RC et al. (1980) Hemangioendothelial sarcoma of the liver associated with long-term estrogen therapy in a man. Dig Dis Sci 25: 879

Hartley RA, Boitnott JK, Ibeer FL (1969) Topics in clinical medicine: the liver and oral contraceptives. Johns Hopkins Med J 124:112

Hayashida CY, Duarte AJ, Sato AE, Yomoslura-Kaesboro EH (1991) Neonatal hepatitis and lymphocyte sensitization by placental transfer of propylthiouracil. J Endocrinol Invest 13:937

Heaney RP, Whedon GD (1958) Impairment of hepatic bromosulphalein clearance by two 17-substituted testosterones. J Lab Clin Med 52:169
Helling TS, Wood WG (1982) Oral contraceptives and cancer of the liver: a review with two additional cases. Am J Med 77:504
Henderson BE, Preston-Martin S, Edmondson HA et al. (1983) Hepatocellular carcinoma and oral contraceptives. Br J Cancer 44:437
Hibbard LT (1976) Spontaneous rupture of the liver in pregnancy: a report of eight cases. Am J Obstet Gynecol 126:334
Hill RB Jr (1961) Fatal fat embolism from steroid-induced fatty liver. N Engl J Med 165:318
Hoch-Ligeti C (1978) Angiosarcoma of the liver associated with diethylstilbestrol. JAMA 240:1510
Ingelmo M, Vivanias J, Brugero M et al. (1980) Angitis por hypersensibiladad hepatitis granulomatosa indicuda a por glibenclamide: a propositon de un casro. Med Clin 75:306
Ishak KG (1979) Hepatic neoplasms associated with contraceptive and anabolic steroids. In: Rentchnick P, Horfarth C, Senn HJ (eds) Recent results in cancer research, vol 66. Springer, Berlin Heidelberg New York, p 73
Ishak KG (1988) Benign tumors and pseudotumors of the liver. Appl Pathol 6:82
Ishak KG, Rabin L (1975) Benign tumors of the liver. Med Clin North Am 59: 995
Ishak KG, Zimmerman HJ (1987) Hepatotoxic effects of the anabolic/androgenic steroids. Semin Liver Dis 7:230
Iverson D-E, Thoresen SO (1986) Oral contraceptives and hepatocellular carcinoma. Br Med J 292:1668
Jacobs MB (1984) Hepatic infarction related to oral contraceptive use. Arch Intern Med 144:642
Jones JP, Engleman EP, Najarian JS (1965) Systemic fat embolism after renal homotransplantation and treatment with corticosteroids. N Engl J Med 273: 1453
Kang H, Cho JD, Jung IG et al. (1990) A case of methimazole-induced acute hepatic failure in a patient with chronic hepatitis B carrier. Korean J Intern Med 5:69
Kappas S, Granick S (1968) Experimental hepatic porphyria: studies with steroids of physiological origin in man. Ann NY Acad Sci 151:842
Karasawa T, Shikata T, Smith RD (1979) Peliosis hepatis. Report of nine cases. Acta Pathol Jpn 29:457
Keeffe EB, Blankenship NM, Scharschmidt BF (1980) Alteration of rat liver plasma membrane fluidity and ATPase activity by chlorpromazine hydrochloride and its metabolites. Gastroenterology 79:222
Keifer WS, Scott JC (1977) Liver neoplasms and the oral contraceptives. J Obstet Gynecol 128:448
Kerlin P, Davis GL, McGill DB et al. (1983) Hepatic adenoma and focal nodular hyperplasia: clinical, pathologic, and radiologic features. Gastroenterology 84:994
Kirtley WR (1957) Occurrence of sensitivity and side reactions following carbutamide. Diabetes 6:72
Klaassen CD, Watkins JB (1984) Mechanisms of bile formation, hepatic uptake and biliary excretion. Pharmacol Rev 36:1
Klatskin G (1977) Hepatic tumors. Possible relationship to use of oral contraceptives. Gastroenterology 73:386
Kobayashi M, Higashiyama S, Nagakiri S et al. (1981) A case of drug-induced liver injury with positive LE phenomenon caused by meraczole. Acta Hematol Jpn 22:1453
Kohigashi K, Fukuda Y, Imura H, Nakano H (1986) Promotive effect of estrogen on hepatocarcinogenesis and estrogen receptor in male rats. Acta Hepatol Jpn 27:220
Konturri M, Sotaniemi E, Ahlgvist J (1972) Liver damage and estrogen therapy of prostatic cancer. Scand J Urol Nephrol 6:289

Kory RC, Bradley MH, Watson RN et al. (1959) Six month evaluation of anabolic drug, norethandrolone in underweight persons. II. Bromsulfalein (BSP) retention and liver function. Am J Med 26:243
Kositchek RJ, Cullen RA (1970) Hemangiomatosis of the liver with thrombosis following use of an oral contraceptive. Calif Med 113:70
Koszalka MF (1957) Medical obstructive jaundice: report of a death due to methylestosterone. Lancet 77:51
Kreek MJ (1987) Female sex steroids and cholestasis. Semin Liver Dis 7:8
Langlands AD, Martin WM (1975) Jaundice associated with norethisterone-acetate treatment of breast cancer. Lancet I:584
Leevy CM, Cherrick GR, Davidson CS (1961) Observations of norethandrolone-induced abnormalities in plasma decay of sulfobromophthalein and indocyanine green. J Lab Clin Med 57:918
Leissner KH, Wedel H, Scherstein T (1977) Comparison between the use of oral contraceptives and the incidence of surgically confirmed gallstone disease. Scand J Gastroenterol 12:893
Lewis JH, Tice HL, Zimmerman HJ (1983) Budd-Chiari syndrome associated with oral contraceptive steroids. Review of treatment of 47 cases. Dig Dis Sci 28:673
Liaw YF, Huang MJ, Fan KD et al. (1993) Hepatic injury during propylthiouracil therapy in patients with hyperthyroidism. A cohort study. Ann Intern Med 118:424
Lieberman DA, Keeffe EB, Stenzel P (1984) Severe and prolonged oral contraceptive jaundice. J Clin Gastroenterol 6:145
Lipstate LK, Stromeyer FW, Welsh RA (1981) Benign hepatocellular tumors: a regional survey. South Med J 74:397
Littlewood ER, Barrison IG, Murray-Lyon IM, Paradinas FJ (1980) Cholangiocarcinoma and oral contraceptives. Lancet II:310
Loomus GN, Ameja P, Bota RA (1983) A case of peliosis hepatis in association with tamoxifen therapy. Am J Clin Pathol 80:881
Lowdell CP, Murray-Lyon IM (1985) Reversal of liver damage due to long term methyltestosterone and safety of non-17 α-alkylated androgens. Br Med J 291:637
Mach B, Field RA, Taft E (1959) Metahexamide jaundice. Report of a case. N Engl J Med 261:438
Machin DG, Crosbie RB (1986) Hepatic mesenchymoma in an adult. Br Med J 292:450
Maddrey WC (1987) Hepatic vein thrombosis (Budd-Chiari syndrome): possible association with the use of oral contraceptives. Semin Liver Dis 7:32
Maggiori G, Larizza D, Lorini R et al. (1989) Propylthiouracil hepatotoxicity mimicking autoimmune chronic active hepatitis in a girl (letter). J Pediatr Gastroenterol Nutr 8:547
Martinez-Manautou J, Aznar-Ramos R, Bautista-O'Farril J, Gonzales-Angulo A (1970) The ultrastructure of liver cells in women under steroid therapy. II. Contraceptive therapy. Acta Endocrinol (Copenh) 65:207
McGaughan GW, Bilous MJ, Gallagher ND (1985) Long-term survival with tumor regression in androgen-induced liver tumors. Cancer 56:2622
Meijers WH, Willemse PHB, Sleijfer D, Mulder NH, Grond J (1986) Hepatocellular damage by cyproterone acetate. Eur J Cancer Clin Oncol 22:1121
Melamed I, Bujanover Y, Hammer J, Spirer Z (1982) Hepatoblastoma in an infant born to a mother after hormonal treatment for sterility. N Engl J Med 307:820
Metreau JM, Dhumeaux D, Berthelot P (1972) Oral contraceptives and the liver. Digestion 7:318
Mettlin C, Nachimuthu N (1981) Studies on the role of oral contraceptive use in the etiology of benign and malignant liver tumors. J Surg Oncol 18:73
Middleton C, McCaughan GW, Painter DM et al. (1989) Danazol and hepatic neoplasia. A case report. Aust NZ J Med 19:733
Minocha A, Dean HA Jr (1991) Octreotide-induced acute hepatic toxicity (letter). Am J Gastroenterol 86:515

Molleken K (1979) Leberbiosiebefunde nach Einnahme oraler Kontrazeptiva. Zentralbl Allg Pathol Anat 123:195
Monckaton-Capeman PW, Cripps J, Summerly R (1966) Cutaneous hepatic porphyria and oestrogens. Br Med J 1:461
Monroe PS, Riddell RH, Siegler M et al. (1981) Hepatic angiosarcoma: possible relationship to long-term oral contraceptive ingestion. JAMA 246:64
Mosonyi L (1956) Multiple benign hepatomas and virilisation by ovarian tumor. Lancet II:23
Mueller MN, Kappas A (1964) Estrogen pharmacology. I. The influence of estradiol and estriol on hepatic disposal of sulfobromophthalein. J Clin Invest 43:1905
Nadell J, Kosek J (1977) Peliosis hepatis: twelve cases associated with oral androgen therapy. Arch Pathol Lab Med 101:405
Nagasue N, Ito A, Yukaya H, Ogaw Y (1985) Androgen receptors in hepatocellular carcinoma and surrounding parenchyma. Gastroenterology 89:643
Nakajima T, Mizushima N, Matsuda M et al. (1986) Fulminant hepatic failure associated with aplastic anemia after treatment with danazol. Br J Obstet Gynacol 93:1013
Nakao NL, Gelb AM, Stenger R, Sitgel JH (1985) A case of chronic liver disease due to tolazamide. Gastroenterology 89:192
Namahisa T, Yamagudi K, Kitami N (1975) Der Lymphozyten Transformationstest bei allergischen Arzeneimittelshaden de Leber. Leber Magen Darm 5:73
Nand S, Gordon LI, Brestan E et al. (1982) Benign hepatic cyst in a patient on antiestrogen therapy for metastatic breast cancer. Cancer 50:1882
Nesher G, Dolberg L, Zimran A, Hershko A (1985) Hepatosplenic peliosis after danazol and glucocorticoids for ITP. Lancet I:242
Neuberger J, Forman D, Doll R, Williams R (1986) Oral contraceptives and hepatocellular carcinoma. Br Med J 292:1355
Nordsten M (1985) Hemangiosarcoma hepatis asocieret med brug of androgene steroider. Ugeskr Laeger 147:2615
O'Sullivan JP, Rosswick RP (1976) Oral contraceptives and malignant hepatic tumors. Lancet I:1124
Ohsawa T, Iwaskito S (1986) Hepatitis associated with danazol (letter). Drug Intell Clin Pharmacol 20:889
Olsson R, Tyllstrom J, Zettergren L (1983) Hepatic reactions to cyclofenil. Gut 24:260
Orellana-Alcade JM, Deminquez JP (1966) Jaundice and oral contraceptive drugs. Lancet II:1278
Orlandi F, Jezequel AM (1966) Pathogenesis of the cholestasis induced by C-17 alkylated steroids: ultrastructural and functional changes of the liver cells during treatment. Rev Int Hepat 16:331
Paumgartner G, Reichen J, Von Bergmann K, Preisig R (1976) Elaboration of hepatocytic bile. Bull NY Acad Med 51:455
Pecking A, Lelloy JM, Najean Y (1980) Hepato-toxicite des androgenes au cour du traitment des aplasies medullaires. Nouv Rev Fr Hematol 22:257
Pelletier G, Frija J, Szekely A-M et al. (1984) L'adenome du foie chez l'homme. Gastroenterol Clin Biol 8:269
Perez V, Gorodisch S, DeMartire J et al. (1969) Oral contraceptives: long-term use produces fine structural changes in liver mitochondria. Science 165:805
Perez-Mera RA, Shields CE (1962) Jaundice associated with norethindrone acetate therapy. N Engl J Med 267:1137
Peterson IM, Neumann CH (1984) Focal hepatic infarction with bile lake formation. Am J Roentgenol 142:1155
Phillips M, Oda M, Funatsu K (1978) Evidence for microfilament involvement in norethandrolone-induced intrahepatic cholestasis. Am J Pathol 93:729
Phillips MJ, Poucell S, Oda M (1986) Biology of disease: mechanisms of cholestasis. Lab Invest 54:593

Pitot HC (1988) Hepatic neoplasia: chemical induction. In: Arias IM, Jacoby WB, Popper H, Schachter D, Schafritz DA (eds) The liver. Biology and pathobiology. Raven, New York, pp 1125–1146 (letter) (JAMA 253:1457, 1985)
Plaa GL, Priestly BG (1977) Intrahepatic cholestasis induced by drugs and chemicals. Pharmacol Rev 28:207
Porter JB, Jick H, Ylvisaker JT (1981) Malignant liver tumor associated with oral contraceptive use. Pharmacotherapy 1:160
Porter LE, van Thiel DH, Eagon PK (1987) Estrogens and progestins as tumor inducers. Semin Liver Dis 7:24
Poulsen H, Winkler K (1973) Liver disease with periportal sinusoidal dilatation. Digestion 8:441
Rank JM, Olson RC (1989) Reversible cholestatic jaundice caused by acetohexamide. Gastroenterology 96:1607
Reichen J, Simon FRL (1984) Mechanisms of cholestasis. Int Rev Exp Pathol 26: 231
Reyes H (1982) The enigma of intrahepatic jaundice of pregnancy. Lessons from Chile. Hepatology 2:86
Reyes H, Ritalta J, Gonzales-Ceron M (1976) Intrahepatic jaundice of pregnancy in a large kindred. Gut 17:709
Reynolds TB (1987) Budd-Chiari syndromes. In: Schiff L, Schiff ER (eds) Diseases of the liver, 6th edn. Lippincott, Philadelphia, pp 1466–1472
Rifkind AB, Gilette PN, Song CS, Kappas A (1970) Induction of hepatic δ-aminolevulinic acid synthetase by oral contraceptive steroids. J Clin Endocrin Metab 30:330
Riipa P, Kauppil A, Sundstrom H et al. (1984) Hepatic impairment during simultaneous administration of medroxyprogesterone acetate and tamoxifen in the treatment of endometrial and ovarian carcinoma. Anticancer Res 4:109
Roman P, Hecker R (1968) The liver toxicity of oral contraceptives, a critical review of the literature. Med J Aust 2:682
Rooks JB, Dry HW, Ishak KG et al. (1979) Epidemiology of hepatocellular adenoma. The role of oral contraceptive use. JAMA 242:644
Rosinus V, Maurer R (1981) Diäthylstilbestrol-induziertes Leberzell Karzinom. Schweiz Med Wochenschr 111:1139
Rossi G, Gabbi E, Serra L (1992) Acute hepatitis induced by cyclofenil: a case report. Ital J Gastroenterol 24:77
Routier G, Corette L, Dannas P (1967) Hepatite severe et progestatifs de synthese. J Sci Med Lillte 85:229
Rowley PT, Kurnick J, Cheville R (1970) Hereditary haemorrhagic telangiectasia: aggravation by oral contraceptives. Lancet I:474
Schaffner F (1966) The effect of oral contraceptives on the liver. JAMA 198:1019
Schaffner F, Raisfeld IH (1969) Drugs and the liver. A review of metabolism and adverse reactions. Adv Intern Med 15:221
Schaffner F, Popper H, Chesrow E (1959) Cholestasis produced by the administration of norethandrolone. Am J Med 26:249
Schaffner F, Popper H, Perez V (1960) Changes in bile canaliculi produced by norethandrolone: electron microscopic study of human and rat liver. J Lab Clin Med 56:623
Schneider HL, Hornbach KD, Kniaz JL, Efrusy ME (1984) Chlorpropamide hepatotoxicity: report of a case and review of the literature. Am J Gastroenterol 79:721
Schonberg LA (1982) Peliosis hepatis and oral contraceptives. J Reprod Med 27: 763
Schreiber AH, Simon FR (1983) Estrogen-induced cholestasis: clues to pathogenesis and treatment. Hepatology 3:607
Seki K, Minami Y, Nishikawa M et al. (1983) Non-alcoholic steatohepatitis induced by massive dose estrogen therapy. Gastroenterol Jpn 18:197

Silva MO, Reddy KR, McDonald T et al. (1989) Danazol-induced cholestasis. Am J Gastroenterol 84:426
Smetana H (1963) The histopathology of drug-induced liver disease. Ann NY Acad Sci 104:821
Song CS, Kappas A (1975) Hormones and hepatic function. In: Schiff L (ed) Diseases of the liver, 4th edn. Lippincott, Philadelphia, pp 163–183
Sotaniemi E, Kreus KE, Scheinin T (1964) Oral contraceptives and liver damage. Br Med J 2:1264
Sontaniemi EA, Alvaikko MJ, Kaipainen WJ (1975) Primary liver cancer associated with long-term oestrogen therapy. Ann Clin Res 7:287
Stricker BHC (1992) Drug induced hepatic injury, 2nd edn. Elsevier, Amsterdam
Stubblefield PG (1984) Oral contraceptives and neoplasia. J Reprod Med 29:524
Sturvetant FM (1979) Oral contraceptives and liver tumors. In: Moghissi KS (ed) Controversies in contraception. Williams and Wilkins, Baltimore, pp 93–150
Tanaka K, Kean EA, Johnson B (1976) Jamaican vomiting sickness: biochemical investigation of two cases. N Engl J Med 295:461
Taniya T, Noguchi M, Taiiri K et al. (1987) A case report of hyperlipenia with giant fatty liver during adjuvant therapy by tamoxifen. Gan No Rinsho 33:300
Tanyol H, Rehfuss ME (1955) Hepatotoxic effect of cortisone in experimental animals. Am J Dig Dis 22:169
Taylor W, Snowball S (1984) The effects of long-term administration of methyltestosterone on the development of liver lesions in BALB/c mice. J Pathol 143:211
Terblanche J, Goldin AR, Campbell JAH et al. (1978) Liver tumors associated with the use of contraceptive pills. S Afr Med J 53:439
Ticktin HE, Zimmerman HJ (1966) Effects of synthetic anabolic agent on hepatic function. Am J Med Sci 251:674
Tuchweber B, Weber A, Roy CC, Yousef IM (1986) Mechanisms of experimentally induced intrahepatic cholestasis. Prog Liver Dis 8:161
Turani H, Levi J, Zevin D et al. (1983) Hepatic lesions in patients on anabolic androgenic therapy. Isr J Med Sci 19:332
Valla D, Casadevall N, Lacombe C et al. (1985) Primary myeloproliferative disorder and hepatic vein thrombosis. Ann Intern Med 103:329
Valla D, Le MG, Poynard T et al. (1986) Risk of hepatic vein thrombosis in relation to recent use of oral contraceptives. A case control study. Gastroenterology 90:807
Van Thiel DH, de Belle R, Mellow M et al. (1974) Tolazamide hepatotoxicity. A case report. Gastroenterology 67:506
Vincens M, Athen N, Daugacies N et al. (1984) Augmentation des transaminases lor de trailment pae le clanazol ches des maleates li pagues. Therapie 39:541
Weill BJ, Menkes CJ, Cormier C et al. (1988) Hepatocellular carcinoma after danazol therapy. J Rheumatol 15:1447
Weinstein A, Massie R, Scoville AB (1963) The use of azepinamide in the management of diabetes mellitus, with a report of jaundice as a complication, and comments relative to the use of oral hypoglycemic agents. Am J Med Sci 245:432
Werner SC (1947) Clinical syndromes associated with gonadal failure in man. Am J Med 3:52
Werner SP, Hanger FM, Kritzler RA (1950) Jaundice during methyltestosterone therapy. Am J Med 8:325
Westaby D, Williams R (1981) Androgen and anabolic steroid-related tumors. In: Davis M, Trediger JM, Williams R (eds) Drug reactions and the liver. Pitman, Bath pp 284–289
Wilder EM (1962) Death due to liver failure following the use of mephandrosterone. Can Med Assoc J 87:768
Wilson JHP (1982) Oral contraceptives and hepatic tumors. Agressologie 23:21
Wongpactoon V, Russell RF, Mills PR, Patrick RS (1981) Intrahepatic cholestasis and cutaneous bullae associated with glibenclamide therapy. Postgrad Med J 57:244
Wynn V (1977) Metabolic effects of danazol. J Int Med Res 5:25

Zafrani ES, Pinadeau Y, Dhumeaux D (1983) Drug-induced vascular lesions of the liver. Arch Intern Med 143:495
Zimmerman HJ (1963) Clinical and laboratory manifestations of hepatotoxicity. Ann NY Acad Sci 104:954
Zimmerman HJ (1978) Hepatotoxicity adverse effects of drugs and other chemicals in the liver. Appleton Century Croft, New York
Zimmerman HJ, Lewis JH (1987) Drug-induced cholestasis. Med Toxicol 2:112
Zimmerman HJ, Maddrey WC (1987) Toxic and drug-induced hepatitis. In: Schiff L, Schiff ER (eds) Diseases of the liver, 6th edn. Lippincott, Philadelphia, pp 591–667

CHAPTER 24

Hepatotoxicity of Immunomodulating Agents

R.J. FINGEROTE and G.A. LEVY

A. Introduction

Immunomodulation, which is defined as the stimulation or suppression of the immune system through the use of biological or pharmacological agents, has become increasingly important in modern medicine. Immunostimulatory agents are currently being used in cancer chemotherapy and chronic viral hepatitis while immunosuppressive agents have become indispensable in solid organ and bone marrow transplantation with an expanding role in the management of patients with autoimmune diseases, allergies, infectious diseases and certain malignancies.

In addition to their beneficial effects, immunomodulating agents are capable of causing four broad categories of liver injury: cytotoxic, cholestatic, steatotic and vascular (Table 1) (SHERLOCK 1986). Cytotoxic injury, resulting from the direct toxicity of a drug or its metabolite, is usually dose dependent. In the acute form, clinical features are similar to those of acute viral hepatitis and are associated with elevations of serum transaminases. Chronic cytotoxic liver injury may result in the development of cirrhosis and clinical features of chronic liver failure. Cytotoxic liver injury secondary to a drug hypersensitivity reaction is not dose related, usually occurs within 4 weeks of initiation of therapy and has a presentation similar to acute viral hepatitis with the additional features of fever, rash and eosinophilia. Cholestatic liver injury is characterized by elevations of bilirubin and alkaline phosphatase accompanied by jaundice and pruritus. In addition to evidence of cholestasis, there may be features of cytotoxic injury present (hepatocanalicular cholestasis). Steatosis is a histologic diagnosis in which accumulation of fat droplets within the cytoplasm of hepatocytes can be demonstrated on liver biopsy. In macrovesicular steatosis, the fat droplets are large and the nucleus is displaced towards the cell border, whereas in microvesicular steatosis the intracytoplasmic fat droplets are small without associated displacement of the nucleus. Patients with macrovesicular steatosis, which has been associated with immunomodulatory drug therapy, usually present with mildly elevated serum aminotransferases. Typically, these patients are asymptomatic, although they may present with right upper quadrant abdominal pain. Vascular disorders which have been associated with immunomodulating drug therapy include veno-occlusive disease, sinusoidal dilatation/peliosis hepatis and hepatoportal sclerosis/

Table 1. Patterns of immunomodulating drug-induced liver injury

Type	Drug
Cytotoxic	
Direct	Methotrexate
	Cyclophosphamide
	Recombinant interleukin-2
	Interferons
	Azathioprine
	Cyclosporine
	FK-506
Hypersensitivity	Azathioprine
Cholestatic	Cyclosporine
	Interferons
	Recombinant interleukin-2
	Azathioprine
Vascular	Azathioprine
Steatotic	Corticosteroids
	Methotrexate
	Interferons

perisinusoidal fibrosis. Patients with these liver injuries commonly present with symptoms of portal hypertension, hepatosplenomegaly and ascites.

In patients receiving immunomodulating drugs, other causes of liver injury must be considered. In liver transplant patients, elevated serum transaminases may be indicative of rejection while the development of jaundice may be the first indication of vascular or biliary tract complications. In cancer patients, the underlying malignancy, radiation injury to the liver, graft versus host disease following bone marrow transplantation, parenteral nutrition or concurrently administered medications may contribute to liver injury. A thorough diagnostic workup, which may include liver biopsy, is indicated in all cases in which immunomodulating-drug-related liver injury is suspected.

In this chapter, a classification of both immunostimulatory and immunosuppressive agents will be presented and a review of the mechanisms of injury, clinical features, management and prevention of liver injury related to therapy with individual agents will be provided.

B. Immunostimulatory Agents

I. Classification

Immunostimulatory agents, which are defined as agents capable of enhancing immunocompetence, can be classified into two fundamental categories: im-

Table 2. Classification of immunostimulatory agents

1. Immune-system-derived biologicals
Interferons
Interleukin-2
Tumor necrosis factor
Leukotrienes
2. Immunostimulatory pharmaceutical agents
Levamisole
Ampligen
Isoprinosine

mune-system-derived biologicals and immunostimulatory pharmaceutical agents (Table 2).

1. Immune-System-Derived Biologicals

Immune-system-derived biologicals are molecules which have been identified as being active in cellular immune responses and which, using recombinant DNA technology, have been sequenced, cloned and expressed. Examples of such molecules include the interferons, interleukin-2 and tumor necrosis factor. Both the interferons and interleukin-2 are being used in cancer chemotherapy while interferons are being used in the management of patients with chronic hepatitis B and C viral infections.

2. Immunostimulatory Pharmaceutical Agents

Immunostimulatory pharmaceutical agents include the antiparasite compound levamisole, which is capable of augmenting lymphocyte, macrophage and neutrophil proliferation, secretion and motility; the mismatched double-stranded RNA compound ampligen, which induces the production of cytokines such as the interferons and tumor necrosis factor; and isoprinosine, which induces T-lymphocyte differentiation and potentiates the effects of antigens and lymphokines on lymphocytes and macrophages (HADDEN et al. 1990). Of these three agents, only levamisole is currently in clinical use, in the management of pediatric nephrotic syndrome (British Association for Paediatric Nephrology 1991) and in cancer chemotherapy (STEVENSON et al. 1991).

II. Hepatotoxicity of Specific Immunostimulatory Agents

1. Interleukin-2

a) Introduction

Interleukin-2 is a glycoprotein produced by T lymphocytes during immune responses which induces T-cell proliferation and differentiation and generation of lymphokine activated natural killer (LAK) cells which are capable of lysing tumor cells. The availability of interleukin-2 in recombinant form (rIL-2) has made possible the development of new immunotherapies for patients with cancer. In LAK therapy, lymphocytes are harvested by lymphocytophereses from patients with disseminated or nonresectable malignancy, treated with rIL-2 to produce LAK cells and reinfused into the patients. In combination with intravenous infusions of rIL-2, this regimen has proven beneficial in the treatment of nonresectable and disseminated malignancies (ROSENBERG and LOTZE 1986).

Therapy with rIL-2 has been associated with the development of dose-related, reversible cytotoxic and cholestatic liver injury. These side effects of rIL-2 therapy will be reviewed in this section.

b) Mechanisms of Injury

MATORY et al. (1985) demonstrated, in a rat model, that high-dose intravenous rIL-2 induced hepatocellular necrosis associated with periportal lymphocyte infiltration and elevated serum aminotransferases. Indeed, liver injury was the dose-limiting factor in these studies. GATELY et al. (1988) subsequently determined that, in mice treated with rIL-2, the lymphocytes surrounding the portal triads and central veins and within sinusoids were LAK-like effector cells which were 74%–98% Thy-1$^+$ and 55%–83% asialo-GM_1 (ganglio-*n* tetrosylceramide)$^+$. The critical role of these LAK-like effector cells in rIL-2-related toxicity was demonstrated by the observations that the toxic effects of rIL-2 could be abolished by pretreating mice with X-irradiation, administering corticosteroids during rIL-2 therapy or treating rIL-2-treated mice with anti asialo-GM-1 γ-globulin. Thus, rIL-2-related liver injury was most likely mediated by the generation, proliferation and tissue localization in the liver of rIL-2-activated lymphocytes and not a direct effect of rIL-2. Potential mechanisms for this lymphocyte-mediated liver injury include cytolysis of host endothelium and hepatocytes with subsequent development of capillary leak syndrome and hepatocellular injury or proteolysis of subendothelial basement membranes (ANDERSON et al. 1988). It has also been suggested that rIL-2-mediated cellular injury may occur secondary to vasoactive lymphokines secreted by rIL-2-activated lymphocytes (ROSENSTEIN et al. 1986).

The liver injury associated with low-dose rIL-2 therapy in man is predominantly cholestatic rather than cytotoxic (FISHER et al. 1989). Hepatic engorgement related to rIL-2-induced increased hepatic capillary permeability may result in bile stasis and decreased canalicular bile flow. Alternatively, rIL-2-stimulated cytokine production may cause hepatic production of acute-phase reactants which alter bile flow by interfering with hepatocyte membrane transport processes, altering cytoskeletal organization or function, or interfering with bilirubin reabsorption by altering the permeability of the paracellular pathway.

c) *Clinical and Pathological Features*

In a series of 261 cancer patients, therapy with rIL-2 was associated with jaundice, right upper quadrant abdominal tenderness, hepatomegaly, nausea, anorexia and pruritus (FISHER et al. 1989) in association with elevations in alkaline phosphatase and total bilirubin as well as lesser increases in serum aminotransferases. Bilirubin levels correlated with total rIL-2 dose and increases in alkaline phosphatase, body weight and aspartate transaminase levels. In all cases, abnormal liver function tests returned to normal following cessation of rIL-2 therapy. Computerized hepatobiliary nuclear scans in patients who developed cholestasis demonstrated delays in uptake and excretion of technetium-99m-labeled disofenin while hepatic ultrasound demonstrated no evidence of biliary duct dilation, consistent with intrahepatic cholestasis.

Similar results have been reported in other studies. ROSENBERG et al. (1993) noted that reversible hyperbilirubinemia developed in 233 of 262 courses of therapy in patients receiving either rIL-2 plus lymphokine-activated killer cells (LAK) (123/137 courses) or rIL-2 alone (110/125 courses). FISHER et al. (1988) noted bilirubin levels of between five and ten times normal in 11% of a cohort of 35 renal cell carcinoma patients receiving rIL-2 and LAK with significantly elevated aspartate transaminase occurring in 48%. PARKINSON et al. (1990a) noted hyperbilirubinemia and elevated alkaline phosphatase in 17% of a cohort of 47 patients being treated for metastatic malignant melanoma. In a second series of 47 patients with metastatic renal cell carcinoma being treated with rIL-2 and LAK, hyperbilirubinemia was observed in 8% of the patients and elevated aspartate transaminase levels in 46% of patients (PARKINSON et al. 1990b).

Histological studies in a patient receiving rIL-2 who developed cholestasis demonstrated preservation of liver architecture. However, periportal necrosis and moderate to severe infiltration of lymphocytes in the portal, periportal and sinusoidal areas was present with immunohistochemistry, demonstrating the presence of $CD2^+$, $CD3^+$ and $CD45^+$ and $CD22^-$ lymphocytes (PUNT et al. 1990).

d) *Management and Prevention of rIL-2-Related Liver Injury*

Liver injury may be avoided by employing the lowest possible dose for the shortest period of time and limiting therapy following the development of weight gain or increases in alkaline phosphatase or aspartate transaminase. It is now recommended that therapy be discontinued in the presence of bilirubin levels exceeding 6–10 mg/dl (FISHER et al. 1989).

2. Interferons

a) *Introduction*

The interferons are proteins, produced by nucleated cells in response to viruses, bacteria, double-stranded RNA, mitogens and antigens, which have antiviral, antitumor and immunoregulatory effects (PESTKA et al. 1987). Three general types of interferon have been isolated, sequenced and genetically engineered; interferon-α (leukocyte derived), -β (fibroblast derived) and -γ (lymphocyte derived). These agents are being used in the management of chronic viral infections such as hepatitis B and C (HOOFNAGLE 1990; DAVIS 1990) and disseminated solid organ and hematological malignancies such as ovarian carcinoma, renal cell carcinoma, chronic myelogenous leukemia and hairy cell leukemia (BORDEN 1992).

Following exposure to interferons, patients commonly develop an influenza-like illness consisting of fever, chills, tachycardia, malaise, myalgias and headaches. Less frequently, they develop depression, hemolytic anemia, thrombocytopenia, diarrhea, proteinuria, alopecia and autoantibodies associated with the development of autoimmune thyroiditis (MANNERING and DELORIA 1986). Both cytotoxic and cholestatic liver injury have been described following interferon therapy and will be reviewed in this section.

b) *Mechanisms of Injury*

In a study of newborn mice, high-dose subcutaneous injections of interferon caused 100% mortality (GRESSER et al. 1975). At postmortem examination, the livers of these mice appeared gray and pale and, on histologic examination, demonstrated acellular hepatocellular necrosis with accumulation of fat and decreased glycogen in hepatocytes associated with swelling of both the mitochondria and rough endoplasmic reticulum on electron microscopy examination. No toxic effects were seen at similar doses when therapy was initiated after the 6th day of life. ZWINGELSTEIN et al. (1985) subsequently reported in newborn mice that interferon therapy was associated with modifications in the lipid composition of the liver. GRESSER et al. (1987) suggested that interferon-related liver injury in immature animals may be secondary to alterations in lipid biosynthesis and hepatocyte membrane viscosity.

In isolated mouse hepatocytes, it has been demonstrated that interferon-γ stimulates nitric oxide synthase activity and decreases intracellular ATP levels (ADAMSON and BILLINGS 1993). When hepatocytes were exposed to tumor necrosis factor-α in addition to interferon-γ, these effects increased beyond a merely additive effect. Furthermore, exposure of these cells to both cytokines resulted in significant cytotoxicity whereas neither agent alone produced toxicity. Thus, interferon-γ may increase tumor necrosis factor-α-related liver injury by potentiating intracellular oxidative stress, inhibiting energy metabolism and increasing cytotoxicity.

Interferons and interferon inducers inhibit the hepatic cytochrome P-450 drug-metabolizing systems (MANNERING et al. 1980). Thus, interferons may potentiate the effects of certain xenobiotics by interfering with their metabolism (STANLEY et al. 1991). KALABIS and WELLS (1990) have shown that modulation of cytochrome P-450 activity can be biphasic with inhibition of activity being followed by induction. In their study, the interferon inducer polyinosinic-polycytidylic acid (Poly I-C) inhibited the hepatotoxicity of acetaminophen given within 8 days of Poly I-C administration, whereas toxicity was enhanced when acetaminophen was given after this time.

The mechanisms by which interferons affect cytochrome P-450 activity are unclear. GHEZZI et al. (1985) demonstrated that interferon and interferon inducers increase hepatic xanthine oxidase activity and therefore concluded that interferon induces generation of reactive oxygen intermediates which cause oxidative damage to cytochrome P-450. Indeed, they speculated that other toxic effects of interferon, such as hepatic injury in newborn mice and cardiotoxicity, occur secondary to interferon-related induction of xanthine oxidase and free oxygen radical generation. In a later study, MANNERING et al. (1988) showed that induction of xanthine oxidase and the loss of cytochrome P-450 following interferon therapy were coincidental. They, therefore, suggested that interferon-induced depression of hepatic cytochrome P-450 occurs secondary to decreased synthesis and increased degradation of cytochrome P-450 apoprotein.

c) *Clinical and Pathological Features*

In a series of 1019 cancer patients treated with recombinant interferon-α 2-a, 77% developed elevated aspartate aminotransaminase while increased alkaline phosphatase and bilirubin were noted in 48% and 31% of patients, respectively (JONES and ITRI 1986). In a second study, aspartate transaminase levels correlated with the dose of interferon being administered (QUESADA and GUTTERMAN 1983; QUESADA et al. 1986). Although liver function abnormalities in these two studies were not associated with clinical liver disease, fulminant hepatic failure has been reported in cancer patients treated with interferon (KLOKE et al. 1992; WANDL et al. 1992; DURAND et al. 1991).

KELLOKUMPU et al. (1989) described three patients treated with interferon-α in combination with vinblastine who developed elevated liver enzymes and, in one case, hyperbilirubinemia temporally related to the administration of acetaminophen. The authors speculated that these enzyme changes were secondary to a drug interaction involving acetaminophen and they therefore suggested that in patients undergoing therapy with interferons, acetaminophen should be avoided or, if used simultaneously, liver function should be monitored. Acetylsalicylic acid was suggested as an alternative to acetaminophen.

Histologically, interferon therapy has been associated with steatosis (QUESADA and GUTTERMAN 1983), cholestasis with evidence of septal fibrosis and irregular cirrhotic transformation (WANDL et al. 1992) and centrilobular zonal necrosis associated with mild portal and periportal inflammation (DURAND et al. 1991). ITOH et al. (1989) demonstrated, in a 65-year-old man with hairy cell leukemia, that interferon-α therapy was associated with steatosis, the development of enlarged or vacuolated nuclei in hepatocytes and hepatocellular necrosis. Ultrastructurally, hepatocytes exhibited cytoplasmic vacuoles and weakly stained glycogen particles, a reduced number of mitochondria and decreased endoplasmic reticulum which appeared dilated and vacuolar.

d) Management and Prevention of Interferon-Related Liver Injury

Therapy with interferons requires close monitoring of liver function tests. Abnormalities in liver function tests may indicate the exacerbation or development de novo of autoimmune liver disease (SILVA et al. 1991; VENTO et al. 1989; PAPO et al. 1992). Therapy should be discontinued in the presence of persistently abnormal liver biochemistry or clinical evidence of liver injury.

C. Immunosuppressive Agents

I. Classification

Immunosuppressive agents can be divided into six distinct groups: antilymphocyte products, immunophilin-binding agents, cytotoxic agents, sterols, immunosuppressive antibiotics and arachidonic acid metabolites (Table 3).

Table 3. Classification of immunosuppressive agents

1. Antilymphocyte products
Polyclonal preparations
Antithymocyte globulin
Antilymphocyte globulin
Monoclonal preparations
OKT3
2. Immunophilin-binding agents
Cyclosporine
FK-506
Rapamycin
3. Cytotoxic agents
Nonselective
Cyclophosphamide
Azathioprine
Methotrexate
Lymphocyte selective
mycophenolate mofetil (CellCept)
Bredinin (Mizorbine)
Brequinar
4. Corticosteroids
5. Immunosuppressive antibiotics
15-Deoxyspergualin
6. Arachidonic acid metabolites
Prostaglandin E analogues

1. Antilymphocyte Products

Antilymphocyte products are commonly used following solid organ transplantation for both induction and rescue to combat acute rejection (Drews 1990). These agents achieve immunosuppression by either inducing T-cell destruction by cytolysis or blocking T-cell activity by interfering with functional molecules on their cellular membrane (Koene 1992). Included in this category are the polyclonal antibody preparations, such as antilymphocyte globulin and antithymocyte globulin, in which the clinically active components are antibodies against one or more T-cell antigens and monoclonal antibodies in which antibodies, produced by hybridomas, are directed against targets involved in T-lymphocyte immune recognition. The only monoclonal antibody currently in clinical use, OKT3, is a mouse monoclonal IgG directed at the T3 (CD3) antigen which is present on T cells.

2. Immunophilin-Binding Agents

Immunophilins are cytosolic-binding proteins that play important roles in signal transduction and T-cell proliferation (Galat 1993). The immunophilin-binding agents, cyclosporine, FK-506 and rapamycin, are prodrugs which become active when they bind to immunophilins. Although they bind to different immunophilins, cyclosporine binding to cyclophilin and FK-506 and rapamycin binding to the FK506-binding protein (FKBP), their effects are similar in that they block the calcium-induced translocation of a component of nuclear factor of activated T cells (NF-AT) and inhibit the calcium-activated protein phosphatase, calcineurin (Schreiber and Crabtree 1992). Immunosuppression subsequently occurs as a result of impaired T-cell activation (Shevach 1985). Both FK-506 and rapamycin are investigational at present. Cyclosporine is currently being used in the management of patients undergoing solid organ or bone marrow transplantation as well as in patients with autoimmune diseases (Kahan 1989; Feutren and von Graffenried 1992).

3. Cytotoxic Agents

Cytotoxic agents exert immunosuppressive effects by eliminating immunologically competent cells. Currently available agents, such as the alkylating agent cyclophosphamide, the folic acid antagonist methotrexate and the cytotoxic purine analog azathioprine, exert nonselective cytotoxicity against all actively replicating cells, including leukocytes and mucosal epithelial cells (Thomson et al. 1992). These agents are used in solid organ and bone marrow transplantation and in the management of autoimmune and rheumatological disorders.

Cytotoxic agents with greater selectivity for lymphocytes have been synthesized and are undergoing intensive examination in controlled studies. Mycophenolate mofetil (cellcept), which is a semisynthetic derivative of mycophenolic acid, blocks the de novo pathway for synthesis of guanine nucleotides by inhibiting inosine monophosphate (IMP) dehydrogenase. This effect is selective for T and B lymphocytes which are more dependent on this pathway for purine synthesis than other actively replicating cells. Bredinin (mizorbin), like mycophenolate mofetil, achieves an immunosuppressive effect by inhibiting IMP dehydrogenase. Brequinar is a carboxylic acid derivative which inhibits dihydro-orotate dehydrogenase and thereby blocks de novo pyrimidine synthesis (Makowka and Cramer 1992).

4. Sterols

The term sterols refers to a diverse group of organic compounds derived from cholesterol. Steroid hormones are one such group and include androgens, estrogens, progestogens, adrenal corticosteroids and diuretics. Synthetic analogs and antagonists of these compounds have been synthesized and are currently in wide use in medical practice (Di Cyan 1987).

Adrenal corticosteroids and their synthetic analogs have immunosuppressive properties which have resulted in their use in patients following solid organ and bone marrow transplantation as well as in patients with autoimmune, rheumatological and allergic disorders. The rationale for their use was the observation that glucocorticoid receptors are present on all cells but particularly so on T lymphocytes. Following binding to these receptors, corticosteroids induce apoptosis (Cohen and Duke 1984). Thus, these agents induce peripheral lymphopenia which is more pronounced for T lymphocytes than other immunologically active cell populations. In addition, corticosteroids inhibit cytokine gene transcription by binding to a nuclear protein receptor that blocks a regulator segment on the 5′ region of cytokine genes (Strom 1992).

5. Immunosuppressive Antibiotics

The antibiotic 15-deoxyspergualin is currently being investigated for use in solid organ transplantation. Its predominant effect appears to be on cells of monocyte/macrophage lineage, resulting in reduced expression of IL-1 and MHC class II antigens as well as decreased phagocytotic activity and oxygen free radical production. Decreased clonal expansion, production of cytokines and cytokine responsiveness in other immunologically active cell lines have been reported following therapy with this compound (Thomson et al. 1992).

6. Arachidonic Acid Metabolites

The arachidonic acid metabolite prostaglandin E and its analogs decrease antibody synthesis and the ability of T lymphocytes to proliferate in response to allogeneic stimulation. In addition, they inhibit IL-2 release, antigen- and mitogen-induced lymphocyte proliferation and class II antigen expression by macrophages (Sinclair and Levy 1990). They are currently being studied in the management of patients with fulminant hepatic failure (Sinclair et al. 1989) as well as in patients with primary graft nonfunction (Greig et al. 1989) and recurrent hepatitis B infection post liver transplantation (FLOWERS et al. 1994).

II. Hepatotoxic Effects of Specific Immunosuppressive Agents

1. Methotrexate

a) Introduction

Discovered over 40 years ago, methotrexate is an effective inhibitor of dihydrofolate reductase. This results in impaired production of tetrahydrofolic acid which, in turn, inhibits transfer of 1-carbon units and production of purine and pyrimidine bases, ultimately leading to decreased cellular synthesis of DNA and RNA (JOLIVET et al. 1983). Methotrexate has been used extensively in the treatment of solid organ and hematological malignancies (JOLIVET et al. 1983). In addition, it has proven beneficial in the management of rheumatoid arthritis, psoriasis, sarcoidosis and asthma and is being studied for possible beneficial effects in primary sclerosing cholangitis and inflammatory bowel disease.

Within a few years of its introduction, an association between methotrexate therapy and hepatic fibrosis was described in children undergoing chemotherapy for acute leukemia (HUTTER et al. 1960). Subsequent studies, which will be reviewed in this section, have confirmed an association between methotrexate therapy and the development of hepatic fibrosis and cirrhosis. Methotrexate therapy has also been associated with the development of chronic active hepatitis (CLEGG et al. 1989; KUJALA et al. 1990) and liver failure requiring liver transplantation (GILBERT et al. 1990).

b) Mechanisms of Injury

Noting that methotrexate therapy related hepatic fibrosis is predominantly periportal, SHERLOCK (1986) has suggested that methotrexate hepatotoxicity is secondary to the effects of a toxic liver-derived metabolite. Indeed, BREMNES has incriminated the methotrexate metabolite 7-hydroxy methotrexate in hepatotoxicity following high-dose methotrexate therapy (BREMNES et al. 1989, 1991a,b). HALL et al. (1991) demonstrated in rats that, following administration of oral methotrexate for 6 weeks, necrosis and lysis of zone 3 hepatocytes occurs in association with ceroid-laden macrophages, lymphocytes and focal areas of fibrosis. They speculated that methotrexate-related hepatic fibrosis was secondary to induction of cytokine synthesis and peptide growth factors release from inflammatory cells stimulating Ito cells (fat-storing cells) to undergo morphological and functional transition to collagen-producing transitional cells or myofibroblasts.

TUMA et al. (1975) have demonstrated in a rat model that methotrexate blocks the de novo synthesis of choline and methionine, potentiates choline deficiency related fatty liver and inhibits the lipotropic effects of vitamin B_{12}. Thus, they suggested, methotrexate-related liver injury may be secondary to inhibition of methionine and choline biosynthesis, resulting in impaired lipid transport due to interference with hepatic one-carbon transfer reactions.

c) Clinical and Pathological Features

In a series of 37 patients with psoriasis who had been treated with methotrexate for up to 73 months, cirrhosis and hepatic fibrosis were present in 7 and 10 patients, respectively (DAHL et al. 1971). Hepatomegaly was seen in 7 of these 17 patients, while splenomegaly was seen in 3 patients with cirrhosis and 1 patient with fibrosis. Ascites was present in two cirrhotic patients. Abnormal liver function tests were seen during treatment in all 17 patients, although abnormalities in several cases were slight and transitory. In the remaining 20 patients, only 3 had normal liver biopsies; all other patients had nonspecific reactive hepatitis.

Methotrexate-associated liver injury has been associated with several risk factors including alcohol abuse (WHITING-O'KEEFE et al. 1991), obesity (NEWMAN et al. 1989), diabetes mellitus (SHERGY et al. 1988), large cumulative doses (DAHL et al. 1971; WHITING-O'KEEFE et al. 1991) and a dosing regimen of frequent small doses rather than large intermittent doses (DAHL et al. 1972). In patients with rheumatoid arthritis, methotrexate-related liver injury has been associated with advanced age at initiation of therapy (PHILLIPS et al. 1992; WALKER et al. 1993). Liver biochemistry has not been found useful in predicting the development of methotrexate-related liver injury and, therefore, liver biopsies are necessary to determine whether patients are developing hepatotoxicity (REYNOLDS and LEE 1986; SHERGY et al. 1988).

Histologic liver abnormalities attributed to methotrexate include macrovesicular steatosis, piecemeal necrosis and hepatic fibrosis. As methotrexate-related injury becomes more advanced, fibrosis, which in early lesions is periportal, develops into partial, and then whole, fibrous septa extending between portal tracts and central veins. Ultimately, micronodular cirrhosis may be seen. Methotrexate-associated portal inflammatory cell infiltration is usually of only moderate severity and consists of lymphocytes, macrophages and neutrophils. Nuclei of injured hepatocytes are usually hyperchromatic, pleomorphic and vacuolated (ZIMMERMAN 1978). The histologic findings of methotrexate-related liver injury can be divided into five major grades (Table 4). This grading system has achieved widespread use in the classification of methotrexate-induced liver injury.

Unfortunately, the above-noted findings are not pathognomonic of methotrexate-related liver injury. Indeed, many of these abnormalities have been described in the liver biopsies of psoriasis patients obtained prior to initiation of methotrexate therapy (KEVAT et al. 1988; NYFORS and POULSEN 1976).

Table 4. Classification of histologic findings on liver biopsy in patients receiving methotrexate therapy (modified from ROEGNIGK et al. 1988)

	Steatosis	Nuclear variability	Inflammation ± necrosis	Fibrosis	Cirrhosis
Grade 0	–	–	–	–	–
Grade I	+	+	+	–	–
Grade II	++	++	++	–	–
Grade IIIa				+	–
Grade IIIb				++	–
Grade IV					+/++

–, absent; +, mild; ++, moderate to severe.

d) Prevention and Management of Methotrexate-Related Liver Injury

Guidelines for methotrexate therapy in psoriasis have been established (ROEGNIGK et al. 1982, 1988). In these guidelines, relative contraindications to the use of methotrexate in psoriasis included significant abnormalities in renal function or liver chemistry, active or recent hepatitis, cirrhosis and excessive alcohol consumption. Liver biopsy was recommended after a cumulative methotrexate dosage of 1.5g in patients with normal liver chemistry, normal physical examination and no risk factors for liver disease. In the absence of significant abnormalities, repeat liver biopsies were recommended after patients had received an additional 1.0–1.5g methotrexate. In the presence of normal liver chemistry values, history and physical examination, a pretreatment liver biopsy was considered discretionary. In patients with significant abnormalities on liver chemistry or risk factors for liver disease, liver biopsy was recommended following every 1.0g of cumulative methotrexate dose. It was suggested that patients with grade I or II liver histology abnormalities could safely continue therapy whereas patients with grade IIIa liver abnormalities should have repeat biopsies every 6 months. Patients with higher grades of abnormality should discontinue treatment.

The risk of liver injury in patients with rheumatoid arthritis being treated with methotrexate is significantly lower than the risk in patients with psoriasis (KEVAT et al. 1988; SHERGY et al. 1988; WHITING-O'KEEFE et al. 1991; WALKER et al. 1993). Thus, liver biopsies prior to initiation of therapy should only be carried out in rheumatoid arthritis patients with a history of significant alcohol consumption, liver disease or jaundice (KREMER 1992; KREMER et al. 1994). Liver biopsies during therapy should be carried out in the presence of persistently elevated aspartate transaminase or depressed albumin without regard to the cumulative dose of methotrexate.

e) Management and Prevention of Methotrexate-Related Liver Injury

Liver injury associated with the use of methotrexate does not correlate well with liver function test abnormalities. Thus, liver biopsies are indicated to confirm the diagnosis and severity of liver injury. Therapy with this agent should be avoided in patients with risk factors for liver injury such as regular alcohol consumption. Advanced fibrosis or cirrhosis on liver biopsy are indications to discontinue therapy.

2. Corticosteroids

a) Introduction

Corticosteroids are the most widely used agents for the control of immunological reactions. At the molecular level, they act by passively entering target lymphocytes and binding to intracellular, cytoplasmic sterol receptors, thereby forming steroid-receptor complexes. These complexes undergo conformational changes that allow them to bind to nuclear acceptor sites which influence expression of mRNA for various cytokines, including interleukin-1, interleukin-2 and interferon-γ (BEHRENS and GOODWIN 1988). As corticosteroid receptors are also present in neutrophils, eosinophils and monocytes, corticosteroids have major anti-inflammatory as well as immunoregulatory properties.

An association between corticosteroid therapy and reversible fat infiltration of the liver was first reported over 40 years ago (STEINBERG et al. 1952). This association will be reviewed in this section.

b) Mechanisms of Injury

Corticosteroids have multiple metabolic effects including inhibition of synthesis and acceleration of catabolism of protein and RNA. In adipose tissue, these agents increase lipolysis while, in the liver, they stimulate gluconeogenesis and glycogen deposition (BAXTER and FORSHAM 1972). Lipolysis in adipose tissue results in increased circulating levels of lipids which stimulate hepatic uptake of free fatty acids (HILL et al. 1965). PESSAYRE (1992) has postulated that the main mechanism leading to macrovesicular steatosis is impaired hepatic release of lipids resulting from decreased synthesis of the apoprotein required for triglyceride transport. In addition, intrahepatic lipid accumulation may occur secondary to corticosteroid-mediated inhibition of hepatic esterification of fatty acids (JEANRENAUD 1967).

c) Clinical and Pathological Features

In 1952, STEINBERG et al. reported a case of reversible fatty infiltration of the liver associated with hepatomegaly in a patient treated with cortisone. More recently, IANCU et al. (1986) documented asymptomatic reversible hepatomegaly occurring in 7 of 122 patients treated with 2 mg/kg per day prednisone and in 12 of 18 patients treated with 4 mg/kg per day prednisone for periods of less than 10 days. Although abnormal liver function tests were not noted in this study, in 80% of a group of 25 patients undergoing therapy with ≥10 mg prednisone daily for over 4 months, WALD and FARR (1991) noted mild, but statistically significant elevations in one or more of four liver enzymes (alkaline phosphatase, alanine transaminase, aspartate transaminase or lactic acid dehydrogenase).

These studies suggested that corticosteroid-related fatty liver infiltration is a benign condition. However, HILL (1961) and JONES et al. (1965) each reported a case of fatal fat embolism occurring in a patient with fatty liver secondary to corticosteroid therapy. JONES et al. (1965) described a 25-year-old renal transplant recipient managed with azathioprine and high-dose prednisone who died following the development of small bowel ischemia. At autopsy, hepatomegaly and steatosis were found with systemic evidence of fat embolism. The authors suggested that the origin of the fat emboli was the fatty liver.

Liver biopsies of patients with corticosteroid-related fatty liver have demonstrated that fat deposition is macrovesicular and predominantly centrilobular in distribution (STEINBERG et al. 1952; JONES et al. 1965). IANCU et al. (1986) found preserved liver architecture, distended hepatocytes, moderate sinusoidal compression and coarse parenchymal cell membranes in biopsies from patients who were treated with prednisone for short periods of time. Electron microscopy demonstrated that the hepatocytes were distended with glycogen. There was no evidence of parenchymal or sinusoidal cell damage or increased collagen formation.

d) Management and Prevention of Corticosteroid-Related Liver Injury

In addition to causing reversible steatosis and hepatomegaly, corticosteroid therapy may result in the development of myopathy, psychosis, osteoporosis, cataracts, poor wound healing, hypertension or diabetes mellitus (KIRKHAM and PANAYI 1992). The risk of side effects can be minimized by reducing or stopping corticosteroid therapy. Azathioprine may be used as a substitute for corticosteroids in the management of chronic autoimmune hepatitis (KRAWITT 1994). Favorable results have been reported for long-term immunosuppression without the use of corticosteroids in liver (BELLI et al. 1994) as well as heart (PRICE et al. 1992) and renal transplant recipients (BRY et al. 1991). Potentially, in the future, new immunosuppressive agents will be developed which may allow the management of patients without the use of corticosteroids.

3. Azathioprine

a) Introduction

Azathioprine, a methylnitroimidazole-substituted derivative of the immunosuppressive agent 6-mercaptopurine, is an inhibitor of hypoxanthine-phosphoribosyl transferase. Inhibition of this enzyme results in reduced de novo purine and, thus, DNA synthesis. Ultimately, production of rapidly replicating cells including T and, to a lesser extent, B lymphocytes is suppressed, resulting in impaired cell-mediated immunity and antibody production (WOLBERG 1988). This agent is used in solid organ and bone marrow transplant patients as part of a triple immunosuppressive regimen which also incorporates cyclosporine and prednisone (SLAPAK et al. 1991). In addition, its use is well established in patients with autoimmune chronic active hepatitis, rheumatoid arthritis, chronic inflammatory polyneuropathy, myasthenia gravis, dermatomyositis and polymyositis.

The most important toxicity of azathioprine is dose-related bone marrow suppression (CHAN et al. 1987). Azathioprine has been incriminated in the development of cytotoxic and cholestatic liver injury as well as in hypersensitivity reactions involving the liver. In addition, focal nodular hyperplasia and the hepatic vascular disorders veno-occlusive disease, peliosis hepatis and sinusoidal dilatation have been described in patients receiving azathioprine. These forms of liver injury associated with azathioprine therapy will be reviewed in this section.

b) Mechanisms of Injury

HABOUBI et al. (1988) and STERNECK et al. (1991) have suggested that azathioprine hepatotoxicity and vascular injuries such as peliosis hepatis and veno-occlusive disease occur secondary to injury of the endothelial cells lining the hepatic sinusoids and terminal venules. On electron microscopy, HABOUBI et al. demonstrated degeneration of sinusoidal endothelial cells in patients with nodular regenerative hyperplasia and peliosis hepatis secondary to azathioprine therapy. Many endothelial cells were edematous and demonstrated fatty infiltration and cytoplasmic fragmentation while other endothelial cells were completely sloughed off, leaving hepatocytes directly exposed to the sinusoidal lumen. As a consequence of endothelial cell injury, extravasation of red blood cells into the space of Disse associated with perisinusoidal and perivenular fibrosis was noted. The authors speculated that inadequate perfusion of adjacent hepatocytes resulted in atrophy and death of some cells and compensatory hyperplasia of other cells leading to the development of focal nodular hyperplasia. Portal hypertension ensued secondary to fibrosis-related narrowing of the hepatic sinusoids, capillarization of the sinusoids following endothelial cell injury and compression of the sinusoids by regenerating nodules.

Azathioprine has been associated with hypersensitivity-related liver injury (DAVIS et al. 1980; MEYS et al. 1992; JEURISSEN et al. 1990; COOPER et al. 1986). Noting that its major metabolite 6-mercaptopurine is not associated with hypersensitivity reactions, DAVIS et al. (1980) have suggested that the hypersensitivity reaction attributed to azathioprine is secondary to the effects of the imidazole side chain rather than the 6-mercaptopurine component of the azathioprine molecule.

c) Clinical and Pathological Features

Azathioprine has been reported to cause both hepatocellular injury and cholestasis (SPARBERG et al. 1969; ZARDAY et al. 1972; DEPINHO et al. 1984; KISSEL et al. 1986). However, in a series of 24 renal transplant patients who were treated with azathioprine and developed liver disease, as demonstrated clinically by the presence of jaundice or hepatomegaly or biochemically by the presence of either elevated total bilirubin or elevated transaminases associated with elevated alkaline phosphatase, IRELAND et al. (1973) demonstrated no correlation between the course of liver disease and azathioprine administration or withdrawal. Thus, they suggested, withdrawal of azathioprine was not indicated in the presence of evidence of post-transplant liver disease.

Nodular regenerative hyperplasia (NHP) has been reported following azathioprine therapy in renal, cardiac and bone marrow transplant patients (OLSEN et al. 1991; DUVOUX et al. 1991; JONES et al. 1988; BUFFET et al. 1988; HABOUBI et al. 1988; XERRI et al. 1989) as well as in patients with multiple sclerosis (MION et al. 1991) and inflammatory bowel disease (DUVOUX et al. 1991). Patients with NHP presented with evidence of portal hypertension such as hematemesis and ascites.

Peliosis hepatis, which is defined histologically by blood-filled cavities bordered by hepatic plates distributed at random through the hepatic parenchyma (DEGOTT et al. 1978), has been reported in renal transplant recipients receiving azathioprine (DEGOTT et al. 1978; HANKEY and SAKER 1987) as well as a patient who was being treated with azathioprine for dermatomyositis (LORCERIE et al. 1990). DEGOTT et al. (1978) reported this condition in 12 patients presenting up to 17 months post renal transplantation. The authors differentiated major from minor peliosis. In major peliosis, blood-filled cavities were large and often confluent with the lesions affecting a large proportion of the hepatic lobules. All six patients with major peliosis exhibited hepatomegaly with symptoms of portal hypertension present in five patients. Patients with minor peliosis, in which only part of the liver lobule was affected by small lesions, were asymptomatic and none demonstrated hepatomegaly.

GERLAG and VAN HOOFF (1987) described four patients being treated with azathioprine post renal transplantation who developed hepatic sinusoidal dilatation associated with portal hypertension. Azathioprine was discontinued in all patients with resultant reduction of midzonal and pericentral sinus dilatation in follow-up liver biopsies. Nonetheless, follow-up liver biopsy demonstrated cirrhosis in three of these patients, with NHP developing in the fourth patient.

Hepatic veno-occlusive disease is an uncommon disorder characterized histologically by hepatic congestion associated with nonthrombotic occlusion of centrilobular venules, perivenular necrosis and fibrosis and perisinusoidal fibrosis with sinusoidal dilatation (LEMLEY et al. 1989). It has been described in patients receiving azathioprine following renal transplantation (ADLER et al. 1987; READ et al. 1986; KATZKA et al. 1986; LIAÑO et al. 1989) and in a patient being treated with azathioprine for rheumatoid arthritis (LEMLEY et al. 1989). Patients with this condition typically are male and present with jaundice and portal hypertension (KATZA et al. 1986).

d) Management and Prevention of Azathioprine-Related Liver Injury

Liver biopsy should be considered in any patient who is receiving azathioprine and develops abnormal liver function tests. Improvement in both biochemistry and histological abnormalities have been documented in patients with symptomatic NHP (DUVOUX et al. 1991; HABOUBI et al. 1988; BUFFET et al. 1988) as well as veno-occlusive disease (KATZKA et al. 1986; LEMLEY et al. 1989; ADLER et al. 1987; READ et al. 1986) following discontinuation of azathioprine. However, in some patients, there may be no improvement following discontinuation of azathioprine, probably due to the late identification of liver injury (OLSEN et al. 1991).

4. Cyclosporine

Cyclosporine is a neutral, lipophilic, cyclic polypeptide first isolated in 1970 from the fungi *Tolypocladium inflatum* Gams. Within 2 years of its discovery, the immunosuppressive properties of this compound were established (BOREL 1982) and, in 1978, the first reports of its successful use in the management of bone marrow (POWLES et al. 1978) and renal (CALNE et al. 1978) transplant patients were published. In addition, it has been proven beneficial in the management of patients with autoimmune disorders such as rheumatoid arthritis, autoimmune uveitis, idiopathic nephrotic syndrome, systemic lupus erythematosis and primary biliary cirrhosis, chronic inflammatory bowel disease and dermatological disorders such as psoriasis, pemphigus and pyoderma gangrenosum (KAHAN 1989; FEUTREN and VON GRAFFENRIED 1992).

The mechanism of action of cyclosporine is uncertain. It has been postulated that cyclosporine is a prodrug which becomes activated following binding to the immunophilin protein cyclophilin. The cyclophilin-cyclosporine complex binds and inhibits the Ca^{2+}- and calmodulin-dependent protein phosphatase, calcineurin. Inhibition of this enzyme prevents translocation across the nuclear membrane of the cytoplasmic subunit of the nuclear factor of activated T cells (NF-AT) which, in turn, prevents transcription of the interleukin-2 (IL-2) gene. This results in the loss of IL-2-driven T- and B-cell proliferation, reduced production of T-cell cytokines such as macrophage migration inhibition factor, γ-interferon and granulocyte-macrophage colony-stimulating factor and, ultimately, impaired antibody- and cell-mediated immunity (SHEVACH 1985; SCHREIBER and CRABTREE 1992; WONG et al. 1993).

Cyclosporine has many side effects which limit its widespread application. In a series of 3859 renal transplant patients treated with cyclosporine, the most frequent adverse events during the 1st year of surveillance were renal disfunction (57%), hypertension (47%), hypertrichosis (43%), tremor (25%), gingival hypertrophy (20%) and liver enzyme abnormality (19%) (COCKBURN et al. 1988). Both cholestatic and cytotoxic liver injury have been described in patients receiving cyclosporine and will be reviewed in this section.

a) Mechanisms of Injury

NICCHITTA et al. (1985) demonstrated, in isolated rat hepatocytes, that vasopressin-induced calcium flux across the cellular plasma membrane and total cellular calcium content increased following treatment with cyclosporine. These increases were dose dependent and associated with progressive increases in the endoplasmic reticulum and mitochondrial calcium pools. Thus, they suggested, cyclosporine induces intracellular accumulation of calcium at levels toxic to hepatocytes.

BACKMAN et al. (1986) studied the properties of hepatocyte intracellular membranes isolated from rats exposed in vivo to cyclosporine. They established that cyclosporine interfered with cellular functions in selective ways. Increased volumes and vacuolization of the endoplasmic reticulum were noted. Moreover, decreases in B oxidation of fatty acids and reduced catalase and urate activities in isolated peroxisomes were noted. In a subsequent study, this group demonstrated both in vitro, in a cell-free suspension of rat liver microsomal and supernatant fractions, and in vivo that cyclosporine inhibited hepatocyte protein synthesis in a dose-dependent fashion (BACKMAN et al. 1988). They suggested that cyclosporine and/or its metabolites directly inhibited protein synthesis at the level of ribosomal translation and that interference with protein synthesis could be a mechanism whereby cyclosporine caused liver injury (BACKMAN et al. 1986, 1988).

In vivo studies in rats by ROMAN et al. (1990) and STONE et al. (1987) have determined that cyclosporine causes dose-dependent cholestasis concomitant with decreases in the biliary secretion of bilirubin and increases in the serum levels of bile acid and bilirubin. In these studies, cyclosporine interfered with both bile-salt-dependent and bile-salt-independent bile flow.

The mechanisms by which cyclosporine affects biliary flow and induces cholestasis are unclear. STONE et al. (1988) speculated that, since cyclosporine is extremely hydrophobic and is preferentially distributed to lipid membranes, it might induce cholestasis by altering membrane fluidity and $Na^{+}K^{+}$ adenosine triphosphatase (ATP) activity. In support of this theory, KADMON et al. (1993) demonstrated in vitro in rat and human liver plasma membrane vesicles that cyclosporine inhibited ATP-dependent transport of the bile acid taurocholic acid. Thus, cholestasis in patients receiving cyclosporine may develop secondary to inhibition of ATP-dependent export carriers responsible for membrane transport of bile salts.

Animal studies have demonstrated that animals treated with cyclosporine have increased serum and urine levels of endothelin (BENIGNI et al. 1991; KON et al. 1990). BLUHM et al. (1993) demonstrated that endothelin 1, endothelin 3 and cyclosporine caused reductions of bile flow when infused individually into an isolated perfused rat liver. When cyclosporine and endothelin 1 were infused together at doses that were not cholestatic for either compound alone, cholestasis was evident. Thus, interaction between endothelin and cyclosporine may produce or potentiate cholestasis under certain conditions.

b) Clinical and Pathological Features

Early clinical studies demonstrated a high frequency of abnormal liver function tests in transplant patients receiving cyclosporine (CALNE et al. 1978; POWLES et al. 1978). In pilot clinical studies of cyclosporine in seven renal transplant patients, CALNE et al. (1978) noted elevated bilirubin and alkaline phosphatase in all patients with elevations of aspartate transaminase in three patients. Changes in liver function developed within 1 week of initiating therapy and normalized upon reduction of cyclosporine dosage. In a subsequent study by STARZL et al. (1980), elevated bilirubin, serum transaminases, alkaline phosphatase and prothrombin times were noted in 6 of 22 renal transplant patients treated with cyclosporine at a dose of 17 mg/kg. All patients were asymptomatic and abnormalities resolved when the dose was decreased below 10 mg/kg.

In bone marrow transplant patients receiving cyclosporine, ATKINSON et al. (1983) noted elevated bilirubin levels post-transplant in 18 of 21 patients. In 34% of these patients, the hyperbilirubinemia was attributed to cyclosporine therapy; acute graft versus host disease, hemolysis and sepsis were considered the most likely cause in 45% while multiple factors were considered causative in the remaining 21%. Cyclosporine-related hyperbilirubinemia was associated with a moderate increase in alanine transaminase and a minimal rise in alkaline phosphatase and occurred either following an early, marked and rapid increase in cyclosporine trough serum levels or a gradual increase in the cyclosporine trough serum concentration. Liver function abnormalities were completely reversible upon either reducing the dosage or discontinuing cyclosporine. LORBER et al. (1987), in a series of 466 renal transplant patients, similarly reported that cyclosporine-related liver injury was related to the trough serum levels and reversible following reduction in cyclosporine dose.

The histologic features of cyclosporine-related liver injury have been examined. WISECARVER et al. (1990) demonstrated that cyclosporine therapy in renal transplant recipients was associated with the presence of foamy material within the hepatic sinusoids, apoptosis, nonduct-directed portal inflammation and hypertrophy of bile duct epithelium. Ultrastructural abnormalities consisted of membrane-bound structures within the hepatic sinusoids that contained glycogen and small organelles and appeared to be derived from surrounding hepatocytes. Within hepatocytes, enlarged endoplasmic reticulum cysternae were noted. Abnormalities correlated with tissue levels of cyclosporine and its metabolites.

In liver transplant patients, cyclosporine-related liver injury was characterized by isometric vacuolization of the hepatocytes and endothelial cells, often accompanied by centrilobular fatty change and/or centrilobular necrosis (PALAZZI et al. 1993). The degree of isometric vacuolization correlated with trough blood levels of cyclosporine.

c) *Management and Prevention of Cyclosporine-Related Liver Injury*

In managing patients being treated with cyclosporine, it is critical to maintain plasma levels within therapeutic ranges to avoid liver injury. LAUPACIS et al. (1981) have suggested that cyclosporine-induced hyperbilirubinemia may occur when trough levels exceed 400 ng/ml and 2 h postdose blood levels exceed 1000 ng/ml. Cyclosporine is metabolized almost exclusively by the hepatic monooxygenase system, in particular, cytochrome P-450. Thus, drugs inhibiting this system, such as cimetidine, erythromycin and ketoconazole, will increase plasma levels of cyclosporine while inducers of cytochrome P-450, such as rifampicin, phenobarbitol and phenytoin, will result in decreased cyclosporin levels (COCKBURN and KRUPP 1989). In such circumstances, cyclosporine doses will need to be adjusted in order to maintain plasma levels within therapeutic ranges.

Alternative causes for liver injury in patients being treated with cyclosporine need to be considered. Liver transplant patients may develop hepatic dysfunction secondary to acute rejection, cholestasis, cholangitis, viral or bacterial infection or recurrence of the original disease requiring transplantation. Hepatic dysfunction in bone marrow transplant patients may occur secondary to graft versus host disease, hepatic veno-occlusive disease or infection of bacterial or viral origin.

Once cyclosporine-related liver injury has been diagnosed, adjustment in dosages is indicated. Potentially, cholestasis associated with the use of cyclosporine may respond to therapy with ursodeoxycholic acid (KALLINOWSKI et al. 1991).

5. FK-506

Currently undergoing clinical trials, FK-506 is an immunomodulating agent which, like cyclosporine, is believed to exert an immunomodulatory effect by virtue of its ability to bind and inhibit an immunophilin, in this case FK-binding protein. In preliminary studies, hepatotoxicity for this agent has been described in the cynomolgus monkey (WIJNEN et al. 1991) and rat (FARGHALI et al. 1991) while histologic changes, consisting of prominent perivenular hepatocellular dropout and necrosis, were seen in liver biopsies from liver transplant patients treated with FK-506 (HYTIROGLOU et al. 1993). Recently, the Japanese FK-506 study group has reported, in a series of 104 renal transplant patients, that therapy with FK-506 was associated with a frequency of hepatic dysfunction of 9.6% (Japanese FK506 Study Group 1994). As experience with this drug accumulates, the hepatotoxicity associated with its use will become clearer.

D. Conclusion

Immunomodulating agents are now used widely for treatment of a multitude of diseases, and are a common cause of hepatotoxicity. They cause four broad categories of liver injury: cytotoxic, cholestatic, steatotic and vascular. The clinical spectrum of disease associated with their use ranges from mild abnormalities of liver function tests in asymptomatic patients to severe hepatic necrosis and life-threatening liver failure.

In patients receiving immunomodulatory therapy, abnormal liver function tests are an indication for aggressive investigation which frequently will include liver biopsy. In the presence of persistently abnormal liver function tests or histologic abnormalities on liver biopsy, either reductrion of dose or discontinuation of potentially hepatotoxic immunomodulatory therapy is required.

Acknowledgements. This work was supported by a program project grant (PG 11810) from the Medical Research Council of Canada. R.J.F. is a recipient of a Medical Research Council of Canada Fellowship. We thank Ms. Charmaine Mohamed for her help in the preparation of this manuscript and Ms. Linda Wein BSc (Pharmacy) for her editorial assistance.

References

Adamson GM, Billings RE (1993) Cytokine toxicity and induction of NO synthase activity in cultured mouse hepatocytes. Toxicol Appl Pharmacol 119:100–107

Adler M, Delhaye M, Deprez C, Hardy N, Gelin M, De Pauw L, Vereerstraeten P (1987) Hepatic vascular disease after kidney transplantation: report of two cases and review of the literature. Nephrol Dial Transplant 2:183–188

Anderson TD, Hayes TJ, Gately MK, Bontempo JM, Stern LL, Truitt GA (1988) Toxicity of human recombinant interleukin-2 in the mouse is mediated by interleukin-activated lymphocytes. Lab Invest 59:598–612

Atkinson K, Biggs J, Dodds A, Concannon A (1983) Cyclosporine-associated hepatotoxicity after allogeneic marrow transplantation in man: differentiation from other causes of posttransplant liver disease. Transplant Proc 15:2761–2767

Bãckman L, Appelkvist E-L, Brunk U, Dallner G (1986) Influence of cyclosporin A treatment on intracellular membranes of hepatocytes. Exp Mol Pathol 45:31–43

Bãckman L, Appelkvist E-L, Ringdèn O, Dallner G (1988) Effects of cyclosporine A on hepatic protein synthesis. In: Kahan BD (ed) Cyclosporine: therapeutic use in transplantation. Grune and Stratton, Philadelphia, pp 853–858

Baxter JD, Forsham PH (1972) Tissue effects of glucocorticoids. Am J Med 53:573–589

Behrens TW, Goodwin JS (1988) Glucocorticosteroids. In: Bray MA, Marley J (eds) The Pharmacology of lymphocytes. Springer, Berlin Heidelberg New York, pp 425–439 (Handbook of experimental pharmacology, vol 85)

Belli LS, De Carlis L, Rondinara GF, Romani F, Alberti A, Pirotta V, Sansalone CV, Riolo F, Rossetti O, Slim OA, Aseni P, Ideo G, Belli L (1994) Prospective randomized trial of steroid withdrawal in liver transplant patients: preliminary report. Transplant Int 7 [Suppl 1]:S88–S90

Benigni A, Perico N, Ladny JR, Imberti O, Bellizzi L, Remuzzi G (1991) Increased urinary excretion of endothelin-1 and its precursor, big endothelin-1, in rats chronically treated with cyclosporine. Transplantation 52:175–177

Bluhm RE, Frazer MG, Vore M, Pinson CW, Badr KF (1993) Endothelins 1 and 3: potent cholestatic agents secreted and excreted by the liver that interact with cyclosporine. Hepatology 18:961–968

Borden EC (1992) Interferons: pleiotropic cellular modulators. Clin Immunol Immunopathol 62:S18–S24

Borel JF (1982) The history of cyclosporin A and its significance. In: White DJG (ed) Cyclosporin A: proceedings of an international conference on Cyclosporin A. Elsevier Biomedical, Amsterdam, pp 5–17

Bremnes RM, Slordal L, Wist E, Aarbakke J (1989) Dose-dependent pharmacokinetics of methotrexate and 7-hydroxymethotrexate in the rat in vivo. Cancer Res 49:6359–6364

Bremnes RM, Smeland E, Huseby N-E, Eide TJ, Aarbakke J (1991a) Acute hepatotoxicity after high-dose methotrexate administration to rats. Pharmacol Toxicol 69:132–139

Bremnes RM, Smeland E, Slordal L, Wist E, Aarbakke J (1991b) The effect of vindesine on methotrexate hydroxylation in the rat. Biochem Pharmacol 42:1561–1568

British Association for Paediatric Nephrology (1991) Levamisole for corticosteroid-dependent nephrotic syndrome in childhood. Lancet 337:1555–1557

Bry W, Warvariv V, Bohannon L, Feduska N, Straube B, Collins G, Levin B (1991) Cadaveric renal transplant without prophylactic prednisone therapy. Transplant Proc 23:994–996

Buffet C, Cantarovitch M, Pelletier G, Fabre M, Martin E, Charpentier B, Etienne JP, Fries D (1988) Three cases of nodular regenerative hyperplasia of the liver following renal transplantation. Nephrol Dial Transplant 3:327–330

Calne RJ, White DJG, Thiru S, Evans DB, McMaster P, Dunn DC, Craddock GN, Pentlow DB, Rolles K (1978) Cyclosporin A in patients receiving renal allografts from cadaver donors. Lancet II:1323–1327

Chan GLC, Canafax DM, Johnson CA (1987) The therapeutic use of azathioprine in renal transplantation. Pharmacotherapy 7:165–177

Clegg DO, Furst DE, Tolman KG, Pogue R (1989) Acute, reversible hepatic failure associated with methotrexate treatment of rheumatoid arthritis. J Rheumatol 16:1123–1126

Cockburn I, Gõtz E, Gũlich A, Krupp P (1988) An interim analysis of the on-going long-term safety study of cyclosporine in renal transplantation. In: Kahan BD (ed) Cyclosporine: therapeutic use in transplantation. Grune and Stratton, Philadelphia, pp 519–529

Cockburn ITR, Krupp P (1989) An appraisal of drug interactions with Sandimmun. Transplant Proc 21:3845–3850

Cohen JJ, Duke RC (1984) Glucocorticoid activation of a calcium-dependent endonuclease in thymocyte nuclei leads to cell death. J Immunol 132:38–42

Cooper C, Cotton DWK, Minihane N, Cawley MID (1986) Azathioprine hypersensitivity manifesting as acute focal hepatocellular necrosis. J R Soc Med 79:171–173

Dahl MGC, Gregory MM, Scheurer PJ (1971) Liver damage due to methotrexate in patients with psoriasis. Br Med J 1:625–630

Dahl MGC, Gregory MM, Scheurer PJ (1972) Methotrexate hepatotoxicity in psoriasis – comparison of different dose regimens. Br Med J 1:654–656

Davis GL (1990) Recombinant a-interferon treatment of non-A, non-B (type C) hepatitis: review of studies and recommendations for treatment. J Hepatol 11:S72–S77

Davis M, Eddleston ALWF, Williams R (1980) Hypersensitivity and jaundice due to azathioprine. Postgrad Med J 56:274–275

Degott C, Rueff B, Kreis H, Duboust A, Potet F, Benhamou JP (1978) Peliosis hepatis in recipients of renal transplants. Gut 19:748–753

DePinho RA, Goldberg CS, Lefkowitch JH (1984) Azathioprine and the liver: evidence favoring idiosyncratic, mixed cholestatic-hepatocellular injury in humans. Gastroenterology 86:162–165

Di Cyan E (1987) Steroid hormones and other steroidal synthetics. In: Weast RC, Astle MJ, Beyer WH (eds) CRC handbook of chemistry and physics. CRC Press, Boca Raton, pp C682–C698

Drews J (1990) Antibodies as immunopharmacological agents. In: Drews J (ed) Immunopharmacology. Springer, Berlin Heidelberg New York, pp 92–128

Durand JM, Kaplanski G, Portal I, Scheiner C, Berland Y, Soubeyrand J (1991) Liver failure due to recombinant alpha interferon. Lancet 338:1268–1269

Duvoux C, Kracht M, Lang P, Vernant J-P, Zafrani E-S, Dhumeaux D (1991) Hyperplasie nodulaire règènèrative du foie associèe á la prise d'azathioprine. Gastroenterol Clin Biol 15:968–973

Farghali H, Sakr M, Gasbarrini A, Venkataramanan R, Gavaler J, Starzl TE, Van Thiel DH (1991) Effect of FK-506 chronic administration on bromosulphthalein hepatic excretion in rats. Transplant Proc 23:2802–2804

Feutren G, von Graffenried B (1992) Cyclosporin A: pharmacology and therapeutic use in autoimmune disease. In: Rugstad HE, Endresen L, Forre O (eds) Immunopharmacology in autoimmune diseases and transplantation. Plenum, New York, pp 159–173

Fisher B, Keenan AM, Garra BS, Steinberg SM, White DE, DiBisceglie AM, Hoofnagle JH, Yolles P, Rosenberg SA, Lotze MT (1989) Interleukin-2 induces profound reversible cholestasis: a detailed analysis in treated cancer patients. J Clin Oncol 7:1852–1862

Fisher RI, Coltman CA, Doroshow JH, Raynor AA, Hawkins MJ, Mier JW, Wiernik P, McMannis JD, Weiss GR, Margolin KA, Gemlo BT, Hoth DF, Parkinson DR, Paietta E (1988) Metastatic renal cancer treated with interleukin-2 and lymphokine-activated killer cells: a phase II trial. Ann Intern Med 108:518–523

Flowers M, Sherker A, Sinclair SB, Greig PD, Cameron R, Phillips MJ, Blendis L, Chung SW, Levy GA (1994) Prostaglandin E in the treatment of recurrent hepatitis B infection after orthotopic liver transplantation. Transplantation 58:183–191

Galat A (1993) Peptidylproline cis-trans-isomerases: immunophilins. Eur J Biochem 216:689–707

Gately MK, Anderson TD, Hayes TJ (1988) Role of asialo-GM_1-positive cells in mediating the toxic effects of recombinant IL-2 in mice. J Immunol 141:189–200

Gerlag PGG, van Hooff JP (1987) Hepatic sinusoidal dilatation with portal hypertension during azathioprine treatment: a cause of chronic liver disease after kidney transplantation. Transplant Proc 19:3699–3703

Ghezzi P, Bianchi M, Gianera L, Landolfo S, Salmona M (1985) Role of reactive oxygen intermediates in the interferon-mediated depression of hepatic drug metabolism and protective effect of N-acetylcysteine in mice. Cancer Res 45:3444–3447

Gilbert SC, Klintmalm G, Menter A, Silverman A (1990) Methotrexate-induced cirrhosis requiring liver transplantation in three patients with psoriasis: a word of caution in light of expanding use of this "steroid sparing" agent. Arch Intern Med 150:889–891

Greig PD, Woolf GM, Sinclair SB, Abecassis M, Strasberg SM, Taylor BR, Blendis LM, Superina RA, Glynn MFX, Langer B, Levy GA (1989) Treatment of primary liver graft nonfunction with prostaglandin E_1. Transplantation 48:447–453

Gresser I, Tovey MG, Maury C, Chouroulinkov I (1975) Lethality of interferon preparations for newborn mice. Nature 258:76–78

Gresser I, Woodrow D, Moss J, Maury C, Tavernier J, Fiers W (1987) Toxic effects of recombinant tumor necrosis factor in suckling mice: comparisons with interferon α/β. Am J Pathol 128:13–18
Haboubi NY, Ali HA, Whitwell HL, Ackrill P (1988) Role of endothelial cell injury in the spectrum of azathioprine-induced liver disease after renal transplant: light microscopy and ultrastructural observations. Am J Gastroenterol 83:256–261
Hadden JW, Renoux G, Chirigos M (1990) The characterization of immunotherapeutic agents. In: Hadden JW, Szentivanyi A (eds) Immunopharmacology reviews, vol 1. Plenum, New York, pp 1–64
Hall PDeLa, Jenner MA, Ahern MJ (1991) Hepatotoxicity in a rat model caused by orally administered methotrexate. Hepatology 14:906–910
Hankey GJ, Saker BM (1987) Peliosis hepatis in a renal transplant recipient and in a hemodialysis patient. Med J Aust 146:102–104
Hill RB Jr (1961) Fatal fat embolism from steroid-induced fatty liver. N Engl J Med 265:318–320
Hill RB Jr, Droke WE, Hays AP (1965) Hepatic lipid metabolism in the cortisone-treated rat. Exp Mol Pathol 4:320–327
Hoofnagle JH (1990) α-Interferon therapy of chronic hepatitis B. Current status and recommendations. J Hepatol 11:S100–S107
Hutter RVP, Shipkey FH, Tan CTC, Murphy ML, Chowdhury M (1960) Hepatic fibrosis in children with acute leukemia: a complication of therapy. Cancer 13:288–307
Hytiroglou P, Lee R, Sharma K, Theise ND, Schwartz M, Miller C, Thung SN (1993) FK506 versus cyclosporine as primary immunosuppressive agent for orthotopic liver allograft recipients: histologic and immunopathologic observations. Transplantation 56:1389–1394
Iancu TC, Shiloh H, Dembo L (1986) Hepatomegaly following short-term high-dose steroid therapy. J Pediatr Gastroenterol Nutr 5:41–46
Ireland P, Rashid A, von Lichtenberg F, Cavallo T, Merrill JP (1973) Liver disease in kidney transplant patients receiving azathioprine. Arch Intern Med 132:29–37
Itoh S, Matsuo S, Shimoji K, Oda T, Sasaki I, Katayama I (1989) The effect of α-interferon on the liver in a patient with hairy cell leukemia: light and electron microscopic studies. Am J Gastroenterol 84:942–947
Japanese FK 506 Study Group (1994) Two year follow-up study of the efficacy and safety of FK 506 in kidney transplant patients. Transplant Int 7 [Suppl 1]:S247–S251
Jeanrenaud B (1967) Effect of glucocorticoid hormones on fatty acid mobilization and reesterification in rat adipose tissue. Biochem J 103:627–633
Jeurissen MEC, Boerbooms AMTH, Van de Putte LBA, Kruijsen MWM (1990) Azathioprine induced fever, chills, rash, and hepatotoxicity in rheumatoid arthritis. Ann Rheum Dis 49:25–27
Jolivet J, Cowan KH, Curt GA, Glendeninn NJ, Chabner BA (1983) The pharmacology and clinical use of methotrexate. N Engl J Med 309:1094–1104
Jones GJ, Itri LM (1986) Safety and tolerance of recombinant interferon alfa-2a (Roferon-A) in cancer patients. Cancer 57:1709–1715
Jones JP, Engleman EP, Najarian JS (1965) Systemic fat embolism after renal homotransplantation and treatment with corticosteroids. N Engl J Med 273:1453–1458
Jones MC, Best PV, Catto GRD (1988) Is nodular regenerative hyperplasia of the liver associated with azathioprine therapy after renal transplantation? Nephrol Dial Transplant 3:331–331
Kadmon M, Klünemann C, Böhme M, Ishikawa T, Gorgas K, Otto G, Herfarth C, Keppler D (1993) Inhibition by cyclosporin A of adenosine triphosphate-dependent transport from the hepatocyte into bile. Gastroenterology 104:1507–1514
Kahan BD (1989) Cyclosporine. N Engl J Med 321:1725–1738
Kalabis GM, Wells PG (1990) Biphasic modulation of acetaminophen bioactivation and hepatotoxicity by pretreatment with the interferon induced polyinosinic-polycytidylic acid. J Pharmacol Exp 255:1408–1419

Kallinowski B, Theilmann L, Zimmerman R, Gams E, Kommerell B, Stiehl A (1991) Effective treatment of cyclosporine-induced cholestasis in heart transplanted patients treated with ursodeoxycholic acid. Transplantation 51:1128

Katzka DA, Saul SH, Jorkasky D, Sigal H, Reynolds JC, Soloway RD (1986) Azathioprine and hepatic venoocclusive disease in renal transplant patients. Gastroenterology 90:446–454

Kellokumpu P, Iisalo E, Nordman E (1989) Hepatotoxicity of paracetamol in combination with interferon and vinblastine. Lancet I:1143

Kevat S, Ahern M, Hall P (1988) Hepatotoxicity of methotrexate in rheumatic diseases. Med Toxicol 3:197–208

Kirkham BW, Panayi GS (1992) Steroids. In: Rugstad HE, Endresen L, Forre O (eds) Immunopharmacology in autoimmune diseases and transplantation. Plenum, New York, pp 103–121

Kissel JT, Levy RJ, Mendell JR, Griggs RC (1986) Azathioprine toxicity in neuromuscular disease. Neurology 36:35–39

Kloke O, Wandl U, Opalka B, Moritz T, Nagel-Hiemke M, Franz T, Becher R, Hirche H, Seeber S, Niederle N (1992) A prospective randomized comparison of single-agent interferon (IFN)-alpha with the combination of IFN-alpha and low-dose IFN-gamma in chronic myelogenous leukemia. Eur J Haematol 48:93–98

Koene RAP (1992) Immunosuppression by T cell antibodies in renal transplantation. Nephron 61:383–392

Kon V, Sugiura M, Inagami T, Harvie BR, Ichikawa I, Hoover RL (1990) Role of endothelin in cyclosporine-induced glomerular dysfunction. Kidney Int 37:1487–1491

Krawitt EL (1994) Autoimmune hepatitis: classification, heterogeneity, and treatment. Am J Med 96 [Suppl 1A]:23S–26S

Kremer JM (1992) Liver biopsies in patients with rheumatoid arthritis receiving methotrexate: where are we going? J Rheumatol 19:189–191

Kremer JL, Alarcon GS, Lightfoot RW Jr, Willkens RF, Furst DE, Williams HJ, Dent PB, Weinblatt ME (1994) Methotrexate for rheumatoid arthritis: suggested guidelines for monitoring liver toxicity. Arthritis Rheum 37:316–328

Kujala GA, Shamma'a JM, Chang WL, Brick JE (1990) Hepatitis with bridging fibrosis and reversible hepatic insufficiency in a woman with rheumatoid arthritis taking methotrexate. Arthritis Rheum 33:1037–1041

Laupacis A, Keown PA, Ulan RA, Sinclair NR, Stiller CR (1981) Hyperbilirubinaemia and cyclosporin A levels. Lancet II:1426–1427

Lemley DE, Delacy LM, Seeff LB, Ishak KG, Nashel DJ (1989) Azathioprine induced hepatic veno-occlusive disease in rheumatoid arthritis. Ann Rheum Dis 48:342–346

Liaño F, Moreno A, Matesanz R, Teruel JL, Redondo C, Garcia-Martin F, Orte L, Ortunõ J (1989) Veno-occlusive hepatic disease of the liver in renal transplantation: is azathioprine the cause? Nephron 51:509–516

Lorber MI, Van Buren CT, Flechner SM, Williams C, Kahan BD (1987) Hepatobiliary and pancreatic complications of cyclopsorine therapy in 466 renal transplant recipients. Transplantation 43:35–40

Lorcerie B, Grobost O, Lalu-Fraisse A, Piard F, Camus P, Portier H, Martin F (1990) Peliose hepatique au cours d'une dermatomyosite traitee par azathioprine et corticoides. Rev Med Interne 11:25–28

Makowka L, Cramer DV (1992) Brequinar sodium: a new immunosuppressive drug for transplantation. Transplant Sci 2:50–54

Mannering GJ, Deloria LB (1986) The pharmacology and toxicology of the interferons: an overview. Annu Rev Pharmacol Toxicol 26:455–515

Mannering GJ, Renton KW, el Azhary R, Deloria LB (1980) Effects of interferon-inducing agents on hepatic cytochrome P-450 drug metabolizing systems. Ann NY Acad Sci 350:314–331

Mannering GJ, Deloria LB, Abbott V (1988) Role of xanthine oxidase in the interferon-mediated depression of the hepatic cytochrome P-450 system in mice. Cancer Res 48:2107–2112

Matory YL, Chang AE, Lipford III EH, Braziel R, Hyatt CL, McDonald HD, Rosenberg SA (1985) Toxicity of human recombinant interleukin-2 in rats following intravenous infusion. J Biol Respir Modif 4:377–390

Meys E, Devogelaer J-P, Geubel A, Rahier J, Nagant de Deuxchaisnes C (1992) Fever, hepatitis and acute interstitial nephritis in a patient with rheumatoid arthritis. Concurrent manifestations of azathioprine hypersensitivity. J Rheumatol 19:807–809

Mion F, Napoleon B, Berger F, Chevallier M, Bonvoisin S, Descos L (1991) Azathioprine induced liver disease: nodular regenerative hyperplasia of the liver and perivenous fibrosis in a patient treated for multiple sclerosis. Gut 32:715–717

Newman M, Auerbach R, Feiner H, Holzman RS, Shupack J, Migdal P, Culubret M, Camuto P, Tobias H (1989) The role of liver biopsies in psoriatic patients receiving long-term methotrexate treatment: improvement in liver abnormalities after cessation of treatment. Arch Dermatol 125:1218–1224

Nicchitta CV, Kamoun M, Williamson JR (1985) Cyclosporine augments receptor-mediated cellular Ca^{2+} fluxes in isolated hepatocytes. J Biol Chem 260:13613–13618

Nyfors A, Poulsen H (1976) Liver biopsies from psoriatics related to methotrexate therapy: findings in 123 consecutive non-methotrexate treated patients. Acta Pathol Microbiol Scand [A] 84:253–261

Olsen TS, Fjeldborg O, Hansen HE (1991) Portal hypertension without liver cirrhosis in renal transplant recipients. APMIS [Suppl] 23:13–20

Palazzi P, Parenti M, Rivolta R, Lucianetti A, Romito R, Gridelli B (1993) Fine-needle aspiration biopsy and hepatotoxicity of cyclosporin A in orthotopic liver transplantation. In: Galmarini D, Fassati LR, Paoletti R, Sherlock S (eds) Drugs and the liver: high risk patients and transplantation. Kluwer Academic/Fondazone Giovanni Lorenzini, Dordrecht, pp 171–176

Papo T, Marcellin P, Bernuau J, Durand F, Poynard T, Benhamou JP (1992) Autoimmune chronic active hepatitis exacerbated by interferon-alpha. Ann Intern Med 116:51–53

Parkinson DR, Abrams JS, Wiernik PH, Rayner AA, Margolin KA, Van Echo DA, Sznol M, Dutcher JP, Aronson FR, Doroshow JH, Atkins MB, Hawkins MJ (1990a) Interleukin-2 therapy in patients with metastatic malignant melanoma: phase II study. J Clin Oncol 8:1650–1656

Parkinson DR, Fisher RI, Rayner AA, Paietta E, Margolin KA, Weiss GR, Mier JW, Sznol M, Gaynor ER, Bar MH, Gucalp R, Boldt DH, Mills B, Hawkins MJ (1990b) Therapy of renal cell carcinoma with interleukin-2 and lymphokine-activated killer cells: phase II experience with a hybrid bolus and continuous infusion interleukin-2 regimen. J Clin Oncol 8:1630–1636

Pessayre D (1992) Drug-induced liver disease. In: Prieto J, Rodés J, Shafritz DA (eds) Hepatobiliary diseases. Springer, Berlin Heidelberg New York, pp 697–728

Pestka S, Langer JA, Zoon KC, Samuel CE (1987) Interferons and their actions. Annu Rev Biochem 56:727–777

Phillips CA, Cera PJ, Mangan TF, Newman ED (1992) Clinical liver disease in patients with rheumatoid arthritis taking methotrexate. J Rheumatol 19:229–233

Powles RL, Barrett AJ, Clink H, Kay HEM, Sloane J, McElwain TJ (1978) Cyclosporin A for the treatment of graft-versus-host disease in man. Lancet II:1327–1331

Price GD, Olsen SL, Taylor DO, O'Connel JB, Bristow MR, Renlund DG (1992) Corticosteroid free maintenance immunosuppression after heart transplantation: feasibility and beneficial effects. J Heart Lung Transplant 11:403–414

Punt CJA, Henzen-Logmans SC, Bolhuis RLH, Stoter G (1990) Hyperbilirubinaemia in patients treated with recombinant human interleukin-2 (rIL-2). Br J Cancer 61:491

Quesada JR, Gutterman JU (1983) Clinical study of recombinant DNA-produced leukocyte interferon (clone A) in an intermittent schedule in cancer patients. J Natl Cancer Inst 70:1041–1046

Quesada JR, Talpaz M, Rios A, Kuzrock R, Gutterman JU (1986) Clinical toxicity of interferons in cancer patients: a review. J Clin Oncol 43:234–245
Read AE, Wiesner RH, LaBrecque DR, Tifft JG, Mullen KD, Sheer RL, Petrelli M, Ricanati ES, McCullough AJ (1986) Hepatic veno-occlusive disease associated with renal transplantation and azathioprine therapy. Ann Intern Med 104:651–655
Reynolds FS, Lee WM (1986) Hepatotoxicity after long-term methotrexate therapy. South Med J 79:536–539
Roegnigk HH Jr, Auerbach R, Maibach HI, Weinstein GD (1982) Methotrexate guidelines: revised. J Am Acad Dermatol 6:145–155
Roegnigk HH Jr, Auerbach R, Maibach HI, Weinstein GD (1988) Methotrexate in psoriasis: revised guidelines. J Am Acad Dermatol 19:145–155
Roman ID, Monte MJ, Gonzalez-Buitrago JM, Esteller A, Jiminez R (1990) Inhibition of hepatocytary vesicular transport by cyclosporin A in the rat: relationship with cholestasis and hyperbilirubinemia. Hepatology 12:83–91
Rosenberg SA, Lotze MT (1986) Cancer immunotherapy using interleukin-2 and interleukin-2-activated lymphocytes. Annu Rev Immunol 4:681–709
Rosenberg SA, Lotze MT, Yang JC, Topalian SL, Chang AE, Schwartzentruber DJ, Aebersold P, Leitman S, Linehan WM, Seipp CA, White DE, Steinberg SM (1993) Prospective randomized trial of high-dose interleukin-2 alone or in conjunction with lymphokine-activated killer cells for the treatment of patients with advanced cancer. J Natl Cancer Inst 85:622–632
Rosenstein M, Ettinghausen SE, Rosenberg SA (1986) Extravasation of intravascular fluid mediated by systemic administration of recombinant interleukin 2. J Immunol 137:1735–1742
Schreiber SL, Crabtree GR (1992) The mechanism of action of cyclosporin A and FK506. Immunol Today 13:136–142
Shergy WJ, Polisson RP, Caldwell DS, Rice JR, Pisetsky DS, Allen NB (1988) Methotrexate-associated hepatotoxicity: retrospective analysis of 210 patients with rheumatoid arthritits. Am J Med 85:771–774
Sherlock S (1986) The spectrum of hepatotoxicity due to drugs. Lancet II:440–444
Shevach EM (1985) The effects of cyclosporin A on the immune system. Annu Rev Immunol 3:397–423
Silva MO, Reddy KR, Jeffers LJ, Hill M, Schiff ER (1991) Interferon-induced chronic active hepatitis. Gastroenterology 101:840–842
Sinclair SB, Greig PD, Blendis LM, Abecassis M, Roberts EA, Phillips MJ, Cameron R, Levy GA (1989) Biochemical and clinical response of fulminant viral hepatitis to administration of prostaglandin E: a preliminary report. J Clin Invest 84:1063–1069
Sinclair S, Levy G (1990) Eicosanoids and the liver. Ital J Gastroenterol 22:205–213
Slapak M, Dihgard N, Wise M, Setakis N (1991) Triple therapy. Transplant Proc 23:2186–2188
Sparberg M, Simon N, Del Greco F (1969) Intrahepatic cholestasis due to azathioprine. Gastroenterology 57:439–441
Stanley LA, Adams DJ, Balkwill FR, Griffin D, Wolf CR (1991) Differential effects of recombinant interferon α on constitutive and inducible cytochrome P450 isozymes in mouse liver. Biochem Pharmacol 42:311–320
Starzl TE, Weil R, Iwatsuki S, Klintmalm G, Schroter GPJ, Koep LJ, Iwaki T, Terasaki PI, Porter KA (1980) The use of cyclosporin A and prednisone in cadaver kidney transplantation. Surg Gynecol Obstet 151:17–26
Steinberg H, Webb WM, Rafsky HA (1952) Hepatomegaly with fatty infiltration secondary to cortisone therapy: case report. Gastroenterology 21:304–309
Sterneck M, Wiesner R, Ascher N, Roberts J, Ferrell L, Ludwig J, Lake J (1991) Azathioprine hepatotoxicity after liver transplantation. Hepatology 14:806–810
Stevenson HC, Green I, Hamilton JM, Calabro BA, Parkinson DR (1991) Levamisole: known effects on the immune system, clinical results, and future applications to the treatment of cancer. J Clin Oncol 9:2052–2066

Stone B, Udani M, Sanghvi A, Warty V, Plocki K, Bedetti CD, Van Thiel D (1987) Cyclosporin A-induced cholestasis: the mechanism in a rat model. Gastroenterology 93:344–351

Stone B, Warty V, Dindzans V, Van Thiel D (1988) The mechanism of cyclosporine-induced cholestasis in the rat. In: Kahan BD (ed) Cyclosporine: therapeutic use in transplantation. Grune and Stratton, Philadelphia, pp 841–844

Strom TB (1992) Molecular immunology and immunopharmacology of allograft rejection. Kidney Int 42 [Suppl 38]:S182–S187

Thomson AW, Woo J, Cooper M (1992) Mode of action of immunosuppressive drugs with particular reference to the molecular basis of macrolide-induced immunosuppression. In: Thomson AW (ed) The molecular biology of immunosuppression. Wiley, New York, pp 154–179

Tuma DJ, Barak AJ, Sorrell MF (1975) Interaction of methotrexate with lipotropic factors in rat liver. Biochem Pharmacol 24:1327–1331

Vento S, Di Perri G, Garofano T, Dosco L, Concia E, Ferraro T, Bassetti D (1989) Hazards of interferon therapy for HBV-seronegative chronic hepatitis. Lancet II:926

Wald JA, Farr RS (1991) Abnormal liver-function rests associated with long-term systemic corticosteroid use in subjects with asthma. J Allergy Clin Immunol 88:277–278

Walker AM, Funch D, Dreyer NA, Tolman KG, Kremer JM, Alarcon GS, Lee RG, Weinblatt ME (1993) Determinants of serious liver disease among patients receiving low-dose methotrexate for rheumatoid arthritis. Arthritis Rheum 36:329–335

Wandl UB, Kloke O, Niederle N (1992) Liver failure due to recombinant alpha interferon for chronic myelogenous leukaemia. Lancet 339:123–124

Whiting-O'Keefe QE, Fye KH, Sack KD (1991) Methotrexate and histologic hepatic abnormalities: a meta-analysis. Am J Med 90:711–716

Wijnen RMH, Ericzon BG, Tiebosch ATGM, Beysens AJ, Groth CG, Kootstra G (1991) Toxicity of FK 506 in the cynomolgus monkey: noncorrelation with FK 506 serum levels. Transplant Proc 23:3101–3104

Wisecarver JL, Earl R, Haven M, Timmons P, Markin R (1990) Histological manifestations of cyclosporine therapy in liver allografts (abstract). Am J Clin Pathol 93:436

Wolberg G (1988) Antipurines and purine metabolism. In: Bray MA, Marley J (eds) The pharmacology of lymphocytes. Springer, Berlin Heidelberg New York, pp 517–533 (Handbook of experimental pharmacology, vol 85)

Wong RL, Winslow CM, Cooper KD (1993) The mechanisms of action of cyclosporin A in the treatment of psoriasis. Immunol Today 14:69–74

Xerri L, Payan MJ, Choux R, Gros N, Hassoun J, Chamlian A, Blin D, Monties JR (1989) An exceptional 18-year follow-up after cardiac transplantation. How can malignancies occur during immunosuppressive therapy? Cancer 63:1697–1699

Zarday Z, Veith FJ, Gliedman ML, Soberman R (1972) Irreversible liver damage after azathioprine. JAMA 222:690–691

Zimmerman HJ (1978) Antineoplastic agents. In: Zimmerman HJ (ed) Hepatoxicity: the adverse effects of drugs and other chemicals on the liver. Appleton-Century-Crofts, New York, pp 523–543

Zwingelstein G, Meister R, Malak NA, Maury C, Gresser I (1985) Interferon alters the composition and metabolism of lipids in the liver of suckling mice. J Interferon Res 5:315–325

CHAPTER 25

Alcohol-Induced Liver Injury

Y. Israel and E. Rubin

A. Epidemiology

The prevalence of cirrhosis in population correlates well with per capita consumption of ethanol, regardless of the type of beverage consumed (Grant et al. 1988; Parrish et al. 1991). Moreover, it has been shown that the risk of developing cirrhosis increases with the total amount of ethanol consumed over a lifetime (Lelbach 1974, 1975). An individual who consumes about 200 g ethanol (about 20 oz of 86 proof whisky) a day for 20 years has a 50% chance of manifesting cirrhosis (Lelbach 1974, 1975).

Since the half-life of liver cell constituents is in the range of minutes to months, rather than in decades, it is necessary to postulate that alcoholic liver cirrhosis follows the alteration of several processes in series, each with a long half-life. Alternatively, that the continuous exposure to alcohol renders hepatotoxic a randomly occurring factor that is otherwise innocuous. Such a secondary factor could be present at different times in the life of an individual. The combination of the two above mechanisms is also conceivable.

To facilitate the analysis of data, we will differentiate between morphological changes (injury or lesion) and functional changes (alcoholic liver disease or dysfunction) induced by ethanol. The term "dysfunction" is used to imply a physiological change associated with an increased risk of mortality.

Supporting the concept that a secondary factor is required for the production of liver dysfunction are studies showing that following wine rationing in France during World War II cirrhosis mortality was reduced by 60% in only 1 year (Pequinot and Cyrulnik 1970). By the 2 year, cirrhosis mortality had been reduced by 75%. These data indicate that the irreversible alterations seen in liver morphology do not always translate into liver dysfunction leading to death. These irreversible alterations may, nevertheless, increase the pathogenicity of a secondary factor; after discontinuation of wine rationing, cirrhosis mortality increased by 60% in 1 year. Thus, the combination of the two types of mechanisms indicated above is likely to occur.

This chapter initially provides an overview of (a) the pathophysiological and (b) the morphological changes that occur in alcoholic liver disease in humans. Animal models of alcoholic liver injury and mechanisms are subsequently discussed in detail.

B. Liver Dysfunction in Alcoholic Liver Disease

Patients with alcoholic liver disease die of two main causes: (a) hemodynamic problems and (b) hepatic failure; in most cases, these two factors reinforce each other.

I. Hemodynamic Alterations

Mortality related to hemodynamic dysfunction derives principally from portal hypertension (see REYNOLDS 1975; GROSZMANN et al. 1988), a condition in which intrahepatic resistance to portal blood flow is markedly increased. An increased portal pressure is one of the mechanisms responsible for the accumulation of ascitic fluid in the peritoneal cavity of the alcoholic liver disease patient. At high portal pressures, blood flows through collateral pathways which return the portal blood to the systemic circulation, thereby bypassing the liver. Increased blood flow through these pathways leads to the enlargement of collateral vessels, especially the lower esophageal and gastric coronary veins. The resulting collaterals have a tendency to rupture, causing death by exsanguination. An important consequence of collateral circulation is a reduction in the clearance of toxins of bacterial origin, such as endotoxin, produced in the gut (see RUBIN and FARBER 1994).

Portal hypertension in alcoholic cirrhosis has been attributed to an increased resistance to blood flow of either sinusoidal or of postsinusoidal origin (REYNOLDS 1975; GROSZMANN et al. 1988). Whereas the former mechanism should be accompanied by sinusoidal compression, the latter is expected to result in an increased (or normal) sinusoidal caliber, for example, in conditions in which the diameter of the terminal hepatic venule is reduced, backing-up sinusoidal flow. Unlike the observation in cirrhosis of nonalcoholic etiology, in which sinusoidal caliber is generally normal, in alcoholic liver disease the size of the sinusoid is markedly reduced, on average by about 80% (VIDINS et al. 1985). Under these circumstances, sinusoids appear to become resistance vessels (VIDINS et al. 1985). It is now clear that the main site of regulation of blood flow through the liver resides in the sinusoid itself (see MCCUSKEY and REILLY 1993).

A marked increase in hepatocyte volume has been associated with a reduced sinusoidal caliber and an increased intrahepatic and portal pressure (ISRAEL et al. 1982b; BLENDIS et al. 1982; VIDINS et al. 1985). While increases in hepatocyte volume are seen in patients with alcoholic hepatitis, the largest increases are found in patients presenting cirrhosis, in agreement with the general knowledge that portal hypertension is mainly seen in cirrhotics. In alcoholic cirrhotics presenting intrahepatic pressures above 30 mmHg (which correlates with portal and wedge pressures with r values exceeding 0.9; VIDINS et al. 1985), mean hepatocyte cross-section is two- to threefold larger than that in patients with normal portal pressures, below 10 mmHg (BLENDIS et al. 1982). Alcoholic cirrhotics with normal portal pressures have small hepatocytes (BLENDIS et al. 1982).

A role for hepatocyte volume expansion in portal hypertension in alcoholic cirrhosis is further suggested by the observation that marked reductions in portal pressure are observed in cirrhotics following a few weeks of alcohol withdrawal and hospitalization (REYNOLDS et al. 1960). Although there are no studies on the half-life of collagen in alcoholic cirrhosis in humans, in rats the half-life of collagen in carbon tetrachloride induced cirrhosis in the rat is of the order of 1 year (HUTTERER et al. 1970), compared to the half-life of alcohol-induced hepatomegaly of 1 week (ISRAEL and ORREGO 1981).

Recent studies have suggested that swelling of Kupffer cells and endothelial cells may also lead to the narrowing of the sinusoidal lumen, primarily in conditions of endotoxemia (MCCUSKEY and REILLY 1993).

II. Liver Failure

In liver failure, hepatic encephalopathy is characterized by the progressive loss of cognitive function leading to coma. In such a condition the liver is unable to detoxify a number of noxious substances generated by normal physiological processes, such as ammonia, and toxic products generated by the intestinal flora which subsequently affect brain function (see RUBIN and FARBER 1994). Associated with this condition are reduced levels of serum albumin and prothrombin (and other clotting factors) which are produced exclusively by the liver (see ORREGO et al. 1981b, 1985). Low albumin levels reduce plasma oncotic pressure, contributing to edema and aggravating ascites; while a low prothrombin level increases the clotting time and contributes to hemorrhage. Liver dysfunction is also apparent in number of other hepatic functions; the liver also fails to transport, conjugate and excrete bilirubin, which accumulates in the circulation, seen externally as jaundice (RUBIN and FARBER 1994). Abnormalities in the levels of albumin, prothrombin and bilirubin have the highest prognostic value in relation to mortality in alcoholic liver disease (ORREGO et al. 1983, 1985). Minor increases in serum transaminases, indicative of focal cell necrosis, are observed but their prognostic value in relation to mortality is low (ORREGO et al. 1983).

A number of studies have shown that the cytokines tumor necrosis-α, interleukin-1 and interleukin-6, generated by monocyte/macrophages, are greatly elevated – often up to tenfold – in the plasma of patients with alcoholic hepatitis and cirrhosis (MCCLAIN et al. 1993; FELVER et al. 1990; BIRD et al. 1990; DEVIVERE et al. 1990; KHORUTS et al. 1991). The levels of plasma tumor necrosis factor-α were found to correlate highly with mortality (FELVER et al. 1990; BIRD et al. 1990; SHERON et al. 1991). Tumor necrosis factor is a potent inducer of the synthesis of interleukin-1 and interleukin-6 and is also an autocrine inducer of its own production (DECKER 1990; GRILLI et al. 1993). While tumor necrosis factor-α is produced almost exclusively by monocytes/ macrophage, interleukin-1 and interleukin-6 are generated by a number of cell types, including monocyte/macrophages (DECKTER 1990; ANDUS et al. 1991). Tumor necrosis factor, interleukin-1 and interleukin-6 may be responsible for a number of the clinical manifestations of alcoholic hepatitis, such as muscle wasting, hypermetabolism, fever, anorexia, neutrophilia, decreased albumin and decreased bile flow/cholestasis (see MCCLAIN et al. 1993).

The mechanism of hepatotoxicity of cytokines released by monocytes and tissue macrophages (in the liver, Kupffer cells) is not clear. Low levels of tumor necrosis factor-α are actually required for cell proliferation (AKERMAN et al. 1992). However, a number of studies indicate that, when greatly elevated, tumor necrosis factor-α is a major mediator in experimentally induced hepatotoxicity. Administration of antitumor necrosis factor-α antibodies markedly inhibits liver damage induced by endotoxin (NAGAKAWA et al. 1990) and by ischemia reperfusion (COLETTI et al. 1990). While the administration of tumor necrosis per se does not induce liver damage, it markedly increases the hepatotoxicity induced by very small doses of galactosamine (TIEGS et al. 1989). Depletion of Kupffer cells virtually suppressed the liver injury induced by carbon tetrachloride (EDWARDS et al. 1993), acetaminophen (LASKIN et al. 1995), endotoxin (BAUTISTA et al. 1994) and chronic ethanol administration (ADACHI et al. 1994). Kupffer cell activation appears also to play a role in liver failure following cold storage prior to transplantation (LINDELL et al. 1994).

Peripheral blood moncoytes of patients with alcoholic liver disease generate tumor necrosis factor-α, interleukin-1 and interleukin-6 at rates that are three to six times those of monocytes from controls (MCCLAIN and COHEN 1989; DEVIERE et al. 1990). They also display markedly increased lipopolysaccharide-induced release of tumor necrosis factor when compared to monocytes of control subjects (MCCLAIN and COHEN 1989). Endotoxin and its active lipopolysaccharide moiety are produced by gram-negative bacteria, often present in the gastrointestinal tract. Endotoxin is one of the most powerful activators of cytokine production by monocyte/macrophages (DECKER 1990).

Increases in plasma endotoxin have been reported to occur in 50%–90% of patients with alcoholic hepatitis and cirrhosis (BODE et al. 1987; BIGATELLO et al. 1987; KHORUTS et al. 1991). Other studies, while confirming marked increases in plasma tumor necrosis factor-α and interleukin-6 in alcoholic hepatitis, observed that these did not correlate with endotoxemia (BIRD et al. 1990; KHORUTS et al. 1991; SHERON et al. 1991). Nevertheless, increases in circulating endotoxin due to blood shunting, bacterial sepsis or increased absorption from the gastrointestinal tract would potentiate other mechanisms which increase the production of cytokines (see below).

A good correlation between plasma interleukin-6 levels and mortality has also been reported (KHORUTS et al. 1991; SHERON et al. 1991). Interleukin-6 normalized in parallel with clinical recovery. However, the levels of tumor necrosis factor-α and of interleukin-6 were not significantly correlated. Interleukin-6, generated by many cell types, is cleared from the plasma by the liver (CASTELL et al. 1988). Thus, increases in interleukin-6 generation would be potentiated by the liver dysfunction per se, and might rather be indicative of the terminal disease stages (see SHERON et al. 1991; KHORUTS et al. 1991). Recent studies also indicate that plasma interleukin-8, a cytokine which induces neutrophil chemotaxis and neutrophil respiratory burst, is also markedly increased in alcoholic hepatitis (HILL et al. 1993). Interleukin-8 production by hepatocytes is also stimulated by tumor necrosis factor-α (THORNTON et al. 1992).

C. Alcoholic Liver Injury: Morphological Studies

The literature in this field traditionally divides the hepatic lesion(s) induced by chronic alcohol consumption into three types: (a) fatty liver, (b) alcoholic hepatitis and (c) cirrhosis (RUBIN and FARBER 1994), although all these alterations may coexist. While this classification system has provided the pathologist with a standard nomenclature to communicate with the clinician, for the scientist interested in the pathogenesis of alcoholic liver disease it may give an exaggerated notion of simplicity. For example, cirrhosis, which is generally considered as the most severe lesion, can also exist in a form that is clinically silent (HALLEN and NORDEN 1964; LUDWIG et al. 1970; BRUGUERA et al. 1977; RANKIN et al. 1978). The prognosis of inactive cirrhosis (i.e., the absence of necrosis and inflammation) in the relation to mortality is not different from that of fatty liver (ORREGO et al. 1987). On the other hand, alcoholic hepatitis, in the absence of cirrhosis, carries a substantial mortality (LISCHNER et al. 1971; ORREGO et al. 1987).

While an experimental pathologist would prefer to develop, in an animal model, a lesion that reproduces all the morphological abnormalities seen in humans, whether such is necessary to understand hepatic dysfunction is, however, not clear. In consideration of the above, we initially describe the different morphological abnormalities in alcoholic liver injury in humans without clustering these into the three classical categories. The morphological changes accompanying alcoholic liver disease have been covered extensively (CHEDID et al. 1991; FRENCH et al. 1993b; RUBIN and FARBER 1994; LIEBER 1994). Clustering is discussed subsequently; in this regard the reader is referred to the work of the INTERNATIONAL GROUP REVIEW (1981) and to RUBIN and FARBER (1994).

I. Hepatocytes

Fat accumulation in hepatocytes is initially seen in small droplets that can coalesce forming large droplets. Hepatocyte enlargement, or cell ballooning, is prominent. In some cases hepatocyte cross-section is doubled or tripled. As will be discussed further, hepatocyte ballooning and fat accumulation are not synonymous. Hepatocyte necrosis, when present, is focal, mainly involving one to three hepatocytes, and is observed almost exclusively in the vicinity of the terminal hepatic venule. Mallory bodies, eosinophilic inclusions of intermediate filaments, can be observed but they do not always accompany necrosis. By electron microscopy, additional changes observed are enlarged mitochondria with a reduction in mitochondrial cristae, and a marked proliferation of smooth endoplasmic reticulum.

II. Inflammation

Neutrophil (polymorphonuclear leukocyte) infiltration is seen in apposition with necrotic cells and in some cases with cells containing Mallory bodies. Neutrophil infiltration, the hallmark of the alcoholic liver lesion, is seen primarily around the terminal hepatic veins. Limited mononuclear leukocytic infiltration can also be observed in later stages of the disease, involving the portal tracts and extending to several areas of the lobule.

III. Collagen Deposition

Collagen fibrils are initially seen surrounding the terminal hepatic veins (central vein sclerosis). In extreme cases, collagen deposition markedly reduces the caliber of the vessel. This lesion has been proposed to precede the generalized formation of collagenous septa. In later stages, such septa link portal hepatic venules with terminal hepatic venules forming nodules. In severe fibrosis and cirrhosis, a band of collagen can be seen by electron microscopy (EM) in the space of Disse, where if forms a basal membrane (capillarization).

IV. Nonparenchymal Cells (EM Studies)

1. Ito Cells

Alterations in Ito cells (also referred to as fat-storing cells, hepatic lipocytes or perisinusoidal stellate cells) have also been shown. In alcoholic liver injury, these cells display a marked reduction in the number of lipid droplets and an increase in endoplasmic reticulum. The term transitional cells has been used to refer to these cells which acquire myofibroblast-like phenotypic characteristics. Collagen fibrils are often found in the extracellular matrix around transitional Ito cells. Intracellular collagen fibrils are sometimes observed.

2. Endothelial Cells

A reduction in fenestration is seen in alcoholic liver injury, often associated with collagen deposition in the space of Disse. However, alterations in fenestral morphology have also been observed following ethanol in rat models in which collagen deposition does not develop.

3. Kupffer Cells

Data on the morphology of the Kupffer cell, the resident hepatic macrophage, are surprisingly scarce, and contrast with the relevance of Kupffer cell action in the production of hepatocellular necrosis and fibrosis in several models of alcoholic, drug and ischemic liver injury (see below).

D. Clustering

The reader is referred to RUBIN and FARBER (1994) and to the work of the INTERNATIONAL REVIEW GROUP (1981).

I. Fatty Liver

The most conspicuous morphological changes in this condition is the accumulation of fat in droplets, which can coalesce, and cell ballooning. Most pathologists will accept the presence of minor fibrosis, primarily in the terminal hepatic vein area. However, necrosis, inflammation and Mallory bodies and fibrous septa must be absent. (Enlarged mitochondria and increased endoplasmic reticulum are observed by EM in this condition).

II. Alcoholic Hepatitis

Alcoholic hepatitis is characterized by (a) necrosis of hepatocytes predominantly around the terminal hepatic venule; (b) neutrophil inflammation mainly in the areas of necrosis and around hepatocytes presenting Mallory bodies; (c) perivenular fibrosis, which in severe cases may obliterate some of the terminal hepatic venules; and (d) Mallory bodies. The presence of Mallory bodies is not required for the diagnosis of alcoholic hepatitis, but the diagnosis is strengthened by this abnormality. By EM, transformed Ito cells are observed and collagen fibrils appear in the space of Disse and in apposition with transformed Ito cells.

III. Alcoholic Cirrhosis

Cirrhosis is defined as a "diffuse process characterized by fibrosis and a conversion of normal architecture into structurally abnormal nodules." The hallmark of cirrhosis is the existence of fibrous septa surrounding hepatocellular nodules. The diagnosis of cirrhosis does not require necrosis, inflammation, Mallory bodies or hepatocellular regeneration. Some investigators have used the term "inactive cirrhosis" to describe the condition in which these other abnormalities are absent. Nevertheless, necrosis, inflammation, hepatocyte ballooning and fat accumulation usually coexist with cirrhosis.

E. Pathogenesis of Alcohol-Induced Liver Injury

I. Liquid Diet Model

Lieber and coworkers (LIEBER et al. 1989, 1994) developed a semisynthetic liquid diet that contained approximately 5% alcohol and provided 36% of calories as ethanol. The diet provided adequate levels of proteins, fat and carbohydrates to maintain growth and was nutritionally balanced in terms of vitamins, salts and lipotropic agents. The liquid diet overcomes the natural aversion of rats to consume large amounts of alcohol. Control animals are pair-fed this diet, where alcohol was replaced isocalorically by carbohydrates, and display normal hepatic histology. In the rat, this model showed the production of fatty liver, limited hepatocyte ballooning, increased endoplasmic reticulum and mitochondrial enlargement. Animals fed alcohol chronically with this diet also demonstrate increased rates of ethanol metabolism (metabolic tolerance). However, no necrosis, inflammation or fibrosis develop in this rat model.

The liquid diet model contributed most importantly to the demonstration that fatty liver induced by ethanol is not caused by a nutritional deficiency but rather by a direct effect of ethanol (LIEBER 1994). Upon chronic ethanol administration fat, mainly in the form of triglycerides, accumulates in the hepatocytes. Several mechanisms may be involved in the generation of alcoholic fatty liver. In the presence of ethanol, mitochondria oxidizes mainly the NADH generated in the metabolism of ethanol by alcohol dehydrogenase. The alcohol dehydrogenase pathway is, quantitatively, the most important pathway in the oxidation of ethanol (LIEBER et al. 1994).

$$CH_3\text{-}CH_2OH + NAD^+ \rightarrow CH_3\text{-}CHO + NADH$$
(alcohol dehydrogenase: cytosol)

$$NADH + O_2 \rightarrow NAD^+ + H_2O$$ (respiratory chain: mitochondria)

The mitochondrial oxidation of fatty acids is markedly reduced in the presence of ethanol, leading to fat accumulation. Most of the triglycerides that accumulate following the chronic administration of ethanol are of dietary origin. Other factors contributing to fat accumulation are an increased esterification of fatty acids into triglycerides and a reduced secretion of triglycerides, in the form of lipoproteins, from the hepatocyte (see LIEBER 1994).

II. Cytochrome P450 2E1

The liquid diet model also allowed investigators to understand the relevance of the increased endoplasmic reticulum (RUBIN et al. 1968) and cytochrome P450 2E1 levels (LIEBER and DECARLI 1970; OHNISHI and LIEBER 1977; KOOP et al. 1982) following chronic ethanol administration. Ethanol was found to be a substrate for the microsomal cytochrome P450 2E1 system (LIEBER and DECARLI 1970; TESCHKE et al. 1972):

$$CH_3\text{-}CH_2OH + NADPH + O_2 \rightarrow CH3\text{-}CHO + NADP^+$$
(endoplasmic reticulum)

Acetaldehyde, generated both via alcohol dehydrogenase and by the cytochrome P450 2E1 system, is metabolized into acetate mainly by a low K_m

mitochondrial acetaldehyde dehydrogenase (TIPTON 1985; SVANAS and WEINER 1985; CAO et al. 1988).

$$CH3\text{-}CHO + NAD + \rightarrow CH3\text{-}COOH + NADH \text{ (mitochondria)}$$

Most of the acetate produced from ethanol in the liver is metabolized extrahepatically (LUNDQUIST et al. 1962).

Ethanol was shown to posttranslationally increase cytochrome P450 2E1 levels by inhibiting its degradation (ELIASSON et al. 1988; see KOOP and TIERNEY 1990). Under experimental conditions, and in alcoholics, where high blood ethanol concentrations are attained, increases in the levels of cytochrome P450 2E1 mRNA are also observed (DIEHL et al. 1991; BADGER et al. 1993; TAKAHASHI et al. 1991). Recent work shows that Kupffer cells also contain cytochrome P450 2E1, the levels of which are increased up to 15-fold by chronic ethanol treatment (KRANER et al. 1993).

Cytochrome P450 2E1 is able to oxidize a number of other drugs, including some procarcinogens and acetaminophen (KOOP 1992). The latter, a commonly used nonprescription drug, is metabolized into a reactive toxic radical which combines with hepatic glutathione, and binds covalently to cell macromolecules, triggering processes which result in hepatocellular necrosis (see Chap. 2, this volume). Rats fed alcohol chronically, in which the levels of hepatic cytochrome P450 2E1 can be increased up to tenfold (EKSTROM and INGELMAN-SUNDBERG 1989), and alcoholics, are highly susceptible to acetaminophen hepatotoxicity (LIEBER 1994).

The liquid diet model also contributed the demonstration of the role of the cytochrome P450 2E1 in the generation oxygen radicals and lipoperoxidation following chronic ethanol administration (CEDERBAUM 1989; EKSTROM and INGELMAN-SUNDBERG 1989; DAI et al. 1993). Cytochrome P450 2E1 has been shown to generate superoxide ions, hydrogen peroxide and hydroxyl radicals (see CEDERBAUM 1989; NORDMANN et al. 1992). Lipid peroxidation, in turn, results from the action of these radicals and other intermediates of the cytochrome P450 chain, on polyunsaturated fatty acids (CEDERBAUM 1989). As will be seen below, lipoperoxidation products can activate the production of fibrogenesis by Ito cells.

Recent studies have also shown that hydroxyl radicals produced in the cytochrome P450 2E1 system react with ethanol, generating hydroxyethyl radicals which bind covalently to proteins (ALBANO et al. 1993; MONCADA et al. 1994). The adducts were found to be neoantigenic, generating antibodies against hydroxyethyl radical-protein adducts (MONCADA et al. 1994).

III. Acetaldehyde Adducts

As indicated above, acetaldehyde is generated both by the alcohol dehydrogenase and the cytochrome P450 2E1 reactions. Acetaldehyde binds covalently to proteins, also generating adducts (STEVENS et al. 1981; TUMA et al. 1984), which are also immunogenic (STEINBRECHER et al. 1984; ISRAEL et al. 1986; NIEMELÄ et al. 1987; HOERNER et al. 1988). Acetaldehyde adducts with cytochrome P450 and with some cytosolic proteins, for example, a cytosolic 37-kDa protein, have been shown in rats fed alcohol-containing liquid diets (BEHRENS et al. 1988; LIN and LUMENG 1989). Intracellular acetaldehyde adducts have been shown by immunofluorescent techniques in hepatocytes surrounding the terminal hepatic venules (periacinar) in rats fed ethanol chronically and in the liver of patients with active liver disease (NIEMELÄ et al. 1994). The production of acetaldehyde adducts should more likely occur in the periacinar zone; cytochrome P450 2E1 is highly concentrated in periacinar hepatocytes (INGELMAN-SUNDBERG et al. 1988), while acetaldehyde, contributed by hepatocytes along the sinusoidal length, is expected to be most concentrated at the venular end of the sinusoid.

Antibodies against acetaldehyde-protein adducts have been reported to exist in the serum of patients with alcoholic liver disease displaying hepatocellular necrosis but not in patients with fatty liver or inactive cirrhosis (NIEMELÄ et al. 1987; WORRALL et al. 1990; KOSKINAS et al. 1992; TEARE et al. 1993). It is not known, however, if these antibodies are involved in the pathogenesis of necrosis or actually result from necrosis per se. Nevertheless, these antibodies may contribute to perpetuating a preexistent lesion. In rats and mice, chronic alcohol consumption leads to only minor increases in antibodies against acetaldehyde adducts (ISRAEL et al. 1986; WORRALL et al. 1991). On the other hand, guinea pigs immunized with acetaldehyde adducts formed in vitro and administered to the animals develop hepatocellular necrosis when fed alcohol chronically (YOKOYAMA et al. 1993).

It has been proposed that when acetaldehyde adducts formed on the external surface of the hepatocyte membrane are recognized by anti-adduct antibodies, cell necrosis would ensue via complement activation or antibody-dependent cell-mediated cytotoxicity (ISRAEL et al. 1987). Cell necrosis via antibody-dependent cell-mediated cytotoxicity (ADCC) occurs when antibodies in the membrane of neutrophils recognize cells that expose the specific epitopes (ROITT et al. 1989). Upon antigen-antibody recognition, neutrophils are activated, leading to the generation of oxygen radicals of strong oxidants and the release of proteolytic enzymes which result in cell necrosis (WEISS 1989). An immunological mechanism of cell damage would be potentiated by mechanisms that attract neutrophils. It has been shown that hepatocytes metabolizing ethanol generate neutrophil chemoattractants (ROLL et al. 1991). As indicated earlier, neutrophil infiltration in the centrilobular zone is the hallmark of alcoholic hepatitis.

IV. Hepatocyte Ballooning and Hepatomegaly

Chronic administration of ethanol to rats in liquid diets results in moderate increases in liver weight (normally 15%–40%) with no increases in total DNA, indicating an increase in cell size rather than an increase in the number of hepatocytes (BARAONA et al. 1975; ISRAEL et al. 1982a,b). Studies on the mechanism of cell ballooning show that fat accumulation induced by ethanol accounts for only a fraction (25%) of the increase in hepatocyte and liver size. Most (50%–60%) of the increase in cell size is accounted for by an increase in intracellular water, balanced iso-osmotically with intracellular potassium (ISRAEL et al. 1982; ISRAEL and ORREGO 1983). The livers also show an increase in soluble intracellular proteins, which may contribute, in part, to water retention in the hepatocytes (BARAONA et al. 1975). It has nevertheless been estimated that the osmotic pressure contributed by proteins is too small to account for the accumulation of water (ISRAEL and ORREGO 1983).

An increased hepatocyte volume induced by chronic alcohol consumption is accompanied by a reduction in extracellular space per unit liver weight (ISRAEL et al. 1982). Such a reduction in extracellular volume suggests that hepatocyte expansion compresses the sinusoidal caliber and that the liver capsule expansion cannot fully accommodate the increases in hepatocyte volume. This finding is consistent with the marked reduction in sinusoidal caliber in alcoholic liver disease (VIDINS et al. 1985). In rats fed alcohol by the liquid diet method, intrahepatic pressure is generally not increased. However increases in intrahepatic pressure (equivalent to sinusoidal pressure) have been reported for animals in which hepatomegaly exceeds 50% (ORREGO et al. 1990). Marked hepatomegaly, of the order of 80%, develops with the alcohol intragastric infusion model (TSUKAMOTO et al. 1992), but portal or intrahepatic pressures have not been examined in these animals.

V. Hepatic Oxygen Consumption

In vitro, in the presence of exogenously added ADP, liver mitochondria of rats fed alcohol chronically utilize oxygen at lower rates than those of control animals (RUBIN et al. 1972; THAYER and RUBIN 1981). However, when tissue respiration is determined in perfused livers, chronic alcohol consumption administered by liquid diets leads to 30%–60% increases in hepatic oxygen consumption (hypermetabolic state) (BRITTON et al. 1984; RACHAMIN et al. 1985). The existence of a hypermetabolic state has also been observed in vivo in rats fed alcohol chronically (TSUKAMOTO and XI 1989; CARMICHAEL et al. 1993), where oxygen consumption rates are increased by 40%–160%. The hypermetabolic state is likely to result from a reduction in the ATP/ADP × Pi ratio (BERNSTEIN et al. 1973; MIYAMOTO and FRENCH 1988), which controls the mitochondrial respiration in the intact cell.

The hypermetabolic state has also been observed in perfused livers following the in vivo administration of one single large dose of ethanol. Perfused livers of animals killed 2–3h after ethanol administration use oxygen at rates that are 50%–80% higher than controls. This latter condition is referred to as SIAM, the acronym for "swift increase in ethanol metabolism," which reflects the increased rate of ethanol metabolism that is seen in the hypermetabolic condition (YUKI and THURMAN 1980; YUKI et al. 1982). Recent studies show that the liver hypermetabolic state induced by ethanol administration is fully prevented in animals in which Kupffer cells are destroyed (BRADFORD et al. 1993). It has recently been pointed out that cytokines produced by Kupffer cells typically produce a hypermetabolic state in the whole animal (MCCLAIN et al. 1993).

VI. Liver Hypoxia

In the presence of ethanol in the blood, the liver hypermetabolic state induced by the chronic administration of ethanol does not result in hepatic oxygen deficiency since oxygen delivery to the liver is also increased (CARMICHAEL et al. 1993). An increased oxygen delivery is the result of an increased portal blood flow induced by adenosine, a powerful vasodilator generated in the metabolism of acetate (ORREGO et al. 1988). However, upon alcohol withdrawal, acetate production ceases and liver blood flow returns to normal. The hypermetabolic state is long lived, generating a state of relative oxygen deficiency, evidenced by a reduction in hepatic vein oxygen tensions (CARMICHAEL et al. 1993).

Rats fed ethanol chronically by liquid diets, and withdrawn from alcohol, develop hepatocellular necrosis when exposed to low oxygen tensions (ISRAEL et al. 1975; FRENCH et al. 1984) or they are subjected to experimental anemia (ISRAEL et al. 1979). Necrosis and neutrophil inflammation are seen surrounding the terminal hepatic venule, where oxygen tensions are lowest, only in the ethanol chronically fed animals.

Low oxygen levels in the hepatic vein have also been reported in withdrawn alcoholics with liver disease (KESSLER et al. 1954; HADANGUE et al. 1988). Hepatic vein oxygen tensions are significantly lower in alcoholics with hepatocellular necrosis than in alcoholics in which no necrosis is observed (ITURRIAGA et al. 1980). In baboons fed alcohol chronically and withdrawn, no increases in oxygen utilization are seen, while minor reductions in hepatic vein oxygen tension are observed, mainly due to reduced hepatic blood flow in the ethanol-treated animals (JAUHONEN et al. 1982).

In alcoholic liver disease in humans, the prognosis of low hemoglobin values in relation to mortality is very high and similar to that of low prothrombin levels (ORREGO et al. 1985). The 1-year risk of mortality of alcoholic liver disease patients with hemoglobin levels below 75% of normal is 79%; that for patients with hemoglobin in the range of 75%–90% of normal is 47%. Patients with normal hemoglobin values have a mortality risk of 11%. Nevertheless, the cause-effect relationship between low hemoglobin levels and alcoholic liver disease remains to be established. In alcoholics a number of conditions of reduced oxygen delivery exist, including anemia, smoking, respiratory dysfunction and sleep apnea (ISRAEL et al. 1979; FRENCH et al. 1984). Epidemiological studies show that cigarette smoking confers a very marked increase in the risk of alcoholic cirrhosis mortality (KLATSKY and ARMSTRONG 1992).

VII. Intragastric Infusion Model

TSUKAMOTO, FRENCH and associates developed a model of alcoholic liver injury in the rat in which a liquid diet containing ethanol or isocaloric carbohydrate is continuously infused via an intragastric cannula (TSUKAMOTO et al. 1986; FRENCH 1993; FRENCH et al. 1993a; MORIMOTO et al. 1994) In this model, ethanol is infused to match the rate of ethanol elimination by the animal and to keep high ethanol concentrations. Minor changes in the rate of ethanol elimination in a system of constant infusion result in marked periodic fluctuations in blood ethanol levels, mimicking the situation in humans. This method results in oscillating blood alcohol concentrations with an average in the 100- to 300-mg/dl range (TSUKAMOTO et al. 1985; RONIS et al. 1993; ADACHI et al. 1994). Animals fed alcohol chronically for up to 6 months develop lesions which vary in severity but can include marked fatty accumulation, ballooning, centrilobular focal hepatocellular necrosis, neutrophil inflammation, perivenular fibrosis with bridging and, in some animals, cirrhosis. Serum transaminases are elevated two- to threefold (MORIMOTO et al. 1994) by ethanol treatment. Animals fed alcohol by this technique develop centrilobular necrosis following minor episodes of experimental hypoxia (FRENCH et al. 1984). In this model, hepatic oxygen extraction is increased by about 160% in the ethanol-fed animals, an increase that is not compensated by an increased oxygen delivery (60%), thus resulting in a marked reduction (40%) in the mean oxygen tension in the hepatic vein (TSUKAMOTO and XI 1989).

It has been proposed that hypoxic episodes induced by chronic ethanol treatment in this model may result in cell death by the same mechanisms involved in cell necrosis in ischemia-reperfusion models (INGELMAN-SUNBERG et al. 1993; see also JAESCHKE and FARHOOD 1991; JAESCHKE et al. 1992a, 1993b). Kupffer cells respond to hypoxia-reoxygenation with marked increases in the production of oxygen radicals (RYMSA et al. 1991; DE GROOT 1992). Oxidative stress is known to activate nuclear factor kappa-B, a gene transcription factor for many cytokines produced in Kupffer cells, including tumor necrosis factor-α and transforming growth factor-β (GRILLI et al. 1993; KOPP and GHOSH 1994); tumor necrosis factor promotes neutrophil accumulation and is an autocrine activator of nuclear factor kappa-B (DECKER 1990; GRILLI et al. 1993). Recent studies suggest that tumor necrosis factor-α can induce apoptosis of sinusoidal endothelial cells (TAKEI et al. 1994). Transforming growth factor-β promotes fibrogenesis by Ito cells (MATSUOKA and TSUKAMOTO 1990; BACHEM et al. 1992) and may contribute to hepatocyte apoptosis (GRESSNER and MANNHERZ 1994).

Factors other than hypoxia-reoxygenation, which can also activate Kupffer cells, include activated complement products (LASKIN et al. 1988; JAESCHKE et al. 1993), antigen-antibody complexes (LATOCHA et al. 1989) and lipopolysaccharide, the active component of endotoxin (DECKER 1990; MCCLAIN et al. 1993).

VIII. Modulation of Alcohol-Induced Liver Injury

The production of liver necrosis and fibrosis in this ethanol intragastric infusion model can be influenced by at least four factors: (a) the production of Kupffer cell products (ADACHI et al. 1994), (b) the intestinal flora of the animals (IIMURO et al. 1994; NANJI et al. 1994c), (c) the caloric percentage of fats and the degree of unsaturation of fats in the diet (NANJI et al. 1989; 1993; MORIMOTO et al. 1994) and (d) the amount of iron in the diet (TSUKAMOTO et al. 1992).

Recent studies (ADACHI et al. 1994) show that the destruction of Kupffer cells fully suppresses the production of necrosis and inflammation and the increases in serum transaminases induced by chronic alcohol treatment in the intragastric infusion model. The destruction of Kupffer cells also prevented the hypermetabolic state induced by the ethanol administration (BRADFORD et al. 1993). These studies indicate a central role for Kupffer cell activation in alcoholic liver injury. However, since a number of factors can activate Kuppffer cells, Occam's parsimony rule should be reconsidered. It is more likely that a combination of factors act in synergy.

Animals fed alcohol chronically by the continuous infusion method display elevated levels of endotoxin, a Kupffer cell activator, and of tumor necrosis factor, both of which correlate with the severity of liver damage (NANJI et al. 1993a, 1994b). Thus, in this model, in which high ethanol levels are continuously present in the gastrointestinal tract, absorption of endotoxin generated by gastrointestinal bacteria may play an important role in the production of liver damage. Studies in humans have shown that the presence of ethanol in the gastrointestinal tract promotes the absorption of large molecular weight substances from the gut (ROBINSON et al. 1981; BJARNASON et al. 1984).

A recent report showed that antibiotic treatment aimed at reducing intestinal flora and endotoxin production in animals fed alcohol by the intragastric infusion method fully prevented the production of alcohol-induced liver damage in this animal model (IIMURO et al. 1994). Similar protection against liver injury was reported following the intragastric administration of lactobacillus, which reduced endotoxemia in rats fed alcohol chronically by the intragastric infusion system (NANJI et al. 1994c). As pointed out earlier, alcoholic liver disease in humans can occur in the presence or absence of endotoxemia. When present, endotoxemia could potentiate other mechanisms of Kupffer cell activation.

Studies have shown that in rats chronic administration of ethanol in liquid diets sensitizes the liver to the hepatotoxic effects of bacterial endotoxin (BHAGWANDEEN et al. 1987; HANSEN et al. 1994). Ethanol-fed animals respond to low levels of endotoxin with marked elevations in tumor necrosis factor-α, when compared to control animals, and display significantly elevated serum transaminase levels, both of which correlate strongly (HONCHEL et al. 1992; HANSEN et al. 1994). Focal hepatocellular necrosis and neutrophilic infiltration are observed in ethanol-treated animals given small doses of endotoxin (BHAGWANDEEN et al. 1987; HANSEN et al. 1994). These changes were seen in the absence of changes in lipopolysaccharide clearance (HANSEN et al. 1994), confirming an increased sensitivity of the monocyte/macrophage(Kupffer) series. Monocytes of patients with alcoholic liver disease show elevated tumor necrosis factor-α production when stimulated by lipopolysaccharide (MCCLAIN and COHEN 1989). In the absence of endotoxin, Kupffer cells isolated from chronically ethanol fed animals present five- to tenfold elevations in tumor necrosis factor-α mRNA levels (EARNEST et al. 1993).

It should be noted that when the production of tumor necrosis factor is maximally stimulated by lipopolysaccharide, ethanol in vitro, or acutely administered, inhibits the production of tumor necrosis factor-α by monocytes/macrophages and splenocytes (NELSON et al. 1989; D'SOUZA et al. 1989; CHEN et al. 1993; VERMA et al. 1993). Whether this occurs when Kupffer cells are not exogenously activated by lipopolysaccharide is unlikely; the acute administration of ethanol to rats markedly increases the production of superoxide radicals by isolated Kupffer cells (BAUTISTA and SPITZER 1992). An increase in superoxide ion production is also seen in perfused livers of animals administered ethanol in vivo (BAUTISTA and SPITZER 1992).

Epidemiological studies indicate that, when adjusted for per capita alcohol consumption, countries in which mainly saturated fats are consumed have lower rates of cirrhosis than countries in which unsaturated fat consumption predominates (NANJI and FRENCH 1985, 1986). A similar observation has been made in rats fed ethanol by the intragastric infusion route (NANJI et al. 1989; FRENCH et al. 1993, 1993b; MORIMOTO et al. 1994). In the ethanol-fed animals the production of fibrosis was high when unsaturated fats were given (corn oil or fish oil), but was virtually nonexistent when the ethanol-fed animals were administered saturated fats (beef fat). Rats fed ethanol plus unsaturated fats but not those fed ethanol plus saturated fats show increased liver tumor necrosis factor-α mRNA levels (NANJI et al. 1994).

A strong correlation between lipoperoxidation products and fibrosis has also been reported (KAMIMURA et al. 1992). Recent work has suggested that an increased lipoperoxidation requires both increased cytochrome P450 2E1 levels and the feeding of unsaturated or polyunsaturated fats (NANJI et al. 1993; MORIMOTO et al. 1994). The lipoperoxidation products, malondialdehyde, 4-hydroxynonenal – both aldehydes – have been reported to activate the production of collagen by fibroblasts and Ito cells (CHOJKIER et al. 1989; TSUKAMOTO 1994). Acetaldehyde per se has also been reported to increase collagen gene transcription in rat Ito cells in vitro (CASINI et al. 1991). These products could potentiate the stimulatory effect of transcription growth factor-β on collagen gene transcription in Ito cells (TSUKAMOTO 1994; WEINER et al. 1994). Data suggest that increases in tumor necrosis factor-α induced in rat liver by chronic ethanol treatment precede the changes in transforming growth factor-β (NANJI et al. 1994).

Mechanisms other than cytochrome P450 2E1 may also generate oxygen radicals and have lipoperoxidative potential. These include (a) the oxidation of acetaldehyde by aldehyde oxidase (SHAW and JAYATILLEKE 1990, 1992); (b) the increased availability of xanthine and hypoxanthine, substrates for the xanthine oxidase reaction (KATO et al. 1990), substrates which are produced in the ATP-mediated conversion of acetate, generated from acetaldehyde, into acetyl-CoA; (c) an increased mobilization of bound iron into free iron induced by ethanol (SHAW 1989); and (d) an increased generation of reactive oxygen species by mitochondria of ethanol-fed animals (KUKIELKA et al. 1994).

The relevance of reactive oxygen intermediates and of lipoperoxidation in the development of alcohol-induced fibrosis is further suggested by studies in which the diets infused intragastrically were supplemented with carbonyl iron. Supplementation with iron, known to promote oxygen radical generation and lipoperoxidation, markedly increased the development of fibrosis in the ethanol-treated animals (TSUKAMOTO et al. 1992).

A central issue in the alcoholic liver disease field is whether fibrosis and the production of cirrhosis can occur in the absence of cell necrosis per se. An analysis of the pathogenesis of cirrhosis by a wide variety of mechanisms, including viral hepatitis, hemochromatosis, Wilson's disease, α_1-antitrypsin accumulation and experimental cirrhosis such as carbon tetrachloride or choline and lipotropic deficiency indicates that in all these conditions necrosis is seen to occur (RUBIN and FARBER 1994). The superimposition of conditions which could accentuate fibrogenesis with limited necrosis is, however, conceivable.

IX. Glutathione

Glutathione, a cysteine-containing tripeptide, is an essential molecule in cell protection against reactive oxygen intermediates, primarily hydrogen peroxide. Superoxide ion radical, produced in a number of oxidation reactions, is rapidly converted into hydrogen peroxide by the action of superoxide dismutase. In turn, glutathione reacts with hydrogen peroxide in a reaction mediated by glutathione peroxidase (KAPLOWITZ and OOKHTENS 1985). It is therefore surprising that 80%–90% of glutathione produced by the liver is actually not utilized in the hepatocyte but exported into the sinusoids (LAUTERBERG et al. 1984; SPEISKY et al. 1985). Glutathione is present in the hepatocyte at concentrations of 5–8 mM, about 3 orders of magnitude that in plasma 8–10 μM). Efflux of glutathione from the hepatocyte is carrier dependent QOKHTENS et al. 1985). Recent studies suggest that efflux of glutathione into the sinusoid may constitute a mechanism of protection against oxygen radicals liberated by nonparenchymal cells into the sinusoidal space. Glutathione efflux into the sinusoidal space is greatly activated following ischemia-reperfussion conditions (JAESCHKE et al. 1993), an effect that may be mediated by tumor necrosis factor-α (RAIFORD et al. 1994).

Acute administration of ethanol markedly increases the efflux of hepatic glutahione (SPEISKY et al. 1985), increases the levels of circulating glutathione and reduces hepatic glutathione (VIDELA et al. 1981; SPEISKY et al. 1985). The chronic administration of ethanol is also characterized by a marked increase in hepatic glutathione efflux (PIERSON and MITCHELL 1985; FERNANDEZ-CHECA et al. 1987). Animals fed for 16 weeks by the intragastric infusion method present minor reductions in total hepatic glutathione but an 85% reduction in mitochondrial glutathione, which comprises about 10% of the total cellular glutathione (HIRANO et al. 1992). Alcoholics presenting liver disease display low levels of hepatic glutathione (VIDELA et al. 1984). The implications of a reduction in mitochondrial glutathione are not clear. However, it is clear that mitochondria which have lost a major proportion of their glutathione will be less protected against oxygen radicals. The radiation injury literature has shown that oxygen radicals are strong mutagens (RUBIN and FARBER 1994). Studies to determine the rate of mutation of mitochondrial DNA in alcoholics would be of interest.

X. Micropig Model of Alcoholic Liver Injury

Recent studies have established a new animal model of alcoholic liver injury (HALSTEAD et al. 1993). Yucatan micropigs (20 kg) voluntarily consume ethanol in the diet. A balanced diet which provided 33% of calories as corn oil and 40% of calories as ethanol was administered for 12 months. Control animals were pair-fed isocaloric carbohydrate. Fatty liver, focal necrosis and inflammation developed in all the ethanol-fed animals(5/5), while 60% (3/5) developed perivenous and interstitial fibrosis. Electron microscopy showed Ito cell transformation and perisinusoidal collagen accumulation. Adducts of acetaldehyde and of malondialdehyde, a product of lipid peroxidation, determined by immunofluorescence, were prominently displayed in centrilobular hepatocytes around the terminal hepatic venule (HALSTEAD et al. 1993; NIEMELÄ et al. 1995). Controls displayed normal histology and no adducts.

XI. Baboon Model of Alcoholic Liver Injury

The liquid diet technique, originally devised for rats by LIEBER and DECARLI (LIEBER et al. 1989), was modified for use with baboons. Animals were administered 7% ethanol in the diet and 50% of calories as ethanol, along with 18% proteins and 21% fat, for up to 5 years. Control animals were pair-fed isocaloric amounts of carbohydrates. Alcohol-fed animals showed fatty liver, alcoholic hepatitis and cirrhosis (RUBIN and LIEBER 1974; LIEBER et al. 1975). Increases in serum transaminases, indicative of necrosis, were also observed in the ethanol-fed animals. Subsequent studies emphasized the production of fibrosis and cirrhosis (POPPER and LIEBER 1980); of 67 baboons fed ethanol, 14 (20%) had developed cirrhosis following 5 years of treatment, and an additional 14 animals had developed septal fibrosis (LIEBER et al. 1994). A number of different approaches have been employed to modify the extent of the lesion produced by ethanol. Choline supplementation did not result in a reduction in the production of fatty liver, fibrosis or cirrhosis (LIEBER et al. 1985), while lecithin, which contains the choline moiety and is not toxic, resulted in a marked reduction in fibrosis (LIEBER et al. 1994). While the mechanism of this effect is not clear, the administration of *S*-adenosylmethionine, which spares choline and generates the glutathione precursor cysteine, attenuated the alcohol-induced liver injury (LIEBER et al. 1990).

Acknowledgement. Work by the authors cited in this review was supported by the National Institute on Alcohol Abuse and Alcoholism. This review is dedicated to Dr. Hector Orrego, Professor Emeritus, scientist, friend and gentleman.

References

Adachi Y, Bradford BU, Gao W, Bojes HK, Thurman RG (1994) Inactivation of Kupffer cells prevents early alcohol induced liver injury. Hepatology 20:453–460

Akerman P, Cote P, Yang SQ et al. (1992) Antibodies to tumor necrosis factor alpha inhibit induction of hepatocyte and non-parenchymal cell proliferation after partial hepatectomy. Am J Physiol 263:G579–585

Albano E, Parola M, Comoglio A, Dianzani MU (1993) Evidence for the covalent binding of hydroxyethyl radicals to rat liver microsomal proteins. Alcohol Alcohol 28:453–459

Andus T, Bauer J, Wolfgang G (1991) Effects of cytokines on the liver. Hepatology 13:364–375

Bachem MG, Meyer D, Melchior R et al. (1992) Activation of rat liver perisinusoidal lipocytes by transforming growth factors derived from myofibroblast-like cells. Potential mechanism of self perpetuation in liver fibrogenesis. J Clin Invest 89:19–27

Badger TM, Huang J, Ronis M, Lumpkin CK (1993) Induction of cytochrome P450 2E1 during chronic alcohol exposure occurs via transcription of the CYP 2E1 gene when blood concentrations are high. Biochem Biophys Res Commun 190:780–785

Baraona E, Leo MA, Borowsky SA, Lieber CS (1975) Alcoholic hepatomegaly: accumulation of protein in the liver. Science 190:794–795

Bautista AP, Spitzer JJ (1992) Acute ethanol intoxication stimulates superoxide anion production by in situ perfused rat liver. Hepatology 15:892–898

Bautista AP, Skrepnikn N, Niesman MR, Begby GJ (1994) Elimination of macrophages by liposome-encapsulated dichloromethylene diphosphonate suppresses the endotoxin-induced priming of Kupffer cells. J Leukoc Biol 55:321–327

Behrens UJ, Hoerner M, Lasker JM, Lieber CS (1988) Formation of acetaldehyde adducts with ethanol-inducible P4502E1 in vivo. Biochem Biophys Res Commun 154:584–590

Bernstein J, Videla L, Israel Y (1973) Metabolic alterations produced in the liver by chronic ethanol administration. Changes related to energetic parameters of the cell. Biochem J 134:515–521

Bhagwandeen BS, Apte M, Manwarring L, Dickerson J (1987) Endotoxin induced hepatic necrosis in rats on an alcohol diet. J Pathol 152:47–53

Bigatello LM, Broitman SA, Fattori L, Di Paoli M, Pontello M, Bevilacqua G, Nespoli A (1987) Endotoxemia, encephalopathy and mortality in cirrhotic patients. Am J Gastroenterol 82:11–15

Bird GLA, Sheron N, Goka AKJ, Alexander GS, Williams RS (1990) Increased plasma tumor necrosis factor in severe alcoholic hepatitis. Ann Intern Med 112:917–920

Bjarnason I, Ward K, Peters TJ (1984) The leaky gut of alcoholism: possible route of entry for toxic compounds. Lancet 1:179–182

Blendis LM, Orrego H, Crossley IR, Blake JE, Medline A, Israel Y (1982) The role of hepatocyte enlargement in hepatic pressure in cirrhotic and noncirrholic alcoholic liver disease. Hepatology 2:539–546

Bode C, Kluger V, Bode JC (1987) Endotoxemia in patients with alcoholic and non alcoholic cirrhosis and in subjects with no evidence of chronic liver disease following acute alcohol excess. J Hepatol 4:8–14
Bradford BU, Misra UK, Thurman RG (1993) Kupffer cells are required for the swift increase in alcohol metabolism. Res Commun Subst Abuse 14:1–6
Britton RS, Videla LA, Rachamin G, Okuno F, Israel Y (1984) Effect of age on metabolic tolerance and hepatomegaly following chronic ethanol administration. Alcohol Clin Exp Res 8:528–534
Bruguera M, Bordas JM, Rodes J (1977) Asymptomatic liver disease in alcoholics. Arch Pathol Lab Med 101:644–647
Cao QN, Tu G-C, Weiner H (1988) Mitochondria as the primary site of acetaldehyde metabolism in beef and pig liver slices. Alcohol Clin Exp Res 12:720–724
Carmichael FJ, Orrego H, Saldivia V, Israel Y (1993) Effect of propylthiouracil on the ethanol-induced increase in liver oxygen consumption in awake rat. Hepatology 18:415–421
Casini A, Cunningham M, Rojkind M, Lieber CS (1991) Acetaldehyde increases procollagen type I and fibronectin gene transcription in cultures of rat fat-storing cells through a protein synthesis-dependent mechanism. Heapatology 13:758–765
Castell JV, Geiger T, Gross V, Andus T, Walter E, Hirano T, Kishimoto T, Heinrich PCSO (1988) Plasma clearance, organ distribution and target cells of interleukin 6/hepatocyte stimulating factor in the rat. Eur J Biochem 177:237–246
Cederbaum AI (1989) Oxygen radical generation by microsomes. Role of iron and implications for ethanol metabolism and toxicity. Free Radint Biol Med 7:559–567
Chedid A, Mendenhall CL, Garside P, French SW, Chen T, Rabin L (1991) The VA Cooperative Group. Am J Gastroenterol 82:210–216
Chen G-J, Huang DS, Watzl B, Watson RR (1993) Ethanol modulation of tumor necrosis factor and gamma interferon production by murine splenocytes and macrophages. Life Sci 52:1319–1326
Chojkier M, Houlglum K, Solis-Herruzo J, Brenner DA (1989) Stimulation of collagen gene expression by ascorbic acid in cultured human fibroblasts: a role for lipid peroxidation. J Biol Chem 264:16957–16962
Coletti LM, Remick DG, Burtch GD, Kunkel SL, Streter RM, Campbell DA Jr (1990) Role of tumor necrosis factor-α in the pathophysiologic alterations after ischemia/reperfusion injury in the rat. J Clin Invest 85:1936–1943
Dai Y, Rashba-Step J Cederbaum AI (1993) Stable expression of human P450 2E1 in Hep G2 cells; characterization and catalytic activities and production of reactive oxygen intermediates. Biochemistry 32:6928–6973
Decker K (1990) Biologically active products of stimulated liver macrophages (Kupffer cells). Eur J Biochem 192:245–261
de Groot H (1992) Isolated cells in the study of the molecular mechanisms of reperfusion injury. Toxicol Lett 63:111–125
Deviere J, Content J, Denys C, Vandenbussche P, Schandene L, Wybran L, Dupont E (1990) Excessive in vitro bacterial lipopolysaccharide-induced production of monokines in cirrhosis. Hepatology 11:628–634
Diehl AM, Bisgaard HC, Kren BT, Steer CJ (1991) Ethanol interferes with regeneration-associated changes in biotransforming enzymes: a potential mechanism underlying ethanol's carcinogenicity? Hepatology 13:722–727
D'Souza NB, Bagby GJ, Nelson S, Spitzer JJ (1989) Acute infusion suppresses endotoxin-induced serum tumor necrosis factor. Alcohol Clin Exp Res 13:295–298
Earnest DL, Abril ER, Jolley CS, Martinez F (1993) Ethanol and diet-induced alterations in Kupffer cell function. Alcohol Alcohol 28:73–83
Edwards MJ, Keller BJ, Kauffman FC, Thurman RG (1993) The involvement of Kupffer cells in carbon tetrachloride. Toxicol Appl Pharmacol 119:275–279
Ekstrom G, Ingelman-Sundberg M (1989) Rat liver microsomal NADPH-supported activity and lipid peroxidation dependent on ethanol inducible cytochrome P450. Biochem Pharmacol 58:1313–1319

Eliasson E, Johansson I, Ingelman-Sundberg M (1988) Ligand-dependent maintenance of ethanol-inducible cytochrome P-450 in primary rat hepatocyte cell cultures Biochem Biophys Res Commun 150:436–443

Felver ME, Mezey E, McGuire M, Mitchell MC, Herlong F, Veech GA, Veech RL (1990) Plasma tumor necrosis factor-α predicts long term survival in severe alcoholic hepatitis. Alcohol Clin Exp Res 14:255–259

Fernandez-Checa JC, Ookhtens M, Kaplowitz N (1987) Effect of chronic ethanol feeding on hepatocyte glutathione: compartmentation, efflux and response to intubation with ethanol. J Clin Invest 80:57–62

French SW (1993) Nutrition in the pathogenesis of alcoholic liver disease. Alcohol Alcohol 28:97–109

French SW, Benson NC, Sun PS (1984) Centrilobular liver necrosis induced by hypoxia in chronic ethanol-fed rats. Hepatology 4:912–917

French SW, Wong K, Jui L, Albano E, Hagbork A-L, Ingelman-Sungberg M (1993a) Effect of ethanol on cytochrome P450 2E1, lipid peroxidation and serum protein adduct formation in relation to liver pathology. Exp Mol Pathol 58:61–75

French SW, Nash J, Shitabata P, Kachi K, Hara C, Chedid A, Mendenhall CL, VA cooperative study group 119 (1993b) Semin Alcohol Liver Dis 13:154–169

Grant BF, Dufour MC, Harford TC (1988) Epidemiology of alcoholic liver disease. Semin Liver Dis 8:12–25

Gressner AM, Mannherz H-O (1994) Myofibroblasts induce TGF-β-mediated apoptosis of hepatocytes which increase their mitogenic potential for fat-storing cells. Hepatology 20:291A

Grilli M, Chiu J-S, Lenardo MJ (1993) NF-kB and rel: participants in a multiform transcriptional regulatory system. Int Rev Cytol 143:1–62

Groszmann RJ, Blei AT, Atterbury CE (1988) Portal hypertension. In: Arias IM et al. (eds) The liver: biology and pathobiology, 2nd edn. Raven, New York, pp 1147–1159

Hadangue A, Moreau R, Lee SS, Gaudin C, Rueff B, Lebrec D (1988) Liver hypermetabolism during alcohol withdrawal in humans: role of sympathetic overactivity. Gastroenterology 94:1047–1052

Hallen J, Norden J (1964) Liver cirrhosis unsuspected during life: a series of 79 cases. J Chronic Dis 17:951

Halstead CH, Villanueva J, Chandler CJ, Ruebner B, Munn RJ, Parkkila S, Niemela O (1993) Centrilobular distribution of acetaldehyde and collagen in ethanol-fed micropig. Hepatology 18:954–960

Hansen J, Cherwitz DL, Allen JI (1994) The role of tumor necrosis factor-α in acute endotoxin-induced hepatotoxicity in ethanol-fed rats. Heapatology 20:461–474

Hill DB, Marsano LS, McClain GJ (1993) Increased plasma interleukin 8 concentrations in alcoholic hepatitis. Hepatology 18:576–580

Hirano T, Kaplowitz N, Tsukamoto H, Kamimura S, Fernandez-Checa JC (1992) Hepatic mitochondrial depletion and progression of experimental alcoholic liver disease in rats. Hepatology 16:1423–1427

Hoerner M, Behrens UJ, Worner T, Lieber CS (1988) Humoral immune response to acetaldehyde adducts. Hepatology 8:569–574

Hutterer F, Eisenstadt M, Rubin E (1970) Turnover of hepatic collagen in reversible and irreversible fibrosis. Experientia 26:244

Iimuro Y, Adachi Y, Moore LE, Bradford BU, Gao W, Thurman RG (1994) Liver injury following chronic ethanol exposure to rats is prevented by antibiotics. Hepatology 20:316A

Ingelman-Sundberg M, Johansson I, Penttila KE, Glaumann H, Lindros KO (1988) Centrilobular expression of ethanol inducible cytochrome P450(IIE1) in rat liver. Biochem Biophys Res Commun 157:55–60

Ingelman-Sundberg M, Johansson I, Yin Hu, Terelius Y, Eliasson E, Clot P, Albano E (1993) Ethanol-inducible cytochrome P4502E1: genetic polymorphism, regulation and possible role in the etiology of alcohol-induced liver disease. Alcohol 10:447–452

International Group Review (1981) Alcoholic liver disease: morphological manifestations. Lancet March 28:707–711
Israel Y, Orrego H (1981) Liver oxygen demand and hepatocyte enlargement: their possible role in the pathogenesis of alcoholic liver disease. In: Lautt WW (ed) Hepatic circulation in health and disease. Raven, New York, pp 351–375
Israel Y, Orrego H (1983) On the characteristics of alcohol-induced liver enlargement and its possible hemodynamic consequences. Pharmacol Biochem Behav 18 [Suppl 1]:433–437
Israel Y, Kalant H, Orrego H, Khanna JM, Phillips JM (1975a) Experimental alcohol-induced hepatic necrosis: suppression by propylthiouracil. Proc Natl Acad Sci USA 72(3):1137–1141
Israel Y, Videla L, Bernstein J (1975b) Liver hypermetabolic state after chronic ethanol consumption: hormonal interrelations and pathogenic implications. Fed Proc 34:2052–2059
Israel Y, Kalant H, Orrego H, Khanna JM, Phillips MJ, Stewart DJ (1979) Hypermetabolic state, oxygen availability, and alcohol-induced liver damage. In: Majchrowicz E, Noble EP (eds) Biochemistry and pharmacology of ethanol, vol 1. Plenum, New York, pp 433–444
Israel Y, Britton RS, Orrego H (1982a) Liver cell enlargement induced by chronic alcohol consumption: studies on its cause and consequences. Clin Biochem 15:189–192
Israel Y, Orrego H, Colman JC, Britton RS (1982b) Alcohol-induced hepatomegaly: pathogenesis and role in the production of portal hypertension. Fed Proc 41:2472–2477
Israel Y, Hurwitz E, Niemelä O, Arnon R (1986) Monoclonal and polyclonal antibodies against acetaldehyde containing epitopes in acetaldehyde-protein adducts. Proc Natl Acad Sci USA 83:7923–7927
Israel Y, Niemelä O, Khanna J, Orrego H (1987) Antibodies against acetaldehyde-modified epitopes: a new perspective. In: Goedde HW, Agarwal DP (eds) Genetics and alcoholism. Liss, New York, pp 283–289
Iturriaga H, Ugarte G, Israel (1980) Hepatic vein oxygenation, liver blood flow and the rate of ethanol metabolism in recently abstinent alcoholic patients. Eur J Clin Invest 10:211–218
Jaeschke H, Farhood A (1991) Neutrophil and Kupffer cell-induced oxidant stress and ischemia-reperfusion injury in rat liver. Am J Physiol 260:G355–G362
Jaeschke H, Farhood A, Smith CW (1992) Neutrophil-induced liver cell injury in endotoxin shock is a CD11b/CD18-dependent mechanism. Am J Physiol 261:G1051–G1056
Jaeschke H, Bautista AP, Spolarics Z, Spitzer JJ (1992) Superoxide generation by neutrophils and Kupffer cells during in vivo reperfusion after hepatic ischemia in rats. J Leukoc Biol 52:377–382
Jaeschke H, Farhood A, Bautista AP, Spolarics Z, Spitzer JJ (1993) Complement activates Kupffer cells and neutrophils during reperfusion after hepatic ischemia. Am J Physiol 264:G801–G809
Jauhonen P, Baraona E, Miyakawa H, Lieber CS (1982) Mechanism for selective perivenular hepatotoxicity. Alcohol Clin Exp Res 6:350–357
Kamimura S, Gaal K, Britton RS, Bacon B, Triadafilopoulos G, Tsukamoto H(1992) Increased 4-hydroxynonenal levels in experimental alcoholic liver disease: association of lipid peroxidation with fibrogenesis. Hepatology 16:448–453
Kaplowitz N, Ookhtens M (1985) The regulation of hepatic glutathione. Annu Rev Pharmacol Toxicol 25:715–744
Kato S, Kawase T, Alderman J, Inatomi N, Lieber CS (1990) Role of xanthine oxidase in ethanol-induced lipid peroxidation in rats. Gastroenterology 98:203–210
Kessler BJ, Liebler JB, Brofin GJ, Sasso M (1954) The hepatic blood flow and splanchnic oxygen consumption in alcohol fatty liver. J Clin Invest 33:338–345

Khoruts A, Stanke L, McClain CF, Logan G, Allen JI (1991) Circulating tumor necrosis factor, interleukin-1 and interleukin 6 concentrations in chronic alcoholic patients. Hepatology 13:267–276

Klatsky AL, Armstrong MA (1992) Alcohol, smoking, coffee and cirrhosis. Am J Epidemiol 136:1248–1257

Koop DR (1992) Oxidative and reductive metabolism of cytochrome P450 2E1. FASEB Journal 6:724–730

Koop E, Ghosh S (1994) Inhibition of NF-kB by sodium salicylate and aspirin. Science 265:956–959

Koop DR, Tierney DJ (1990) Multiple mechanism in the regulation of ethanol inducible cytochrome P450 2E1. Bioassays 12:429–435

Koop DR, Morgan ET, Tarr GE, Coon MJ (1982) Purification and characterization of a unique isozyme of cytochrome P450 isozyme 3a isolated from microsomes of ethanol treated rabbits. J Biol Chem 257:8472–8480

Koskinas J, Kenna JG, Bird GL, Alexander GJM, Williams R (1992) Immunoglobulin A antibody to a 200-kilodalton cytosolic acetaldehyde adduct in alcoholic hepatitis. Gastroenterology 103:1860–1867

Kraner J, Eskelson C, Abril E, Jolley C, Jalpert J, Earnest D (1993) Kupffer cell expression of cytochrome P-4502E1 and metabolism of ethanol is induced by ethanol feeding. Hepatology 18:120A

Kukielka E, Dicker E, Cederbaum AI (1994) Increased production of reactive oxygen species by rat liver mitochondria after chronic ethanol treatment. Arch Biochem Biophys 309:377–386

Laskin DL, Sirak AA, Pilaro AM, Laskin JD (1988) Functional and biochemical properties of rat Kupffer cells and peritoneal macrophages. J Leukoc Biol 44:71–78

Laskin BL, Gardner CR, Price VF, Jollow DJ (1995) Modulation of macrophage functioning abrogates the acute hepatotoxicity of acetaminophen. Hepatology 21:1045–1050

Latocha G, Dieter P, Schulze-Specking A, Decker K (1989) F_c receptors mediate prostaglandin and superoxide synthesis in cultured Kupffer cells. Biol Chem 370:1055–1061

Lauterburg BH, Smith CV, Mitchell JR (1984) Hepatic glutathione homeostasis in the rat: efflux accounts for turnover. Hepatology 4:586–590

Lelbach WK (1974) Organic pathology related to volume and pattern of alcohol use. In: Gibbins RJ, Israel Y, Kalant H, Popham RE, Schmidt W, Smart RG (eds) Research advances in alcohol and drug problems, vol 1. Wiley, New York, pp 93–167

Lelbach WK (1975) Cirrhosis in the alcoholic and its relationship to the volume of alcohol abuse. Ann NY Acad Sci 252:85–105

Lieber CS (1994) Alcohol and the liver: 1994 Update. Gastroenterology 106:1085–1105

Lieber CS, DeCarli LM (1970) Hepatic ethanol oxidixing system: in vitro characteristics and adaptive properties in vivo. J Biol Chem 245:2505–2512

Lieber CS, DeCarli LM, Rubin E (1975) Sequential production of fatty liver, hepatitis and cirrhosis in subhuman primates fed ethanol with adequate diets. Proc Natl Acad Sci USA 72:437–441

Lieber CS, Leo MA, Mak KM, DeCarli LM, Sato S (1985) Choline fails to prevent liver fibrosis in ethanol-fed baboons but causes toxicity. Hepatology 5:561–572

Lieber CS, DeCarli LM, Sorell MF (1989) Experimental methods of ethanol administration. Hepatology 10:501–510

Lieber CS, Casini A, DeCarli LM, Kim C, Lowe N, Sasaki R, Leo MA (1990) S-Adenosylmethionine attenuates alcohol induced liver injury in the baboon. Hepatology. 11:165–172

Lieber CS, Robins S, Li J, DeCarli LM, Mak KM, Fasulo JM, Leo MA (1994) Phosphatidyl choline protects against fibrosis and cirrhosis in the baboon. Gastroenterology 106:152–159

Lin RC, Lumeng L (1989) Further studies on the 37kD liver protein-acetaldehyde adduct that forms in vivo during chronic alcohol ingestion. Hepatology 10:807–814

Lindell SL, Southard JH, Vreugdenhill P, Belzer FO (1994) Kupffer cells depress hepatocyte protein synthesis on cold storage of the rat liver. Transplantation 58:869–874

Lischner MW, Alexander JF, Galambos JT (1971) Natural history of alcoholic hepatitis. I. The acute disease. Am J Dig Dis 16:481–494

Ludwig J, Garrison CO, Baggentoss AH (1970) Latent hepatic cirrhosis: a study of 95 cases. Gastroenterology 15:7–15

Lundquist F, Tygstrup K, Winkler K, Mellemgaard K, Munk-Petersen S (1962) Ethanol metabolism and production of free acetate in the human liver. J Clin Invest 41:955–961

Matsuoka M, Tsukamoto H (1990) Stimulation of hepatic lipocyte collagen production by Kupffer cell derived transforming factor beta: implications for a pathogenic role in alcoholic liver fibrogenesis. Hepatology 11:599–506

McClain CJ, Cohen DA (1989) Increased tumor necrosis factor production by monocytes in alcoholic hepatitis. Hepatology 9:349–351

McClain C, Hill D, Schmidt J, Diehl AM (1993) Cytokines and alcoholic liver disease. Semin Liver Dis 13:170–182

McCuskey RS, Reilly FD (1993) Hepatic microvasculature: dynamic structure and its regulation. Semin Liver Dis 13:1–12

Miyamoto K, French SW (1988) Hepatic adenosine nucleotide metabolism measured in vivo in rats fed ethanol and a high fat-low protein diet. Hepatology 8:53–60

Moncada C, Torres V, Varghese G, Albano E, Israel E (1994) Ethanol-derived immunoreactive species formed by free radical mechanisms. Mol Pharmacol 46:786–791

Morimoto M, Zern MA, Hagbjork AL, Ingelman-Sundberg M, French SW (1994) Fish oil, alcohol and liver pathology: role of cytochrome P450 2E1. Proc Soc Exp Biol Med 207:197–205

Nagakawa J, Hishinuma I, Hirota K, Miyamoto K, Yamanaka T, Tsukidate K, Katayama K, Yamatsu I (1990) Involvement of tumor necrosis factor-α in the pathogenesis of activated macrophage-mediated hepatitis in mice. Gastroenterology 99:758–765

Nanji AA, French SW (1985) Relationship between pork consumption and cirrhosis. Lancet I:681–683

Nanji AA, French SW (1986) Dietary factors and alcoholic cirrhosis. Alcohol Clin Exp Res 10:271–273

Nanji AA, Mendenhall CL, French SW (1989) Beef fat prevents alcoholic liver disease in the rat. Alcohol Clin Exp Res 13:15–19

Nanji AA, Khettry U, Sadrzadeh SMH, Yamanaka T (1993a) Severity of liver injury in experimental alcoholic liver disease. Am J Pathol 142:367–373

Nanji AA, Zhao S, Lamb RG, Sardrzareh SMH, Dannenberg AJ, Waxman DJ (1993b) Changes in microsomal phospholipases and arachidonic acid in experimental alcoholic liver injury: relationship to cytochrome P450 2E1 induction and conjugate d diene formation. Alcohol Clin Exp Res 17:598–603

Nanji AA, Zhao SP, Sadrzadeh SMH, Dannenberg AJ, Tahan SR, Waxman DJ (1994a) Markedly enhanced cytochrome P450 2E1 induction and lipid peroxidation is associated with severe liver injury in fish oil-ethanol-fed rats. Alcohol Clin Exp Res 18:1280–1285

Nanji AA, Zhao S, Sadrzadeh H, Waxman D (1994b) Use of reverse transcription-polymerase chain reaction to evaluate in vivo cytokine gene expression in rats fed ethanol for long periods. Hepatology 19:1483–1487

Nanji AA, Khettry U, Sadrzadeh SM (1994c) Lactobacillus feeding reduces endotoxemia and severity of experimental alcoholic liver disease. Proc Soc Exp Biol Med 205:243–247

Nelson S, Bagby G, Bainton BG, Summer WR (1989) The effects of acute and chronic alcoholism on tumor necrosis factor and the inflammatory response. J Infect Dis 160:422–429
Niemelä O, Klajner F, Orrego H, Vidins E, Blendis L, Israel Y (1987) Antibodies against acetaldehyde-modified protein epitopes in human alcoholics. Hepatology 7:1210–1214
Niemelä O, Parkkila S, Ylä-Herttuala S, Halsted C, Witztum JL, Lança AJ, Israel Y (1994) Covalent protein adducts in the liver as a result of ethanol metabolism and lipid peroxidation. Lab Invest 70:537–546
Niemelä O, Parkkila S, Ylä-Herttuala S, Villanueva J, Reubner B, Halsted CH (1995) Sequential acetaldehyde production, lipid peroxidation and fibrogenesis in micropig model of alcohol-induced liver disease. Hepatology 22:1208–1214
Nordmann R, Ribière C, Rouach H (1992) Implication of free radical mechanisms in ethanol-induced cellular injury. Free Radiat Biol Med 12:219–240
Ohnishi K, Lieber CS (1977) Reconstitution of the microsomal ethanol-oxidizing system: qualitative and quantitative changes of cytochrome P450 after chronic alcohol consumption. J Biol Chem 252:7124–7131
Ookhtens M, Hobdy K, Corvasce MC, Aw YU, Kaplowitz H (1985) Sinusoidal efflux of glutathione in the perfused liver. Evidence for a carrier mediated process. J Clin Invest 75:258–265
Orrego H, Blendis LM, Crossley IR, Medline A, Macdonald A, Ritchie S, Israel Y (1981a) Correlation of intrahepatic pressure with collagen in the Disse space and hepatomegaly in humans and in the rat. Gastroenterology 80:546–556
Orrego H, Israel Y, Blendis LM (1981b) Alcoholic liver disease: information in search of knowledge? Hepatology 1(3):267–283
Orrego H, Israel Y, Blake JE, Medline A (1983) Assessment of prognostic factors in alcoholic liver disease: toward global quantitative expression of severity. Hepatology 3:896–905
Orrego H, Blake JE, Medline A, Israel Y (1985) Interrelation of the hypermetabolic state, necrosis, anemia and cell enlargement as determinants of severity in alcoholic liver disease. Acta Med Scand [Suppl] 703:81–95
Orrego H, Blake JE, Blendis LM, Medline A (1987) Prognosis of alcoholic cirrhosis in the presence and absence of alcoholic hepatitis. Gastroenterology 92:208–214
Orrego H, Carmichael FJ, Saldivia V, Giles HG, Sandrin S, Israel Y (1988) Ethanol induced increase in portal blood flow: role of adenosine. Am J Physiol 254:G495–501
Orrego H, Blendis LM, Israel Y (1990) Hepatomegaly and portal pressure (correspondence). Hepatology 12:1457–1458
Parrish KM, Higuchi S, Dufour MC (1991) Alcohol consumption and the risk of developing cirrhosis: implications for future research. J Subst Abuse 3:325–335
Pequinot G, Cyrulnik F (1970) Chronic disease due to overconsumption of alcoholic drinks. In: International encyclopedia of pharmacology and therapeutics. Alcohols and derivatives, vol III. Pergamon, London, pp 375–412
Pierson JL, Mitchell MC (1986) Increased hepatic efflux of glutathione after chronic ethanol feeding. Biochem Pharmacol 35:1533–1537
Popper H, Lieber CS (1980) Histogenesis of alcoholic fibrosis and cirrhosis in the baboon. Am J Pathol 98:695–716
Rachamin G, Okuno F, Israel Y (1985) Inhibitory effect of propylthiouracil on the development of tolerance to ethanol. Biochem Pharmacol 34:2377–2383
Raiford DS, Smith RM, Thigpen MC (1994) Non-parenchymal cell-hepatocyte interactions influence hepatic sinusoidal efflux of glutathione. Hepatology 20:179A
Rankin JGD, Orrego Matte H, Deschenes J, Medline A, Findlay JE, Armstrong AIM (1978) Alcoholic liver disease: the problem of diagnosis. Alcohol Clin Exp Res 2:327–338
Reynolds TB (1975) Portal hypertension. In: Schiff L (ed) Diseases of the liver. Lippincott, Philadelphia, pp 330–367
Reynolds TB, Geller HM, Kuzma OT et al. (1960) Spontaneous decrease in portal pressure with clinical improvement in cirrhosis. N Engl J Med 263:734–739

Robinson GM, Orrego H, Israel Y, Devenyi P, Kapur BM (1981) Low molecular weight polyethylene glycol as a probe of gastrointestinal permeability after alcohol ingestion. Dig Dis Sci 26:971–977
Roitt IM, Brostoff J, Male DK (1989) Immunology, 2nd edn. Harper and Row, New York
Roll FJ, Alexander AM, Cua D, Swanson W, Perez HD (1991) Metabolism of ethanol by rat hepatocytes results in generation of lipid chemotactic factor: studies using a cell-free system and role of oxygen-derived free radicals. Arch Biochem Biophys 287:218–224
Ronis MJ, Huang J, Crouch J, Mercado C, Irby D, Valemtine CR, Lumpkin CK, Ingelman-Sundberg M, Badger TM (1993) Cytochrome P450 CYP2E1 induction during chronic alcohol exposure occurs by a two step mechanism associated with blood alcohol concentrations. J Pharmacol Exp Ther 264:944–950
Rubin E, Farber JL (1994) The liver and biliary system. In: Rubin E, Farber JL (eds) Pathology, 2nd edn. Lippincott, Philadelphia, pp 735–740
Rubin E, Lieber CS (1974) Fatty liver, alcoholic hepatitis and cirrhosis produced by alcohol in primates. N Engl J Med 290:128–135
Rubin E, Hutterer F, Lieber CS (1968) Ethanol increases hepatic smooth endoplasmic reticulum and drug metabolizing enzymes. Science 155:1459–1470
Rubin E, Beattie S, Toth A, Lieber CS (1972) Structural and functional effects of ethanol on hepatic mitochondria. Fed Proc 31:131–140
Rymsa B, Wang J-W, de Groot H (1991) O_2-release by activated Kupffer cells upon hypoxia-reoxygenation. Am J Physiol 261:G602–G607
Shaw S (1989) Lipid peroxidation, iron mobilization and radical generation induced by alcohol. Free Radiat Biol Med 7:541–547
Shaw S, Jayatilleke E (1990) The role of aldehyde oxidase in ethanol-induced hepatic liquid peroxidation in the rat. Biochem J 268:579–583
Shaw S, Jayatilleke E (1992) The role of cellular and catalytic iron in the pathogenesis of ethanol-induced liver injury. Life Sci 50:2045–2052
Sheron N, Bird G, Goka J, Alexander G, Williams R (1991) Elevated plasma interleukin-6 and increased severity and mortality in alcoholic hepatitis. Clin Exp Immunol 84:499–453
Speisky HA, MacDonald G, Giles G, Orrego H, Israel Y (1985) Increased loss and decreased synthesis of hepatic glutathione after acute ethanol administration: turnover studies. Biochem J 225:565–572
Steinbrecher UP, Fisher M, Witztum JL, Curtiss LK (1984) Immunogenicity of homologous low density lipoprotein after methylation, ethylation, acetylation, or carbamylation: generation of antibodies specific for derivatized lysine. J Lipid Res 25:1109–1116
Stevens VJ, Fantl WJ, Newman CG, Sims RV, Cerami A, Peterson CM (1981) Acetaldehyde adducts with hemoglobin. J Clin Invest 67:361–369
Svanas GW, Weiner H (1985) Aldehyde dehydrogenase as the rate limiting factor for acetaldehyde metabolism in rat liver. Biochem Pharmacol 34:1197–1202
Takahashi H, Wong K, Jui L, Nanji AA, Mendenhall CS, French SW (1991) Effect of dietary fat on Ito cell activation by chronic ethanol intake: a long-term serial morphometric study on alcohol-fed and control rats. Alcoholism: Clin Exp Res 15:1060–1066
Takei Y, Kawano S, Goto M, Nishimura Y, Nagai H, Chen SS, Fusamoto H, Kamada T, Kawada N, Kaneda K (1994) Activated Kupffer cells induce apoptosis in sinusoidal endothelial cells by juxtacrine mechanism. Hepatology 20:191A
Teare JP, Carmichael AJ, Burnett FR, Rake MO (1993) Detection of antibodies to acetaldehyde-albumin conjugates in alcoholic liver disease. Alcohol Alcohol 28:11–16
Thayer WS, Rubin E (1981) Molecular alterations in the respiratory chain of rat liver after chronic ethanol consumption. J Biol Chem 256:6090–6097
Teschke R, Hasumura Y, Joly JG, Lieber CS (1972) Microsomal ethanoloxidizing system (MEOS): purification and properties of a rat liver system free of catalase and alcohol dehydrogenase. Biochem Biophys Res Commun 49:1187–1193

Thornton AJ, Ham J, Kunkel SL (1992) Kupffer cell-derived cytokines induce the synthesis of a leukocyte chemotactic peptide, interleukin-8, in human hepatoma and primary hepatocyte cultures. Hepatology 15:1112–1122

Tiegs G, Wolter M, Wendel A (1989) Tumor necrosis factor is a terminal mediator in galactosamine/endotoxin-induced hepatitis in mice. Biochem Pharmacol 38:627–631

Tipton DF (1985) Aldehyde dehydrogenase. In: Flynn TG, Weiner H (eds) Enzymology of carbonyl metabolism 2: aldehyde dehydrogenase, aldo-keto reductase and alcohol dehydrogenase. Liss, New York, pp 1–13

Tsukamoto H (1994) Activation of fat storing cells in alcoholic liver fibrosis: role of Kupffer cells and lipid peroxidation. In: Surrenti C, Casini A, Milani S, Pinzzani M (eds) Fat-storing cells and liver fibrosis. Falk symposium no 71. Kluwer Academic, Dordrecht, pp 189–195

Tsukamoto H, Xi XP (1989) Incomplete compensation of enhanced hepatic oxygen consumption in rats with alcoholic centrilobular liver necrosis. Hepatology 9:302–306

Tsukamoto H, French SW, Reidelberger RD, Largman C (1985) Cyclical pattern of blood alcohol levels during continuous intragastric ethanol infusion in rats. Alcohol Clin Exp Res 9:31–37

Tsukamoto H, Towner SJ, Ciofalo LM, French SW (1986) Ethanol-induced liver fibrosis in rats fed high fat diet. Hepatology 6:814–822

Tsukamoto H, Kaminura S, Yeager S, Chen HY, Highman TJ, Luo ZZ, Kim CW, Brittenham GM (1992) Hepatic cirrhosis in rats fed a liquid diet with added alcohol and iron. Hepatology 16:113A

Tuma DJ, Donohue TM, Medina VA, Sorrell MF (1984) Enhancement of acetaldehyde-protein adduct formation by L-ascorbate. Arch Biochem Biophys 234:377–381

Verma BK, Fogarasi M, Szabo G (1993) Down-regulation of tumor necrosis factor α activity by acute ethanol treatment in human peripheral blood monocytes. J Clin Immunol 13:8–22

Videla LA, Fernandez V, Fernandez N, Valenzuela A (1981) On the mechanism of glutathione depletion induced in the liver by acute ethanol ingestion. Subst Alcohol Actions Misuse 2:153–156

Videla L, Iturriaga H, Pino ME, Bunout D, Valenzuela A, Ugarte G (1984) Content of hepatic reduced glutathione in chronic alcoholic patients: influence of the length of abstinence and liver necrosis. Clin Sci 66:283–290

Vidins EI, Britton RS, Medline A, Blendis LM, Israel Y, Orrego H (1985) Sinusoidal caliber in alcoholic and nonalcoholic liver disease: diagnostic and pathogenic implications. Hepatology 5:408–414

Weiss SJ (1989) Tissue destruction by neutrophils. N Engl J Med 320:365–376

Weiner FR, Degli Esposti S, Zern MA (1994) A role for transforming growth factor-b in hepatic fibrogenesis. In: Surrenti C, Casini A, Milani S, Pinzzani M (eds) Fat-storing cells and liver fibrosis. Falk symposium no 71. Kluwer Academic, Dordrecht

Worrall S, de Jersey J, Shanley BC, Wilce PA (1990) Antibodies against acetaldehyde-modified epitopes: presence in alcoholic, non-alcoholic liver disease and control subject. Alcohol Alcohol 25:509–517

Worrall S, de Jersey J, Shanley BC, Wilce PA (1991) Detection of stable acetaldehyde-modified proteins in the livers of ethanol-fed rats. Alcohol Alcohol 26:437–444

Yokoyama H, Ishii H, Nagata S, Kato S, Kamegaya K, Tsuchiya M (1993) Experimental hepatitis induced by ethanol after immunization with acetaldehyde adducts. Hepatology 17:14–19

Yuki T, Thurman RG (1980) The swift increase in alcohol metabolism. Biochem J 186:119–126

Yuki T, Thurman RG, Israel Y (1982) The swift increase in alcohol metabolism: inhibition of propylthiouracil. Biochem Pharmacol 31:2403–2407

CHAPTER 26

Antiepileptic Drugs

H.J. ZIMMERMAN and K.G. ISHAK

The frequent, concurrent use of several drugs has hampered the evaluation of the hepatotoxic potential of individual anticonvulsants. Nevertheless, it has been possible to characterize the hepatic injury associated with the commonly used anticonvulsive agents. Although at least 30 drugs have seen use as anticonvulsants, only 3 have drawn attention as important causes of hepatic injury (ZIMMERMAN and MADDREY 1993). These include phenytoin, carbamazepine, and valproic acid. While this chapter will focus on these three agents, reference will be made to other anticonvulsants that have been implicated in hepatic injury (Table 1). The hepatic injury produced by anticonvulsants is quite uniform. That associated with phenytoin and valproic acid is predominately hepatocellular. Rare instances of phenytoin-induced injury have been cholestatic, and carbamazepine jaundice may be either hepatocellular or cholestatic.

A. Phenytoin

This classic anticonvulsant has been in clinical use for more than half a century. Introduced to clinical medicine in 1938 (MERRITT and PUTMAN 1938), it quickly found extensive application. Within a few years reports of hepatic injury appeared (MANDELBAUM and KANE 1941; RITCHIE and KOLB 1942; VAN WYK and HOFFMAN 1948). During the subsequent 50 years, at least 100 cases of hepatic injury have been reported (PARKER and SHEARER 1979; MULLICK and ISHAK 1980; TING and DUNSKY 1982; GRAM and BENTSEN 1983; JEAVONS 1983); and we have encountered at least 25 unreported cases. Nevertheless, relative to the millions of patients who have taken the drug, the incidence must be judged to be very low.

I. Type of Hepatic Injury

The injury produced by phenytoin is a composite of hepatocyte damage accompanied by systemic responses reflective of immunologic response. This combination is seen in the histologic changes in the liver and in the clinical manifestations (Table 2).

Table 1. Anticonvulsants reported to cause hepatic injury

Agents	Presumed incidence	Type of mechanism	Injury
Carbamazepine (Tegretol)	VL	HS[a]	Hepatocellular, granuloma cholestasis
Mephenytoin (Mesantoin)	VVL	HS	Hepatocellular
Paramethadione (Paradione)	VL	HS	Hepatocellular, mixed
Phenacemide (Phenurone)	2%	HS	Hepatocellular, mixed
Phenobarbital	VVL	HS[a]	Hepatocellular, cholestasis
Phenytoin (Diphenylhydantoin, Dilantin)	VL	HS[a]	Hepatocellular, cholestasis, granulomas
Primidone	VVL	MI	No cases in man, hepatic injury in dogs
Progabide	>15%	MI	Hepatocellular
Thiantoin	VL	HS or MI	Hepatocellular
Trimethadione (Tridione)		HS	Hepatocellular, mixed
Valproic acid (Depakene)	<0.2%	MI	Hepatocellular (microvesicular steatosis, necrosis in some instances)

HS, hypersensitivity; MI, metabolic idiosyncrasy.
[a] Injury has prominent features of hypersensitivity but also evidence for relevance of genetic metabolic idiosyncrasy, namely defective detoxication of active intermediate (see text).

II. Clinical Manifestations

The clinical features are very uniform (Table 2). Fever, rash, and lymphadenopathy mark onset of injury, appearing in over 90% of the reactions between 1 and 5 weeks of starting intake of the drug. These features are followed promptly by jaundice. Usually accompanying the lymphadenopathy is leukocytosis with a relative and absolute lymphocytosis which includes atypical lymphocytes. Indeed, the constellation of lymph node enlargement, lymphocytosis, and atypical lymphocytes yields a syndrome that mimics infectious mononucleosis and serum sickness (BRAVERMAN and LEVIN 1963; KLECKNER et al. 1975; SIEGAL and BERKOWITZ 1981; BROWN and SCHUBERT 1986).

This constellation of systemic features, which has been dubbed (TOMSICK 1983) the "phenytoin syndrome," characteristically dominates the clinical picture. The cutaneous changes are often dramatic, ranging from a mild morbilliform rash to a severe, potentially fatal erythema multiforme reaction, which may lead to exfoliation and the full-blown Stevens-Johnson syndrome.

Table 2. Phenytoin (DPH) jaundice

	Susceptibility	
Age:	Adult (80% > 20 years; 90% > 10 years)	
Sex:	No clear difference	
Race:	Some reports suggest racial differences in susceptibility. Genetically determined impaired detoxification of active metabolites plays an important role in susceptibility	
	Clinical features	
Duration: DPH therapy:	1–5 weeks	
Signs and symptoms:	Fever:	90%
	Rash:	90%
	Lymph nodes[a]:	80%
	Hepatomegaly:	80%
	Splenomegaly:	30%
	Laboratory values	
Leukocytosis:	80%	
Lymphocytosis:	60% (some atypical)	
Eosinophilia:	80%	
Bilirubin:	Variable	
AST (SGOT):	300–>3000 IU	
ALT (SGPT):	< = > AST (SGOT)	
	Histology	
Degeneration, necrosis, inflammation		
Necrosis can be massive		
Inflammation can be granulomatous		
	Prognosis	
Case-fatality rate ~30%		
Fatalities usually to severe manifestation of immunologic response (e.g., Steven-Johnson syndrome) combined with liver failure		

[a] General enlargement.

Severity of hepatic injury may range from modest to severe hepatic damage and fulminant hepatic failure. Jaundice may be deep. Rare instances have been described as cholestatic; and even when the disease is clearly hepatocellular, cholestatic features may be prominent. Evidence of hepatic injury usually appears several days after the systemic manifestations begin. Other dramatic clinical manifestations may accompany the hepatic disease and the "phenytoin syndrome." These include interstitial nephritis (Kleckner et al. 1975), "hypersensitive pneumonia" (Bayer et al. 1976; Michael and Rudin 1981), myositis (Michael and Mitch 1976), eosinophilic fasciitis (Buchanan et al. 1980), lupus erythematosus-like syndrome (Easton 1972), and rhabdomyolysis (Engel et al. 1986). Pseudolymphoma (Salsztein and Ackerman 1959), other pseudoneoplastic syndromes, and even true neoplastic syndromes have been attributed to phenytoin (Wolf et al. 1985). Indeed, even when the hepatic injury is severe, the systemic manifestation may dominate the clinical picture.

III. Biochemical Features

The biochemical pattern of hepatic injury is mainly hepatocellular, although there may also be prominent cholestatic features. Aminotransferase levels usually resemble those of acute viral hepatitis with values for ALT (GPT) and AST (GOT) that are 10–100 times normal. Values for alkaline phosphatase (ALP) may be only twice normal or as high as eight times normal, yielding patterns of mixed-hepatocellular-cholestatic injury. Indeed, occasional instances of mainly cholestatic jaundice have been reported (DHAR et al. 1974; WEEDON 1975; SPECHLER et al. 1981; TAYLOR et al. 1984); although in one of those (DHAR et al. 1974) the designation of "cholestatic" seems belied by the development of severe hepatic failure with hepatic coma as evidence of a severe hepatocellular component.

IV. Histopathology

The histologic changes in most cases are those of severe hepatocellular injury accompanied by a prominent inflammatory response (Figs. 1–3). Degeneration of hepatocytes, "free" (sinusoidal) acidophilic bodies and necrosis are prominent. The inflammation is generally lymphocytic. Indeed, the "beading" pattern of lymphocytes in sinusoids, the hepatocellular injury, the frequent mitotic figures in hepatocytes, and the granulomatoid inflammatory response (Figs. 1, 2) yield a morphologic pattern remarkably similar to that of infectious mononucleosis (MULLICK and ISHAK 1980), an intriguing similarity in view of the similarities in clinical picture. A characteristic difference from infectious mononucleosis, however, is the frequency of prominent aggregates of eosinophils (MULLICK and ISHAK 1980). The frequent severity of phenytoin-associated liver disease, with 15% or more of cases showing submassive or massive necrosis (Fig. 3), also differs from that of infectious mononucleosis, where the liver disease is usually relatively mild. The severe necrosis of fatal cases may be mainly in zone 3 or panacinar.

Cholestasis with bile casts in zone 3 has been prominent in some of the cases with hepatocellular injury. Indeed in about 10% of reported cases studied at biopsy, the lesion has been described as mainly cholestatic (BRAVERMAN and LEVIN 1963; SPECHLER et al. 1981). In one case of cholestatic jaundice which showed histologic features, mimicking those of extrahepatic obstruction, there had been an extraordinarily long period of taking the drug and an apparent dose relationship in the production of the hepatic injury (TAYLOR et al. 1984). For the most part, however, cholestasis, even when prominent, has been accompanied by hepatocellular injury as a "mixed" pattern rather than as the predominant lesion. One case has been reported to show changes of chronic active hepatitis (RIERA VELASCO et al. 1986).

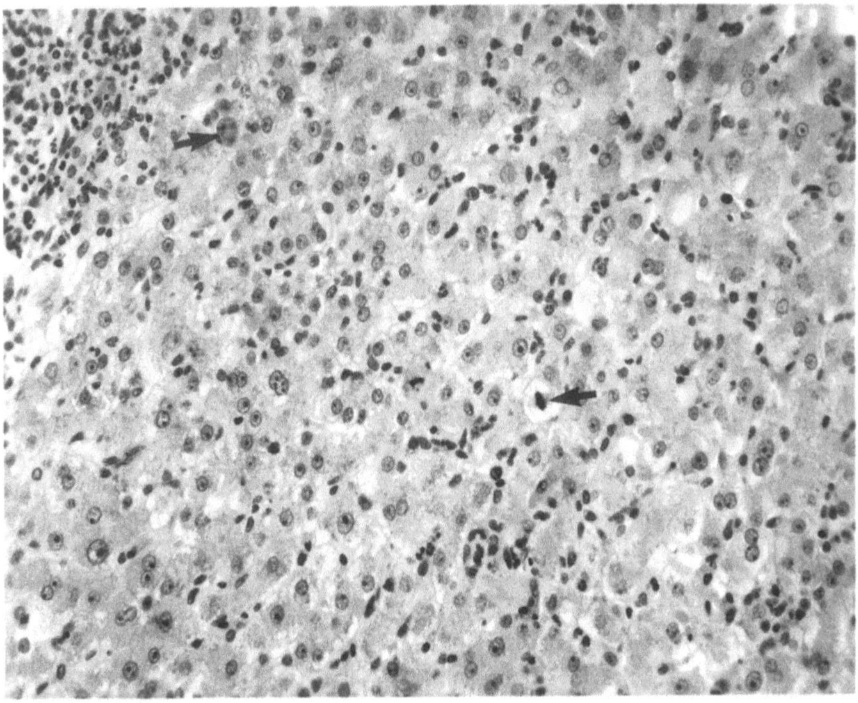

Fig. 1. Diffuse hepatocellular injury in patients taking phenytoin. Acute acidophilic ("apoptotic" body) and mitosis (*arrows*) as well as sinusoidal beading similar to hepatic involvement in infectious mononucleosis. H&E, ×250

A granulomatous or granulomatoid inflammatory response may occur (Figs. 2, 4). Pseudogranulomatous aggregates of Kupffer cells, macrophages, and lymphocytes are characteristic and, in about 15% of patients coming to biopsy, granulomas either in association with hepatocellular injury or as the main lesion are seen.

V. Prognosis

The outlook for the syndrome is guarded. Approximately one-third of the cases recorded in the literature have had a fatal outcome, with many of the deaths in hepatic failure. In many of the fatal cases, the accompanying syndrome of severe hypersensitivity disease with exfoliative dermatitis and the Stevens-Johnson syndrome or even polyarteritis nodosa have contributed importantly to the fatal outcome or have been responsible for it (Gram and Bentsen 1983; Ritchie and Kolb 1942; Van Wyk and Hoffmann 1948; Gropper 1956; Braverman and Levin 1963; Jeavons 1983).

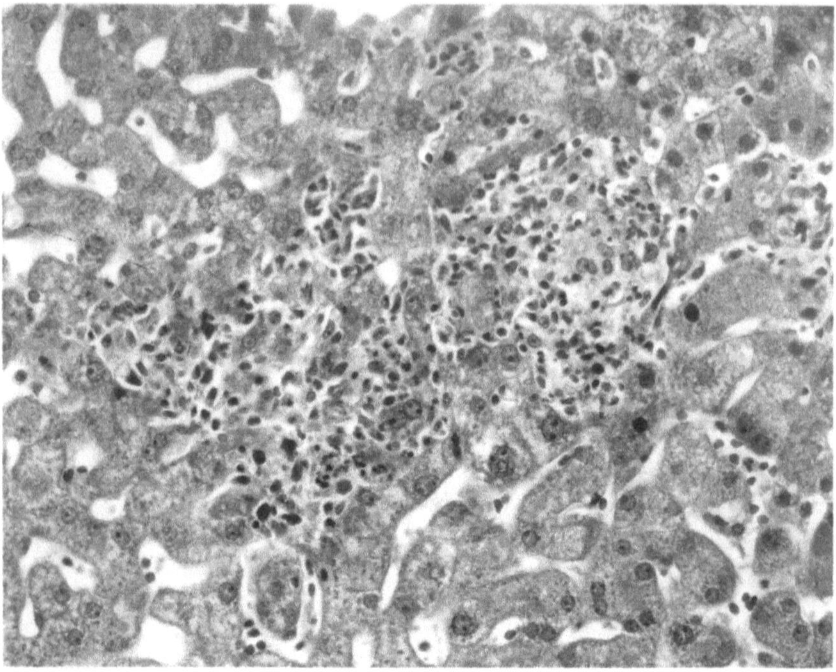

Fig. 2. Focal necrosis with granulomatoid inflammatory response in a patient taking phenytoin. H&E, ×200

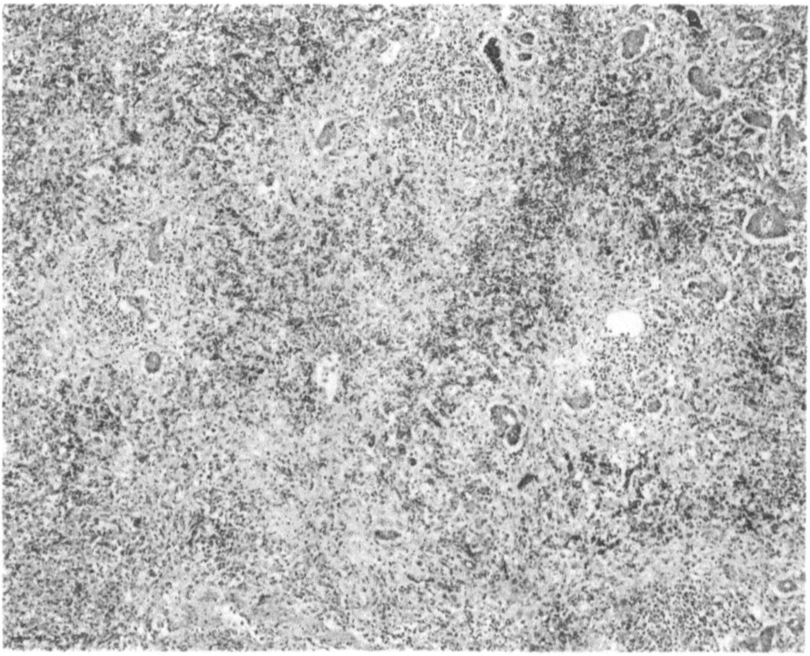

Fig. 3. Massive necrosis in a fatal reaction to phenytoin. H&E, ×60

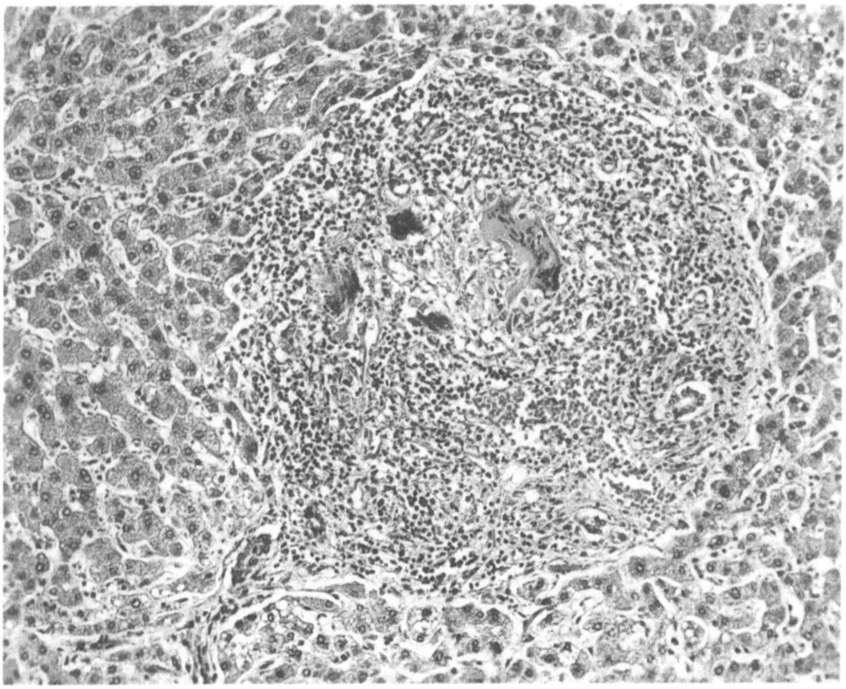

Fig. 4. Portal area granuloma showing giant cells in a patient taking phenytoin. H&E, ×600

VI. Mechanism

There seems little doubt that the hepatic injury reflects immunologic responses. The syndrome of fever, rash, lymphadenopathy, blood and tissue eosinophilia, granulomatous lesions, and the fixed, relatively brief, period of exposure prior to development of injury, all point strongly to hypersensitivity as the mechanism. The demonstration of lymphoblastic transformation of lymphocytes from recovered patients supports this view; although lymphoblastic transformation as evidence for drug-induced hepatic disease offers technical problems and may be misleading. Nevertheless, the demonstration (Kleckner et al. 1975) of antibodies to phenytoin in patients with severe hepatic injury and systemic features of the serum sickness type also support the view of an immunologic pathogenesis of the injury.

The precipitation of other syndromes that have strong immunologic overtones add support to the immunologic basis of phenytoin-induced hepatic disease. Erythema multiforme (Ritchie and Kolb 1942), the systemic lupus erythematosus (SLE) syndrome (Easton 1972), polyarteritis nodosa (Gram and Bentsen 1983), pseudolymphoma (Chaiken et al. 1950; Saltzstein and Ackerman 1959), true lymphoma (Anthony 1970), and immunoblastic lymphadenopathy (Lapes et al. 1976) are dramatic examples of bizarre immunologic accidents provoked by the drug.

Readministration of the drug usually leads to recurrence of fever, rash, and eosinophilia, which may be accompanied by hepatic injury, also offering support for the importance of immunologic mechanisms in pathogenesis. However, administration of a "challenge" dose of a drug which has led to overt, generalized hypersensitivity may lead to disastrous recurrence of the syndrome.

There is also evidence that phenytoin may have intrinsic toxic potential. Studies by several groups (ANDREASEN et al. 1973; AIGES et al. 1980; DEUTSCH et al. 1986) have shown elevated aminotransferase levels in patients taking phenytoin. Mean levels of ALT and AST have been higher than those of control groups (DEUTSCHE et al. 1986), and individual patients have shown a 17% (AIGES et al. 1980) – 25% (ANDREASEN et al. 1973) incidence of elevated values for those enzymes. Studies of individual patients with such elevated values have reported focal necrosis as evidence of hepatic injury (JACOBSEN et al. 1976; NORDIN et al. 1982), or only proliferation of smooth endoplasmic reticulum as evidence of induction of the mixed function oxidase (AIGES et al. 1980; DEUTSCH et al. 1986; JACOBSEN et al. 1976; NORDIN et al. 1982; JEZEQUEL and ORLANDI 1976).

The enzyme induction is also reflected in the elevated serum levels of γ-glutamyl transferase found in almost all patients taking phenytoin (KEEFFE et al. 1986). Indeed, ANDREASSON and associates (1973) have suggested that mild hepatic injury, reflected by the elevated aminotransferase levels, may be a manifestation of the ultimate, adverse effect of enzyme induction. A similar formulation was offered earlier by HUTTERER et al. (1968), who characterized the late stage of induction as "hypoactive, hyperplastic endoplasmic reticulum" and considered it to be early toxicity. In any event the possibility that mild hepatotoxicity of phenytoin combined with hypersensitivity accounts for the overt hepatotoxicity warrants consideration. This hypothesis is consistent with the studies of SPIELBERG et al. (1981) and SHEAR et al. (1988). They have provided evidence that phenytoin toxicity depends on conversion of the drug to an arene oxide which, in genetically susceptible individuals, cannot be adequately converted to the nontoxic dihydrodiol (Fig. 5). The same metabolite, the arene oxide, could act both as a hapten, provoking immunologic factors leading to hypersensitivity, and as a reactive radical, leading to hepatic injury by covalent binding to hepatocyte molecules (SPIELBERG et al. 1981; SHEAR et al. 1988).

Elevated values for alkaline phosphatase (ALP) may occur in up to 30% of patients taking phenytoin and be unaccompanied by evidence of hepatic injury (KAZAMATSURI 1970; FRAME 1971; OFFERMANN 1981). These elevations appear to reflect bone changes secondary to relative deficiency of vitamin D sterol that have been attributed to enhanced inactivation of the vitamin (KAZAMATSURI 1970), in turn due to induction of the cytochrome P450 by phenytoin. While evidence for the role of enhanced metabolism of vitamin D remains scanty, there is good evidence that the elevated ALP levels in patients taking phenytoin are usually of osseous origin (FRAME 1971; OFFERMANN

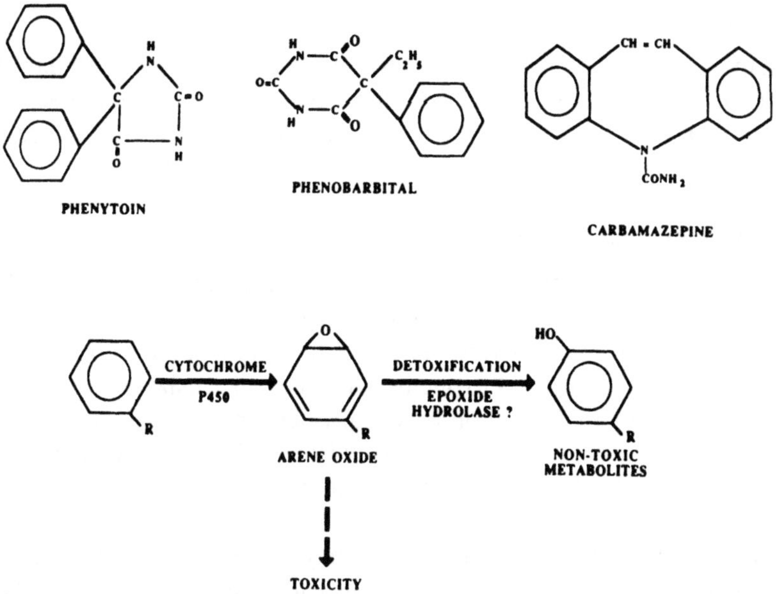

Fig. 5. Structure of phenytoin, phenobarbital, and carbamazepine showing pathway for formation of arene oxide and detoxification under catalytic influence of epoxide hydrolase. Susceptibility to hepatotoxic effects of these anticonvulsants appears to depend on genetically defective conversion of toxic arene oxide to nontoxic hydrodiol. [From SHEAR et al. (1988) with permission. Reproduced from the *Journal of Clinical Investigation* 82: 1826–1832 (1988) (Fig. 1) by copyright permission of the American Society for Clinical Investigation]

1981). Only when accompanied by other evidence of hepatic injury is an elevated ALP level likely to be of hepatic origin.

VII. Other Hydantoins

1. Mephenytoin

Mephenytoin (methylphenylhydantoin) (MARTINDALE 1982) and thiantoin (MARTINDALE 1982; PRYLES et al. 1952; BUTSCHER and GALLAGER 1952) also are credited with being likely to produce hepatocellular injury. Ethiotoin (ethylphenylhydantoin), a weak anticonvulsant, has been relatively little clinical use and has not been reported to produce hepatic injury.

2. Acetylurea Derivatives

Phenurone (GIBBS et al. 1949; CARTER et al. 1950; LEVY et al. 1950) and acetoxyphenurone (SCHNABEL and LAKL 1964) have led to instances of a syndrome that resembles that of phenytoin. The hepatic injury, in several patients, presented as fatal, subacute, rather than acute, hepatic necrosis. Indeed, the severe hepatic toxicity is the chief reason that the use of phenurone was abandoned.

3. Oxazolidinediones

Trimethadione (tridione) has led to several *instances* of hepatocellular injury as part of a syndrome of generalized hypersensitivity (LEARD and KAUFMAN 1949). Renal injury, especially the nephrotic syndrome, is a much more characteristic side effect of trimethadione than is hepatic injury.

4. Barbiturates and Primidone

Phenobarbital has led to rare instances of hepatic injury, hepatocellular or cholestatic, less than ten cases having been reported (SHAPIRO et al. 1980). SHEAR et al. (1988) have provided evidence that immunologic idiosyncrasy to phenobarbital resembles that to phenytoin and to carbamazepine. The hepatic injury also appears to depend on genetically determined inadequate detoxification of the arene oxide by the epoxide hydrolase (Fig. 5). Indeed, they found considerable overlap between clinical sensitivity to phenobarbital, phenytoin, and carbamazepine.

Primidone is an anticonvulsant that may be regarded as a congener of phenobarbital with two hydrogen atoms instead of the carbonyl group. While, to our knowledge, there are no published reports of hepatic injury in humans, there are convincing accounts of hepatic injury in dogs receiving primidone (BUNCH et al. 1985). The injury is hepatocellular. Both acute necrosis and chronic hepatitis have been reported.

B. Carbamazepine

Carbamazepine, a drug structurally related to the phenothiazines and to the tricyclic antidepressants, has been employed as an anticonvulsant and for the treatment of tic douloureux. Since the first instance of hepatic injury was reported more than a quarter century ago (SPILLANE 1964), there have been at least 50 individual cases reported. Furthermore, the report of HADZIE et al. (1990) has cited 499 instances of adverse reactions involving the liver, of which about 50% showed only biochemical abnormality. The estimate of about 250 cases of clinically evident hepatic injury included 18 deaths. Mild to moderate elevations of ALT levels occur in up to 22% of recipients of the drug, and of γ-glutamyl transferase and alkaline phosphatase more frequently than of ALT (STRICKER 1992).

I. Susceptibility

The likelihood of development of carbamazepine-induced hepatic injury appears to be modified by age but not by sex. The majority of patients have been adults over 40 years of age. Males and females seem equally susceptible (WILLIAMS et al. 1986). Studies by SHEAR et al. (1988) suggest that patients who develop hepatic injury have defective detoxification of the active metabolite of carbamazepine. The role of other anticonvulsants or other agents in provoking of modifying carbamazepine-associated hepatic injury, as enzyme inducers or inhibitors or as cotoxic agents, warrants consideration, but is not ascertainable at present.

II. Clinical Features

The syndrome provoked by carbamazepine has much in common with that caused by phenytoin (Table 3). Onset of injury is during the first 8 weeks of taking the drug in 80% of patients (Elitsur 1990; Jaffe 1989) and during the first 4 weeks in over 60% of patients. Among the 20% of patients with duration of exposure greater than 8 weeks, periods as long as 3 months (Fellows 1969), 6 months (Brukher and Joustra 1966; Zucker et al. 1977), and even 4 years (Hopen et al. 1981) have been recorded. The hepatic injury is often accompanied by fever, rash, and eosinophilia (Gram and Bentsen 1983); although the severe hypersensitivity syndrome of the Stevens-Johnson type appears to be less frequent than in phenytoin reactions.

III. Biochemical Features

Hyperbilirubinemia has been of modest degree, ranging from 1.3 to 12 mg/dl. The aminotransferase and ALP levels have yielded an hepatocellular pattern

Table 3. Hepatic injury associated with carbamazepine (CBZ)

Incidence:	Unknown. Over 50 published cases	
Susceptibility:	Most cases involve adults	
	No sex differences apparent	
	May be genetic factors. Impaired detoxification of active metabolite	
	Cross-reactions with phenytoin	
Duration of therapy:	<4 weeks 60%	
	<8 weeks 80%	
Hallmarks of hypersensitivity:	Fever, rash, eosinophilia, frequent	
Hepatic injury:		
	Hepatocellular:	25%
	Cholestatic:	25%
	Mixed:	10%
	Indeterminate:	40%
	Granulomas in 35% of patients with other injury	
	Elevated levels of ALT occur in up to 20% of recipients	
Prognosis:	Case-fatality rate:	~12%
	Chronic cholestasis in at least two cases	
Mechanism:	Immunologic and metabolic idiosyncrasy probably both involved	
	Drug also has some intrinsic toxic potential	

of injury in about 25% of reported cases, a cholestatic one in a similar proportion, and a mixed pattern in about 10% of reported cases. In the remaining published reports the pattern has been consistent with mild hepatocellular or cholestatic injury, or the available data have not been sufficient to permit categorization of the pattern of injury.

IV. Histopathology

The morphologic features also show hepatocellular injury in some patients, cholestatic injury in others and a mixed pattern in some. Necrosis has been massive or submassive in a few patients and of lesser degree in several. Cholestasis has been recorded in a number of others; several have shown cholangitis (LEVY et al. 1981; MITCHELL et al. 1981; LARREY et al. 1987). More than one-third of reported cases have had granulomas (VAN WYK and HOFFMAN 1948; LEVANDER 1980; SOFFER et al. 1983), in association with cholestatic injury, with hepatocellular lesions, or as the only hepatic lesion.

V. Prognosis

The prognosis of carbamazepine jaundice is also somewhat less threatening than that of phenytoin. Of approximately 50 individually reported patients, 6 have died. Four had severe hepatocellular injury and the other two had aplastic anemia and hepatic injury, to give a recorded case-fatality rate of 12%. Were the approximately 250 cases of jaundice in recipients of carbamazepine and the deaths of 18 (HADZIE et al. 1990) all accepted as attributable to the drug, a case-fatality rate of 7% would apply. At least one patient, a child with fulminant hepatic failure, has undergone successful orthotopic liver transplantation (DREIFUSS et al. 1989). The lesser incidence of extensive hepatic necrosis and of the Stevens-Johnson type of systemic response appears to account for a mortality figure seemingly lower than that of phenytoin. Nevertheless, prognosis is guarded in those with a severe, febrile-cutaneous reaction and with hepatocellular injury. Patients with granulomatous disease and cholestasis usually survive (WILLIAMS et al. 1986; LEBLANC and FELDMAN 1961). Rare instances of carbamazepine-induced cholestasis may fail to subside and the syndrome of prolonged cholestasis resembling primary biliary cirrhosis may emerge. We have seen one such instance which ended fatally. Another case of prolonged cholestasis with disappearance of interlobular bile ducts has been reported ("vanishing bile duct syndrome") (FORBES et al. 1992).

VI. Mechanism

Development of injury may be presumed to involve hypersensitivity in view of the high frequency of rash, fever, and eosinophilia and of the relatively short uniform period of exposure to the drug prior to the appearance of injury. Nevertheless, the associated role of intrinsic toxicity of carbamazepine or a metabolite (BERTRAM and TAYLOR 1980) warrants consideration, especially in view of the hepatotoxic effects of large doses of the drug (LUKE et al. 1986).

SHEAR et al. (1988) have found that patients who manifest generalized hypersensitivity to carbamazepine with or without hepatic injury have genetically determined inadequate detoxification of the arene oxide (Fig. 5). The defect appears to be ineffective epoxide hydrolase activity, permitting the epoxide to act as a hapten or a toxic moiety. Indeed, these authors have found the same defect involved in the development of hypersensitivity to phenytoin, carbamazepine, and phenobarbital. All three apparently lead to hypersensitivity in patients whose formation of the dihydrodiol is inadequate. This accounts for the frequency of cross-reactions between these drugs and the need to proceed carefully in substituting one of them for another in individuals who have had reactions.

C. Valproic Acid

This aniconvulsant differs strikingly from those already cited in structure, mechanism of anticonvulsive activity, and hepatic injury. It is an organic acid with anticonvulsant activity apparently dependent on increasing brain levels of γ-aminobutyric acid (BROWNE 1980). Valproate-associated hepatic injury first came to notice in 1978, and by 1990 at least 100 fatal instances of hepatic injury had come to attention (JEAVONS 1982, 1983, 1984; DREIFUSS and SANTILLI 1986; DREIFUSS et al. 1989; ZIMMERMAN 1991). At least 25 reversible cases of hepatic injury have also been reported (ZIMMERMAN 1991).

Three syndromes of hepatic disease have been described:

1. Slowly evolving obtundation and chronic liver failure
2. Acute Reye's syndrome
3. Hyperammonenia with obtundation but without other evidence of liver disease

Most frequent is chronically evolving liver failure with obtundation. Much less frequent is hyperammonemic obtundation with little other evidence of hepatic injury. Even less frequent is a rapidly developing syndrome similar to Reye's syndrome.

I. Incidence of Injury

Overt, serious hepatic disease, usually fatal, has been estimated to be as infrequent as 1 in 37000 patients (JEAVONS 1982, 1983, 1984) or as frequent as 1 in 500 (DREIFUSS et al. 1989). A recent analysis has come up with the figure of 1 in 5000 patients (SCHEFFNER 1988). DREIFUSS and SANTILLI (1986) have drawn attention to a sharp drop in the apparent incidence of valproic acid-associated hepatic injury which they attributed to more selective prescribing and avoidance of use in infants less than 2 years old. Minor abnormalities, i.e., elevated aminotransferase levels, have been recorded in 7%–44% of patients (ZIMMERMAN 1991). Most of these abnormalities do not progress or may even subside despite continuation of the drug.

II. Susceptibility

Children and infants appear to be more susceptible than adults (ZIMMERMAN and ISHAK 1982; JEAVONS 1984; DREIFUSS and SANTILLI 1986; DREIFUSS et al. 1989). While only 50% of the prescriptions have been written for patients below the age of 20 years, almost 90% of the patients with valproic acid injury have been in that age group (JEAVONS 1984); over 70% of them have been under the age of 11 years and a published mean age for patients with hepatic injury is 8.4 years (JEAVONS 1984). Indeed, DREIFUSS and SANTILLI (1986) have reported that the incidence of fatal hepatotoxicity is 1 in 500 in patients younger than 2 years taking valproic acid with other anticonvulsants. A role for genetic factors is suggested by reports of at least two families with more than one case (POWELL et al. 1984). Indeed, there are clinical and experimental reports suggesting that the inborn metabolic errors of ornithine carbamoyl transferase deficiency (ZAFRANI and BERTHELOT 1982; BUCHI et al. 1984; COULTER 1984; SUGIMOTO et al. 1987; OHTANI et al. 1982; TAKEUCHI et al. 1988), and perhaps carnitine deficiency (ZAFRANI and BERTHELOT 1982; BUCHI et al. 1984; COULTER 1984; SUGIMOTO et al. 1987a; OHTANI et al. 1982; TAKEUCHI et al. 1988), may enhance susceptibility to valproic acid toxicity. However, the role of carnitine deficiency has been discounted (MELEGH et al. 1990; LAUB et al. 1986; ROZAS et al. 1990). Even the possible association of α_1-antitrypsin deficiency has been mentioned (MOORE et al. 1984). Other anticonvulsants, taken concurrently, have been suspected of enhancing the toxicity of valproic acid.

III. Clinical Features

Age at presentation has ranged from $2\frac{1}{2}$ months to 67 years. Duration of treatment prior to onset of illness has been as short as 3 days and as long as 2 years, and in 70% of patients has ranged from 4 to 16 weeks. The great majority of patients had been taking other anticonvulsants. Doses of valproic acid have ranged from <20 mg/kg per day to >51 mg/kg per day (ZIMMERMAN 1991).

The most common early symptoms have been anorexia, nausea, vomiting, and ultimately somnolence, often accompanied by increased convulsions (Table 4). Thereafter jaundice, coagulation disorders, and coma develop. There may be ascites and hypoglycemia. While coma is characteristically a reflection of slowly progressive hepatic failure, there are instances of obtundation associated with elevated blood ammonia levels without other evidence of hepatic injury. Most reported cases (approximately 100) have

Table 4. Hepatic injury associated with valproic acid syndrome of chronic hepatic failure

Incidence:	Estimated 0.02% (1 in 5000 patients) overall 0.2% (1 in 500 patients) in infants below 2 years
Susceptibility:	Infants and children far more susceptible than adults Genetic factors Inborn metabolic error may predispose
Duration of treatment:	3 days to 2 years
Sign and symptoms:	Nausea, vomiting Somnolence Jaundice Coagulopathy Coma Ascites ± Abdominal pain
Hepatic injury:	Microvesicular steatosis Necrosis Cirrhosis
Mechanism:	Metabolic idiosyncrasy. Probably toxic effects of product of ω-pathway (14-en-valproic acid) on mitochondria
Prognosis:	Fatality rate among recognized cases 75% (?)

been fatal. However, at least 25 patients have been reported to survive (ZIMMERMAN 1991).

Jaundice has been of modest degree in most patients but very deep in a few, and has been recorded in only 62% of reported cases (JEAVONS 1984). Even in the fatal cases, however, jaundice may not appear. Ascites has been described in about 40% of fatal cases. Fever and hypoglycemia have been noted in an almost equal number. Initial complaints are similar in fatal and in surviving cases. Only in the evolution of the syndrome to jaundice and coma were there differences.

Abdominal pain has been variably prominent. The multiple reports (CAMPBELL et al. 1977; PARKER et al. 1981; MURPHY et al. 1981; WILLIAMS et al. 1983) of valproic acid-associated pancreatitis suggest that the abdominal pain accompanying valproic acid hepatic injury may reflect pancreatitis.

A few children have presented with an abrupt and anicteric syndrome resembling Reye's syndrome (POWELL 1984; GERBER et al. 1979; SUCHY et al. 1979; KEENE et al. 1982; SUGMALA et al. 1983). The syndrome evolves rapidly with anorexia, vomiting, and lethargy presenting abruptly, accompanied by fever, followed by clinical evidence of cerebral edema and coma.

Symptomatic hyperammonemia without overt evidence of liver disease has been reported in at least 22 patients (ZIMMERMAN 1991). All but five of them have been below the age of 14 years; the five ranged in age from 20 to 51 years. This syndrome has been characterized by confusion, stupor, and coma, usually accompanied by ataxia.

IV. Biochemical Features

Bilirubin levels have ranged from the normal to values as high as 36 mg/dl. Aminotransferase levels have been only mildly elevated in more patients. In only 15% of patients have values exceeded 25-fold elevations (1000 u). Values for AST and ALT are approximately equal to those for ALT. Values for ALP have been increased less than threefold. Prothrombin time has ranged up to threefold normal, and in almost all patients has been significantly prolonged. Hyperammonemia has been found in 75% of those with overt hepatic disease as well as in patients with only obtundation as the clinical manifestation.

V. Histopathology

The most frequent lesion has been microvesicular steatosis, often accompanied by necrosis (ZIMMERMAN and ISHAK 1982; POWELL et al. 1984). About 20% of a group of fatal cases showed only necrosis and the remainder showed microvesicular steatosis alone or with necrosis and cirrhosis (ZIMMERMAN and ISHAK 1982) (Figs. 6–9). In one of the fatal cases we studied, the patient had veno-occlusive disease (ZIMMERMAN and ISHAK 1982).

The lesion produced in rats (LEWIS et al. 1982) and mice (POWELL et al. 1984) by valproic acid is also microvesicular steatosis, suggesting that the steatosis is the pure valproic acid lesion in man. Nevertheless, in the cases studied, necrosis multifocal, zone 3 or massive) has accompanied the steatosis or has been the main lesion in half of the cases (ZIMMERMAN 1991). Since almost all of the patients had also been taking other anticonvulsants, the role of valproic acid per se in the lesions remains unclear. Specifically, it is possible that necrogenic effects of other drugs or alterations by them of metabolism of

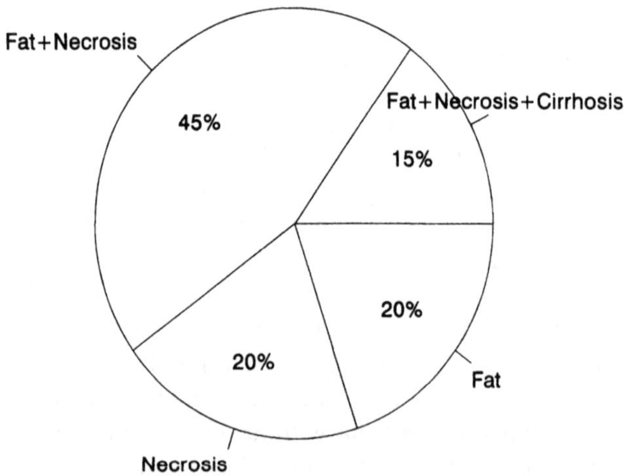

Fig. 6. Distribution of lesions in valproic acid toxicity. Figures based on study of ZIMMERMAN and ISHAK (1982). Since most patients who take valproic acid also take other anticonvulsants, their role in injury attributed to valproic acid is not clear

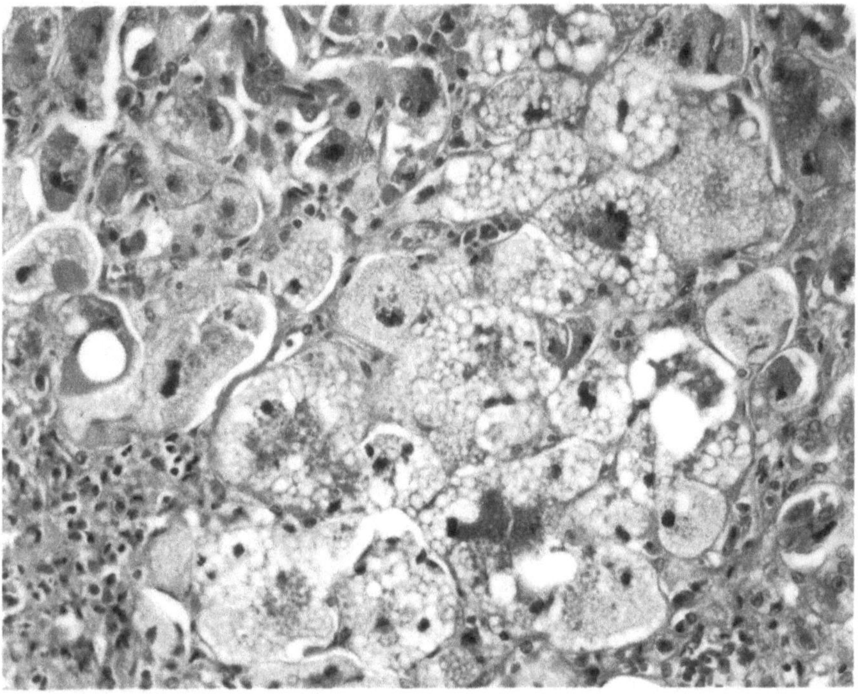

Fig. 7. Microvesicular steatosis due to valproic acid. H&E, ×300

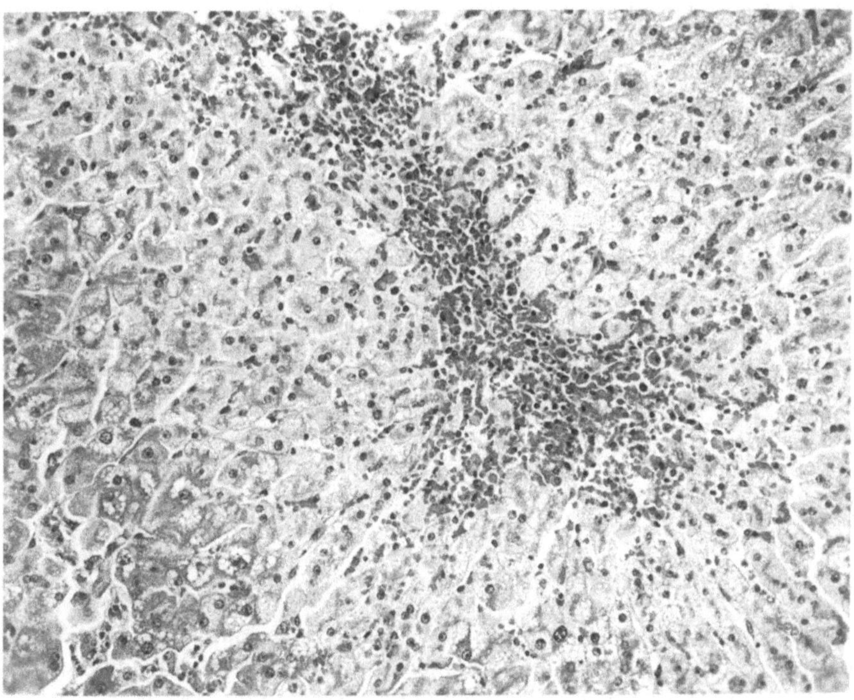

Fig. 8. Lower magnification of case shown in Fig. 7, showing microvesicular steatosis in zones 1 and 2 and perivenous hemorrhagic necrosis. H&E, ×160

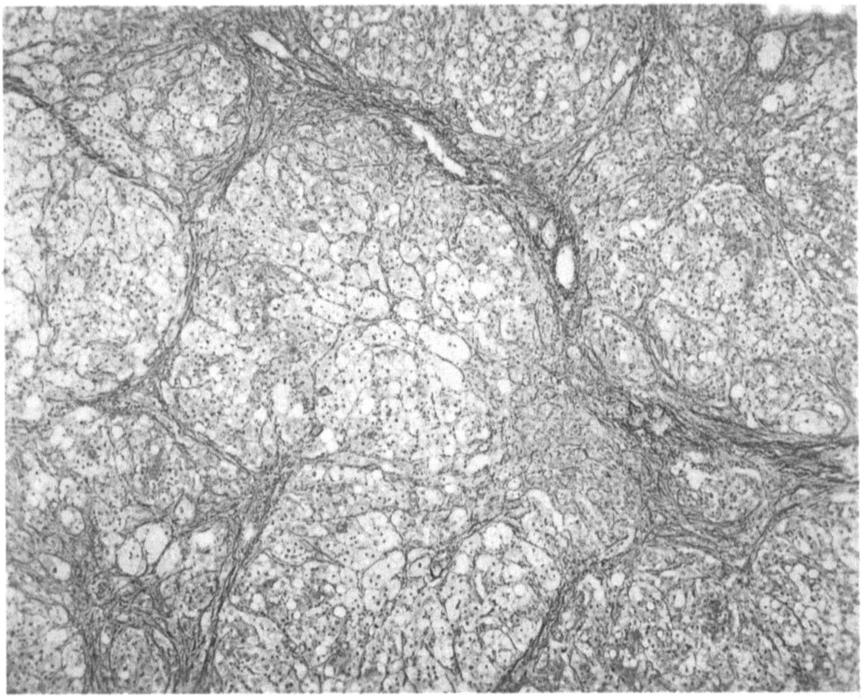

Fig. 9. Cirrhosis in patient taking valproic acid. H&E, ×460

valproic acid, leading to necrogenic metabolites, might account for the necrosis (ZIMMERMAN and ISHAK 1992).

VI. Prognosis

The hepatotoxicity of valproic acid is clearly a grave syndrome. While no useful figure for the case fatality rate can be offered, since there is no denominator for the total number of patients with identifiable, clinically significant hepatic injury, the mortality rate appears to be high. Summation of an estimated 100 fatal with approximately 25 reversible cases provides a dramatic case-fatality figure of 80%. Presumably, milder reversible cases are overlooked. Whatever the correct figure, the outlook for patients with the full syndrome is quite bleak.

VII. Mechanism of Injury

An idiosyncratic reaction is clearly the basis for the serious hepatic injury. The very low incidence of overt injury demonstrates the role of individual susceptibility. That the idiosyncrasy is metabolic is implicit in the lack of hallmarks of hypersensitivity, in the nature of the morphologic lesion, and in the delayed onset of hepatic disease (ZIMMERMAN and ISHAK 1982). Rash, eosinophilia, or early fever are not seen. Steatosis, which is the characteristic lesion, is not the type of injury associated with hypersensitivity; and onset delayed for months after the drug has been started is more characteristic of metabolic, than of immunologic, idiosyncrasy (BOWDLE et al. 1979). The microvesicular steatosis that is a characteristic abnormality of valproic acid toxicity and the associated clinical features comprise a syndrome that resembles Jamaican vomiting sickness (JVS) (BOWDLE et al. 1979; TANAKA et al. 1976) and Reye's syndrome, as well as the experimental equivalent of those lesions reproduced by 4-pentanoic acid (GLASGOW and CHASE 1975). Accordingly, it is of great interest that products of the ω-pathway of valproic acid metabolism are 4-en-valproic acid and 3-en-valproic acid (Fig. 10). These compounds are remarkably similar to a product of hypoglycin A, the agent responsible for JVS, and to 4-pentanoic acid, the compound that produces microvesicular steatosis in rats, considered an experimental model of Reye's syndrome (Fig. 10) (GLASGOW and CHASE 1975). Furthermore, administration of 4-en-valproic acid leads to microvesicular steatosis in rats and to injury to hepatocytes in vitro (KESTERSON et al. 1984). It is our opinion (ZIMMERMAN and ISHAK 1982) and that of others (SUGIMOTO et al. 1983; KESTERSON et al. 1984; GRANNEMAN et al. 1984) that the toxic metabolites are 4-en-valproic acid and 3-en-valproic acid and that the probable mechanism for valproic acid hepatic injury is the enhanced metabolism along the ω-pathways.

The observation that phenobarbital pretreatment of rats (LEWIS et al. 1982) enhances the production in them of steatosis by valproic acid, and the demonstration (KESTERSON et al. 1984; GRANNEMAN et al. 1984; KINGSLEY et al. 1983) that the 4-en-valproic acid is hepatotoxic, confirms this view. The recent demonstration (RETTIE et al. 1986) that microsomes from phenobarbital-pretreated rats catalyze the conversion of valproic acid to 4-en-valproic acid, deduced to reflect cytochrome P450 induction, offers additional support for that view.

The metabolic lesion imposed by valproic acid has appeared to be inhibition of fatty acid metabolism by blockade of β-oxidation (BUCHI et al. 1984; BJORGE and BAILLIE 1985). While 4-en-valproic acid can effect this block, 4-en-pentanoic acid seems a less effective inhibitor; yet it produces similar injury. The precise mechanism by which valproic acid leads to hepatic injury is incompletely established, but metabolic idiosyncrasy seems clearly incriminable.

Irrespective of the precise molecular instigator of the injury, the site of damage appears to be the mitochondrion (MURPHY et al. 1985; BONAZZI et al. 1986; JIMENEZ-RODRIGUEZVILA et al. 1985; COUDE et al. 1983a,b; JEZEQUEL et al. 1984). Structural change consists of distortion and disappearance of cristae, electron-dense deposits, fat inclusion, and deformation of the mitochondria (KESTERSON et al. 1984; JEZEQUEL et al. 1984). Functional injury is suggested by some, albeit controversial, evidence of carnitine deficiency in patients taking valproic acid (MURPHY et al. 1985; COULTER 1984), the inhibition by valproic acid of *N*-acetylglutamate activity and consequent inhibition of carbamoyl

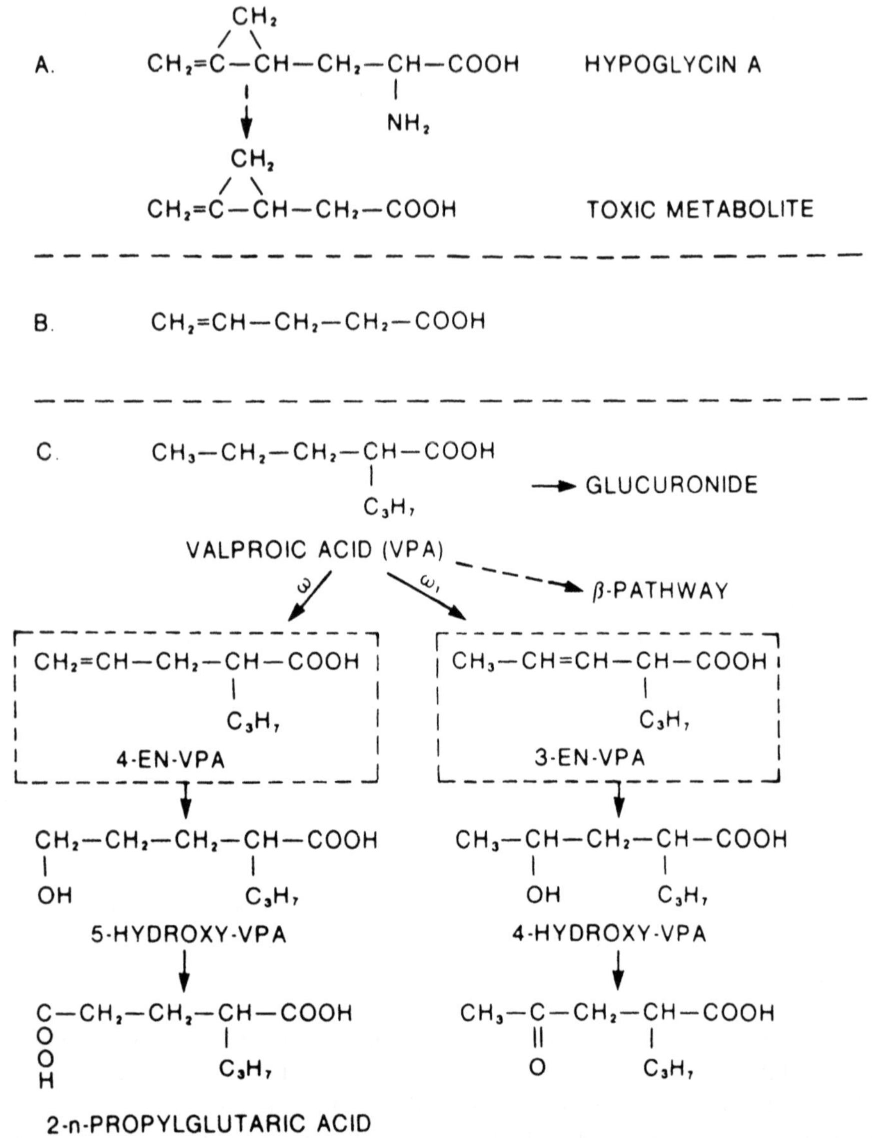

Fig. 10. Structure of **A** hypoglycin A, the cause of Jamaican vomiting sickness and its presumed toxic metabolic product. **B** 4-Pentanoic acid and **C** valproate and the metabolic products formed by metabolism along the ω- and ω_2-pathways. Note structural similarity of metabolite of valproate (4-en-VPA) to the toxic product of hypoglycin and 4-pentanoic acid. All can lead to hepatic steatosis. [From ZIMMERMAN and ISHAK (1982) with permission]

phosphate synthesis leading to hyperammonemia and the resemblance of valproic acid hyperammonemia to the ornithine transcarbamyl deficiency syndrome (TRIPP et al. 1981; HJELM et al. 1986; OURESHI et al. 1985; GRANNEMAN et al. 1984; KINGSLEY et al. 1983; BUCHI et al. 1984; MURPHY et al. 1985; BONAZZI et al. 1986; JIMENEZ-RODRIGUEZVILA et al. 1985; COUDE et al. 1983 b).

The mild intrinsic toxicity, expressed as mildly elevated levels of aminotransferase in 7%–44% of patients (WILLMORE et al. 1978; VINING et al. 1979; SHERARD et al. 1980; SUSSMAN and MCLAIN 1979; COULTER et al. 1980), may reflect the same qualitative lesion produced by valproic acid, but to a much lesser degree. It may be proposed that most patients adapt to this satisfactorily, perhaps by adaptive diversion of metabolism to other pathways. Only those with metabolic predisposition perhaps genetic, or with susceptibility enhanced by other drugs or factors, produce the damaging metabolite in sufficient quantity to produce overt injury.

VIII. Prevention

Recognition that infants are particularly vulnerable to valproic acid hepatic injury (DREIFUSS and SANTILLI 1986; DREIFUSS et al. 1989) and that patients with mental retardation, structural brain damage (POWELL et al. 1984), or metabolic disorders, such as ornithine carbamoyl transferase (TRIPP et al. 1981; HJELM et al. 1986; QUERESHI et al. 1985) or carnitine deficiency (MURPHY et al. 1985; COULTER 1984), also are especially susceptible, should alert the physician to be particularly responsive to early manifestation of valproic acid damage. Specifically, the recommendations (GREEN 1984) to monitor aminotransferase levels should be followed. Elevated values for the aminotransferases that continue to rise, or even that do not return to normal on lowering the dose, provide reason to discontinue the drug. Development of lethargy, lassitude, anorexia, nausea, and vomiting make withdrawal of the drug mandatory.

References

Aiges HW, Daum F, Olson M et al. (1980) The effects of phenobarbital and diphenylhydantoin on liver function and morphology. J Pediatr 97:22

Andreasen PB, Lyngbye J, Trolle E (1973) Abnormalities in liver function tests during long-term diphenylhydantoin therapy in epileptic out-patients. Acta Med Scand 194:261

Anthony J (1970) Malignant lymphoma associated with hydantoin drugs. Arch Neurol 22:450

Bayer AS, Targan SR, Pitchon HE, Guze LB (1976) Dilantin toxicity: miliary pulmonary infiltrates and hypoxemia. Ann Intern Med 85:475

Bertram PD, Taylor RJ (1980) Carbamazepine hepatotoxicity: clinical and histopathological features. Am J Gastroenterol 74:78

Bjorge SM, Baillie TA (1985) Inhibition of medium-chain fatty acid β-oxidation in vitro by valproic acid and its unsaturated metabolic, 2-n-propyl-4-pentenoic acid. Biochem Biophy Res Comm 132:245

Bonazzi P, Novelli G, Macarri G et al. (1986) Effect of drug pretreatment on the interaction of valproic acid with the liver cell: functional and ultrastructural data. Ital J Gastroenterol 18:79

Bowdle TA, Patel IH, Wilensky AJ et al. (1979) Hepatic failure from valproic acid (letter). N Engl J Med 301:435

Braverman IM, Levin J (1963) Dilantin-induced serum sickness: case report and inquiry into its mechanisms. Am J Med 35:418

Brown M, Schubert T (1986) Phenytoin hypersensitivity hepatitis and mononucleosis syndrome. J Clin Gastroenterol 4:469

Browne TR (1980) Valproic acid. Med Intell 302:661

Brukher AB, Joustra UH (1966) Leberbeschadiging door carbamazepine. Ned Tijdochr Genesked 110:1181
Buchanan RRC, Gordon DA, Muckle TJ et al. (1980) The eosinophilic fascitis syndrome after phenytoin (dilantin) therapy. J Rheumatol 7:733
Buchi KN, Gray PD, Rollins DE (1984) Protection against sodium valproate injury in isolated hepatocytes by α-tocopherol and N,N'-diphenyl-p-phenylenediamine. J Clin Pharmacol 24:148
Bunch SE, Castleman WL, I aldwin BH et al. (1985) Effects of long-term primidone and phenytoin administration on canine hepatic function and morphology. Am J Vet Res 46:105
Butscher WC, Gallager HS (1952) Fatal hepatic necrosis occurring during therapy with phethenylate sodium. JAMA 148:535
Campbell CB, McGuffie C, Weedon AP, Powell LW (1977) Cholestatic liver disease associated with diphenylhydantoin therapy. Am J Dig Dis 22:255
Carter S, Scearra D, Merritt HH (1950) Phenylacetylurea in the treatment of convulsive seizures. Dis Nerv Sys 11:139
Chaiken BH, Goldberg BI, Segal JP (1950) Dilantin sensitivity: report of a case of hepatitis with jaundice, pyrexia and exfoliative dermatitis. N Engl J Med 242:897
Coude FX, Grimber G, Pelet A et al. (1983a) Action of the antiepileptic drug valproic acid on fatty acid oxidation in isolated rat hepatocytes. Biochem Biochys Res Commun 115:730
Coude FX, Grimber G, Parvy P et al. (1983b) Inhibition of ureagenesis by valproate in rat hepatocytes. Biochem J 216:233
Coulter DL (1984) Carnitine deficiency: a possible mechanism for valproate hepatotoxicity. Lancet 1:689
Coulter DL, Wu H, Allen RJ (1980) Valproic acid therapy in childhood epilepsy. JAMA 244:785
Deutsch J, Fritsch G, Golles J, Semmelrock HJ (1986) Effects of anticonvulsive drugs on the activity of gammaglutamytransferase and aminotransferases in serum. J Pediatr Gastroenterol Nutr 542
Dhar GJ, Pierach CA, Ahamed PN, Howard RB (1974) Diphenylhydantoin-induced hepatic necrosis. Postgrad Med 56:128
Dreifuss FE, Santilli N (1986) Valproic acid hepatic fatalities: analysis of United States cases. Neurology 36 [Suppl 1]:175
Dreifuss FE, Langer DH, Moline KA, Maxwell JE (1989) Valproic acid hepatic fatalities. II. US experience since 1984. Neurology 39:201
Easton JD (1972) Potential hazards of hydantoin use. Ann Intern Med 77:998
Elitsur Y (1990) Pemoline (Cylert)-induced hepatotoxicity (letter). J Pediatr Gastroenterol Nutr 11:143
Engel JN, Mellul VG, Goodman DBP (1986) Phenytoin hypersensitivity: a case of severe acute rhabdomyolysis. Am J Med 81:928
Fellows WR (1969) A case of aplastic anemia and pancytopenia with Tegretol therapy. Headache 9:92
Forbes GM, Jeffrey GP, Shilkin KB, Reed WD (1992) Carbamazepine hepatotoxicity: another case of the vanishing bile duct syndrome. Gastroenterology 102:1385
Frame B (1971) Hypocalcemia and osteomalacia associated with anticonvulsant therapy. Ann Intern Med 74:294
Gerber N, Dickinson RG, Harland RD et al. (1979) Reye-like syndrome associated with valproic acid therapy. J Pediatr 95:142
Gibbs FA, Everett GM, Richards RK (1949) Phenurone in epilepsy. Dis Nerv Sys 10:47
Glasgow AM, Chase HP (1975) Production of the features of Reye's syndrome in rats with 4-pentenoic acid. Pediatr Res 9:133
Gram L, Bentsen KD (1983) Hepatic toxicity of antiepileptic drugs: a review. Acta Neurol Scand [Suppl] 97:81
Granneman CR, Wang S-I, Kesterson JW et al. (1984) The hepatotoxicity of valproic acid and its metabolites in rats. II. Intermediary and valproic acid metabolism. Hepatology 4:1153

Green SH (1984) Sodium valproate and routine liver function tests. Arch Dis Child 59:813

Gropper AL (1956) Diphenylhydantoin sensitivity: report of a case of hepatitis with jaundice, pyrexia and exfoliative dermatitis. N Engl J Med 242:897

Hadzie N, Portmann B, Davies ET et al. (1990) Mieli-Vergani G: acute liver failure induced by carbamazepine. Arch Dis Child 65:315

Hjelm M, De Silva LVK, Seakins IWT (1986) Evidence of inherited urea cycle defect in a case of fatal valproate toxicity. Br Med J 292:23

Hopen G, Nesthus I, Laerum OD (1981) Fatal carbamazepine-associated hepatitis: report of two cases. Acta Med Scand 210:333

Hutterer F, Schaffner F, Klion FM, Popper H (1968) Hypertrophic hypoactive smooth endoplasmic reticulum: a sensitive indicator of hepatotoxicity exemplified by dieldrin. Science 161:1017

Jacobsen NO, Mosekilde L, Myhre-Jensen O et al. (1976) Liver biopsies in epileptics during anticonvulsant therapy. Acta Med Scand 199:345

Jaffe SL (1989) Pemoline and liver function (letter). J Am Acad Adolesc Psychiatry 28:457

Jeavons PM (1982) Valproate toxicity. In: Woodbury DM, Penry JK, Pippenger CE (eds) Antiepileptic drugs. Raven, New York, pp 601–610

Jeavons PM (1983) Hepatotoxicity of antiepileptic drugs. In: Oxley J, Janz D, Meinardi H (eds) Chronic toxicity of antiepileptic drugs. Raven, New York, pp 1–45

Jeavons PM (1984) Non-dose-related side effects of valproate. Epilepsia 25:550

Jezequel AM, Orlandi F (1976) Unusual residual bodies in human liver cells. J Ultrastruct Res 57:87

Jezequel AM, Bonazzi P, Novelli G et al. (1984) Early structural and functional changes in liver of rats treated with single dose of valproic acid. Hepatology 4:1159

Jimemez-Rodriguezvila M, Caro-Paton A, Duenas-Laita A et al. (1985) Histological, ultrastructural and mitochondrial oxidative phosphorylation studies in livers of rats chronically treated with oral valproic acid. J Hepatol 1:453

Jimenez-Rodriguezvila M, Caro-Paton A, Conde M et al. (1986) Side effects of sodium valproate, mainly related to its hepatic and pancreatic toxicity. Int J Clin Pharm Res 6:271

Kazamatsuri H (1970) Elevated serum alkaline phosphatase levels in epilepsy during diphenyldantoin therapy. N Engl J Med 283:1411

Keeffe EB, Sunderland MC, Gabourel JD (1986) Serum gamma-glutamyl transpeptidase activity in patients receiving chronic phenytoin therapy. Dig Dis Sci 31:1056

Keene DL, Humphrey P, Carpenter B, Fletcher JP (1982) Valproic acid producing a Reye-like syndrome. Le J Can Sci Neurol 00:435

Kesterson JW, Granneman GR, Machinist JM (1984) The hepatotoxicity of valproic acid and its metabolites in rats. I. Toxicologic, biochemical and histopathologic studies. Hepatology 4:1143

Kingsley E, Gray P, Tolman KG et al. (1983) The toxicity of metabolites of sodium valproate in cultured hepatocytes. J Clin Pharmacol 23:178

Kleckner HB, Yakulis V, Heller P (1975) Severe Hypersensitivity to diphenylhydantoin with circulating antibodies to the drug. Ann Intern Med 83:522

Lapes MJ, Vivacqua RJ, Antoniades K (1976) Immunoblastic lymphadenopathy associated with phenytoin (diphenylhydantoin). Lancet 1:198

Larrey D, Hadengue A, Pessayre D (1987) Carbamazepine-induced acute cholangitis. Dig Dis Sci 32:354

Laub MC, Paetzke-Brunner I, Jaeger G (1986) Serum carnitine during valproic acid therapy. Epilepsia 27:559

Leard G, Greer WER, Kaufman IC (1949) Hepatitis, exfoliative dermatitis and abnormal bone marrow occurring during tridione therapy; report of case with recovery. N Engl J Med 240:962

Leblanc JL, Feldman A (1961) Trimethadione hepatitis: a case report and review of trimethadione toxicity. Can Med Assos J 85:200

Levander HG (1980) Granulomatous hepatitis in a patient receiving carbamazepine. Acta Med Scand 208:333
Levy M, Goodman MW, Van Dyne BJ, Sumner HW (1981) Granulomatous hepatitis secondary to carbamazepine. Ann Intern Med 95:64
Levy RW, Simmons DJ, Aronson S (1950) Fatal hepatorenal syndrome associated with phenurone therapy. N Engl J Med 242:933
Lewis JH, Zimmerman HJ, Garrett CT, Rosenburg E (1982) Valproate-induced hepatic steatogenesis in rats. Hepatology 2:870
Luke DR, Rocci ML, Schaible DH, Ferguson RK (1986) Acute hepatotoxicity after excessively high doses of carbamazepine on two occasions. Pharmacotherapy 6:108
Mandelbaum H, Kane LJ (1941) Dilantin sodium poisoning: report of a case with dermatitis exfoliative, pyrexia and hepatic and splenic enlargement. Arch Neurol Psychiatr 45:769
Martindale (1982) The extra pharmacopeia, 28th edn. Pharmaceutical Press, pp 437
Melegh B, Kerner J, Acsadi G et al. (1990) L-Carnitine replacement therapy in chronic valproate treatment. Neuropediatrics 21:40
Merritt HH, Putnam TJ (1938) Sodium diphenylhydantoin in the treatment of convulsive disorders. JAMA 111:1068
Michael JR, Mitch WE (1976) Reversible renal failure and myositis caused by phenytoin hypersensitivity. JAMA 36:2773
Michael JR, Rudin ML (1981) Acute pulmonary disease caused by phenytoin. Ann Intern Med 95:452
Mitchell MC, Boitnott JK, Arregue A, Maddrey W (1981) Granulomatous hepatitis associated with carbamazepine therapy. Am J Med 71:733
Moore JR, Williams THC, Talbot FC, Tanner MS (1984) Heterozygous antitrypsin deficiency and valproate hepatotoxicity. Lancet 1:221
Mullick FG, Ishak KG (1980) Hepatic injury associated with diphenylhydantoin therapy: a clinicopathologic study of 20 cases. Am J Clin Pathol 74:442
Murphy JV, Marguardt K (1982) Asymptomatic hyperammonemia in patients receiving valproic acid. Arch Neurol 39:591
Murphy JV, Marquardt KM, Shug AL (1985) Valproic acid associated abnormalities of carnitine metabolism. Lancet 1:820
Murphy MJ, Lyon LW, Taylor JW, Mills G (1981) Valproic acid associated pancreatitis in an adult. Lancet 1:41
Nordin G, Hemdal I, Olsson J-E, Rolny P (1982) Liver damage and anti-epileptic drugs. Acta Neurol Scand 65 [Suppl 90]:199
Offermann G (1981) Chronic antiepileptic drug treatment and disorders of mineral metabolism. In: Oxley J, Janz D, Meinardi H (eds) Chronic toxicity of antiepileptic drugs. Raven, New York, pp 175–184
Ohtani Y, Ebdo F, Matsuda I (1982) Carnitine deficiency and hyperammonemia associated with valproic acid therapy. J Pediatr 101:782
Parker PH, Helineck GL, Guisan FK, Greene HL (1981) Recurrent pancreatitis induced by valproic acid. Gastroenterology 80:826
Parker WA, Shearer CA (1979) Phenytoin hepatotoxicity: a case report and review. Neurology 29:175
Powell PR, Jackson JM, Williams R (1984) Hepatotoxicity to sodium valproate. A review. Gut 25:673
Pryles CV, Burnett JM, Livingston S (1952) Acute hepatic necrosis with death occurring during phethenylate sodium therapy. Report of two cases. JAMA 148:536
Qureshi IA, Letarte J, Tuchweber B et al. (1985) Hepatotoxicity of sodium valproate in ornithine transcarbamylase-deficient mice. Toxicol Lett 25:297
Rettie AE, Rettenmeier AW, Howalk WN, Baille TA (1986) Cytochrome P-450-catalyzed formation of 4-VPA, a toxic metabolite of valproic acid. Science 235:890
Riera Velasco JR, Rodrigo Saez LR et al. (1986) Hepatitis cronica activa por difenilhidantoinas. Med Clin (Barc) 87:214

Ritchie EB, Kolb W (1942) Reaction to sodium diphenylhydantoinate (dilantin sodium): hemorrhagic erythema multiforme terminating fatally. Arch Dermatol Syph 46:856
Rozas I, Camina MF, Paz JM et al. (1990) Effects of acute valproate administration on carnitine metabolism in mouse serum and tissues. Biochem Pharmacol 39:181
Saltzstein SL, Ackerman LV (1959) Lymphadenopathy induced by anticonvulsant drugs and mimicking clinically and pathologically malignant lymphomas. Cancer 12:164
Schnabel R, Lahl R (1964) Leberparenchymnekrosen durch das neue Antiepilepticum alpha-Acetoxyphenuron. Bericht uber tierexperimentelle Untersuchungen und 4 letal verlaufene Falle. Zentralbl Allg Pathal Anat 106:42
Scheffner D (1988) Fatal liver failure in 16 children with valproate therapy. Epilepsia 29:530
Shapiro PA, Antonioli DA, Peppercorn MA (1980) Barbiturate-induced submassive hepatic necrosis: report of a case and review of the literature. Am J Gastroenterol 74:270
Shear NH, Spielberg SP, Cannon M, Miller M (1988) Anticonvulsant hypersensitivity syndrome. In vitro assessment of risk. J clin Invest 82:1826–1832
Sherard ES, Steinman GS, Couri D et al. (1980) Treatment of childhood epilepsy with valproic acid. Neurology 30:31
Siegel S, Berkowitz J (1961) Diphenylhydantoin (dilantin) hypersensitivity with infectious mononucleosis-like syndrome and jaundice. J Allergy 32:447
Soffer EE, Taylor RJ, Bertram PD et al. (1983) Carbamazepine-induced liver injury. South Med J 76:681
Spechler SJ, Sperber H, Doos WG et al. (1981) Cholestasis and toxic epidermal necrolysis associated with phenytoin sodium ingestion: the role of bile duct injury. Ann Intern Med 95:455
Spielberg SP, Gordon GB, Blake DA et al. (1981) Predisposition to phenytoin hepatotoxicity assessed in vitro. N Engl J Med 305:722
Spillane J (1964) The treatment of trigeminal neuralgia: preliminary experience with tegretol. Practitioner 192:71
Stricker BHCH (1992) Drug-induced hepatic injury, 2nd edn. Elsevier, Amsterdam, pp 412–460
Suchy FJ, Balistreri WF, Buchino JJ et al. (1979) Acute hepatic failure associated with the use of sodium valproate: report of two fatal cases. N Engl J Med 300:962
Sugimoto T, Nishida N, Yasuhara A et al. (1983) Reye-like syndrome associated with valproic acid. Brain Dev 5:334
Sugimoto T, Araki A, Nishida N, Kobayashi Y et al. (1987a) Hepatotoxicity in rat following administration of valproate: effect of L-carnitine administration. Epilepsia 28:373–377
Sugimoto T, Woo M, Nishida N et al. (1987b) Hepatotoxicity in rat following administration of valproic acid. Epilepsia 28:142
Sussman NM, McLain LW (1979) A direct hepatotoxic effect of valproic acid. JAMA 242:1173
Takeuchi T, Sugimoto T, Nishida N, Kobayashi Y (1988) Protective effect of d,l-carnitine on valproate-induced hyperammonemia and hypoketonemia in primary cultured rat hepatocytes. Biochem Pharmacol 37:2255
Tanaka K, Kean EA, Johnson B (1976) Jamaican vomiting sickness: biochemical investigation of two cases. N Engl J Med 295:461
Taylor JW, Stein MN, Murphy MJ, Mitros FA (1984) Cholestatic liver dysfunction after long-term phenytoin therapy. Arch Neurol 41:500
Ting S, Dunsky EH (1982) Diphenylhydantoin-induced hepatitis. Ann Allergy 48:331
Tomsick RS (1983) The phenytoin syndrome. Cutis 32:535
Tripp JH, Hargreaves T, Anthony PP et al. (1981) Sodium valproate and ornithine carbamyl transferase deficiencies. Lancet 1:1165

Van Wyk JJ, Hoffmann CR (1948) Periarteritis nodosa. A case of fatal exfoliative dermatitis resulting from "dilantin sodium" sensitization. Arch Intern Med 81:605
Vining EPG, Botsford E, Freeman JM (1979) Valproate sodium in refractory seizures. Am J Dis Child 133:274
Weedon AP (1975) Diphenylhydantoin sensitivity: a syndrome resembling infectious mononucleosis with a morbilliform rash and cholestatic hepatitis. Aust NJ Med 5:561
Williams SJ, Ruppin DC, Grierson JM, Farrell GC (1986) Carbamazepine hepatitis: the clinicopathological spectrum. J Gastroenterol Hepatol 1:159
Williams LHP, Reynolds RP, Emery JL (1983) Pancreatitis during sodium valproate treatment. Arch Dis Child 58:543
Willmore LJ, Wilder BJ, Bruni J et al. (1978) Effect of valproic acid on hepatic function. Neurology 28:961
Wolf R, Kahane E, Sandbank M (1985) Mycosis fungoides-like lesions associated with phenytoin therapy. Arch Dermatol 121:1181
Zafrani ES, Berthelot P (1982) Sodium valproate in the induction of unusual hepatotoxicity. Hepatology 2:648
Zimmerman HJ (1991) Lesions of drug-induced liver disease and valproate toxicity. In: Levy RH, Penry JH (eds) Idiosyncratic reactions to valproate: clinical risk patterns and mechanisms of toxicity. Raven, New York, pp 31–45
Zimmerman HJ, Ishak KG (1982) Valproate induced hepatic injury: analysis of 23 fatal cases. Hepatology 2:591–598
Zimmerman HJ, Maddrey WC (1993) Toxic and drug-induced hepatitis. In: Schiff L, Schiff ER (eds) Diseases of the liver. Lippincott, Philadelphia, pp 707–769
Zucker P, Daum F, Cohen MI (1977) Fatal carbamazepine hepatitis. J Pediatr 91:667

Subject Index

abdominal pain 520, 651
acetaldehyde 189, 191, 618, 625, 626
– adducts 619, 620, 627
acetaminophen 2, 25, 27, 32, 33, 35, 36, 38, 123, 124, 136, 138, 139, 140, 141, 284, 294, 502, 515, 517, 518, 532, 587, 614, 619
– clearance values 353
– hepatotoxicity 355, 422, 424
– metabolism 346
– overdose 451
– protein adduct 136
– toxicity 442
acetate 618
– ATP-mediated conversion of 626
acetic acid 527
acetohexamide 567, 568
acetoxyphenurone 645
acetyl-CoA 188, 626
acetyl-coenzyme A 185
acetyl-*p*-benzoquinoneimine 136
2-acetylaminofluorene 213
acetylator
– phenotype 426
– slow 302
acetylhydralazine 490
acetylsalicyclic acid 530, 587
acetylurea derivatives 645
acid 193
acidophilic (apoptotic) body 640, 641
acidosis 522
– lactic 55, 80, 569
acinus, hepatic 560
acrolein 103
ACTH 187
actinomycin D 193, 200
acyl glucuronide 144
acyl halide 136
acyltransferase activity 60
AD (see also Alzheimer's disease) 395
adenine 5, 61
adenoma 556, 558, 561, 564, 565
– hepatic 544, 556, 562
– hepatocellular 549, 555, 557, 566
– multiple 550
– rupture of 556
adenosine monophosphatase, cyclic 481
adenosyl-S-ethionine 193
adenylate cyclase 187
adipocyte lipase 200
adrenal corticosteroids 590
adriamycin (see also doxorubicin) 112, 305
aflatoxin B_1 81, 129, 193, 197, 212
agents
– antiarrhythmic 503
– antihypertensive 503
– antimicrobial 385, 457
– antiprotozoal 472
– antituberculosis 386
– antiviral 472
– cardiovascular 383
– cytotoxic 588, 589
– hypolipidemic 17
– immunophilin-binding 588, 589
– immunosuppressive 588, 595
– – classification 588
– lipid-lowering 503
– lipotropic 618
– toxic 647
agranulocytosis 492, 570
AH receptor 128
alanine aminotransferase (see also ALT) 520, 595, 600
– activity
– – serum 395
albumin 480, 481, 483, 593, 614
alcohol 103, 120, 234, 622
– abuse 451, 592
– – acute 522
– – chronic 522
– allyl 33, 99, 111
– butylated hydroxytoluene 51
– dehydrogenase 618
– hepatotoxicity 358
alcoholic 296, 516, 518, 522
– cirrhosis 617, 622

alcoholic (*contd.*)
– hepatitis 617, 620
– increased susceptibility 426
alcoholism 519
– chronic 520
– cirrhosis 617, 622
– hepatitis 617, 620
– like hepatitis 477
– liver disease 624
– liver injury 611
– liver lesion 616
– porhyria cutanea tarda 563
aldehyde 198
– dehydrogenase 120
– oxidase 191
– oxygenase 120, 626
alkaline phosphatase (ALP) 155, 240, 480, 481, 483, 484, 486, 489, 492, 493, 494, 498, 500, 520, 532, 546, 554, 568, 570, 581, 585, 587, 595, 597, 600, 640, 644, 646
alkyl group 544
allergic
– disorders 590
– reactions 443
allergies 581
allopurinol 226, 241
alopecia 586
ALP 554, 644, 645, 646, 647, 653
ALT (see also alanine aminotransferase, GP, SGPT) 395, 520, 639, 640
Alzheimer's disease (see also AD) 254, 395
α-amanitin 19, 60, 84, 197
amanita 19
amides, aryloxyalkanoic 59
amino acid
– excitatory 261
– oxydase 57
γ-aminobutyric acid 258, 649
5-aminolevulinic acid 83
δ-aminolevulinic acid synthetase 563
6-aminonicotinamide 107
aminoglycosides 457
aminonucleoside 53
aminopyrine-*N*-demethylase 63, 64
aminotransferase 85, 520, 521, 528, 531, 532, 533, 534, 535, 546, 566, 568, 570, 571, 585, 640, 644, 647, 650, 653, 657
amiodarone 62, 124, 281, 310, 477, 483, 484, 485, 486, 487, 488, 503
amitriptyline 171
ammonia 253, 254, 488, 613, 650
ammonia blood 327
amoxycillin 230
AMP 194
amphetamine 51
amphiphilic drugs 487
ampligen 583
amsacrine 84
amyloidosis 53
anabolic
– agents, icterogenic 563
– effects 565
– steroid 166, 543, 546, 548
– – alkylated 545
– – C–17-alkylated 543
– – nonalkylated 544
anaphylactoid reaction 524
androgen 565, 590
– natural 543
androgenic steroids 158
anemia 478, 622
– aplastic 543, 544, 548, 648
– Fanconi's aplastic 550
– haemolytic 238, 586
– immune drug-induced hemolytic 481
angiosarcoma 550, 560
anicteric
– hepatitis 227
– patient 546
– syndrome 651
animal 482, 488, 498, 519, 524
– experimental 566
– model 344, 362, 615
ANIT (see also α-naphtylisothiocyanate) 158, 165
anorexia 479, 483, 519, 534, 545, 554, 585, 614, 650, 651, 657
anoxia 169
antagonists 590
anthracycline 84
anti asialo-GM–1 γ-globulin 584
antiarrhythmic 477, 501
– agents 503
antibiotics 282
– immunosuppressive 588, 590
antibodies 225, 229, 233
– anti-adduct 620
– anti LKM_1 138, 139
– anti-LKM_2 138, 143
– antinuclear 480
– immunity 598
– monoclonal 589
anticonvulsants 637, 645
antidepressant, tricyclic 171, 646
antidote 522
antiemetics 283
antiepileptic drugs 637
antiestrogens 565
antigen 233, 585
– antibody complex 623
– expression, class II 590
antigonadotropin 565

antihypertensives 477, 496
antihypophysial drugs 565
anti LKM_1 138, 139
anti-inflammatory, nonsteroid 144
anti-LKM_2 138
antilymphocyte
- globulin 588, 589
- products 588, 589
antimicrobial agent 385, 457, 465
antineoplastic drugs 304
antioxidant 192
- enzymes 351
antiprotozoal 472
antipyrine 482
antirheumatics 496
antisense technology 93
α_1-antitrypsin 18
- accumulation 626
- deficiency 650
antitumor effects 586
antitumor necrosis factor-α antibodies 614
antiviral effect 586
ApoA-1 500
apoprotein B 500
apoptosis (see also sinusoidal acidophilic bodies) 10, 11, 13, 84, 86, 92, 222, 546, 590, 600, 623
aprindine, chemical structure 489
arabinoside 13
arachidonic acid metabolites 588, 590
arene oxide 303, 644, 646
arrhythmia 486, 488, 492, 493, 520
arteriography 556
arthritis 479, 598
Arthus reaction 226
arylamidase 491
arylsulfatase 104
ascites 370, 582, 592, 613, 651
asialo-GM_1 584
aspartate aminotransferase (see also AST) 520, 587
aspartate transaminase 585, 593, 595, 600
aspirin 58, 284, 307, 332, 488, 526, 530, 532, 533
AST (see also aspartate aminotransferase, GOT, SGOT) 520, 554, 639, 640, 644, 653
asterixis 250
asthma 591
astrocytes 254
ataxia 651
atorvastatin 496, 500
ATP 60, 157, 194
- dependent 157
- depletion 169
atrophy 596
- brown 17
augmentin 230, 442
autoantibodies 138, 237, 294, 586
autoantigen 138, 237, 238
autocrine inducer 613
autoimmune
- disorders 581, 589
- haemolytic 478
- hepatitis 503
- mechanism 481
- reaction 443
- uveitis 598
5-azacytosine 83
azathioprine 311, 582, 588, 595, 596, 597
- hepatotoxicity 596
azepinamide 568
AZT 56, 80
Azulfidine (see also sulfasalazine) 468

B cell 224, 239, 598
B lymphocyte 222, 224, 481, 590, 596
barbiturates 50, 242, 646
basolateral (sinusoidal) plasma membrane 548
benorilate 527, 532
benoxaprofen 526, 527, 531, 532, 533
benzodiazepine, receptor agonist 265
betaine 61, 211
bezafibrate 58, 496, 498, 499
bicarbonate 157
biguanide 569
bile 155
- canalicular 547, 551
- - flow 584
- canaliculi 44, 546, 564
- cast 546
- flow/cholestasis 551, 557, 584, 614
bile acid 156, 599
- concentration of 564
- pool 564
- synthesis 564
- taurocholic acid 599
bile canaliculus
- pericanalicular 564
- - microfibrillar network 548
bile duct epithelium
- hyperplasia 500
- inflammation 600
- interlobular 648
bile salts 599
- dependent fraction (see also BSDF) 547
- monohydroxy 162
biliary
- cirrhosis 232

biliary (*contd.*)
- disease 536
- duct dilation 585
- spasm 536
bilirubin 228, 479, 481, 483, 484, 486, 490, 493, 500, 503, 520, 532, 545, 546, 554, 564, 581, 584, 585, 587, 597, 599, 600, 613, 639
bioactivation 135, 139
biologicals, immune-system-derived 583
biotransformation 43, 143
bleomycin 83
Blighia sapida 569
bone marrow 589, 598
- suppression 596
- transplantation 589, 590, 596, 597
bowel ischemia 595
brain 649
- damage, structural 657
bredinin 588, 590
brequinar 588, 590
bromobenzene 33, 129, 200
bromotrichloromethane 202
brown atrophy 17
BSDF (see also bile salt dependent fraction) 547
BSIF (see also bile salt independent fraction) 547
BSP 564
- excretion of 551, 553
Budd-Chiari syndrome (see also hepatic vein thrombosis) 310, 449, 543, 553, 561, 564
butylated hydroxytoluene
- alcohol 51
- methyl ether 51
BZ–55 568

C–17 544
- alkyleted anabolic androgen steroids 544
- β-glucuronide 563
C–19 nor-compounds 552
caffeine 61, 128, 187
calcineurin 589, 598
calcium 39, 60, 163, 199, 211, 215, 502
- calmodulin antagonist 502
- channel antagonists 502
- channel blocking agents 384
- homeostasis 169
- intracellular 169
- level 502
calmodulin 598
caloric percentage 624
canaliculi 546, 564
cancer 8
- chemotherapy 581, 583
capillary leak syndrome 584
captopril 137, 501
carbamazepine 226, 241, 303, 637, 638, 645, 646, 647, 649
- hypersensitivity 649
carbimazole 569, 570, 571
carbon
- disulfide 199
carbon tetrachloride 33, 99, 211, 502, 614, 626
- hepatotoxicity of 361, 424
- toxicoxis 502
carboxylesterase 141, 228
carbutamide 566, 568
carcinogen 8, 214
carcinogenecity 500
carcinoma
- hepatic 550, 564
- hepatocellular 544, 549, 550, 558, 566
- ovarian 555
- prostatic 552, 563
cardiolipin 193
cardiomyopathy 486, 488
cardiopulmonary disease 517
cardiotoxicity 587
cardiovascular
- agents 383
- drugs 477, 501, 502, 503
carnitine deficiency 650, 655, 657
carprofen 527
catalase 57, 102, 599
cataracts 595
CCl_4 (see carbontetrachloride) 187, 195, 196
cell
- ballooning 483, 615, 617, 621
- death 10, 11, 16
- - programmed 14
- endothelial 596, 616
- Ito 20, 616
- Kupffer 616, 622
- mesenchymal 480
- necrosis 613, 620
- sinusoidal 480
- transitional 591, 616
- viability 106
cell-mediated immunity 598
cellular
- membrane 589
- protein 144
central nervous system 498, 526
- drugs 384
central vein sclerosis (see also hepatic veins) 616
cephalosporin 63, 457

cerebrum
– cerebral circulatory disorders 492
– cerebral edema 323, 328, 335, 651
– cerebral energy metabolism 256
– cerebrovascular accident 562
cerium 193
ceroid 57
chemoattractants 620
chenodeoxycholic acid 285
children 519, 650, 651
– drug hepatotoxicity in 293
chills 492, 586
chloramphenicol 457
chloroform 61
chlorphentermine 62
chlorpromazine 62, 158, 169, 170, 502, 546
chlorpropamide 567, 568, 569
cholangiocarcinoma 550, 560
cholangitis 20, 501, 601, 648
cholecystitis 556
choledocholithiasis 556
cholelithiasis 564
choleresis 59
cholestasis (see also bile, see also biliary) 20, 45, 62, 155, 158, 165, 166, 477, 480, 482, 489, 491, 493, 503, 533, 536, 543, 544, 546, 563, 568, 570, 585, 587, 597, 599, 600, 601, 640, 648
– canalicular 447
– chronic 464, 568
– hepatocellular 638
cholestasis, intrahepatic (see also bile, see also biliary) 490, 492, 498, 546, 585
– erythromycin estolate 461
– injury 551, 648
– jaundice 543
cholesterol 164, 274, 495, 500, 554, 564, 590
choline 52, 61, 211, 212, 591
– deficiency 38, 215, 592, 626
– supplementation 627
cholylglycylhistamine 159
chronic inflammatory bowel disease 598
cigarette smoking 622
cimetidine 519, 524, 601
ciprofibrate 498
cirrhosis 20, 308, 477, 483, 558, 559, 581, 591, 592, 593, 594, 611, 612, 615, 616, 623, 625, 626, 628, 651, 652, 654
– alcoholic 612, 614, 617, 622
– biliary 554
– carbon tetrachloride induced 613
– decompensated 251
– experimental 626
– inactive 615, 617
– macronodular 568
– micronodular 592
– postnecrotic 483
– primary biliary 547, 598, 648
– renal blood flow in 370
– scarse, coarse 483
clearance models 387
clindamycin 458
clofibrate 17, 58, 60, 201, 496, 498, 499
clofibric acid 60
clometacin 235, 527, 529, 530, 531, 532
clomiphene 565
clotting factors 613
CNS function 265
coagulation abnormalities 558
coagulopathy 651
coarse scars 483
cobalt chloride 63, 140
cocaine 312
codeine 124
colchicine 160, 194
colimycin 458
collagen 591, 595, 613, 625
– accumulation, perisinusoidal 627
– deposition 482, 616
– fibrils 616
– septa 616
collateral vessels, enlargement 612
coma 250, 326, 613, 651
– hepatic 522, 640
compactin 495
complement 623
contraceptive
– oral 549, 559, 561, 562
contraceptive steroids 447, 543
– adverse effects on the liver 553
convulsions 569, 650
Coomb's antiglobulin 478, 480
coralgil 62, 477, 484
corticosteroid 284, 535, 582, 584, 588, 594, 595
cortisone 56, 594
cotinine 128
coumarin 50, 51, 53
Councilman bodies 87
covalent
– adduct 137
– binding 196, 422
– modification 135
creatine phosphokinase 493, 500
CSF 253
(+)-cyanidanol-3 111
cyclofenil 565
cycloheximide 12, 13, 54, 60, 164, 194, 197, 200
cyclophilin 589, 598

cyclophilin-cyclosporine complex 598
cyclophosphamide 582, 589
cyclosporine 170, 582, 588, 589, 596, 598, 599, 600, 601
cyproterone acetate 553
cysteamine 202
cysteine 38, 519
cytochalasin B 159
cytochrome P-450 32, 46, 48, 50, 60, 102, 106, 120, 194, 201, 221, 295, 345, 482, 491, 601, 644
- activity (see also P-450 IIE1) 519
- CYP1 122, 130
- CYP1A 127
- CYP1A1mRNA 122
- CYP1A2 32, 140, 143, 236, 397
- CYP2 130, 132
- CYP2A6 122
- CYP2B6 122
- CYP2C 122, 143
- CYP2C8 122
- CYP2C9 122, 142, 143
- CYP2C10 122
- CYP2C18 142
- CYP2C19 123
- CYP2D 123
- CYP2D6 126, 143, 236
- CYP2E1 32, 123, 128, 140, 142, 143
- CYP3 130
- CYP3A 123, 129
- CYP3A4 140, 143
- CYP450 1A2 236
- CYPB2 142
- drug metabolizing systems 586
- enzymes 484
- inducers of 480, 601
- inhibitors 129
- oxidases 228
cytokine 229, 230, 583, 584, 586, 598, 613, 614, 622, 623
- gene transcription 590
cytokine synthesis induction 591
cytolysis 225, 589
cytometry 55
cytoplasmic organelles (see also organelles) 495
cytosine 13
- arabinose 80
cytosol 199
cytosolic 37-kDa protein 620

D-galactosamine 60, 194, 202
d-penicillamine 221, 227
danazol 549, 565
ddC (see also dideoxycytidine) 56, 80
ddI (see also dideoxyinosine) 56, 80
death 569
debrisoquine 124, 134
dehydrogenase, aldehyde 120
deoxycytosine triphosphate 79
15-deoxyspergualin 588, 590
depakene 638
depression 478, 492, 586
dermatitis, exfoliative 641
dermatological disorder 526, 596, 597, 598
DES (see also diethylstilbestrol) 552, 560, 563
desethylamiodaraone 484, 487
desferrioxamine 111
desipramine 132
detoxication 120, 420, 649
dextromethorphan 124, 134
diabetes 123, 592, 595
diabinese 568
diacetate, 2',7' dichlorodihydrofluorescein 55
diagnostic approach 285
diarrhea 586
diazepam 47, 124
1,2 dibromoethane 195, 196
diclofenac 144, 241, 527, 528, 529, 530, 531, 532, 533, 535
dideoxycytidine (see also ddC) 80
dideoxyinosine (see also ddI) 80
diet 498, 519
- liquid 617, 623
diethyl-dithio-carbamate 12
diethylmaleate 5, 63, 202
diethylnitrosamine 7, 33
diethylstilbestrol (see also DES) 551, 552
diflunisal 532
diflunisol 527
dihydralazine 138, 143, 236, 489, 491
dihydro-orotate dehydrogenase 590
dihydrodiol, nontoxic 644
dihydrofolate reductase 591
dilantin 638
dilatation, sinusoidal 543, 560, 561, 581, 598
diltiazem 125, 502
dimelor 568
2,6-dimethyl acetaminophen 140
3,5-dimethyl acetaminophen 140
dimethylnitrosamine 3, 12, 33, 99, 502
dinitrochlorobenzene 226
diphenyl-*p*-phenylenediamine 12
diphenylhydantoin 242, 638
diphospho-D-galactosamine 194
diptheria toxin 194
disopyramide 501
- chemical structure 489

Disse, space of 119, 596, 616, 617
distribution volume 379
disulfide isomerase 141
disulfiram 124
diuretics 590
DNA
- damage 77, 81, 92, 502
- gyrase 84
- ligase 81
- mitochondrial 627
- polymerase 78
- polymerase α 79
- polymerase γ 79
- repair 81
- replication 81
- synthesis 33, 77, 595
- technology, recombinant 583
- total 620
- turnover 78
doxorubicin (see also adriamycin) 112, 113, 502
drug
- absorption 278
- accumulation 375
- anticonvulsant 517
- antiepileptic 637
- antihypophysial 565
- antithyroid 543, 569, 571
- antituberculous 469
- cardiovascular 477, 502, 503
- drug interactions 388
- elimination rate 375
- high-clearance 279
- hypersensitivity 427, 581
- illicit 450
- interaction 517, 519
- nonsteroidal antiinflammatory 526
drug binding
- plasma proteins 370
drug metabolism 43, 300, 482, 519
drug reaction, cholangiolytic 447
ductular cell proliferation 491
dyslipidemias 495
dyslipoproteinemic patients 499
dyspepsia 479, 481

edema 478, 482, 613
- cerebral 251
elderly subjects 341, 353
electroencephalography 251, 327
electron transport 55
elimination half-life 379
embolism 566
emetin 60
emetine 200
encephalopathy 323
- grade III 522
- hepatic 249, 491, 613
- metabolic 327
endoplasmic reticulum 46, 130, 143, 481, 494, 495, 588, 616, 617, 618
- hypoactive hypertrophic 6
- hypofunctional 49, 63
- hypofunctional smooth 63
- membrane 48
- rough 44
- smooth 44
endothelial cell 596, 613, 616, 644
- damage to 305
- sinusoidal 623
endothelin 600
endotoxemia 613, 614, 624
endotoxin 163, 612, 614, 623, 624
- bacterial 624
- production 624
energy metabolism 586
enflurane 234
enolic acid 527
enzymes
- capacity-limited drugs 378
- drug-metabolizing (see also drug metabolism) 49
- inducers 647
- induction 644
eosinophilia 492, 530, 533, 567, 581, 643, 647, 648, 655
epigastric pain 479, 481
epinephrine 61, 161, 187, 200
epitopes 137
epoxide hydrolase 303, 645
erythema multiforme 638, 643
erythrocyte antigen 481
erythromycin 133, 134, 171, 459, 601
erythromycin estolate 241, 283, 462
erythromycin ethylsuccinate 241
estradiol 163, 545, 551
- 17β-D-glucuronide 167, 170
- valerate 166
estriol 551
- 16α-glucuronide 167
estrogen (see also DES) 158, 161, 273, 552, 562, 564, 590
- receptor 564
estrone 160, 551
ethanol 25, 48, 123, 124, 187, 189, 191, 192, 201, 611, 614, 616, 620, 622, 627
- metabolism 618
ethinyl estradiol 158, 163, 551, 555, 564
ethionine 4, 60, 197
ethiotoin 645
7-ethoxycoumarin 103, 105, 107
etodolac 527, 529
etofibrate 496
etoposide 84

euglycin 568
excision repair 81
extracellular matrix 616
extrapyramidal signs 478

Fabry's disease 487
factor VIII 522
fat 581, 586, 617, 624
- accumulation 615, 617, 618, 623
- embolism 595
- saturated 625
- stains 324
- storing cells 616
- vacuoles 494
fatty acid 48, 594
- esterification of 594
- flux 61
- free 594
- metabolism 655
- β oxidation 599
- oxidation 331
- polyunsaturated 619
fatty change (see also fat) 447, 477, 481, 482, 499, 503, 566, 594, 596
- liver 18, 566, 592, 595, 615, 617, 618, 627, 628
felodipine 129
female sex steroids 543
fenamic acid 527
fenbufen 527
fenofibrate 235, 496, 498, 499
fenoprofen 527, 530, 534
α_1-fetoprotein 274, 550, 558
fever 478, 492, 530, 531, 533, 567, 571, 581, 586, 614, 638, 639, 643, 647, 648, 651
FFAs (see also free fatty acids) 185
fialuridine 55, 56, 80
fibrates 495, 496, 498
fibrosis 20, 480, 483, 484, 536, 558, 587, 591, 592, 594, 597, 598, 616, 617, 620, 624, 625, 626
first-order kinetics 373
first-pass hepatic clearance 381
first-pass metabolism 380
FK—506 588, 589, 601
FKBP 589
floctafenine 527
5-fluorocytosine 83
fluoxetine 124
fluoxymestrone 545
flurbiprofen 534
5-flurouracil 83
flutamide 230
fluvastatin 496, 500
fluvastatin sodium 497
FNH 558
foamy changes 485
focal necrosis 481, 642
folic acid 211, 213
folic acid antagonist 589
free fatty acids (see also FFAs) 185
free radical 63, 136

GABA 253, 258
galactosamine 4, 614
galactosyltransferase 53
gallopamil 502
gallstones 274, 564
ganglio-*n*-tetrosylceramide 584
gemfibrozil 58, 496, 498, 499
genetic factors 519, 548, 650, 651
genotoxic 9
genotyping 145
gentamicin 62
gingival hypertrophy 599
glibenclamide 567, 568
gliburide 567
glibuthiazole 568
glipizide 568
glisoxepide 568
γ-globulin 480, 483, 495
globulin 480, 483
- antilymphocyte 588
- antithymocyte 588, 589
glomerulonephritis 239
glucagon 187
glucocorticoid 187, 543, 566, 590
gluconeogenesis 594
glucose 101
- 6-phosphatase 46, 64
- 6-phosphate dehydrogenase 99
glucotrol 568
glucuronidation 108, 109, 110, 111
glucuronide 518
- conjugates 167
glucuronosyltransferase 108
glutamate 30
- receptor 262
glutamine 30
γ-glutamyl transpeptidase 240, 493, 644, 646
glutathione (see also GSH) 5, 32, 38, 75, 103, 140, 157, 281, 294, 347, 351, 482, 518, 519, 619, 626, 627
glyburide 568
glycerol 185
glycine 168
glycogen 18, 62, 101, 111, 586, 588, 595, 601
glycoprotein 20, 53
glycosyltransferase 53, 54
glymidine 568
glyparamide 568

glypasol 568
Golgi 18, 44, 46, 52, 53, 61, 64, 186, 546
gonadafon 568
GOT (see also AST, transaminases) 520, 554, 639, 644
GPT (see also ALT, transaminases) 395, 520, 639, 640
GR 95030X 500
granulocyte-macrophage colony-stimulating factor 598
granulocytopenia 478
granuloma 232, 490, 494, 495, 565, 567, 569, 638, 641, 648
granulomatous
- hepatitis 477, 494
- reaction 446, 503
griseofulvin 471
GSH (see also glutathione)
- activities, age-related differences 348
- concentration, in the liver with age 351
- transferase 196
guanine 193
- nucleotides 589

hairy cell leukemia 586, 587
hallucination 492
haloalkanes 195
halothane 76, 136, 138, 141, 142, 195, 232, 233, 242, 302
- hepatitis 141, 429
- hepatotoxicity 430
- product TFA-protein adducts 431
hapten 137, 226, 427, 644, 649
- protein conjugate 428
HDL (see also high-density lipoprotein) 500
heat shock proteins 9
hemangioma 553, 560
hematological malignancies 591
heme 48, 130, 132
- oxygenase 49
- thiolate P450s 120
hemochromatosis 83, 626
hemodynamic alterations 612
hemoglobin 622
hemolysis 241, 600
hemolytic anemia 238
hemoperitoneum 556, 561
hemorrhage 491, 556, 562, 613
hepatectomy 36
hepatic
- adenoma 544
- adenomatosis 549
- capillary permeability 584
- clearance 517
- - high 387
- collapse, submassive 483
- coma 487, 522, 640
- damage 639
- endophlebitis 480
- failure 487, 568, 612, 640, 641, 650
- fibrosis 591, 592
- necrosis 482, 534
- - fatal submassive 482
- - focal 532
- oxygen consumption 621
- porphyria 543
- vein thrombosis (see also Budd-Chiari syndrome) 310, 544
hepatic encephalopathy 250
hepatitis 45, 46, 87, 224, 228, 230, 477, 479, 481, 486, 489, 490, 491, 492, 494, 499, 503, 535, 593
- α-methyldopa 479
- acute drug-induced 487
- alcoholic 308, 477, 483, 485, 612, 613, 614, 615, 617, 620
- anicteric 534
- autoimmune 503, 596
- cholestatic 532
- chronic 446, 463, 481, 532, 570, 591, 640, 646
- delta 234
- granulomatous 477, 492, 494
- peliosis 543
- pseudoalcoholic 484, 487
- toxic 491
- viral 410, 568, 581, 583, 626, 640
hepatitis B 138, 570, 586
- infection 560
- recurrent 591
- viral infections 583
hepatitis C 139, 586
hepatoblastoma 565
hepatocellular 531, 566, 570, 637, 639
- atypia 500
- fibrosis 616
- injury 493, 551, 584, 597, 641, 646, 648
- - acute 462, 503
- necrosis 396, 445, 616
hepatocyte 480, 495, 584, 601, 615
- centrilobular 57, 627
- cultures 402, 488
- isolated 100
- necrosis 615
- volume 612, 621
hepatocyte protein synthesis 599
hepatomegaly 493, 498, 585, 594, 595, 597, 613, 621, 639
hepatosplenomegaly 582
hepatotoxicity
- in alcoholics 516

hepatotoxicity (*contd.*)
- dose-dependent 343
- factors influencing 519
- immunologic idiosyncratic 515
- metabolic 515
- modulation 502
- nonsteroidal antiinflammatory 527
hepatotoxin 569
herbal teas 449
hexachromanol 201
high-density lipoprotein (see also HDL) 500
histiocytes 481, 495
HMG-GoA inhibitors 500
hormones 543
- steroid 590
human hepatocytes 295
hyaline (see also Mallory's bodies) 552
hybridomas 589
hydantoin 645
hydralazine (1-hydrazinophthalazine) 221, 227, 238, 489, 503
hydrocarbon, halogenated 195
hydrogen peroxide 619, 626
hydrolase, epoxide 646, 649
hydroperoxides 56
hydropic degeneration 60
β-hydroxybutyrate 104
7-hydroxycoumarin 105
7-hydroxycoumarin glucuronide 109
4- hydroxy-hexenal 198
hydroxyethyl radical-protein adducts 619
8-hydroxyguanosine 58
hydroxylation 48
hydroxyl radicals 619
7-hydroxy methotrexate 591
3-hydroxy-3-methylglutaryl coenzyme A reductase (see also HMG CoA) 495
5-hydroxy-methyl-2'-deoxyuridine 58
4-hydroxy-octenal 198
hydroxyurea 83
hyperammonemia 254, 256, 649, 651, 656
hyperbilirubinemia 155, 165, 170, 520, 552, 585, 587, 600, 601, 647
hyperlipidemia 496, 498, 565
hyperlipoproteinemia 46, 496
hyperplasia 9, 15, 596
- adaptive 8
- diffuse 549
- focal nodular 558, 559
- nodular regenerative 448, 549, 550, 596, 597
hypersensitivity 132, 228, 294, 427, 467, 480, 489, 490, 494, 531, 534, 535, 536, 544, 567, 571, 582, 638, 641, 643, 644, 646, 648, 649, 654, 655
- reaction 429, 443, 480, 492, 493, 571, 596
- - classification of 429
- syndrome drug 296
hypertension 478, 490, 595, 599
- portal 582, 596, 597, 598, 612
hypertransaminemia 415, 487
- asymptomatic 417, 418
- chronic chemical 431
- chronic idiosyncratic 432
- immune-mediated 426
- symptomatic 418
hypertrichosis 599
hypoactive hypertrophic ER 6
hypoalbuminemia 274, 530
hypofunctional smooth ER 63
hypoglycemia 323, 651
hypoglycemic agents
- oral 566
- other oral 568, 569
hypoglycin 299, 655
- toxicity 331
hypoglycin A 325, 656
hypolipidemic agents 17, 56, 477, 495
hypophysectomy 189
hypotension 478
hypoxanthine 626
- phosphoribosyl transferase 595
hypoxia 59
- hepatic 517
- reoxygenation 623

ibufenac 526, 527
ibuprofen 58, 529
icterogenic steroids 544, 551
idiopathic nephrotic syndrome 598
idiosyncrasy 530, 655
- immune-mediated 425
- immunologic 530, 531, 571, 646
- metabolic 425, 467, 530, 531, 571, 638, 651
idiosyncratic 134
- basis 76
- drug reaction 443
- mechanism 519
- reaction 343, 467, 503, 544, 569, 654
- type 344
idiotype 226
IgD 224
IgE 239
IgG 495
IgM 224

IL
- IL–1 (see also interleukin–1) 590, 594, 614
- IL–2 (see also interleukin–2) 224, 583, 590, 594, 598
- IL–5 224
- IL–6 (see also interleukin–6) 614
- IL–8 (see also interleukin–8) 614
- rIL–2 (see also interleukin) 584
- rIL–2 dose 585
- rIL–2-plus lymphokine-activated killer cells (see also LAK) 585
imipramine 132, 171
immune
- reaction 425
- response 428
- system 581
immunity, cell-mediated 434, 596
immunoallergic reaction 293
immunocompetence 582
immunofluorescence 233, 234, 480
- techniques 620
immunoglobulin A 160
immunologic
- changes 503
- factors 644
- response 637, 639, 643
immunomodulating agent 581, 601
immunophilin 589, 601
immunostimulatory 583
immunosuppressive agents 581
IMP dehydrogenase 590
inborn metabolic errors 650, 651
inclusion bodies 487
indomethacin 32, 241, 527, 529, 532, 533
infarction
- hepatic 563
- myocardial 562
infection
- bacterial 601
- related 517
- viral 601
infectious
- diseases 581
- mononucleosis 638
inflammation 20, 482, 532, 587, 616, 617, 627, 639
inflammatory
- bowel disease 591
- cell infiltration 491
- response, granulomatoid 642
influenza-like 586
injury
- cholestatic 567
- hematologic 571
- hepatic 553, 567, 571, 654
- mechanisms of 586, 594, 596, 599, 654
- parenchymal 554, 568
inosine 5
inosine monophospate (IMP) dehydrogenase 590
inositol 211
interferon 582, 583, 585, 586
interferon-α 586, 587
interferon-α 2-a 587
interferon-β 586
interferon-γ 229, 586, 594, 598
interleukin
- IL–1 (see also IL–1) 594, 614
- IL–2 (see also IL–2) 224, 583, 594, 598
- IL–6 (see also IL–6) 614
- IL–8 (see also IL–8) 614
intermediate filaments 615
intestinal
- absorption 156
- flora 613, 624
intracytoplasmic eosinophilic bodies 480
intragastric infusion model 623
intravascular coagulation 520
inulin 166
iron 18, 624, 626
ischemia 12, 59, 614
ischemic
- heart disease 488
- reperfusion model 623
isolated perfused liver 100
isoniazid (INH) 123, 283, 301, 452, 470, 517, 519
- rapid acetylator 470
isoprinosine 583
Ito cell 20, 591, 616, 625

Jamaican vomiting sickness 299, 323, 569, 655
jaundice 46, 232, 285, 479, 487, 493, 520, 531, 545, 552, 570, 581, 593, 598, 613, 638, 648
- sulfonylurea-induced 567
- syndrome contraceptive steroid 553

karyolysis 10, 13
karyorrhexis 10, 13
3-keto-5α-cholanic acid 169
ketoconazole 310, 471, 601
ketoprofen 527, 529, 534
Kupffer cells 111, 224, 481, 494, 613, 614, 616, 619, 622, 623, 624, 625
- proliferation 492
- pseudogranulomatous aggregates 641

L-α-methyl–3,4-dihydroxy-phenylalanine (see also α-methyldopa) 477, 478
L-asparaginase 305
labetalol 501, 503
lactation 478
lactic acid dehydrogenase 595
lactobacillus 624
LAK 584, 585
lamellar bodies 484
lanthanum 192
lasiocarpine 17
lecithin 628
leukotrienes 20, 583
levamisole 583
ligandin 159
lipid
– accumulation 594
– biosynthesis 586
– lowering-agents 498, 503
– metabolism 495
– metabolism, inborn errors of 487
– peroxidation 75, 190, 351
– regulating agents 495
– turnover of 281
lipofuscin 17, 57
lipolysis 594
lipoperoxidation 619
lipopolysaccharide 614, 623, 625
lipoprotein 53, 186, 192, 495, 618
– (LDL)-cholesterol 496
– low density (LDL) 500
lipotropic 212
– deficiency 212, 626
– effects 592
lithocholate 164, 168, 169
lithocholic acid 63
liver 498, 566, 586
– biopsy 28, 396, 592, 593
– damage 502, 567, 624
– enzymes 587
– fatty 18, 185, 188, 195, 200, 323, 595, 617, 618, 627, 628
– hypermetabolic state 622
– isolated perfused 100
– necrosis 624
– phospholipid fatty 487
– rupture 562
– transaminase 500
– transplantation 287, 525, 582, 591
– tumors 498
liver cell (see also hepatocyte)
– injury 45
– necrosis 415
– periportal 57
liver failure 581, 591, 613, 614
– acute 517
– chronic 649
– management 336
liver function tests 275, 481, 600
liver injury (see also hepatocyte, liver cell) 515, 533, 582, 586, 593, 599
– acute 517
– cholestatic 581, 584, 586
– cytotoxic 581
– hypersensitivity 503, 596
– iatrogenic 273
– ischemic 616
– NSAID-associated 528
– pathogenesis 617
lovastatin 125, 495, 496, 497, 500
lupus erythematosus (SLE) 479, 490, 492, 529, 598, 643
– cells 478, 480
– like syndrome 639
lymphadenopathy 227, 570, 638, 643
lymphocytes 12, 233, 480, 483, 495, 536, 571, 583, 584, 585, 591, 592, 594, 643
– $CD2^+$ 585
– CD3 589
– $CD3^+$ 585
– CD4 223
– CD4 T cells 225, 229, 239
– CD8 cytotoxic T cells 229
– $CD22^-$ lymphocytes 585
– $CD45^+$ 585
– CD45RA 223
– CD45RO 223
lymphocytosis 638, 639
lymphokines 583
lysophosphatidylcholine 49
lysosomal
– lamellar bodies 486
– phospholipids, human 488
lysosome-like materials 494
lysosomes 44, 484, 487, 494, 495, 546

macrophage 483, 583, 590, 592, 598, 614
– activates 422
– ceroid-laden 591
– hepatic 616
– migration inhibition 493
– pseudogranulomatous aggregates 641
magnesium trisalicylate 530
malignant melanoma 585
Mallory bodies (see also alcoholic hyaline) 155, 483, 484, 485, 552, 615, 616, 617
malnutrition 53, 517, 519
malonyldialdehyde 190, 625
manganese sulfate 170
mannitol 166

marmosets 63, 500, 501
mast cell
– degranulation 493
maternal-placental-fetal unit 279
meclofenamic acid 527, 529, 534
medroxyprogesterone 565
membrane 46
– assembly 54
– canalicular 170
menadione 112
menstruation 556, 563
mephenytoin 638, 645
mercaptans 257
6-mercaptopurine 595, 596
mercapturic acid 518
mesantoin 638
mestranol 545, 551, 564
metabolic
– idiosyncrasy 293, 467
– tolerance 618
– zonation 30
metabolite 581
– isoniazid 425
– reactive 405, 430
– reactivity 135
metahexamide 566, 567, 568
metalloporphyrin 60
methamphetamine 51
methandrolone 545
methapyrilene 17
methimazole 569, 570, 571
methionine 4, 52, 61, 211, 213, 591
methotrexate 78, 83, 92, 308, 451, 582, 588, 589, 591
methyl 193
– derivatives 50
– ether, butylated hydroxytoluene 51
– isobutyl ketone 169
4-methylcoumarin 50, 51, 53
α-methyldopa (see also L-α-methyl-3,4-dihydroxy-phenylalanine) 477, 478, 479, 503
– hepatitis 479
– metabolites 480, 482
4-methylpyrazole 51
methylcholantrene 50, 127
methyltestosterone 544, 545, 547, 549
methylthiouracil 569, 570
mevastatin 496, 497
mevinolin 495
Mg^{2+} 163
MHC class II antigens 590
microfilament 53, 157
micronase 567, 568
microsome 199
microsome autoantibodies 491
microtubule 53, 62, 157
microvilli 157
mitochondria 10, 44, 55, 60, 64, 186, 199, 298, 300, 328, 331, 494, 499, 554, 586, 588, 615, 617, 618, 621, 626, 655
– acetaldehyde dehydrogenase 619
– calcium 599
– enlargement 618
– gluathione 627
– β-oxidation 299
– Reye's syndrome 332
mizorbin 588, 590
monoamine oxidase 120
monocytes/macrophage 613, 614
monohydroxy bile salts 162
mononuclear
– cells 480
– infiltrates 494
mononucleosis
– infectious 640, 641
– like illness 303
monooxygenase system 601
morphometry 55
mRNA 594
mucin 53
multidrug resistance 45
muscle 498
– myopathy 500, 595
– myositis 639
– wasting 613
mustard 13
mutagens 627
myalgias 586
myasthenia gravis 596
mycophenolic acid 589
myeloproliferative state 562
myofibroblast 591

N-acetylcysteine 38, 295, 521, 523, 524
N-acetylglutamate 655
N-acetyl-*p*-benzoquinone imine (NAPQI) 32, 140, 294, 518
N-acetyl-para-amino-phenol 515
N-acetylprocainamide 492
N-acetyl-semiquinone imine 200
N-acetyltransferase 491
N-methyl derivative 192
N-oxide reductase 120
Na^+K^+adenosine 599
– triphosphatase 599
Na^+-K^+-ATPase 156, 162
– activity 552
nabumetone 527, 529, 534
NAD^+ (see mitochondria) 104
NADH redox 105
$NADP^+$ 103, 104
NADPH 103, 104, 136
nafenopin 17, 59

β-naphtoflavone 33
α-naphtylisothiocyanate (see also ANIT) 62, 158, 165
naproxen 527, 528, 529, 532, 534
narcotic analgesics 385, 536
naringin 129
NAT–2
– acetylation 302
– polymorphic N-acetyltransferase 302
– rapid/slow polymorphism 307
necrosis 3, 11, 12, 25, 38, 45, 196, 230, 481, 549, 568, 616, 617, 622, 626, 638, 639, 640, 651, 652
– absence of 615
– bridging 491, 570
– central 494
– – spotty hepatocellular 494
– centrilobular 490, 491, 520, 533, 623
– – focal hepatocellular 623
– – hepatocyte 500
– distal tubular 520
– factor-α 624
– focal 480, 481, 491, 495, 627, 642
– hepatocellular 415, 445, 483, 500, 518, 586, 616
– massive 446, 642
– – isoniazid therapy 458
– periportal 33, 585
– perivenous 38
– piecemeal 592
neodymium 193
neoplasm 543, 549
– other 550
nephrotic syndrome 646
– pediatric 583
nephrotoxicity 170
neuropsychiatric
– deficits 336
– syndrome 252
neurotoxin, synergistic 257
neurotransmission
– altered 252
– catecholamine 265
– GABAergic 258
neutrophil 481, 592, 594, 620
– accumulation 623
– chemotaxis 614
– infiltration 616
– inflammation 617, 622, 623
– proliferation 583
– respiratory burst 614
neutrophilia 614
NF-AT (see also nuclear factor of activated T cells) 589
NHP 598
niacin 498
nicotinamide 192
nicotine 128
nicotinic acid 495, 496, 498
Niemann-Pick 487
nifedipine 125, 129, 241
niflumic acid 527
nitrites 213
nitrofurans 227
nitrofurantoin 238, 242, 342, 463, 469
nitrosamines 2, 12, 213
nonlinear pharmacokinetics 376
nonsteroidal antiinflammatory drugs (see also NSAIDs) 515, 526
19-nontestosterone 544
norepinephrine 61, 132, 200
norethandrolone 545, 546
norethindrone 553
norethisterone 552
norethyndrol 545
norethynodrel 552
nornicotine 51
norprogestin, ethinylated 552
19-nortestosterone 552
NSAIDs (see also nonsteroidal antiinflammatory drugs) 515, 528, 530, 532
nuclear inclusions 480
nuclear protein receptor 590
nucleophiles 422
nucleoside
– analogue 55
– antiviral 93
nucleosome 79
nutritional deficiency 618

O-deethylation 107
obesity 123, 499
obstruction, extrahepatic 640
octreotide 566
OKT3 588
oleandomycin 194
one-compartment
– model kinetics 375
oral
– bioavailability 387
– contraceptive 274, 544, 555, 557
– hypoglycemic 543
organelle 43
– antibodies 499
– biogenesis 56
– subcellular 499
organic
– acidemias, salicylates 333
– arsenicals 463
organohalogen compounds 50
orinase 568
ornithine carbamoyl transferase 657
orotic acid 56, 60

osteoporosis 595
oxaprozin 527, 529, 534
oxapurinol 241
oxazolidinediones 646
oxidase
- aldehyde 120
- amino acid 57
- monoamine 120
- urate 57
oxidation 130, 186
β-oxidation 59, 655
oxidative
- metabolites 350
- phosphorylation 189
- stress 59, 623
oxidipine 502
oxygen 30
- radicals 201, 590, 619, 620, 627
- reactive intermediates 587
- reactive species 626
oxymetholone 548
oxyphenbutazone 527
oxyphenysatin 499

p-aminosalicylic acid (PAS) 469
P glycoprotein 502
P–1306 568
palmitic 193
pancreatitis 55, 533, 651
pantothenic acid 211
papaverine 235, 491, 492, 499
paracetamol 199, 515
paradione 638
paraformaldehyde 106
paramethadione 638
patch test 241
PBC-like syndrome 567
peliosis 549, 563, 597
- hepatis 448, 543, 548, 553, 581, 596
pemoline 306
pemphigus 598
penicillamine 137
penicillin 63, 137, 462
4-pentanoic acid 655, 656
pentanoic acid 655
pentose 107
peptide growth factors 591
perhexiline 84, 126
- maleate 499
perisinusodial stellate cells 616
peroxidation, lipid (see also lipid) 39
peroxidative injury 518
peroxisome 17, 44, 45, 56, 57, 62, 64, 201, 498, 499, 599
- proliferation 58, 498
- proliferator response element 59
phagocytotic activity 590
phalloidin 160
pharmacokinetic models
- intravenous dosing 371
- linear 371
- one-compartment model 371
phase I 119
- drug metabolism 344
phase II 119
- reactions 346
phenacemide 638
phenacetin 134
phenindione 501
phenobarbital 47, 50, 54, 63, 163, 188, 199, 304, 400, 490, 519, 601, 638, 645, 655
phenol, polyalkyl 50
phenothiazines 646
phenotype 145, 495
phentermine 62
phenurone 638, 645
phenylbutazone 226, 526, 527, 529, 530, 531, 532, 534
α-phenyl-*tert*-butylnitrone 215
phenytoin 47, 127, 227, 284, 296, 490, 601, 637, 638, 641, 642, 643, 644, 645, 646, 647, 648
- antibodies to 643
- (DPH) jaundice 639
- syndrome 638, 639
- toxicity 644
phosphatase acid 46
phosphatidylcholine 49, 52, 64, 164
phosphatidylinositol 193
3'-phosphoadenosine 5'-phosphosulfate 109
phospholipase 488
phospholipase A_2 39, 211
phospholipid 51, 64, 164, 192, 211
- biosynthesis 47
- fatty liver 484
- microsomal 52
phospholipidosis 52, 57, 186, 477, 485, 486
phosphorus 61, 195
phosphorylation, oxidative 481, 530
piperonyl butoxide 140
piroxicam 527, 528, 532, 534, 535
pirprofen 527, 529, 532, 534
polyarthritis 226
polychlorobiphenyl 50
polyclonal preparations 588
polyinosinic-polycytidylic acid (Poly I.C) 587
polymorphism 126, 128, 227, 237, 596
polysomes 5
porphyria 83

porphyria (*contd.*)
- exacerbation 544
- hepatic 563
- provocation 553
porphyrin 563
portosystemic shunts 386
practolol 501
praseodymium 193
pravastatin 496, 497, 500
prednisolone 566
prednisone 594, 596
preeclampsia 562
pregnancy 167, 558, 563
- acute fatty liver 281
- cholestatic jaundice of 544, 551, 552, 555
pregnenolone–16 α carbonitrile 50
primidone 490, 638, 646
probucol 495
procainamide 238, 489, 492, 493
procarcinogen 619
procollagen α_1 202
prodioban 568
progabide 638
progesterone 273, 543, 552, 563
progestin 551, 553
progestogens 590
promethazine 196
propafenone 171
propionic acid 527, 530, 533
propoxyphene 536
propylthiouracil 307, 569, 570
prostaglandin 20
prostaglandin E 588, 590
prostaglandin metabolism 526
protein 16, 617
- binding 380
- binding-insensitive 378
- binding-sensitive 378
- catabolism of 594
- heat shock 9
- irreversible binding 401
- phosphatase 589
- synthesis 13, 18
- thiols, oxidation of 422, 423
- transport 46
proteoglycans 20
proteolytic enzymes 620
prothrombin 487, 520, 600, 613, 622
protoporphyrin 163
pruritus 531, 545, 554, 581, 585
pseudolymphoma 639, 643
pseudoneplastic syndromes 639
psoralen 81
psoriasis 591, 592, 593, 598
purine 83, 595
- analogue azathioprine 589
- bases 591
- synthesis 590
puromycin 54, 61, 194
pyknosis 10, 13
pyoderma gangrenosum 598
pyrazole 51, 201
pyridine nucleotide 102, 189, 190
pyridoxine 211
pyrimidine 83, 591
pyrrolizidine alkaloids 17

quinidine 489, 493, 494, 501, 502
quinone 111, 135, 478, 482

rapamycin 588, 589
rash 226, 530, 531, 533, 567, 571, 581, 638, 639, 643, 647, 655
reaction
- allergic 443
- anaphylatoid 524
- cholestatic 447
- granulomatous 446, 503
- hepatocellular 445
- hepatotoxic 493
- hypersensitivity 443, 596
- idiosyncratic 443, 467, 503, 544, 654
- immunological 594
rejection, acute 601
renal 520, 526
- cell carcinoma 585, 586
- clearance 517
- disfunction 599
- failure 388, 487, 520
- injury 646
- insufficiency 367
- transplant 595
resins 495
reticulum
- collapse 480, 491
- endoplasmic 491, 599, 601
Reye's syndrome 58, 298, 323, 335, 488, 530, 569, 649, 655
rhabdomyolysis 493, 639
rheumatoid factor 478
rhodamine 123 55
ribavirin 85
riboflavin 211
ribosomes 62
rifampicin 601
rifampin 124, 470
ring hydroxylation 63
RNA 16, 19, 594
- double-stranded 583, 585
- polymerase 60, 84
- synthesis 19
- transcription 93
R-p-hydroxylation 127

RS–61443 588, 589, 590

S-adenosyl-L-methionine (see also SAMe) 167, 287, 628
salicylate 527, 529, 530, 532, 535
– intoxication 330
salicylic acid 527
sclerosing cholangitis 591
sclerosis, hepatoportal 581
selenium 140
semiquinone 478, 482
sensitization 234
sepsis 600
SER 201
– membrane 48
serotonin 132
serum
– albumin 613
– ALT 405
– bilirubin 479, 498
– creatinine 522
– dyslipidemias 495
– sickness 638
– transaminase 301, 482, 488, 581, 613, 623
– – peak levels 416
sex hormones 543
– drugs related 565
– female 551, 563
SGOT (see also AST) 639
SGPT (see also ALT) 395, 520, 639, 640
shock, hemorrhagic 556
shunting, portal venous 249
sialyltransferase 53
simvastatin 496, 497, 500
sinusoids 368
– acidophilic bodies (see also apoptosis) 546
– beading 641
– caliber 612, 621
– cell 480
– changes 553
– compression 595
– dilatation 449, 544, 596
– space 626
(S)-mephenytoin 122, 126
SMZ-TMP, Bactrim, Septra (see also sulfamethoxazole-trimethoprim) 468
SOD (see also superoxide dismutase) 351
sodium
– deoxycholate 59
– salicylate 530
solvents 128
somatostatin 566
sorbitol dehydrogenase 189
space of Disse (see also Disse) 119
sparteine 237
sphingomyelin 164
splenomegaly 493, 592, 639
sporidesmin 199
Sr^{2+} 215
statins 496, 500
steatosis 5, 230, 480, 483, 484, 499, 587, 595, 655
– hepatic 80, 566
– macrovesicular 581, 592, 594
– microvesicular 298, 503, 532, 533, 569, 638, 651, 652, 653, 655
steroid 48, 62, 543
– anabolic 549, 550, 564
– anabolic alkylated 554
– C–17-alkylated 549
– contraceptive 551, 552, 555, 560, 561, 563
– gonadal 543
– hormones 590
– progestational 552
– receptor complex 594
sterols 588, 590
Steven-Johnson syndrome 638, 639, 641, 647, 648
stilbestrol 551, 552
stress 187
– oxidative 59
sucrose 166
sulfamethoxazole-trimethoprim (see also SMZ-TMP, Bactrim, Septra) 468
sulfasalazine (see also Azulfidine) 468
sulfatase 109
sulfate conjugation 518
sulfation 107, 159
sulfobromophthalein 159
sulfonamides 306, 468
sulfonylurea 566, 567, 569
– derivatives 567
sulfotransferase 108, 109, 159
sulindac 342, 527, 528, 529, 530, 531, 532, 533
superoxide 188, 626
– anions 482
– dismutase (see also SOD) 351
– ions 619
– radicals 625
systemic bioavailability
– in cirrhotic patients 381
– increased 381

T3 589
tachyarrythmias 483
tachycardia 586

tacrine (see also 1, 2, 3, 4-tetrahydro–9-acridinamine monohydrochloride monohydrate) 395, 396, 399, 405
– binding 401
– hepatotoxicity 395, 406
– metabolic profile 398
tamoxifen 565
taurine 168
taurolithocholate 158, 161
Tay-Sachs 487
TCCD (see also 2,3,7,8-tetrachlorodibenzo-*p*-dioxin) 127
T cells 171, 241, 589, 598
technetium–99m-labeled disofenin 585
tegretol 638
telangiectasia, familial hemorrhagic 553, 560
tenoxicam 527
tenuazonic acid 13
tert-nitrosobutane 215
testosterone 544, 545, 549
– enanthate 549
2,3,7,8-tetrachlorodibenzo-*p*-dioxin (see also TCCD) 127
tetracycline 282, 461
tetradrofolic acid 591
1,2,3,4-tetrahydro–9-acridinamine monohydrochloride monohydrate (see also tacrine) 395
TG synthetase 185
TGFβ_1 202
theobromine 187
theophylline 3, 61, 124, 187
thiabendazole 443
thiantoin 638, 645
thioacetamide 13, 33, 199
thiouracil 569, 570
thiourea 569
thorium dioxide 444
Thorotrast 444
thrombin 481
thrombocytopenia 478, 520, 586
thromboembolism, venous 562
thrombosis 561–563
Thy–1^+ 584
thymidine 241
ticrynofen 235
tienilic acid 136, 142, 143, 235, 238
tight junction 564
tilorone 62
tolazamide 567, 568
tolbutamide 124, 567, 568
tolinase 568
tolmetin 527, 530, 531
toxic
– interactions 43
– liver-derived metabolite 591
– metabolite 297, 298, 420
– products 613
– reaction 442
transaminase (see also ALT, AST, GOT, GPT, SGOT, SGPT) 240, 435, 479, 481, 486, 489, 490, 498, 502, 570, 597
transaminase measurement 435
transforming growth factor-β 623, 625
transitional cells 616
transplantation 614
trichloromethyl 196
tridione 638, 646
trifluoracetyl adduct 136
trifluoroacetic acid 232
triglyceride 18, 64, 185, 500, 618
– levels 495
– secretion 481
– transport 594
trimethadione 638, 646
trimethoprim-sulfamethoxazole 464
trimethylpyrroline (2,5,5-) 202
triton WR 1339 162
Trolox C 200
trypan blue 106, 111
tubulin 160, 186
tumor 543, 555
– associated with drug 444
– benign 549, 553
– malignant 549, 553
– necrosis factor 229, 583
– rupture of 556
tumor necrosis factor-α 586, 613, 614, 623, 626
tumor necrosis factor-α mRNA 625
tumorigenesis 564, 565

UDP-glucuronyltransferase 50
UGT (see also uridine diphosphoglucuronoside glucuronosyl transferases) 228
urase 599
urate oxidase 57
uricosuric 142
uridine 5
– diphosphoglucuronoside glucuronosyl transferases (see also UGT) 228
– triphosphate 60
ursodeoxycholic acid 601

valproate 656
3-en valproic acid 655
4-en-valproic acid 655
4-en-VPA 656
valproic acid 133, 281, 297, 637, 638, 649, 651, 652, 653, 654, 656, 657

vanishing bile duct syndrome 648
vasculitis 226
vasopressin 161
- induced calcium flux 599
vein 584
- hepatic (see also central vein sclerosis) 616, 622
vein, hepatic 617
veno-occlusive disease 305, 448, 561, 581, 596, 652
verapamil 502
vinblastine 587
vinyl chloride 81
viral
- hepatitis 626
- infection 601
- toxin interaction 331
virus infection 517
viruses 585
vitamin 618
vitamin A chronic toxicity 442
vitamin B_{12} 211, 592
vitamin D sterol 644
vitamin E 61, 188, 200, 201
- deficiencies 281
vomiting 479, 519, 520, 534, 650, 651, 657
- acute 569
- occasional 483

water retention 621
Wilson's disease 626
Wolman's disease 187

X-irradiation 584
X-rays 13
xanthine oxidase 191, 626
- hepatic 587
xenobiotic metabolism 45
xenobiotics 11, 99
xylitol 103

Yucatan micropigs 627

zidovudine 80, 296, 517
zomepirac 527
zonal necrosis 445
zonality 25
zone 3 necrosis ketoconazole therapy 459

Springer-Verlag and the Environment

We at Springer-Verlag firmly believe that an international science publisher has a special obligation to the environment, and our corporate policies consistently reflect this conviction.

We also expect our business partners – paper mills, printers, packaging manufacturers, etc. – to commit themselves to using environmentally friendly materials and production processes.

The paper in this book is made from low- or no-chlorine pulp and is acid free, in conformance with international standards for paper permanency.

MIX
Papier aus verantwortungsvollen Quellen
Paper from responsible sources
FSC® C105338

If you have any concerns about our products,
you can contact us on
ProductSafety@springernature.com

In case Publisher is established outside the EU,
the EU authorized representative is:
Springer Nature Customer Service Center GmbH
Europaplatz 3, 69115 Heidelberg, Germany

Printed by Libri Plureos GmbH
in Hamburg, Germany